# CASES IN ADULT CONGENITAL HEART DISEASE

# CASES IN ADULT CONGENITAL HEART DISEASE

**Michael A. Gatzoulis, MD, PhD, FACC, FESC**
Professor of Cardiology and Congenital Heart Disease
Consultant Cardiologist
Head, Adult Congenital Heart Centre
and Centre for Pulmonary Hypertension
Royal Brompton Hospital
National Heart and Lung Institute, Imperial College
London, United Kingdom

**Gary D. Webb, MD, FRCPC, FACC**
Professor of Medicine
Director of the Philadelphia Adult Congenital Heart Center
University of Pennsylvania School of Medicine
The Hospital of the University of Pennsylvania
Philadelphia, Pennsylvania

**Craig S. Broberg, MD**
Assistant Professor
School of Medicine
Director, Adult Congenital Heart Disease Program
Oregon Health & Science University
Portland, Oregon

**Hideki Uemura, MD**
Consultant Cardiac Surgeon
Royal Brompton Hospital
London, United Kingdom

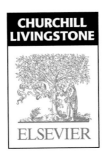

CHURCHILL
LIVINGSTONE

ELSEVIER

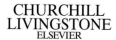

CHURCHILL
LIVINGSTONE
ELSEVIER

1600 John F. Kennedy Boulevard
Suite 1800
Philadelphia, PA 19103-2899

CASES IN ADULT CONGENITAL HEART DISEASE ISBN: 978-0-443-06712-9

---

**Notice**

Knowledge and best practice in this field are constantly changing. As new research and experience broaden our knowledge, changes in practice, treatment and drug therapy may become necessary or appropriate. Readers are advised to check the most current information provided (i) on procedures featured or (ii) by the manufacturer of each product to be administered, to verify the recommended dose or formula, the method and duration of administration, and contraindications. It is the responsibility of the practitioner, relying on their own experience and knowledge of the patient, to make diagnoses, to determine dosages and the best treatment for each individual patient, and to take all appropriate safety precautions. To the fullest extent of the law, neither the Publisher nor the Editors assume any liability for any injury and/or damage to persons or property arising out or related to any use of the material contained in this book.

The Publisher

---

**Library of Congress Cataloging-in-Publication Data**

Cases in adult congenital heart disease : atlas with DVD / [edited by] Michael A. Gatzoulis ... [et al.]. – 1st ed.
      p. ; cm.
   Includes bibliographical references.
   ISBN 978-0-443-06712-9
   1. Congenital heart disease–Case studies–Atlases.   I. Gatzoulis, Michael A.   II. Title.
   [DNLM: 1. Heart Defects, Congenital–Atlases.   2. Heart Defects, Congenital–Case Reports.   3. Adult. WG 17 C338 2009]
   RC687.C375 2009
   616.1'2043–dc22

2009011148

*Executive Publisher:* Natasha Andjelkovic
*Developmental Editor:* Agnes H. Byrne
*Design Direction:* Steven Stave

Printed in China

Last digit is the print number:  9  8  7  6  5  4  3  2  1

*To my late father Athanasios Konstantinos Gatzoulis (1921–2008).*

MAG

*To the patients I have had the privilege of serving in Toronto and Philadelphia, to the excellent colleagues who have helped me care for them, and to all the ACHD patients whose lives we value.*

GDW

*To patients with congenital heart disease throughout the world, who have done the real work represented herein.*

CSB

*To all the patients for whom I have had the privilege of providing care and to all my colleagues and mentors.*

HU

# Contributors

**Dominic J. Abrams, MD, MRCP**
Consultant Cardiologist, St. Bartholomew's and Great Ormond Street Hospitals, London, United Kingdom
*Catheter Ablation for Atrial Arrhythmia*

**William Alazawi, MA (Cantab), MB BChir, PhD, MRCP**
Academic Specialist Registrar, Barts and The London School of Medicine & Dentistry, Queen Mary University of London, London, United Kingdom
*Syncope in a Patient with Noonan Syndrome*

**Dimitrios Alexopoulos, MD**
Professor and Director of Cardiology, Patras University Hospital, Rion, Patras, Greece
*Dyspnea in a Patient with a Loud Murmur*

**Khalid Alnajashi, MD**
Division of Pediatric Cardiology, Prince Sultan Cardiac Center, Riyadh, Saudi Arabia
*Late Outcome Following Systemic Tricuspid Valve Replacement*

**Naser M. Ammash, MD**
Associate Professor of Medicine, Mayo Medical School; Consultant, Division of Cardiovascular Diseases, Department of Internal Medicine, Mayo Clinic, Rochester, Minnesota
*Subaortic Stenosis: Indications for Surgery*

**Kai Andersen, MD, PhD**
Consultant Cardiologist, Rikshospitalet University Hospital, Oslo, Norway
*The Criss-Cross Heart*

**Panagiotis D. Arvanitis, MD**
Honorary Clinical/Research Fellow, Adult Congenital Heart Programme, Royal Brompton Hospital, London, United Kingdom
*Acute Presentation with Cerebral Hemorrhage*

**Sonya V. Babu-Narayan, MBBS, MRCP**
Honorary Clinical Research Fellow, National Heart and Lung Institute, Imperial College London; Specialist Registrar in Adult Cardiology and Adult Congenital Heart Disease, Royal Brompton Hospital, London, United Kingdom
*Timing of Pulmonary Valve Replacement; Management of Tachyarrhythmia in Tetralogy: Ablation versus Surgery; Consideration for Automatic Implantable Cardioverter-Defibrillator in Tetralogy*

**Elisabeth Bédard, MD**
Adult Congenital Heart Centre, Royal Brompton Hospital; Imperial College of Science and Medicine, London, United Kingdom
*Right Heart Enlargement of Uncertain Cause (Sinus Venosus Atrial Septal Defect); Left Atrioventricular Valve Regurgitation: Criteria for Intervention; Late Complications after the Arterial Switch Operation; Intracardiac Thrombus in the Fontan Circulation; Contraception Counseling*

**Lee N. Benson, MD**
Professor of Pediatrics, University of Toronto School of Medicine; Director, Cardiac Diagnostic and Interventional Unit, The Hospital for Sick Children, Toronto, Ontario, Canada
*Catheter Intervention for Baffle Leak or Venous Obstruction*

**Philipp Bonhoeffer, MD**
Professor of Cardiology, Institute of Child Health; Chief of Cardiology, Director of the Cardiac Catheterisation Laboratory, Great Ormond Street Hospital for Children, London, United Kingdom
*Catheter Implantation of Stented Pulmonary Valve*

**Beatriz Bouzas, MD**
Consultant, Cardiology Department, Complejo Hospitalario Universitario Juan Canalejo, Coruña, Spain
*Pregnancy and Fetal Death in a Patient with Ebstein Anomaly; Congenital Pulmonary Stenosis Turned to Pulmonary Regurgitation*

**William Bradlow, BM, BS**
Cardiovascular Magnetic Resonance Unit, Royal Brompton Hospital, London, United Kingdom
*The Role of Pulmonary Vasodilators in Pulmonary Hypertension*

**Craig S. Broberg, MD**
Assistant Professor, School of Medicine; Director, Adult Congenital Heart Disease Program, Oregon Health & Science University, Portland, Oregon
*Straddling of the Tricuspid Valve: Long-Term Outcome; Long-Term Follow-Up of Atrioventricular Septal Defect; Congenital Pulmonary Stenosis Turned to Pulmonary Regurgitation; Pulmonary Atresia with Intact Ventricular Septum; Late Complications after the Arterial Switch Operation; Palliative Mustard for Transposition and Ventricular Septal Defect; The Criss-Cross Heart; Long-Term Survival in Eisenmenger Syndrome; Iron Deficiency in Cyanotic Heart Disease; Pulmonary Artery Thrombosis and Recurrent Hemoptyses in Eisenmenger Syndrome; Contraception Counseling*

**Qi-Ling Cao, MD**
Associate Professor, Department of Cardiology, Rush Medical College, Rush Center for Congenital and Structural Heart Disease, Rush University Medical Center, Chicago, Illinois
*Catheter Closure of Ventricular Septal Defects*

**Pedro A. Catarino, MD**
Department of Cardiothoracic Surgery, Royal Brompton Hospital, London, United Kingdom
*Successful Tricuspid Valve Repair of Ebstein Anomaly*

**Aikaterini Chamaidi, MD**
Consultant Cardiologist, University Hospital Larissa, Larissa Medical School, Larissa, Greece
*Long-Term Outcome after Rastelli Repair*

**Joseph Y.S. Chan, MRCP**
Associate Consultant, Division of Cardiology, Department of Medicine and Therapeutics, Prince of Wales Hospital, Hong Kong
*Transcatheter Options for Atrial Arrhythmia after the Mustard Procedure*

**Jonathan B. Choy, MD, FRCPC, FACC**
University of Alberta; Director, Adult Echocardiography Laboratory, Associate Clinical Professor of Medicine, University of Alberta Hospital, Edmonton, Alberta, Canada
*Anomalous Left Coronary Artery from the Pulmonary Artery*

**Louise Coats, PhD, MRCP**
Clinical Research Fellow, Institute of Child Health; Clinical Research Fellow, Great Ormond Street Hospital for Children, London, United Kingdom
*Catheter Implantation of Stented Pulmonary Valve*

**Andrew Crean, BM, MRCP, MSc, FRCR, MPhil**
Assistant Professor, University of Toronto; Staff Cardiologist and Radiologist, Toronto Congenital Cardiac Centre for Adults, Toronto General Hospital, Toronto, Ontario, Canada
*Cor Triatriatum; Recoarctation: Criteria for Intervention*

**Piers E. F. Daubeney, MA, DM, MRCP, MRCPCH**
Honorary Senior Lecturer, National Heart and Lung Institute, Imperial College London; Consultant Paediatric and Fetal Cardiologist, Royal Brompton Hospital, London, United Kingdom
*Pulmonary Atresia with Intact Ventricular Septum*

**Periklis A. Davlouros, MD**
Senior Lecturer in Cardiology, Patras University Hospital, Rion, Patras, Greece
*Dyspnea in a Patient with a Loud Murmur*

**Barbara J. Deal, MD**
Professor of Pediatrics, Northwestern University Feinberg School of Medicine; Marvin E. Wodika Research Professor of Cardiology and Division Head, Cardiology, Children's Memorial Hospital, Chicago, Illinois
*Arrhythmia Intervention at the Time of Total Cavopulmonary Conversion*

**Joseph A. Dearani, MD**
Consultant, Division of Cardiovascular Surgery; Director, Thoracic Surgery Resident; Consultant, Division of Surgery; Professor of Surgery, Mayo Clinic, Rochester, Minnesota
*Subaortic Stenosis: Indications for Surgery*

**Gerhard-Paul Diller, MD**
Imperial College, London, United Kingdom; University Hospital, Muenster, Germany
*Atrial Septal Defect Associated with Pulmonary Hypertension— Cause and Effect; Erythrocytosis with Normal Oxygen Saturation*

**Konstantinos Dimopoulos, MD, MSc, PhD**
Consultant and Senior Fellow, Adult Congenital Heart Centre for Pulmonary Hypertension, Royal Brompton Hospital and National Heart and Lung Institute, London, United Kingdom
*Ebstein Anomaly and Sudden Cardiac Death*

**Richard M. Donner, MD**
Clinical Professor of Pediatrics, University of Pennsylvania School of Medicine; Senior Cardiologist, The Children's Hospital of Philadelphia, Philadelphia, Pennsylvania
*Recoarctation: Criteria for Intervention; Cyanosis in Ebstein Anomaly and Catheter Closure of Atrial Septal Defect*

**Nigel E. Drury, BM (Hons), MRCS**
Fellow in Congenital Cardiology, Wessex Cardiothoracic Centre, Southampton General Hospital, Southampton, United Kingdom
*Right Ventricular Outflow Obstruction in a Pregnant Woman*

**Mark J. Earley, MD, MRCP**
Consultant Cardiologist, St. Bartholomew's Hospital, London, United Kingdom
*Catheter Ablation for Atrial Arrhythmia*

**Michael A. Gatzoulis, MD, PhD, FACC, FESC**
Professor of Cardiology and Congenital Heart Disease, Consultant Cardiologist; Head, Adult Congenital Heart Centre and Centre for Pulmonary Hypertension, Royal Brompton Hospital, National Heart and Lung Institute, Imperial College London, United Kingdom
*Aortic Stenosis and Endocarditis during Pregnancy; Extraanatomic Bypass Graft Repair of Coarctation; Transcatheter Options for Atrial Arrhythmia after the Mustard Procedure*

**Deborah R. Gersony, MD**
Assistant Professor of Clinical Medicine, Department of Medicine and Pediatrics, Columbia University Medical Center, New York, New York
*Pregnancy and the Systemic Right Ventricle*

**Marc Gewillig, MD, PhD**
Professor of Pediatric Cardiology, University Leuven, Leuven, Belgium
*Protein-Losing Enteropathy*

**Derek G. Gibson, MB, FRCP**
Royal Brompton Hospital, London, United Kingdom
*Pericardial Constriction after Relief of Subaortic Stenosis*

**Omer Goktekin, MD**
Adult Congenital Heart Centre, Royal Brompton Hospital, London, United Kingdom
*Extraanatomic Bypass Graft Repair of Coarctation*

**Massimo Griselli, FRCS**
Adult Congenital Heart Centre, Department of Cardiac Surgery, Royal Brompton Hospital, London, United Kingdom
*Long-Term Outcome after Rastelli Repair*

**Maarten Groenink, MD**
Associate Professor, Department of Cardiology, Academic Medical Center, Amsterdam, The Netherlands
*Recurrent Aortic Dissection in Marfan Syndrome*

**Sheila G. Haworth, MD, FRCP, FRCPATH, FRCPCH, FMedSci**
Professor of Developmental Cardiology, Institute of Child Health, University College London; Honorary Consultant in Paediatric Cardiology, Great Ormond Street Hospital for Children, London, United Kingdom
*Pulmonary Hypertension after Repair of Congenital Diaphragmatic Hernia*

**Howard C. Herrmann, MD**
Professor of Medicine; Director, Interventional Cardiology and Cardiac Catheterization Laboratories, University of Pennsylvania Medical Center, Philadelphia, Pennsylvania
*Cyanosis in Ebstein Anomaly and Catheter Closure of Atrial Septal Defect*

**Ziyad M. Hijazi, MD, MPH, FSCAI, FACC**
Professor of Pediatrics and Internal Medicine; Director, Rush Center for Congenital and Structural Heart Disease, Rush University Medical College, Chicago, Illinois
*Catheter Closure of Ventricular Septal Defects*

**Eric M. Horlick, MD, FRCPC**
Assistant Professor of Medicine, Toronto General Hospital, Toronto, Ontario, Canada
*Catheter Closure of a Patent Ductus Arteriosus*

**Emmeline F. Hou, MD**
Cardiologist, The Permanente Medical Group, Inc., Roseville, California
*Scimitar Syndrome; Endocarditis in a Young Man; Long-Term Survival in Eisenmenger Syndrome*

**Ross J. Hunter, MRCP**
Research Fellow, Cardiology Research Department, St Bartholomew's Hospital, London, United Kingdom
*Arrhythmia and Syncope in a Patient with a Childhood Murmur*

**Toru Ishizaka, MD, PhD**
Chief Cardiovascular Surgeon, Higashi Takarazuka Satoh Hospital, Takarazuka City, Hyogo, Japan
*Atrial Septal Defect with Cyanosis: The Hypoplastic Right Ventricle; Ventricular Septal Defect and the Aortic Valve; Total Cavopulmonary Conversion: When and How*

**Bengt Johansson, MD, PhD**
Cardiovascular Magnetic Resonance Unit, Royal Brompton Hospital; Imperial College of Science and Medicine, London, United Kingdom
*Intracardiac Thrombus in the Fontan Circulation*

**Sofian Johar, MB BChir, PhD, MRCP**
Specialist Registrar in Cardiology, Royal Brompton Hospital, London, United Kingdom
*Aortic Stenosis and Endocarditis during Pregnancy*

**Lesley Jones**
Clinical Nurse Specialist, Adult Congenital Heart Centre, Royal Brompton Hospice, London, United Kingdom
*Contraception Counseling*

**Henryk Kafka, MD, FRCPC, FACP, FACC**
Departments of Cardiology and Radiology, Queen's University, Kingston, Ontario, Canada
*Late Repair of Tetralogy of Fallot; Assessment of Systemic Right Ventricle Function; The Criss-Cross Heart*

**Thomas K. Kaltsas, MD**
Clinical and Research Fellow, Department of Adult Congenital Heart Disease, Royal Brompton Hospital, London, United Kingdom
*Outflow Tract Obstruction after Atrioventricular Septal Defect Repair*

**Ageliki A. Karatza, DS**
Senior Lecturer in Paediatric Cardiology, Patras University Hospital, Rion, Patras, Greece
*Dyspnea in a Patient with a Loud Murmur*

**Omar Khalid, MD**
The University of Chicago Pritzker School of Medicine, Chicago, Illinois
*Catheter Closure of Ventricular Septal Defects*

**Sachin Khambadkone, MBBS, DCH, MD, DNB, MRCP(UK), CCT**
Honroary Senior Lecturer, Institute of Child Health; Consultant Paediatric Cardiologist, Cardiothoracic Unit, Great Ormond Street Hospital for Children, London, United Kingdom
*Catheter Implantation of Stented Pulmonary Valve*

**Arif Anis Khan, FCPS**
Research Fellow, Cardiology Department, Royal Brompton & Harefield NHS Trust, London, United Kingdom
*Patent Foramen Ovale with Transient Ischemic Attack; Arrhythmia and Syncope in a Patient with a Childhood Murmur; Pulmonary Atresia with Intact Ventricular Septum; Late Complications after the Arterial Switch Operation*

**Christoph Kiesewetter, MD**
Kings College London; Consultant Cardiologist, Guy's and St Thomas's NHS Foundation Trust, London, United Kingdom
*Right Ventricular Outflow Obstruction in a Pregnant Woman*

**Philip J. Kilner, MD, PhD**
Reader in CMR, Imperial College London; Consultant in CMR, Royal Brompton Hospital, London, United Kingdom
*Consideration for Automatic Implantable Cardioverter-Defibrillator in Tetralogy*

**Igor Knez, MD**
Professor of Cardiovascular Surgery, Medical University of Graz; Clinical Department of Cardiac Surgery, University Clinic of Surgery, Graz, Austria
*Congenitally Corrected Transposition of the Great Arteries with Pulmonary Stenosis and Ventricular Septal Detect: When to Intervene*

**Masahiro Koh, MD**
Clinical Fellow, Paediatric Cardiac Surgery, Royal Brompton Hospital, London, United Kingdom
*Partial Anomalous Pulmonary Venous Return; Ebstein Anomaly and Wolff-Parkinson-White Syndrome; Complications of Ventricular Septation in a Patient with a Single Ventricle*

**George Krasopoulos, MD, PhD, FRCS-CTH**
Consultant Cardiac Surgeon, Liverpool Heart & Chest NHS Trust, Liverpool, United Kingdom
*Successful Tricuspid Valve Repair of Ebstein Anomaly*

**Yat-Yim Lam, MRCP**
Associate Professor, Division of Cardiology, Department of Medicine and Therapeutics, Prince of Wales Hospital, The Chinese University of Hong Kong, Hong Kong
*Transcatheter Options for Atrial Arrhythmia after the Mustard Procedure*

**Astrid E. Lammers, MD**
University College London; Fellow, Pulmonary Hypertension, Great Ormond Street Hospital for Children, London, United Kingdom
*Pulmonary Hypertension after Repair of Congenital Diaphragmatic Hernia*

**Wei Li, MD, PhD**
Adult Congenital Heart Disease Centre, Royal Brompton Hospital; National Heart Lung Institute, Imperial College School of Science and Medicine
*Right Heart Enlargement of Uncertain Cause (Sinus Venosus Atrial Septal Defect); Rationale for Septal Defect Closure in the Elderly*

**Per Lunde, MD**
Senior Consultant Cardiologist, University Hospital of Northern Norway, Tromsø, Norway
*Long-Term Follow-Up of Atrioventricular Septal Defect; Pacemaker Infection in a Cyanotic Patient; Iron Deficiency in Cyanotic Heart Disease*

**Jonathan Lyne, MRCP**
Royal Brompton Hospital, Cardiovascular Magnetic Resonance Unit, London, United Kingdom
*Ventricular Arrhythmia Following a Ross Procedure*

**Vaikom S. Mahadevan, MD, MRCP (UK)**
Consultant Cardiologist, Manchester Heart Centre, Manchester Royal Infirmary, Manchester, United Kingdom
*Catheter Closure of a Patent Ductus Arteriosus; Recoarctation: Criteria for Intervention; Catheter Intervention for Baffle Leak or Venous Obstruction*

**Constantine Mavroudis, MD**
Professor of Surgery, Case Western Reserve University School of Medicine; Ross Professor of Surgery, Chairman of Pediatric and Congenital Heart Surgery, Cleveland Clinic Foundation, Cleveland, Ohio
*Arrhythmia Intervention at the Time of Total Cavopulmonary Conversion*

**Peter R. McLaughlin, MD, FRCP(C)**
Clinical Adjunct Professor of Medicine, University of Toronto; Chief of Staff, Peterborough Regional Health Centre, Peterborough, Ontario, Canada
*Catheter Closure of a Patent Ductus Arteriosus; Catheter Intervention for Baffle Leak or Venous Obstruction*

**Victor Menashe, MD**
Department of Pediatrics, Oregon Health and Science University, Portland, Oregon
*Scimitar Syndrome; Endocarditis in a Young Man; Long-Term Survival in Eisenmenger Syndrome*

**David B. Meyer, MD**
Cardiothoracic Surgery, Schneider Children's Hospital, New Hyde Park, New York
*Considerations for the Ross Procedure*

**Shelley D. Miyamoto, MD**
Assistant Professor of Pediatrics, University of Colorado Denver Health Sciences Center; Director, Cardiomyopathy and Heart Failure Program, The Children's Hospital, University of Colorado, Denver, Colorado
*Timing and Merits of Transplantation in a Fontan Patient*

**Barbara J.M. Mulder, MD**
Professor of Cardiology, Academic Medical Center, Amsterdam, The Netherlands
*Recurrent Aortic Dissection in Marfan Syndrome*

**Michael J. Mullen, MD, FRCP**
Consultant Cardiologist, Cardiology Department, Royal Brompton & Harefield NHS Trust, London, United Kingdom
*Rationale for Septal Defect Closure in the Elderly; Arrhythmia and Syncope in a Patient with a Childhood Murmur*

**Ed Nicol, MD, MRCP**
Cardiology and General (Internal) Medicine Specialist Registrar, John Radcliffe Hospital, Oxford, United Kingdom; Cardiac Imaging Fellow, National Heart and Lung Institute, Royal Brompton Hospital, London, United Kingdom
*Fever in a Patient with a Single Ventricle*

**Elena Nikiphorou, MD**
Royal Brompton Hospital, London, United Kingdom
*Outflow Tract Obstruction after Atrioventricular Septal Defect Repair*

**Koichiro Niwa, MD, PhD**
Director, Department of Adult Congenital Heart Disease, Chiba Cardiovascular Center, Chiba, Japan
*Aortopathy in Tetralogy of Fallot*

**Erwin Oechslin, MD**
Associate Professor, University of Toronto; Director, Toronto Congenital Cardiac Centre for Adults, Toronto, Ontario, Canada
*Management of Acute Hemoptysis*

**George Pantely, MD**
Professor of Medicine (Cardiology), Adult Congenital Heart Disease Program, Oregon Health & Science University, Portland, Oregon
*Scimitar Syndrome; Endocarditis in a Young Man; Long-Term Survival in Eisenmenger Syndrome*

**Sabrina D. Phillips, MD**
Assistant Professor of Medicine, Mayo College of Medicine; Consultant, Cardiovascular Disease and Internal Medicine, Mayo Clinic, Rochester, Minnesota
*Interrupted Aortic Arch in a Patient with DiGeorge Syndrome; Coronary Artery Fistulae and Their Significance*

**Antonia Pijuan-Domenech, MD**
Cardiologist, Hospital Vall d'Hebron, Barcelona, Spain
*Palliative Mustard for Transposition and Ventricular Septal Defect; The Criss-Cross Heart*

**Daniele Prati, MD**
Research Fellow, Adult Congenital Heart Disease Programme, Royal Brompton Hospital, London, United Kingdom
*Palliative Mustard for Transposition and Ventricular Septal Defect*

**Peter J. Pugh, MD, MRCP, FESC**
Consultant Cardiologist, Addenbrooke's Hospital, Cambridge University Hospitals NHS Foundation Trust, Cambridge, United Kingdom
*Liver Dysfunction after the Mustard Procedure*

**Ivan M. Rebeyka, MD, FRCS**
Clinical Professor, Department of Surgery and Pediatrics, University of Alberta; Head, Pediatric Cardiovascular Surgery, Stollery Children's Hospital, Edmonton, Alberta, Canada
*Anomalous Left Coronary Artery from the Pulmonary Artery*

**Andrew N. Redington**
Division Head, Department of Cardiology, Hospital for Sick Children; Senior Associate Scientist, University of Toronto, Toronto, Ontario, Canada
*Late Outcome Following Systemic Tricuspid Valve Replacement*

**Jonathan Rome, MD, FACC**
Associate Professor of Pediatrics, University of Pennsylvania School of Medicine; Director, Cardiac Catheterization Laboratory, The Children's Hospital of Philadelphia, Philadelphia, Pennsylvania
*Recoarctation: Criteria for Intervention*

**Marlon S. Rosenbaum, MD**
Associate Attending, Columbia University College of Physicians & Surgeons; Director, Schneeweiss Columbia Adult Congenital Heart Center, Columbia University Medical Center, New York, New York
*Pregnancy and the Systemic Right Ventricle*

**Jonathon B. Ryan, MBBS, PhD, FRACS**
Department of Cardiac Surgery, Royal Brompton Hospital, London, United Kingdom
*Left Atrioventricular Valve Regurgitation: Criteria for Intervention*

**Richard J. Schilling, MD, MRCP**
Reader, Queen Mary University of London; Consultant Cardiologist, St. Bartholomew's Hospital, London, United Kingdom
*Catheter Ablation for Atrial Arrhythmia*

**Babulal Sethia, FRCS**
Consultant Cardiac Surgeon, Royal Brompton Hospital, London, United Kingdom
*Management of Tachyarrhythmia in Tetralogy: Ablation versus Surgery*

**Mary N. Sheppard, MD**
Royal Brompton Hospital, London, United Kingdom
*Pericardial Constriction after Relief of Subaortic Stenosis*

**Elliot A. Shinebourne, MD, FRCP, FRCPH**
Consultant Paediatric Cardiologist, Royal Brompton Hospital, London, United Kingdom
*Timing of Pulmonary Valve Replacement*

**Darryl F. Shore, FRCS**
Divisional Director, Heart Division, Consultant Cardiac Surgeon, Royal Brompton Hospital and Harefield NHS Trust, London, United Kingdom
*Extraanatomic Bypass Graft Repair of Coarctation; Consideration for Automatic Implantable Cardioverter-Defibrillator in Tetralogy*

**Candice K. Silversides, MD, MS, FRCPC**
Assistant Professor, University of Toronto; Staff Cardiologist, University Health Network, Toronto General Hospital, Toronto Congenital Cardiac Centre for Adults, Toronto, Ontario, Canada
*Cor Triatriatum; Considerations for Tricuspid Valve Replacement in Patients with a Systemic Right Ventricle*

**Thomas L. Spray, MD**
Professor of Surgery, University of Pennsylvania School of Medicine; Chief, Division of Cardiothoracic Surgery, Alice Langdon Warner Endowed Chair, The Children's Hospital of Philadelphia, Philadelphia, Pennsylvania
*Considerations for the Ross Procedure*

**Mark S. Spence, MB BCH, MD, BAO (Hons), MRCP**
Honorary Secior Lecturer, Queen's University Belfast; Consultant Cardiologist, Royal Vistoria Hospital, Belfast Trust, Belfast, Northern Ireland, United Kingdom
*Multiple Aortic-Pulmonary Collaterals: Too Many or Too Few*

**Martin St. John Sutton, MB, FRCP**
John W. Bryfogle Professor of Medicine, University of Pennsylvania School of Medicine; Director, Cardiovascular Imaging; Director, Cardiovascular Fellowship Program, The Hospital of the University of Pennsylvania, Philadelphia, Pennsylvania
*Cyanosis in Ebstein Anomaly and Catheter Closure of Atrial Septal Defect*

**Philip J. Steer, MBBS, MD, FRCOG**
Emeritus Professor of Obstetrics, Imperial College London; Consultant Obstetrician, Chelsea and Westminster Hospital, London, United Kingdom
*Pregnant Patient with Unoperated Truncus Arteriosus*

**Nilesh Sutaria, MD, MRCP**
Consultant Cardiologist, Imperial College Healthcare NHS Trust, London, United Kingdom
*Pericardial Constriction after Relief of Subaortic Stenosis*

**Lorna Swan, MB ChB, MD, MRCP**
Senior Lecturer, National Heart & Lung Institute, Imperial College; Consultant Cardiologist, Royal Brompton & Harefield NHS Trust, London, United Kingdom
*Ebstein Anomaly and Prepregnancy Counseling*

**Jonathan Swinburn, MBBS, MD**
Consultant Cardiologist, Royal Berkshire Hospital, Reading, United Kingdom
*Left Atrial Isomerism*

**Ju-Le Tan, MBBS, MRCP**
Senior Consultant Cardiologist, Adult Congenital Heart Disease, National Heart Centre, Singapore
*Right Heart Enlargement of Uncertain Cause (Sinus Venosus Atrial Septal Defect); Rationale for Septal Defect Closure in the Elderly*

**Judith Therrien, MD**
Assistant Professor of Medicine, McGill University; Adult Congenital Heart Disease Fellowship Director, MAUDE Unit and Beth Raby Adult Congenital Heart Disease Clinic, Jewish General Hospital, Montreal, Quebec, Canada
*Management of Systemic Ventricular Failure*

**Eapen Thomas, MD**
Grown-Up Congenital Heart Disease Unit, Queen Elizabeth Hospital, Edgbaston, Birmingham, United Kingdom
*Anticoagulation in a Pregnant Patient with a Mechanical Valve; Early Appraisal of Adults with Norwood Correction*

**Sara Thorne, MBBS, MD**
Honorary Senior Lecturer, Consultant Cardiologist, University of Birmingham, Birmingham, United Kingdom
*Anticoagulation in a Pregnant Patient with a Mechanical Valve; Early Appraisal of Adults with Norwood Correction*

**Jan Till, MD**
Consultant Electrophysiologist, Royal Brompton Hospital, London, United Kingdom
*Management of Tachyarrhythmia in Tetralogy: Ablation versus Surgery; Left Atrial Isomerism*

**Filippos Triposkiadis, MD, FESC, FACC**
Professor of Cardiology, University of Thessaly Medical
School; Director, Department of Cardiology, Larissa
University Hospital, Larissa, Greece
*Long-Term Outcome after Rastelli Repair*

**Etsuko Tsuda, MD**
Staff, Department of Pediatrics, National Cardiovascular
Center, Suita, Osaka, Japan
*Long-Term Management of Kawasaki Disease*

**Tomohiro Tsunekawa**
National Cardiovascular Center, Suita City, Osaka, Japan
*Ventricular Septal Defect and the Aortic Valve*

**Anselm Uebing, MD**
Fellow in Adult Congenital Heart Disease, Royal Brompton
Hospital and Harefield NHS Trust, Adult Congenital Heart
Disease Unit, London, United Kingdom
*Pregnancy-Related Complications in Coarctation; Fontan and
Pregnancy; Pregnant Patient with Unoperated Truncus Arteriosus;
Left Coronary Artery Arising from the Right Coronary Sinus*

**Hideki Uemura, MD**
Consultant Cardiac Surgeon, Royal Brompton Hospital,
London, United Kingdom
*Atrial Septal Defect with Cyanosis: The Hypoplastic Right
Ventricle; Partial Anomalous Pulmonary Venous Return;
Ventricular Septal Defect and the Aortic Valve; Left
Atrioventricular Valve Regurgitation: Criteria for Intervention;
Ebstein Anomaly and Wolff-Parkinson-White Syndrome; Successful
Tricuspid Valve Repair of Ebstein Anomaly; Total Cavopulmonary
Conversion: When and How; Complications of Ventricular
Septation in a Patient with a Single Ventricle; Long-Term
Management of Kawasaki Disease*

**Gruschen R. Veldtman, MB ChB, MRCP, Dip
Obstet**
Consultant Cardiologist, Congenital Cardiac Unit, University
of Southampton, Southampton University Hospital,
Southampton, United Kingdom
*Right Ventricular Outflow Obstruction in a Pregnant Woman*

**Isabelle F. Vonder Muhll, MD**
Assistant Professor, University of Alberta; Staff Cardiologist,
Department of Medicine, University of Alberta Hospital,
Edmonton, Alberta, Canada
*Anomalous Left Coronary Artery from the Pulmonary Artery*

**Gary D. Webb, MD, FRCPC, FACC**
Professor of Medicine, Director of the Philadelphia Adult
Congenital Heart Center, University of Pennsylvania School
of Medicine, The Hospital of the University of Pennsylvania,
Philadelphia, Pennsylvania
*Considerations for Tricuspid Valve Replacement in Patients with a
Systemic Right Ventricle; Recurrent Aortic Dissection in Marfan
Syndrome*

**Tom Wong, MRCP**
Consultant Electrophysiologist, Royal Brompton and
Harefield Hospitals, London, United Kingdom
*Ventricular Arrhythmia Following a Ross Procedure*

**Toshikatsu Yagihara, MD**
Deputy Director and Chairman, Cardiovascular Surgery,
National Cardiovascular Surgery Center, Osaka, Japan
*Partial Anomalous Pulmonary Venous Return; Ebstein Anomaly
and Wolff-Parkinson-White Syndrome; Complications of
Ventricular Septation in a Patient with a Single Ventricle; Long-
Term Management of Kawasaki Disease*

**Steve M. Yentis, MBBS, FRCA, MD, MA**
Honorary Senior Lecturer, Imperial College; Consultant
Anaesthetist, Chelsea and Westminster Hospital NHS
Foundation Trust, London, United Kingdom
*Pregnant Patient with Unoperated Truncus Arteriosus*

**Anji T. Yetman, MD**
Professor of Pediatrics, Adjunct Professor of Internal
Medicine, University of Utah; Director, Adult Congenital
Cardiology Program, University Hospital; Director, Adult
Congenital Cardiology Program, Primary Children's Medical
Center, Salt Lake City, Utah
*Timing and Merits of Transplantation in a Fontan Patient*

**Panayiotis Zarvos, MD, FCP-SA**
Director, Pediatric Department, Arch. Makarios Hospital,
Medical Health Services, Nicosia, Cyprus
*Outflow Tract Obstruction after Atrioventricular Septal Defect
Repair*

# Foreword

We live in an era of rapid advances in medicine, including cardiology and cardiac surgery. Because of that, life expectancy of patients born with congenital heart disease has increased steadily in the past four decades. The result of this is a growing population of adults living with congenital heart disease. Every day, teens and young adults with congenital heart disease are transitioning from the care of dedicated pediatric cardiologists into the uncertain world of adulthood. All over the world, specialized medical centers and groups are being formed to provide care appropriate for their complex and ongoing medical needs.

The most common reason patients join the Adult Congenital Heart Association is to find others living with the same condition in the hope of finding others with these rare diagnoses who have shared their particular experiences and struggles. For most of us, survival was dependent on whatever treatments were available at the time and place of our birth. As medicine advanced, treatments were constantly evolving. Over time, all the stents, patches, valves, and pacemakers have changed the structure of our hearts, further affected by the process of aging and the specifics of our life and health.

What does it mean to be an adult living with congenital heart disease? As president of the Adult Congenital Heart Association, I am asked this question every day. A patient facing surgery asks, "Am I likely to feel better?" A newlywed asks, "Do you think I should have children?" A parent of an infant asks, "Can my child live a normal life?" When patients ask me questions about what they might expect from life with their defect, my first answer is always, "I don't know." Each person's journey is dependent on the unique specifics of his or her anatomy, history of care, coexisting medical conditions, and the wild card of luck. The person best equipped to help answer these questions is the patient's own adult congenital heart specialist.

Drs. Gatzoulis, Webb, Broberg and Uemura have been at the forefront of advances in care of adult congenital heart disease for many years and have edited or contributed to numerous textbooks for medical professionals. This new book, however, is the first to focus on specific cases. It includes 85 cases from first presentation to the latest follow-up, and discusses the specific challenges in each patient. By choosing to focus on individual cases, the editors fully explore all aspects of the congenital heart picture and illustrate the array of trajectories that comprise life with congenital heart disease. By creating *Cases in Adult Congenital Heart Disease*, the editors have created a unique and essential tool to help ensure that these patients find the care they seek. They guide the medical professional to a much richer understanding of the complexity one must master to help ensure that each of us, patient by patient, gets the life and health care we deserve.

**Amy Verstappen**
**President and CEO**
**Adult Congenital Heart Association**

# Preface

Training opportunities for congenital heart disease—the most common inborn defect—and in particular its adult aspect of care, remain scarce. This, sadly, is mirrored by major gaps in care provision globally. In the meantime, the number of adults with congenital heart disease (ACHD) continues to increase. Despite advances in our understanding and management of this growing patient cohort, much of the practice is still based on personal experiences and limited or uncontrolled data. Furthermore, the complexity of the various lesions and the multitude of challenges that ACHD patients face call for a multidisciplinary approach to care. This is indeed the essence of good ACHD practice and the very focus of this training/educational book. For cardiology trainees and those who are interested in the ACHD field who desire additional opportunities to expose themselves to this fascinating and evolving field, our book is a forum for such exposure.

We submit that each ACHD patient is very different from another because of the range of anatomy and physiology, the continuously evolving palliative or reparative procedures available, and the different life circumstances that adults encounter. While the list of cases herein is not exhaustive, we have chosen the case mix in such a way to give the reader a good balance and flavor on current topics and areas of debate in ACHD.

The reader will find that the cases demonstrate the realities of the ACHD field, including incomplete medical histories, challenging or even suboptimal imaging, difficult decision making, and even, at times, poor outcome. Each case represents real experiences from real patients. At times, we have supplemented or editorialized the cases to maximize their educational value. This includes the addition of imaging studies, sometimes from similar patients, that, although not necessary from a case management standpoint, were included to demonstrate or clarify teaching points made.

The book can be read as a stand-alone text. There is also a web-based electronic version to facilitate accessibility and add value from cine imaging that cannot be printed. The latter, we hope, will enhance its training and educational value; individual imaging modalities can be played alone, thus facilitating a teaching session on any topic, for example ECG interpretation or CMR.

The format and table of contents follows closely the table of contents of our original textbook, *Diagnosis and Management of Adult Congenital Heart Disease*. It was our intention to provide a companion book that would stimulate further reading and welcome newcomers in one of the most exciting and rewarding areas of cardiology and indeed of medicine.

Michael A. Gatzoulis
Gary D. Webb
Craig S. Broberg
Hideki Uemura

# Abbreviations

| | | | | | |
|---|---|---|---|---|---|
| ACE | Angiotensin-converting enzyme | IPAH | Idiopathic pulmonary arterial hypertension | PV | Pulmonary vein |
| ACHD | Adult congenital heart disease | | | PVC | Premature ventricular contraction |
| AI | Aortic insufficiency | IRB | Institutional Review Board | PVR | Pulmonary vascular resistance |
| ALCAPA | Anomalous left coronary artery from the pulmonary artery | IVC | Inferior vena cava | Qp | Pulmonary blood flow |
| | | IVS | Intact ventricular septum | Qs | Systemic blood flow |
| AP | Anteroposterior (CXR projection) | JVP | Jugular venous pulse/pressure | RA | Right atrium |
| AR | Aortic valve regurgitation | LA | Left atrium | RAO | Right anterior oblique |
| AS | Aortic valve stenosis | LAO | Left anterior oblique | RAVV | Right atrioventricular valve |
| ASD | Atrial septal defect | LAVV | Left atrioventricular valve | RBBB | Right bundle branch block |
| AV | Atrioventricular | LPA | Left pulmonary artery | RPA | Right pulmonary artery |
| AVR | Aortic valve replacement | LV | Left ventricle | RV | Right ventricle |
| AVSD | Atrioventricular septal defect | LVEDd | LV end-diastolic dimension/diameter | RVOT | Right ventricular outflow tract |
| BAV | Bicuspid aortic valve | LVESd | LV end-systolic dimension/diameter | SSFP | Steady-state free precession (standard cine imaging technique by MRI) |
| BP | Blood pressure | LVOT | Left ventricular outflow tract | | |
| BSA | Body surface area | MAPCA | Major aortopulmonary collateral artery | SV | Stroke volume |
| BT | Blalock-Taussig (i.e., aortopulmonary shunt) | MCV | Mean corpuscular volume | SVC | Superior vena cava |
| | | MPA | Main pulmonary artery | SVi | Stroke volume index |
| CCTGA | Congenitally corrected transposition of the great arteries | MR | Mitral regurgitation | SVR | Systemic vascular resistance |
| | | MRI | Magnetic resonance imaging | TA | Tricuspid atresia or truncus arteriosus |
| CMR | Cardiac magnetic resonance | MS | Mitral stenosis | TCPC | Total cavopulmonary connection |
| CT | Computed tomography | NYHA | New York Heart Association | TEE | Transesophageal echocardiogram |
| CXR | Chest X-ray | PA | Pulmonary atresia or pulmonary artery | TGA | Transposition of the great arteries |
| ECG | Electrocardiogram | | | TOF | Tetralogy of Fallot |
| EDV | End-diastolic volume | PA | Posteroanterior (CXR projection) | TR | Tricuspid regurgitation |
| EDVi | End-diastolic volume index | PAH | Pulmonary arterial hypertension | TS | Tricuspid stenosis |
| EF | Ejection fraction | PCV | Packed cell volume | TV | Tricuspid valve |
| ESV | End-systolic volume | PDA | Patent ductus arteriosus | VA | Ventriculoarterial |
| ESVi | End-systolic volume index | PFO | Patent foramen ovale | Ve/Vco$_2$ | Ventilation/$CO_2$ production relationship (slope of ventilatory efficiency) |
| HLHS | Hypoplastic left heart syndrome | PLE | Protein-losing enteropathy | | |
| HR | Heart rate | PR | Pulmonary valve regurgitation | | |
| ICD | Implantable cardioverter-defibrillator | PRA | Panel reactive antibodies | Vo$_2$ | Oxygen consumption |
| ICE | Intracardiac echocardiography | PS | Pulmonary stenosis | VSD | Ventricular septal defect |

# Contents

## SECTION THREE  Right-Sided Lesions

## SECTION FOUR  Complex Congenital Heart Conditions

# Shunts

Part I

# Atrial Septal Defects/Abnormal Pulmonary Venous Return

# Right Heart Enlargement of Uncertain Cause (Sinus Venosus Atrial Septal Defect)

**Ju-Le Tan, Wei Li, and Elisabeth Bédard**

**Age: 56 years**
**Gender: Female**
**Personal information: Grandmother**
**Working diagnosis: Unexplained shortness of breath for several months**

## HISTORY

The patient had been well all her life. She had given birth to two daughters without any difficulties and more recently had been looking after her two young grandchildren. She had never been hospitalized nor had she required an operation. She was postmenopausal.

During a recent checkup with her general practitioner a murmur was heard. On questioning she admitted to feeling more short of breath with exertion. The patient was subsequently referred for further evaluation.

She had no other risk factors for coronary artery disease. There was no family history of congenital or acquired heart disease.

She does not smoke.

***Comments:*** Although the differential diagnosis for a 56-year-old woman with exertional dyspnea is extremely long, it is not uncommon for a congenital heart defect to present for the first time in the fifth or sixth decade of life. ASDs would be by far the most common among them.

## CURRENT SYMPTOMS

There were no symptoms other than exertional dyspnea, although the patient admitted to "slowing down" in the last few years and to avoiding stairs and hills.

Specifically she denied recent fevers, chest pains, palpitations, and gastrointestinal or vaginal bleeding.

NYHA class:  I–II

## CURRENT MEDICATIONS

None

## PHYSICAL EXAMINATION

BP 124/76 mm Hg, HR 60 bpm, oxygen saturation 100% on room air

Height 160 cm, weight 65 kg, BSA 1.7 m$^2$

Neck veins: Venous waveform was normal and not elevated.

Lungs/chest: Clear

Heart: The rhythm was regular. There was no left parasternal heave on palpation. The pulmonary component of the second heart sound was delayed, but was neither loud nor fixed. There was a soft systolic ejection murmur at the upper left sternal border.

Abdomen: The abdomen was normal with no ascites or organomegaly.

Extremities: The extremities were not edematous.

### PERTINENT NEGATIVES
No clubbing was seen.

***Comments:*** This patient has no obvious clinical signs to suggest right ventricular hypertrophy or dilatation. Patients with an ASD often have fixed splitting of the second heart sound, but its absence does not rule out an ASD, such as a sinus venosus ASD. The absence of a loud pulmonary component of the second heart sound makes pulmonary hypertension unlikely. A soft systolic ejection murmur is very common due to increased pulmonary blood flow in such patients.

## LABORATORY DATA

| | |
|---|---|
| Hemoglobin | 14 g/dL (11.5–15.0) |
| Hematocrit/PCV | 41% (36–46) |
| MCV | 90 fL (83–99) |
| Platelet count | $191 \times 10^9$/L (150–400) |
| Sodium | 138 mmol/L (134–145) |
| Potassium | 4.0 mmol/L (3.5–5.2) |
| Creatinine | 0.61 mg/dL (0.6–1.2) |
| Blood urea nitrogen | 5.3 mmol/L (2.5–6.5) |

***Comments:*** No abnormalities were seen. Her breathlessness could not be explained by anemia.

## ELECTROCARDIOGRAM

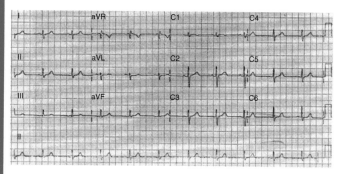

Figure 1-1 Electrocardiogram.

### FINDINGS
Heart rate: 64 bpm

QRS axis: +107°

QRS duration: 84 msec

Sinus rhythm with normal AV conduction. There was an inverted P-wave in lead III and a prominent R in leads V1–2.

***Comments:*** The rightward axis and the R in V1 suggest possible enlargement of the RV, although criteria for RV hypertrophy were not present. This should prompt consideration for an ASD.

The presence of a negative P-wave in lead III as seen in this patient is a typical feature of a sinus venosus ASD. The P-wave vector is approximately –20 degrees, so the term *coronary sinus* or *low atrial* rhythm would be appropriate. The sinus node may also be affected as it lies in the vicinity of the defect or adjacent to the site of an anomalous pulmonary venous connection.

## CHEST X-RAY

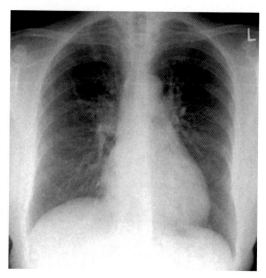

Figure 1-2 Posteroanterior projection.

### FINDINGS
Cardiothoracic ratio: 60%

There is mild cardiomegaly with mild RA dilatation. The central pulmonary arteries are dilated with increased pulmonary vascular markings.

***Comments:*** The CXR findings here combined with the subtle ECG findings are suspicious for right heart enlargement (lateral CXRs are not routinely done at our hospital). Further imaging should focus on a potential source of a left-to-right shunt.

## EXERCISE TESTING

Not performed

## ECHOCARDIOGRAM

### OVERALL FINDINGS
The LV was normal in size and function with a competent mitral valve.

The RV was moderately dilated.

The tricuspid valve was competent. The RA and LA were moderately dilated.

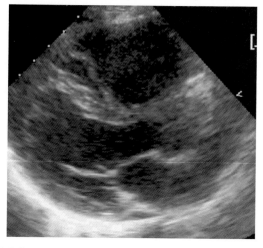

Figure 1-3 Parasternal long-axis view.

## FINDINGS
RV dilatation is seen. The LV and LA were normal.

*Comments:* The RV finding should prompt the sonographer to search extensively for evidence of a left-to-right shunt, most likely across an ASD, and/or for the presence of anomalous pulmonary veins.

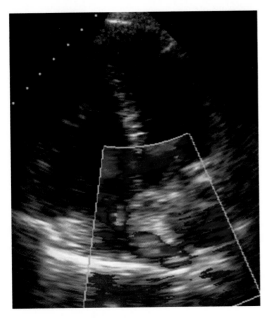

Figure 1-4 Apical four-chamber view.

## FINDINGS
Both the RA and RV were moderately dilated. In addition, there was a 15-mm sinus venosus ASD with a left-to-right shunt.

*Comments:* This shows again the moderately dilated and volume overloaded RV. The cause is a left-to-right shunt through a defect high on the atrial septum (at the bottom of this image).

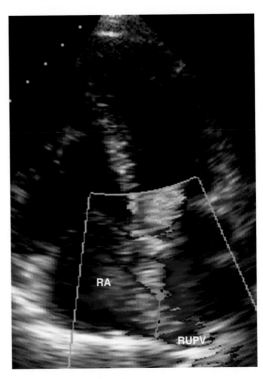

Figure 1-5 Apical four-chamber view.

## FINDINGS
There was an anomalous drainage of the right upper pulmonary vein (RUPV) to the RA. The sinus venosus ASD measured 14 mm.

*Comments:* Sinus venosus ASDs are very commonly associated with partial anomalous pulmonary venous drainage; the anomalous drainage usually involves the RUPV, which often drains into the SVC and RA junction.

# MAGNETIC RESONANCE IMAGING

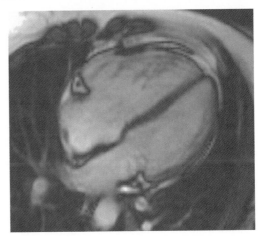

Figure 1-6 Magnetic resonance image.

## Ventricular Volume Quantification

|  | LV | (Normal range) | RV | (Normal range) |
|---|---|---|---|---|
| EDV (mL) | 81 | (52–141) | **187** | (58–154) |
| ESV (mL) | 36 | (13–51) | **87** | (12–68) |
| SV (mL) | 45 | (33–97) | **100** | (35–98) |
| EF (%) | **56** | (59–77) | 53 | (55–79) |
| EDVi (mL/m$^2$) | **48** | (56–90) | **110** | (53–90) |
| ESVi (mL/m$^2$) | 21 | (14–33) | **51** | (11–37) |
| SVi (mL/m$^2$) | **26** | (37–62) | **59** | (17–37) |

## FINDINGS

The RA and RV were dilated with normal RV systolic function. The pulmonary/systemic flow ratio (Qp/Qs) was 2.2:1 based on flow measurements.

**Comments:** Cardiac MRI was primarily performed to clarify the pulmonary venous drainage and confirm the ECG findings. Estimates of ventricular mass, flow, and shunt volume can also be obtained noninvasively from the MRI study. Shunt volume can be calculated by measuring the difference between pulmonary artery (PA) flow and aortic flow. MRI confirmed that the upper right pulmonary vein drains into the SVC at its junction with the RA. Cardiac surgeons would normally inspect the four pulmonary veins during repair; hence it may not be necessary to perform a routine MRI when the diagnosis of sinus venosus ASD has been established. Nevertheless, it is helpful to have complete data on the anomalous pulmonary venous drainage in hand before surgery, as the anomalous vein may occasionally have a longer and tortuous course, draining at a more distal site, which in turn requires a more complex repair.

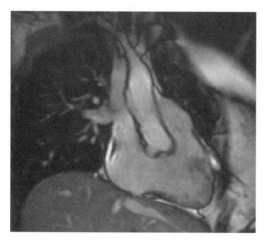

Figure 1-7 Oblique coronal plane.

## FINDINGS

The aortic valve and aorta are in the center of the image. The SVC runs parallel to the aorta. The RUPV can be seen draining into the SVC just as it enters the RA.

**Comments:** Imaging planes such as this that look for specific abnormalities of pulmonary venous drainage are not usually done in a routine study. The imager must know the clinical question at hand to provide useful data. Although not performed in this case, a contrast-enhanced magnetic resonance angiogram is recommended for visualizing all pulmonary veins.

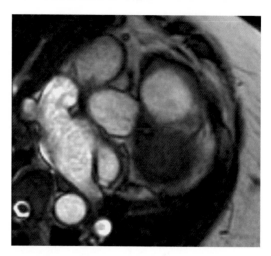

Figure 1-8 Oblique sagittal plane at the level of the high right atrium, viewed from the left ventricular apex.

## FINDINGS

The aortic root is seen in cross section in the center of the image, with the left PA above it. Just below the aorta in this view there is a communication between the atria. This is the location where the upper RA and LA are usually separated by an infolding of the atrial wall, which is absent here.

**Comments:** This demonstrates a sinus venosus ASD. This was associated with anomalous drainage of the RUPV to the SVC (from far left of image). The other pulmonary veins drained normally to the LA. No other defects were found.

Note the relatively small size of the aorta (in short axis) compared to the size of the left PA, reflecting the long-standing low cardiac output and systemic "run-off" ("steal") that this patient has been subjected to throughout her life because of significant left-to-right shunting at atrial level.

## CATHETERIZATION

### HEMODYNAMICS

Heart rate    60 bpm

|  | Pressure | Saturation (%) |
|---|---|---|
| High SVC |  | 66 |
| Low SVC |  | **79** |
| IVC |  | **82** |
| RA | mean 9 | **84** |
| RV | 35/9 | **88** |
| PA | 34/9 mean 19 | **86** |
| PCWP | mean 9 |  |
| LA |  |  |
| LV | 143/11 |  |
| Aorta | 128/77 mean 99 | 97 |

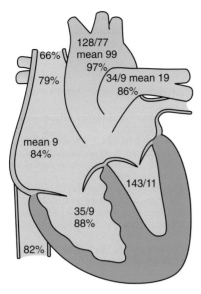

Figure 1-9 Hemodynamic data.

**Calculations**

| | |
|---|---|
| Qp (L/min) | **6.86** |
| Qs (L/min) | 3.05 |
| Cardiac index (L/min/m²) | **1.79** |
| Qp/Qs | **2.25** |
| PVR (Wood units) | 1.17 |
| SVR (Wood units) | 29.53 |

## FINDINGS

Hemodynamic measurements are shown. The coronary angiogram showed no evidence of coronary artery disease.

**Comments:** Diagnostic catheterization was performed to obtain hemodynamic data including pulmonary vascular resistance and also to evaluate the coronary arteries prior to surgery. It was not essential to obtain the hemodynamic data.

Hemodynamic data showed a step-up from high SVC to low SVC, suggesting that the anomalous pulmonary venous connection was nearer the lower SVC or SVC-RA junction.

The RV end-diastolic pressure of 9 mm Hg suggested a compliant RV.

The calculated Qp/Qs of 2.3 confirmed significant left-to-right shunting. There was no significant pulmonary hypertension, as the mean PA pressure was only 19 mm Hg, and pulmonary vascular resistance was not elevated.

### FOCUSED CLINICAL QUESTIONS AND DISCUSSION POINTS

1. What is the diagnosis?

*The patient has a sinus venosus ASD with anomalous drainage of the RUPV near the defect. Anomalous pulmonary venous drainage is commonly associated with superior sinus venosus ASD,[1] which is located superior to the atrial septum and adjacent to the SVC. The true interatrial septum is often intact because the defect is due to the deficiency of infolding of the atrial wall above the septum. Commonly, the upper or middle right pulmonary vein drains directly into the SVC, SVC-RA junction, or into the RA.[1]*

*Routine ECG or MRI can often miss these findings. Even a bubble study may be falsely negative because the shunt is* almost completely left to right. The case illustrates that in patients with evidence of RV enlargement by ECG and no obvious cause, a thorough search for a left-to-right shunt and anomalous pulmonary veins should be specifically conducted.

2. Since the patient was only mildly symptomatic, should the sinus venosus ASD be closed?

*Objectively, there was evidence of right ventricular dilatation and significant left-to-right shunt by ECG, MRI, and cardiac catheterization. Even though only mildly symptomatic at present, the patient is likely to deteriorate further with time. Sinus venosus ASDs with right heart dilatation should be closed regardless of symptoms.[2,3]*

*Because this lesion is not amenable to catheter-based closure, surgery would be required.*

3. What is the risk of atrial arrhythmia after closure of the defect?

*Unfortunately, the risk of atrial arrhythmia is not reduced by surgical closure of an ASD in the older patient.[4] During a mean follow-up of 9 years, atrial fibrillation or flutter was found to have developed in 15% of surgically treated ASD patients.[4] The age at time of surgery (>40 years), the presence of preoperative atrial flutter or fibrillation, and the presence of postoperative atrial flutter or fibrillation or junctional rhythm have been shown to be predictors of late postoperative atrial arrhythmias.[5] Furthermore, patients with superior sinus venosus defects are at risk of sinus node dysfunction because of the proximity of the defect to the sinus node. Thus, patients should be followed longer term for the development of atrial flutter or atrial fibrillation, which puts them at risk for cerebral thromboembolism, or for sinus node dysfunction that may require permanent pacing.*

## FINAL DIAGNOSIS

Secundum ASD, sinus venosus type

Anomalous drainage of the RUPV

## PLAN OF ACTION

Surgical closure of the defect

## INTERVENTION

Open heart surgery, closure of the ASD, and redirection of pulmonary venous drainage

## OUTCOME

The patient underwent closure of her sinus venosus ASD and rerouting of the pulmonary vein to the LA. At surgery the RUPV was seen draining into the RA at the junction with the SVC, and the right lower pulmonary vein drained directly into the RA immediately adjacent to the defect. She developed bilateral pleural effusions postoperatively but had an otherwise uneventful postoperative recovery.

The patient was instructed to take aspirin (75 mg) for 6 months.

Two weeks postoperatively she had made good recovery from her surgery with resolution of her pleural effusions. Transthoracic echocardiography showed no residual shunting across the site of her previous sinus venosus defect, unobstructed pulmonary venous return, and reduction in RA and RV dimensions.

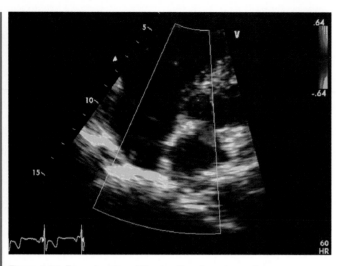

Figure 1-10 Four-chamber, 2D color Doppler echocardiogram.

## FINDINGS

No residual flow from the sinus venosus was visible.

**Comments:** Transthoracic echocardiography showed no residual shunting across the site of her previous sinus venosus defect with reduction in right atrial and ventricular dimensions. Her exercise capacity also improved after surgery, and she was able to climb hills and stairs freely without the dyspnea she had previously experienced. Fortunately, she has not had any cardiac arrhythmias perioperatively or subsequently to this point.

## Selected References

1. Gustafson RA, Warden HE, Murray GF, et al: Partial anomalous pulmonary venous connection to the right side of the heart. J Thorac Cardiovasc Surg 98(5 Pt 2):861–868, 1989.
2. Vogel M, Berger F, Kramer A, et al: Incidence of secondary pulmonary hypertension in adults with atrial septal or sinus venosus defects. Heart 82:30–33, 1999.
3. Webb GD, Gatzoulis MA: Atrial septal defects in the adult: Recent progress and overview. Circulation 114:1645–1653, 2006.
4. Konstantinides S, Geibel A, Olschewski M, et al: A comparison of surgical and medical therapy for atrial septal defect in adults. N Engl J Med 333:469–473, 1995.
5. Gatzoulis MA, Freeman MA, Siu SC, et al: Atrial arrhythmia after surgical closure of atrial septal defects in adults. N Engl J Med 340:839–846, 1999.

## Bibliography

Jost CHA, Connolly HM, Danielson GK, et al: Sinus venosus atrial septal defect: Long-term postoperative outcome for 115 patients. Circulation 112:1953–1958, 2005.
Roess D, Pascoe JK, Oh CA, et al: Diagnosis of sinus venosus atrial septal defect with transesophageal echocardiography. Circulation 94:1049–1055, 1996.

# Rationale for Septal Defect Closure in the Elderly

**Ju-Le Tan, Wei Li, and Michael J. Mullen**

**Age: 88 years**
**Gender: Female**
**Personal information: Grandmother**
**Working diagnosis: Secundum atrial septal defect**

## HISTORY

The patient was healthy throughout her childhood and adult years. She had two uneventful pregnancies, and has two healthy sons and numerous grandchildren.

Mild hypertension was diagnosed 15 years ago, and the patient was treated with medication. Around that same time she developed atrial fibrillation, which was treated with digoxin and aspirin and has been permanent for the last decade.

After the death of her husband several years ago, she managed to live independently. However, over the last few years she noted decreasing effort tolerance and frequent chest infections. She found it difficult to manage housework, shopping, and gardening while living on her own, and therefore moved to a larger city to be nearer her children. On arrival she established medical care with a new general practitioner.

She does not smoke or drink alcohol. There was no family history of congenital or ischemic heart disease.

**Comments:** Although she is now 88 years old the patient has until recently led an active and independent life. Obviously, elderly patients with exertional breathlessness will have ischemic heart disease much more commonly than an ASD, but it is not uncommon for a secundum ASD to present for the first time in an elderly patient.

Although the particular details are unknown, it is surprising that atrial fibrillation did not prompt a more thorough workup including echocardiography, which should have demonstrated her large ASD.

Worsening symptoms in this patient with an ASD are probably due to substantial left-to-right shunting and RV volume overloading (both tend to increase with age because of an increase in left ventricular end-diastolic pressures), and the development of PAH or LV diastolic dysfunction from systolic hypertension.

ASDs can be familial (autosomal dominant); at least three genes have been recently identified in families with ASD.[1]

## CURRENT SYMPTOMS

The patient becomes breathless after walking less than a quarter mile (380 m) on flat ground. She cannot climb one flight of stairs without stopping with dyspnea.

She does not experience exertional chest pain or other cardiac symptoms.

NYHA class: III

## CURRENT MEDICATIONS

Digoxin 125 µg daily

Bendrofluazide 2.5 mg daily (a diuretic used for blood pressure control)

Perindopril 2 mg daily (for blood pressure control)

Aspirin 75 mg daily (presumably for her permanent atrial fibrillation)

**Comments:** Given her atrial fibrillation, hypertension, and age, the role of anticoagulation should be discussed with the patient. She is at risk of stroke (even after ASD repair) and should be advised to take warfarin unless there is a contraindication.[2]

## PHYSICAL EXAMINATION

BP 155/86 mm Hg, HR 70 bpm, oxygen saturation 92% on room air, near sea level

Height 158 cm, weight 53 kg, BSA 1.53 m$^2$

Surgical scars: None

Neck veins: 5 cm above sternal angle, normal waveform

Lungs/chest: Clear

Heart: There was an irregular rhythm, with a right parasternal heave. There was a normal first heart sound and wide splitting of the second sound with a loud pulmonary component (P2). There was also a 3/6 ejection systolic murmur in the third left intercostal space.

Abdomen: The abdominal examination was unremarkable.

Extremities: Extremities were well perfused without edema.

**Comments:** Hypertension may need better control. Her resting ventricular rate response to atrial fibrillation was well controlled. Oxygen saturation was mildly reduced, prompting one to consider why she might have a right-to-left shunt.

The right parasternal heave is indicative of significant RV volume and/or pressure overloading.

The loud P2 indicates elevated pulmonary artery (PA) pressures. The ejection systolic murmur is secondary to increased flow through the RVOT and pulmonary valve. Fixed splitting of the second heart sound would be expected in a patient with a secundum ASD but can be difficult to hear in some patients.

There were no clinical signs of right or left heart failure.

## LABORATORY DATA

| | |
|---|---|
| Hemoglobin | 13.5 g/dL (11.5–15.0) |
| Hematocrit/PCV | 39% (36–46) |
| MCV | 93 fL (83–99) |
| Platelet count | **137 × 10⁹/L** (150–400) |
| Sodium | 141 mmol/L (134–145) |
| Potassium | 4.4 mmol/L (3.5–5.2) |
| Creatinine | 1.0 mg/dL (0.6–1.2) |
| Blood urea nitrogen | **7.3 mmol/L** (2.5–6.5) |

**Comments:** It is important to know whether the renal function is normal (systemic hypertension, on diuretics and an ACE inhibitor), especially if percutaneous intervention is to be considered.

## ELECTROCARDIOGRAM

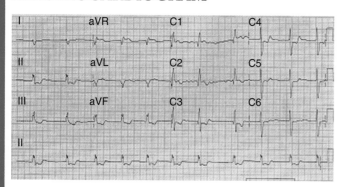

Figure 2-1  Electrocardiogram.

### FINDINGS
Heart rate: 66 bpm

QRS axis: +123°

QRS duration: 133 msec

Atrial fibrillation

Right axis deviation

Right bundle branch block

Nonspecific ST segment depression

**Comments:** RBBB with right axis deviation should immediately prompt consideration of right heart disease. Right axis deviation is commonly associated with a secundum ASD, while RBBB with a leftward axis would be more typical for a primum ASD (see Case 15).

The ST segments in the inferior and anterior chest leads, especially V3–5, are downward sloping, and due to some combination of digoxin effect, RBBB, and RV hypertrophy.

## CHEST X-RAY

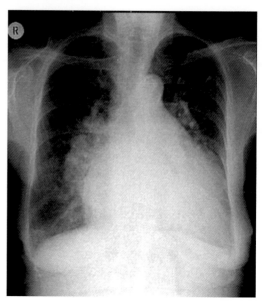

Figure 2-2  Posteroanterior projection.

### FINDINGS
Cardiothoracic ratio: 76%

There is gross cardiomegaly, with prominent central pulmonary arteries and a generally plethoric pulmonary vasculature. There is RA and presumably RV dilation (which would have been better seen on the lateral view, yet is not available).

**Comments:** Most likely, the large cardiac silhouette is mainly due to RA and RV enlargement. Prominent central pulmonary arteries may indicate volume or pressure overload, although the latter is unlikely given the numerous peripheral pulmonary vessels (no "pruning").

## EXERCISE TESTING

Pretest HR: 52, oxygen saturation 94%

Posttest HR: 66, oxygen saturation 87%

Distance walked: 221 m

**Comments:** In elderly patients who are not able to reliably perform maximal exercise testing, the 6MWT is a useful submaximal alternative for functional assessment. It is safe in the older population.[3] The mean walk distance in patients older than 68 years of age is 344 m.

Other information from the test includes the peak heart rate and the oxygen saturation after exercise, which are particularly valuable in congenital heart disease. This test can be easily repeated in the future to monitor for clinical deterioration or improvement after an intervention.

In this patient, the minimal increase in heart rate is not surprising given her medically controlled atrial fibrillation. More important, there was mildly progressive oxygen desaturation after 6 minutes (94% to 87%) suggesting right-to-left shunt during exercise, intrinsic lung disease, or congestive heart failure.

# ECHOCARDIOGRAM

## OVERALL FINDINGS

The RV was severely dilated. The LV was small, with a left ventricular end-diastolic dimension of 42 mm and an end-systolic dimension of 25 mm. The LA was dilated. There was moderate tricuspid regurgitation; otherwise, valve function was normal. The RV size relative to the LV can be seen, as well as LA enlargement.

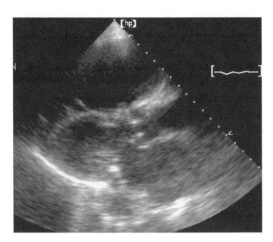

Figure 2-3 Parasternal long-axis view.

**Comments:** The RV enlargement is secondary to the chronic left-to-right shunt. The LA enlargement was probably due to the volume overload, hypertension, and chronic atrial fibrillation itself.

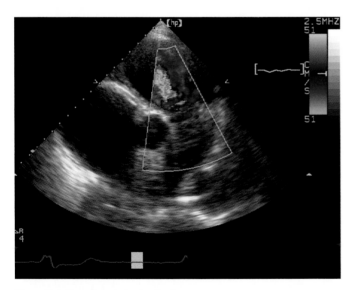

Figure 2-4 Parasternal short-axis view.

## FINDINGS

Dilated main pulmonary artery. Mild to moderate pulmonary regurgitation.

**Comments:** The main pulmonary atery has dilated in response to chronic volume loading, and dilatation of the pulmonary annulus has led to secondary pulmonary regurgitation.

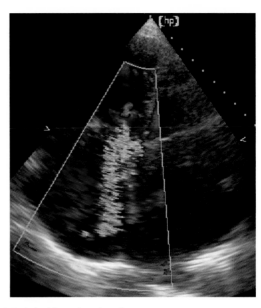

Figure 2-5 Apical four-chamber view.

## FINDINGS

There was severe dilatation of the RA and RV, with moderate central tricuspid regurgitation. The LV was relatively small. Systolic function of both ventricles was normal.

The secundum ASD was large, at least 30 mm in diameter.

**Comments:** The dilatation is secondary to volume overloading of the RA and RV from left-to-right shunting. Tricuspid regurgitation is also secondary to tricuspid annular dilatation and often improves with reverse right heart remodeling after ASD closure.

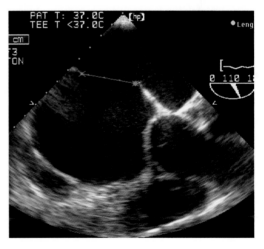

Figure 2-6 Transesophageal echocardiogram.

## FINDINGS

The large secundum ASD measured 34 mm in diameter with left-to-right shunting.

**Comments:** TEE can ensure adequate rim tissue necessary for closure with a transcatheter device.

At times, an atrial defect can be so large that there is not enough remaining septal tissue on which to anchor a closure device. In this patient, although the defect was large, there was a sufficient rim for an ASD closure device to be properly seated. Furthermore, there was a large LA; thus the device would not likely obstruct flow in the pulmonary veins or mitral valve. Therefore, there were no concerns about using a large ASD closure device.

# MAGNETIC RESONANCE IMAGING

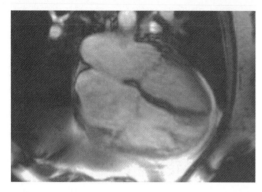

Figure 2-7 Oblique transaxial four-chamber view.

## FINDINGS

The RA and RV were dilated but with normal RV systolic function. The LV was small in comparison. There was mild tricuspid regurgitation. The main pulmonary artery was enlarged. By velocity flow mapping, the pulmonary/systemic flow ratio (Qp/Qs) was 2:1.

**Comments:** MRI is often not necessary if a large defect can be seen by echo. The additional information from an MRI includes volume and mass of the RV, and noninvasive estimates of flow, including Qp/Qs ratio, as well as additional information on the pulmonary venous drainage, which is particularly relevant in patients with sinus venosus ASDs.

In this four-chamber view, the dilatation of the RV is clearly seen (bottom of the image). Interestingly, the ASD is not visible in this view. Instead, the faint impression of the superior rim is visible, which deviates toward the RA when the RV opens and atrial pressure falls.

## Ventricular Volume Quantification

|  | LV | (Normal range) | RV | (Normal range) |
|---|---|---|---|---|
| EDV (mL) | 83 | (52–141) | **171** | (58–154) |
| ESV (mL) | 40 | (13–51) | **82** | (12–68) |
| SV (mL) | 43 | (33–97) | 89 | (35–98) |
| EF (%) | 52 | (60–78) | **52** | (59–83) |
| EDVi (mL/m²) | 54 | (50–84) | **112** | (45–82) |
| ESVi (mL/m²) | 26 | (12–30) | **54** | (6–32) |
| SVi (mL/m²) | **28** | (34–59) | **58** | (14–35) |

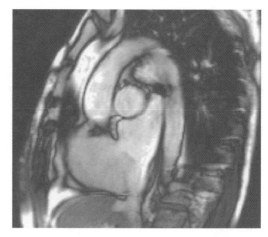

Figure 2-8 Oblique sagittal short axis-view at atrial level.

## FINDINGS

Large secundum ASD, measuring 34 mm in diameter.

**Comments:** The lower portion of the image shows the RA (lower left) and LA (lower right). The IVC can be seen draining upward to the RA, and flow is directed by a Eustachian valve. The ASD is seen above this Eustachian valve.

# CATHETERIZATION

## HEMODYNAMICS

Heart rate     70 bpm

|  | **Pressure** | **Saturation** (%) |
|---|---|---|
| SVC |  | 75 |
| IVC |  | 80 |
| RA | mean 11 | **90** |
| RV | 40/8 | **89** |
| PA | 46/14 mean 23 | **88** |
| PV | mean 14 | 98 |
| LA | mean 9 |  |
| LV | 100/10 |  |
| Aorta | 109/40 mean 64 | **95** |

**Calculations**

| | |
|---|---|
| Qp (L/min) | 7.33 |
| Qs (L/min) | 3.91 |
| Cardiac index (L/min/m²) | 2.56 |
| Qp/Qs | **1.88** |
| PVR (Wood units) | 1.91 |
| SVR (Wood units) | 13.55 |

**Comments:** Cardiac catheterization was performed with the patient under general anesthesia to achieve device closure under TEE guidance. The lower heart rate and blood pressure reflect the anesthesia. It is important to ask the anesthetist to use room air and not supplemental oxygen so that the series of oxygen saturations and the calculations of shunt ratio and pulmonary vascular resistance are accurate.

The patient's hemodynamics showed mildly increased pulmonary artery pressures, reflecting increased pulmonary flow, but the pulmonary vascular resistance was not elevated. The Qp/Qs ratio calculated here agrees with that found by MRI but is surprisingly small considering the size of her heart on CXR.

She also had coronary angiograms to exclude silent coronary artery disease. These showed mid-LAD stenosis of 50% with no other significant lesions.

Despite some previous findings suggesting possible pulmonary vascular disease (such as the loud pulmonary component of the second heart sound and the desaturation with exercise), the pulmonary vascular resistance is low and the operator could continue confidently with ASD closure.

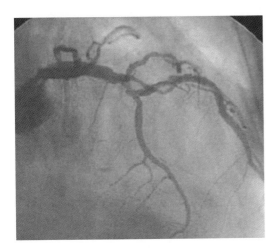

Figure 2-9 Right anterior oblique cranial angiogram.

## FINDINGS

There are diffuse irregularities in the LAD and its branches, including a 50% mid-LAD lesion.

**Comments:** The relevance of these lesions in relation to the patient's symptoms needs to be considered. Often in ACHD too much focus is on the congenital heart defect to the exclusion of other potential comorbidities, cardiovascular or otherwise.

### FOCUSED CLINICAL QUESTIONS AND DISCUSSION POINTS

1. **Should an ASD in an elderly patient be closed?**

*Transcatheter closure of an ASD is a relatively safe procedure; its advantages are obvious, especially improving exercise tolerance and quality of life in a patient who is limited.[4] In the elderly population where comorbidities are common, transcatheter closure conveys additional benefits; it can be performed without the risk of heart surgery and a sometimes prolonged postoperative course. There are limited published data on ASD closure in the elderly population (>65 years old) who have experienced chronic RV overload and reduction in LV preload for decades. However, there is a clear trend toward improved functional capacity following late repair of ASDs in older patients, irrespective of age.*

*A recent publication suggested that in some elderly patients, especially those with systemic hypertension, ASD closure may unmask restrictive LV diastolic dysfunction and lead to pulmonary edema after the procedure.[5] In clinical practice, for the occasional patient felt to be at risk of this complication, a temporary balloon occlusion (10 minutes) of the ASD may allow the operator to assess the hemodynamics, with the defect closed. If the LV end-diastolic pressure increases significantly or the mitral inflow pattern on TEE shows a predominantly restrictive filling during temporary balloon occlusion, the ASD should perhaps not be closed or a fenestrated closure should be considered (for*

*the patient with a very large ASD and marked right heart dilatation).*

2. **Will atrial fibrillation or stroke risk improve after closure of the ASD?**

*Late surgical closure of an ASD does not decrease the risk of late arrhythmia development.[6] In patients with significant atrial dilatation, and in elderly patients with other risk factors for arrhythmia (such as hypertension in this case), return to sinus rhythm after closure would not be expected, unless an arrhythmia-targeting intervention were incorporated around the time of closure. Nevertheless, the hemodynamic response to arrhythmia after ASD closure will be better, and the risk of paradoxical embolus, no matter how small, would be abolished. It should be emphasized, however, that older patients remain at risk of stroke (there has been speculation on the potential pathogenic role of the dilated pulmonary veins) and should be considered for anticoagulation with warfarin for at least 6 months, while reverse remodeling is taking place. Patients with persistent atrial fibrillation after ASD closure should remain on indefinite anticoagulation.*

3. **Could the patient's symptoms be secondary to coronary artery disease?**

*Elderly patients being considered for secundum ASD closure should be tested to exclude coexistent coronary artery disease. This patient had the risk factor of hypertension, and a 50% lesion was found in her LAD. Elsewhere there was no significant coronary artery disease. She denied any angina-like symptoms and experienced none during her 6MWT.*

*In general, coronary artery disease should be treated concurrently with ASD closure, using the same approach used for a similar patient without the congenital defect, including stent deployment before or after ASD closure. In this patient we opted to first pursue medical management of her coronary disease alone. If her exertional dyspnea did not improve significantly following ASD closure, or she developed angina-like symptoms, the LAD lesion could be addressed at a future date. If doubt remained about the cause of her symptoms, assessment of the patient's coronary artery disease with a myocardial perfusion scan and/or a stress echo could guide further management.*

## FINAL DIAGNOSIS

Secundum ASD

Chronic atrial fibrillation

Coronary artery disease

Treated systemic hypertension

## PLAN OF ACTION

Transcatheter closure of the ASD

Medical management of coronary artery disease

## INTERVENTION

At the time of catheterization, TEE showed an adequate rim of tissue for device closure. The defect was measured with a low-pressure occlusive balloon. After 10 minutes of temporary defect closure with the balloon, there was no rise in the LV end-diastolic pressure and the mitral filling pattern did not change. A 36-mm Amplatzer device was selected. The left atrial disc of the Amplatzer device is 16 mm larger than the waist, which may be the limiting factor in some patients with a large defect but small LA. This was not an issue with our patient, as her LA was enlarged. The device was deployed uneventfully and the procedure completed without any complications.

CXR and echo the following day showed good position of the device without a pericardial effusion. She was started on clopidogrel 75 mg daily, to continue for 6 weeks following the procedure. Warfarin was recommended to reduce the thrombo-embolic risk of her chronic atrial fibrillation, but the patient and family refused. Thus she continued on aspirin indefinitely. The patient was advised to practice antibiotic prophylaxis for 6 months after device closure.

## OUTCOME

Six months after device closure, the patient reported marked improvement in her exercise capacity to the extent that she could walk to her local shop without stopping because of breathlessness, and climb a flight of stairs easily. She was able to regain her independence and to look after herself, living on her own.

Objectively, her oxygen saturation at rest was 97% and her 6MWT had improved from 221 m to 382 m, with no desaturation. Her echo showed that her ASD device was well positioned with no residual shunting. Her RV and RA remained moderately dilated, but the estimated pulmonary artery systolic pressure had decreased from 50 mm Hg to 27 mm Hg. She remained in chronic rate-controlled atrial fibrillation.

She developed no chest pain and continued on appropriate medical therapy for coronary artery disease.

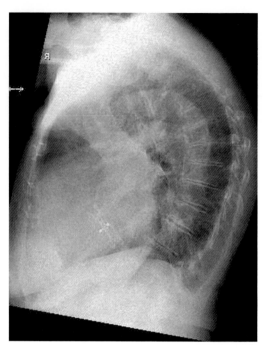

Figure 2-11 Postprocedure lateral projection.

### FINDINGS

Atrial enlargement. ASD occluder device in proper position.

**Comments:** The ASD device is visible in the proper position.

## Selected References

1. Gelb BD: Genetic basis of congenital heart disease. Curr Opin Cardiol 19:110–115, 2004.
2. Gage BF, van Walraven C, Pearce L, et al: Selecting patients with atrial fibrillation for anticoagulation: Stroke risk stratification in patients taking aspirin. Circulation 110:2287–2292, 2004.
3. Enright PL, McBurnie MA, Bittner V, et al: Cardiovascular Health Study: The 6-min walk test: A quick measure of functional status in elderly adults. Chest 123:325–327, 2003.
4. Webb GD, Gatzoulis MA: Atrial septal defects in the adult: Recent progress and overview. Circulation 114:1645–1653, 2006.
5. Ewert P, Berger F, Nagdyman N, et al. Masked left ventricular restriction in elderly patients with atrial septal defects: A contraindication for closure? Cathet Cardiovasc Intervent 52:177–180, 2001.
6. Gatzoulis MA, Freeman MA, Siu SC, et al: Atrial arrhythmia after surgical closure of atrial septal defects in adults. N Engl J Med 340:839–846, 1999.

## Bibliography

Attie F, Rosas M, Granados N, et al: Surgical treatment for secundum atrial septal defects in patients >40 years old: A randomized clinical trial. J Am Coll Cardiol 38:2035–2042, 2001.
Brochu MC, Baril JF, Dore A, et al: Improvement in exercise capacity in asymptomatic and mildly symptomatic adults after atrial septal defect percutaneous closure. Circulation 106:1821–1826, 2002.
Suarez de Lezo J, Medina A, Romero M, et al: Effectiveness of percutaneous device occlusion for atrial septal defect in adult patients with pulmonary hypertension. Am Heart J 144:877–880, 2002.
Sutton MGJ, Tajik AJ, McGoon DC: Atrial septal defect in patients ages 60 years or older: Operative results and long-term post-operative follow-up. Circulation 64:402–409, 1981.

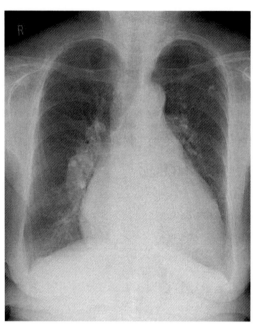

Figure 2-10 Postprocedure posteroanterior projection.

### FINDINGS

Cardiomegaly, prominent right pulmonary artery and branches.

**Comments:** There is reduced cardiac size compared to the preoperative film, although cardiomegaly and dilation of central pulmonary arteries persist. The closure device is not easily visualized in this particular film. It is easier to see in the lateral view.

# Patent Foramen Ovale with Transient Ischemic Attack

**Arif Anis Khan**

Age: 47 years
Gender: Female
Occupation: Staff nurse
Working Diagnosis: Transient ischemic attack

## HISTORY

The patient was completely well until she suddenly developed slurred speech one morning while preparing to go to work. She noted weakness of her right arm and hand at the same time. There was no headache. The symptoms persisted for 1 hour, and her husband brought her to the local hospital.

On examination the patient was in sinus rhythm and had a normal cardiovascular examination. She had mild dysarthria but no drooling, and appreciable but mild weakness in elbow extension, wrist dorsiflexion, and intrinsic hand muscles. No other objective abnormalities were found.

She was admitted to the hospital. A cerebral magnetic resonance angiography suggested thrombosis of the left middle cerebral artery. A duplex ultrasound of her carotid arteries was normal. Her strength gradually returned and she was discharged home. Warfarin therapy was started.

She has a history of migraine with a visual aura that had been treated with ergonovine only when severe. She was on no other medication. She has had no other medical problems including hypertension or diabetes.

She was a chronic smoker.

## CURRENT SYMPTOMS

Asymptomatic

NYHA class: I

## CURRENT MEDICATIONS

Warfarin (target INR 2:3)

## PHYSICAL EXAMINATION

BP 120/70, HR 76 bpm, oxygen saturation 99%

Height: 165 cm, weight 61 kg, BSA 1.67 m²

Surgical scars: None

Neck veins: 2 cm above the sternal angle, with a normal waveform

Lungs/chest: Normal

Heart: Regular rhythm, normal first and second heart sounds, no murmur identified. No abnormalities by palpation.

Abdomen: Normal

Central nervous system: Normal cranial nerves, normal sensory system examination, with very mild residual weakness of right side. Speech was normal, as were her fundi.

## LABORATORY DATA

| | |
|---|---|
| Hemoglobin | 13.1 g/dL (13.0–17.0) |
| Hematocrit/PCV | 39% (36–46) |
| MCV | 93 fL (83–99) |
| Platelet count | $393 \times 10^9$/L (150–400) |
| Sodium | 138 mmol/L (134–145) |
| Potassium | 4.0 mmol/L (3.5–5.2) |
| Creatinine | 0.9 mg/dL (0.6–1.2) |
| Blood urea nitrogen | 3.0 mmol/L (2.5–6.5) |

### OTHER RELEVANT LAB RESULTS
Normal thrombophilia screen

**Comments:** A neurologic assessment and hematologic thrombophilia workup are essential parts of investigating a cryptogenic stroke or transient ischemic attack (TIA).

## ELECTROCARDIOGRAM

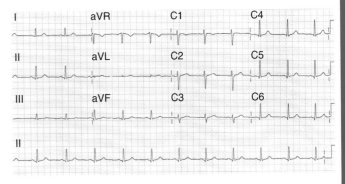

Figure 3-1 Electrocardiogram.

## FINDINGS

Heart rate: 72 bpm

QRS axis: +55°

QRS duration: 90 msec

Normal sinus rhythm

Normal axis

Normal ECG

**Comments:** Possible causes of a cerebral embolus such as atrial fibrillation or a recent myocardial infarction are not seen here.

# CHEST X-RAY

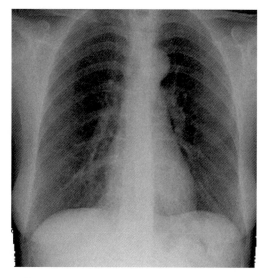

Figure 3-2  Posteroanterior projection.

## FINDINGS

Cardiothoracic ratio: 43%

Normal CXR.

**Comments:** There is no indication of enlarged right or left heart, and the pulmonary arteries are of normal size. Evidence of aortic coarctation is also not seen, which is pertinent given its association with berry aneurysms (see Case 24). The aortic knuckle is more prominent than would be expected in a 47-year-old female.

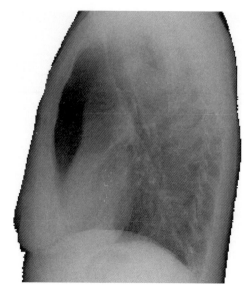

Figure 3-3  Lateral view.

## FINDINGS

Normal

**Comments:** There are no abnormal findings on the lateral CXR.

# EXERCISE TESTING

Not performed

# ECHOCARDIOGRAM

## OVERALL FINDINGS

There was normal LV and RV size and function, and normal RA and LA size. There was no valvular dysfunction. No vegetations were seen.

There was no visible interatrial communication.

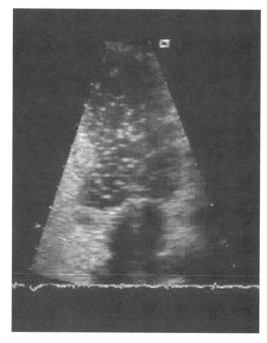

Figure 3-4  Apical four-chamber view showing grade III (right-to-left) shunt at rest with agitated saline contrast study.

# FINDINGS

Positive bubble contrast study (grade III, defined as > 30 bubbles seen in one frame).

**Comments:** Bubble contrast study diagnostic of PFO.

A bubble test with an agitated saline at the end of a sustained Valsalva maneuver (gush of blood filling the right atrium of the empty heart several beats before the left atrium gets filled, thereby opening the foramen) results in excellent sensitivity for the diagnosis of PFO. The sensitivity and specificity for the detection of large shunts, which are more clinically relevant, are surprisingly better with TTE compared to TEE.[1,2]

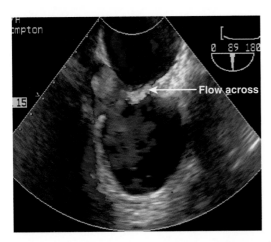

Figure 3-5 Long-axis view transesophageal echocardiogram showing color flow through patent foramen ovale from the left atrium to the right atrium at rest.

# FINDINGS

The interatrial septum was well visualized, and color flow across the septum demonstrated a PFO.

**Comments:** TEE is considered the method of choice for the diagnosis of PFO. However, color flow Doppler is less sensitive at detecting atrial shunts compared to bubble contrast in both TTE and TEE techniques. Release of the Valsalva maneuver increases the RA filling pressure (and thus the apparent size of the shunts) and can unmask PFOs not apparent during quiet breathing. Valsalva maneuvers that are properly timed in relation to the bubble injection are therefore essential during the assessment of cardiac shunts with bubble contrast.

## FOCUSED CLINICAL QUESTIONS AND DISCUSSION POINTS

1. **What is the association between stroke and PFO?**

   *PFO, defined as failure of the flap valve of the oval fossa to fuse with the rim of the atrial septum, is the most frequent interatrial communication (found in one quarter of the normal population).*

   *The following conditions are well known to be associated with PFO:*
   - *Decompression sickness*
   - *Platypnea-orthodeoxia syndrome*

   *PFO has been increasingly recognized as a possible mediator of paradoxical embolism allowing passage of air, thrombus, and fat. Large size and the presence of an atrial septal aneurysm (ASA) have been identified as morphological characteristics of PFO associated with a greater risk of paradoxical embolism.[3]*

   *When other causes of stroke have been excluded (such as cerebral aneurysms or carotid disease), the presence of a PFO or other shunt makes a paradoxical embolus the likely etiology, even if no identifiable source of distal thrombus, such as a deep venous thrombosis, is found. The association of PFO and cryptogenic stroke (odds ratio of stroke with PFO 3:1, 95% confidence interval, 2.3–4.2) has been consistently reported in patients less than 55 years of age.[4] Interestingly, migraine is also more common (35% vs. 12%) in cryptogenic stroke patients with PFO,[5,6] although the literature now contains a range of results.*

2. **What is the risk of a recurrent of stroke in patients with PFO?**

   *Patients with PFO and ASA have an average annual risk of recurrent stroke of 4.4%, and similar stroke rates on medical treatment have been reported from the Lausanne stroke registry.[5]*

   *The percentage of cryptogenic strokes among ischemic strokes (about 75% of all strokes) varies from 8% to 44% with a mean of 31%.[7] A pooled analysis suggests that the presence of a PFO alone increased the risk for recurrent events fivefold, with an even higher risk in the presence of an ASA.[8] The relationship remains controversial in the absence of prospective randomly controlled clinical trials.*

   *Identified risk factors of stroke in patients with a PFO include:*
   - *ASA*
   - *The presence of Eustachian valve directed toward the PFO*
   - *The gap diameter (approximate size) of the PFO*
   - *The number of microbubbles present in the left heart during the first seconds after release of a Valsalva during a bubble test*

3. **What is the evidence to support closure of the PFO in this setting?**

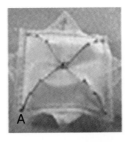

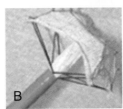

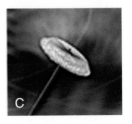

Figure 3-6 **A,** CardioSeal. **B,** STARFlex. **C,** Amplatzer septal occluder.

There are no prospective randomized control studies comparing device closure versus medical therapy at present. However, lower recurrence risks have been observed following catheter closure, and the very low procedural risks combined with the ease of device closure have currently made device closure the treatment of choice in some centers for appropriately selected patients. The following devices have been in use for percutaneous PFO closure (see Fig. 3-6A–C):

• CardioSeal
• STARFlex
• Amplatzer septal occluder

Currently, approved indications for device closure are in patients with recurrent stroke, orthodeoxia syndrome, and scuba divers with decompression syndrome. All other uses, including patients with a single occurrence of a cryptogenic stroke, are not currently approved by the U.S. Food and Drug Administration.

Devices are positioned using a combination of fluoroscopy and TEE and/or intracardiac echocardiogram. Access for closure is almost always via the femoral vein.

The defect is sized in two ways. First, the orifice is measured echocardiographically. Then, after inflation of a static balloon, the stretched diameter is measured, following which an appropriately sized device can be deployed.

Major periprocedural complications occur in 0.9% of patients.[9] Complications may include wire fracture, air embolism, tension pneumothorax, retroperitoneal hemorrhage, perforation of the atrial wall, and allergic reactions to the device.[9]

4. What is the risk of stroke following transcutaneous PFO closure?

The probability of recurrence of stroke or transient ischemic attacks following device closure of the PFO is around 7.8% after 4 years.[10] In a reported comparison of device closure versus medical therapy (aspirin or warfarin), the recurrence rate of embolic events was significantly lower at 0.5% per year in patients with device closure as opposed to 2.9% per year for patients treated with medical therapy.[11]

## FINAL DIAGNOSIS

PFO

Cryptogenic stroke

## PLAN OF ACTION

Transluminal percutaneous closure of PFO

## INTERVENTION

Successful closure of PFO by 23-mm STARFlex device, a self-centering device with flexible nitinol springs that run back and forth between the tips of two umbrellas

## OUTCOME

The patient tolerated the procedure well, and there were no complications. She was discharged the following day and advised to continue 6 months of low-dose aspirin and clopidogrel for 6 weeks.

Two years following deployment she has had no further neurological events.

**Comments:** A TEE probe is visible, which guides measurement and deployment. The sizing balloon shows the waist, which indicates the appropriate diameter to select for the occlusion device. The device is shown being deployed in Figure 3-7B.

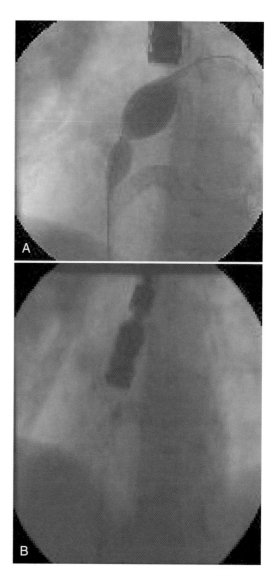

Figure 3-7 **A,** Balloon sizing of patent foramen ovale (PFO); constrain site of the balloon determines PFO diameter and shape. **B,** Implantation of STARFlex device.

## Selected References

1. Ha JW, Shin MS, Kang S, et al: Enhanced detection of right-to-left shunt through patent foramen ovale by transthoracic contrast echocardiography using harmonic imaging. Am J Cardiol 87:669–671, A11, 2001.
2. Madala D, Zaroff JG, Hourigan L, Foster E: Harmonic imaging improves sensitivity at the expense of specificity in the detection of patent foramen ovale. Echocardiography 21:33–36, 2004.
3. Agmon Y, Khandheria BK, Meissner I, et al: Frequency of atrial septal aneurysm in adult patients: A multicenter study using transcatheter and transesophageal echocardiography. Circulation 99:1942–1944, 1999.
4. Carod-Artal FJ, Vilela Nunes S, Portugal D: Thrombophilia and patent foramen ovale in young stroke patients. Neurologia 21:710–716, 2006.
5. Lamy C, Giannesini C, Zuber C, et al: Clinical and imaging findings in cryptogenic stroke patients with and without patent foramen ovale. Stroke 33:706–711, 2002.
6. Reisman M, Christofferson RD, Jesurum J, et al: Migraine headache relief after transcatheter closure of patent foramen ovale. J Am Coll Cardiol 45:493–495, 2005.
7. Windecker S, Meier B: Patent foramen ovale and atrial septal aneurysm: When and how should they be treated. ACC Curr J Rev 11:97–101, 2002.

8. Overell JR, Bone I, Lees KR: Interatrial abnormalities and stroke: A meta analysis of case control studies. Neurology 55:1172–1179, 2000.

9. Post MC, Van Deyk K, Budts W: Percutaneous closure of a patent foramen ovale: Single-centre experience using different types of devices and mid-term outcome. Acta Cardiol 60:515–519, 2005.

10. Windecker S, Wahl A, Nedeltchev K, et al: Comparison of medical treatment with percutaneous closure of patent foramen ovale in patients with cryptogenic stroke. J Am Coll Cardiol 44:750–758, 2004.

11. Mas J-L, Arquizan C, Lamy C, et al: The Patent Foramen Ovale and Atrial Septal Aneurysm Study Group: Recurrent cerebrovascular events associated with patent foramen ovale, atrial septal aneurysm, or both. N Engl J Med 345:1740–1746, 2001.

# Atrial Septal Defect with Cyanosis: The Hypoplastic Right Ventricle

**Toru Ishizaka and Hideki Uemura**

**Age: 40 years**
**Gender: Female**
**Occupation: Housewife**
**Working diagnosis: Atrial septal defect with cyanosis**

## HISTORY

Born small for gestational age (1800 g), the patient was noted to be cyanotic on crying since infancy. Frequent colds and chest infections required treatment, but no cardiac diagnosis was made.

During her elementary school and junior high school life, the patient felt short of breath playing sports, yet recovered readily with rest and hence did not seek medical attention. She began to note clubbing in her teenage years.

At the age of 25 years, a heart murmur and cyanosis were noted when she visited her general practitioner for a common cold. A hole within the heart was suspected, but not pulmonary hypertension. No recommendations were made.

At the age of 34 years, an ASD was diagnosed when she visited another doctor for her pregnancy and delivery. She gave birth to a female baby weighing 1358 g by cesarean section for intrauterine growth retardation (32 weeks' gestation). After this pregnancy, further detailed examinations were recommended, but the patient did not follow this recommendation.

At age 39 years, after contracting a common cold, her dyspnea became more noted and limiting. Eventually, she was referred for a more precise diagnosis and possible treatment. Diuretics were prescribed.

Soon thereafter the patient had a transient ischemic attack probably caused by paradoxical embolism. There was no suspicion of arrhythmia. Warfarin was started.

***Comments:*** Clubbing of fingers appearing as a teenager indicates that she has had moderate or severe cyanosis almost since birth. The fact that she had been able to do sports in her school life suggests that systemic output had been reasonably maintained even in the presence of cyanosis.

The risk of pregnancy is not low in the setting of cyanotic cardiac malformations. Fetal growth retardation can be associated with the maternal cyanotic circulation, and poor fetal outcome is particularly common when resting oxygen saturations are below 85%.

Paradoxical embolism can occur when a right-to-left shunt is present, particularly at the atrial level. This complication can occur even in patients with a small atrial communication such as a PFO. Anticoagulation may reduce the risk, although the evidence is not strong. Current practice would be elective closure of the atrial communication if large.

## CURRENT SYMPTOMS

The patient noted significant dyspnea with minimal effort, such as climbing even one flight of stairs or walking up a slight incline. She did not complain of palpitations.

NYHA class: III

## CURRENT MEDICATIONS

Lasix 40 mg orally twice daily

Potassium chloride 20 mg orally three times daily

Warfarin 2.5 mg orally daily

## PHYSICAL EXAMINATION

BP 100/70 mm Hg, HR 75 bpm and regular, oxygen saturation 61%

Height 151 cm, weight 40.5 kg, BSA 1.30 m$^2$

Surgical scars: A cesarean section scar was present in the lower abdomen

General: Thin woman, with severe cyanosis noted on her lips and cheeks

Neck: JVP was normal.

Lungs/chest: Breath sounds were normal with no rales or crackles

Heart: Regular rate and rhythm, with a grade 2/6 systolic murmur heard at the left sternal border, a single second heart sound of normal intensity, with no gallops

Abdomen: The abdomen was flat and soft. The liver and spleen were not enlarged.

Extremities: Clubbed fingers and toes were noted, with no edema.

***Comments:*** In the absence of a loud second sound, pulmonary hypertension is unlikely.

# LABORATORY DATA

| | |
|---|---|
| Hemoglobin | **18.9 g/dL** (11.5–15.0) |
| Hematocrit/PCV | **61.4%** (36–46) |
| MCV | 88.0 fL (83–99) |
| Platelet count | $211 \times 10^9$/L (150–400) |
| Sodium | 142 mmol/L (134–145) |
| Potassium | 4.4 mmol/L (3.5–5.2) |
| Creatinine | 0.6 mg/dL (0.5–1.0) |
| Blood urea nitrogen | 20 mg/dL (6–24) |
| Uric acid | **9.0 mg/dL** (2.7–6.3) |
| AST | 28 U/L (0–40) |
| ALT | 30 U/L (0–35) |
| T Bil | **2.0 mg/dL** (0.2–1.2) |
| Hb A1c | 5.3% (4.3–5.8) |
| FBS | 77 mg/dL (65–110) |
| Arterial gases: | |
| $Po_2$ | **37 mm Hg** |
| $Pco_2$ | 35 mm Hg |

## OTHER RELEVANT LAB RESULTS

Lung function tests revealed normal vital capacity and normal spirometry.

**Comments:** The secondary erythrocytosis is related to the patient's chronic cyanosis.

Uric acid is often elevated in patients with cyanosis; similarly, gout is not uncommon in such patients.

# ELECTROCARDIOGRAM

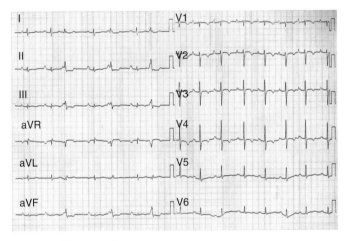

Figure 4-1 Electrocardiogram.

## FINDINGS

Heart rate: 75 bpm

QRS axis: +30°

QRS duration: 90 msec

Regular sinus rhythm with first-degree aortic valve block and frequent premature beats

Tall and especially peaked P-waves noted in V1–3, suggesting RA overload. P-waves are also broad and notched, perhaps reflecting LA overload. Nonspecific, precordial T-wave inversion over the RV leads.

**Comments:** This ECG could be suggestive of right heart disease. The absence of a major right axis shift argues against RV pressure overload.

# CHEST X-RAY

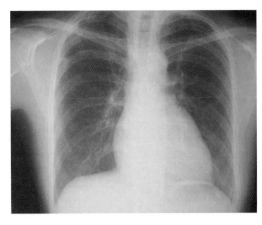

Figure 4-2 Posteran terior projection.

## FINDINGS

Cardiothoracic ratio: 55%

Situs solitus, with mild cardiomegaly, normal pulmonary vascular markings, and normal lung fields.

**Comments:** The cardiac silhouette suggests possible RA dilatation. Despite severe cyanosis, this is a relatively benign X-ray.

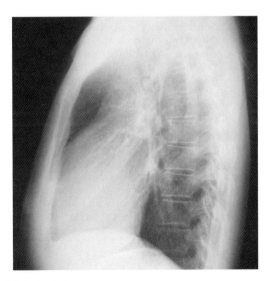

Figure 4-3 Lateral view.

## FINDINGS

Normal chest.

**Comments:** Lateral film shows some retrosternal filling, implying possible enlargement of the RV.

# EXERCISE TESTING

Not employed

# PHYSIOLOGIC TRACINGS

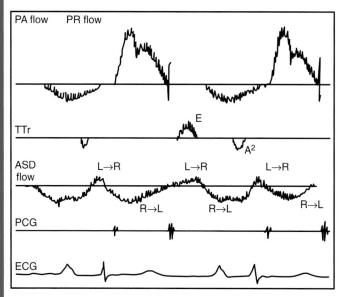

Figure 4-4 Schematic of echo Doppler and other concurrent physiologic tracings.

## FINDINGS

Normal LV was seen with normal function. A moderately large secundum ASD was present with a diameter of 20 mm. Bidirectional shunting was seen, but mainly right-to-left shunting across the defect.

The RV diastolic dimension was normal at 31 mm. All valves appeared normal, and in the presence of trace tricuspid valve regurgitation, all valves functioned normally. The IVC was 9 mm in diameter but did not collapse with inspiration. The tricuspid regurgitation velocity did not suggest an elevated RV systolic pressure.

## DOPPLER SUMMARY

The figure shows (from top to bottom) pulmonary artery (PA) flow, RV inflow, ASD velocity, as well as phonocardiogram and ECG tracing.

The PA tracing shows forward systolic flow, and diastolic flow reversal consistent with regurgitation. The ASD flow curve shows left-to-right shunt during early diastole, then right-to-left shunt, and finally left-to-right shunt again at the end of diastole after the P-wave.

**Comments:** Although the RV had normal systolic function, it appeared small for the moderately sized ASD that would be expected to normally cause RV dilation from predominantly left-to-right shunting. The IVC diameter was also rather small.

The constellation of findings suggests that the RV was actually hypoplastic, and abnormal diastolic function of the RV was responsible for right-to-left shunt through the ASD in mid diastole. Mild pulmonary regurgitation also contributed to early filling of the RV and hence right-to-left shunt.

# MAGNETIC RESONANCE IMAGING

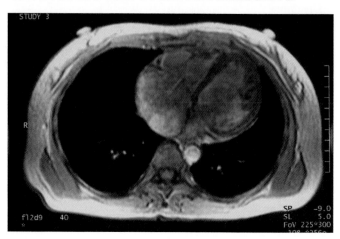

Figure 4-5 Axial steady-state free precession cine image.

## Ventricular Volume Quantification

|  | LV | (Normal range) | RV | (Normal range) |
|---|---|---|---|---|
| EDV (mL) | 103 | (52–141) | 67 | (58–154) |
| ESV (mL) | 49 | (13–51) | 22 | (12–68) |
| SV (mL) | 54 | (33–97) | 45 | (35–98) |
| EF (%) | 52 | (58–76) | 67 | (53–77) |
| EDVi (mL/m$^2$) | 79 | (59–93) | 51 | (57–94) |
| ESVi (mL/m$^2$) | 38 | (16–34) | 17 | (14–40) |
| SVi (mL/m$^2$) | 41 | (39–63) | 35 | (37–61) |
| Mass index (g/m$^2$) | 61 | (48–77) | 9 | (19–39) |

## FINDINGS

The RV wall motion was remarkably hypokinetic. The RV wall was thin. The ventricular septum showed its normal convexity. The stroke volume of the RV was decreased. A right-to-left shunt through an ASD was seen. The RA was large.

**Comments:** MRI assists in quantification of RV size, and in this case reveals the findings that explain the pathophysiology of the patient's cyanosis.

# COMPUTED TOMOGRAPHY

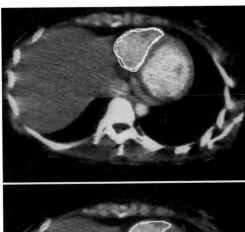

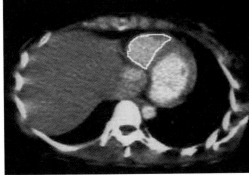

Figure 4-6 Computed tomography scan.

## FINDINGS

Gated CT was performed. Axial plane images were used to define contours of the RV border in diastole and systole.

In the lung field slices, there were multiple linear lines seen originating mainly from the pleura in the bilateral upper lung fields. Pulmonary vascular shadows were rather slender for a patient with a sizable ASD, indicating that there was not increased pulmonary blood flow in this patient. There was no evidence of parenchymal damage, such as thickening of the alveolar wall or the so-called frosted-glass-like appearance. Around the carina and the right bronchus, multiple vascular shadows were present, probably reflecting dilated bronchial arteries.

***Comments:*** The RV demonstrated no dilatation despite the large ASD. The RV end-diostolic volume index was smaller than normal range, as was the RV mass index.

CT and MRI both allow quantification of RV volume. An advantage of CT is the ability to see the lung parenchyma, which is more difficult with MRI since gas does not produce enough signal to construct an image. It should be noted that accurate RV volumes by CT require planning to ensure that adequate contrast is present in the RV at the time of the scan. Also, CT is often done at held inspiration, whereas MRI is often done at end-expiration, and differences may be greater between these, particularly in a case such as this.

## CATHETERIZATION

### HEMODYNAMICS
Heart rate   75 bpm

|  | Pressure | Saturation (%) |
|---|---|---|
| SVC |  | 44 |
| IVC |  | 49 |
| RA | mean 8 | 54 |
| RV | 15/9 | 52 |
| PA | 14/7 mean 10 | 58 |
| PCWP | mean 8 |  |
| LA | mean 7 | 66 |
| LV | 95/7 | 67 |
| Aorta | 92/65 mean 78 | 73 |

**Calculations**

| | |
|---|---|
| Qp (L/min) | **1.31** |
| Qs (L/min) | **1.89** |
| Cardiac index (L/min/m$^2$) | **1.45** |
| Qp/Qs | **0.69** |
| PVR (Wood units) | 2.28 |
| SVR (Wood units) | 36.98 |

### FINDINGS

The catheter study was performed to assess further the hemodynamics, pulmonary vascular resistance, and the degree and direction of shunting.

The patient had a low cardiac output, as evidenced by low systemic venous saturations. There was a borderline/small step-up in oxygen saturations at the PA level. RV and RA pressures were not elevated, nor was there pulmonary stenosis.

Following balloon occlusion of the ASD, the RA pressure did not change (increase). Furthermore, systemic blood pressure was maintained, and arterial saturation increased. Oxygen saturation measurements 5 and 10 minutes after balloon inflation were 83% and 93%, respectively (from 73% at baseline).

***Comments:*** The main concern with this patient is whether the small and hypocontractile RV would be able to function without a decompressing ASD, allowing for right-to-left shunt. The lack of pulmonary vascular disease meant that closure of the ASD may be possible. However, given the small RV cavity, cardiac output, which is already low, could potentially become lower after ASD closure. Balloon occlusion was, therefore, performed.

On the basis of the results of test occlusion, namely stable RA pressures and no fall in cardiac output after 10 minutes, permanent closure to reverse the cyanosis seemed appropriate. Whether 10 minutes of observation is long enough and whether test occlusion at rest will adequately predict RV hemodynamics during exercise is not known.

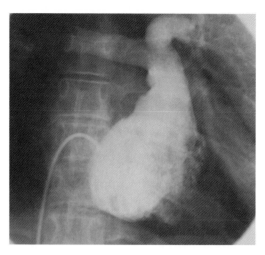

Figure 4-7  Right ventriculogram in posteroanterior projection.

## FINDINGS

The apical portion of the RV was missing. The RV was generally hyperkinetic. There was no obvious obstruction across the RVOT, with a good size pulmonary valve annulus (20 mm in diameter).

**Comments:** The catheter is in the RV, distal to the shunt, so no contrast was seen in the LV or the aorta. The RV is clearly abnormal. The usual morphologic RV contains three portions, namely an inlet, apical, and outlet portion. Here, the apical portion is absent.

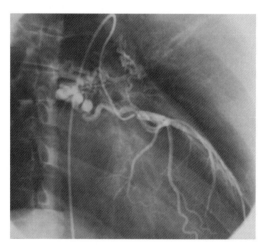

Figure 4-8  Catheterization angiogram.

## FINDINGS

Coronary angiography showed no significant stenoses.

The LAD had a small and tortuous fistula to the PA, an incidental finding.

**Comments:** Coronary fistulae are not uncommon in patients with marked, chronic cyanosis, usually without any hemodynamic impact.

### FOCUSED CLINICAL QUESTIONS AND DISCUSSION POINTS

1. **What is the anatomical diagnosis?**

*The patient has a "hypoplastic" RV with an ASD. In this case, the apical portion of the RV is absent.[1] In more usual circum-*

stances, a small cavity of the RV is associated with a malformed inlet or outlet portion of the chamber. The right ventricular volume generally correlates with the diameter of the tricuspid valve orifice. In this particular patient, the outlet and the inlet portions were of normal size. For example, in hearts with critical pulmonary stenosis or pulmonary atresia and intact ventricular septum, the tricuspid valve is often smaller than normal, and the ventricle can be correspondingly hypoplastic.[2] In this case, the right ventricular cavity was smaller than normal because of the absent apical trabecular component.*

*In addition, the patient has a small coronary to PA fistula. As described in a surgical textbook, the size of fistula is commonly small when connected to this particular site.[3] Sinusoidal fistulous tracts, although somehow different from communication between the coronary artery and the PA, are sometimes seen in patients with pulmonary atresia with intact ventricular septum,[2,4] where the RV is also small. Reasons or mechanisms for their formation are unknown.*

2. **What are the hemodynamic consequences of an ASD with a hypoplastic RV?**

*The absent apical portion obviously reduces the overall RV volume, but also affects filling. The poorly compliant ventricle creates restriction and elevation of the diastolic pressure. This in turn raises RA pressure and favors right-to-left shunt. The low-volume, underfilled RV in turn means that output into the PA is reduced. The Qp/Qs ratio is small, and the patient has not developed pulmonary vascular disease.*

3. **What are the potential consequences of ASD closure in this setting?**

*It is hard to predict whether volume and contractility of the inlet and the outlet components of the RV are capable of pumping all the systemic venous blood into the pulmonary circulation. This can lead to signs of low cardiac output and elevated central venous pressure similar to a Fontan patient relying solely on passive pulmonary blood flow. A similar consideration may be made in patients with Ebstein malformation with an ASD, where the abnormal septal leaflet creates a large atrialized portion of the RA, and a small RV (see Case 30 or 34).[5] The long history of cyanosis implies that diastolic function of the RV has been abnormal, and that the end-diastolic pressure of the RV chamber has been higher than the left.*

*Nevertheless, an obvious benefit of closure would be elimination of right-to-left shunting, which in this patient is considerable, and improved oxygen saturations and oxygen tissue delivery (if systemic cardiac output is not compromised). Furthermore, the risk of paradoxical embolism will be aborted. Closure of the defect ought to be given serious consideration.*

4. **What possible long-term changes may occur after closure of the ASD in this setting?**

*Long-term adaptation of the RV after ASD closure remains somewhat speculative. In theory, the RV may potentially increase its size subsequent to the increase in preload, although this is unlikely given the patient's age. The RV musculature has probably already undergone histopathologic changes because of the long-term cyanosis and underdevelopment such that favorable remodeling may not occur.*

*Persistent pressure overload of the RA can induce atrial flutter. This is even more likely when a surgical scar is present in the atrium that has already accumulated pathologic changes due to the chronically elevated atrial pressure. Sinus nodal dysfunction or atrial flutter would be expected to precipitate clinical symptoms in such patients.*

5. **Should this patient's ASD be closed?**

*On test occlusion of the ASD in the catheterization laboratory, the findings indicated that the RV could maintain a stable output for a short time at rest, without unacceptably raised systemic venous pressure or notably reduced systemic cardiac output. In this respect, it is not unreasonable to consider closure of the defect.*

*This patient presented before routine transcatheter closure was available, and thus closure would require bypass surgery. When considering a surgical procedure, the influence posed by cardiopulmonary bypass must be taken into account. Particularly in patients with abundant systemic-to-pulmonary collaterals developed because of prolonged and severe cyanosis, longer cardiopulmonary bypass running makes the lung congestion or edema worse, and may increase perioperative risks and the level of support required.*

*If the small RV does not cope with the corrected situation and if the superior caval venous pressure exceeds 20 mm Hg with noticeably low cardiac output immediately after coming off bypass, a superior cavopulmonary anastomosis (bidirectional Glenn anastomosis) would be a surgical bailout solution. This additional maneuver provides the so-called one-and-one-half ventricular repair physiology.[6,7,8] The superior caval venous flow is directed to the PA bypassing the RV, and the small RV is used to eject only half the systemic venous return through the inferior caval vein and the coronary sinus. The long-term results with this intermediate physiology between the biventricular and the Fontan circulations remain unclear and controversial.[9,10]*

*Overall, considering the potential benefits and favorable conditions during test closure of the interatrial communication, intervention seems likely the best way forward. The coronary–PA fistula will be closed at the time of surgery as well.*

## FINAL DIAGNOSIS

ASD with a hypoplastic RV causing severe cyanosis

Coronary–PA fistula (incidental)

## PLAN OF ACTION

Surgical closure of the ASD

## INTERVENTION

The ASD at the oval fossa (39 mm × 10 mm) was closed directly (by suture). The coronary arterial fistula (from the left anterior descending artery to the pulmonary trunk) was clipped.

As expected before the operation, massive cardiac return was noted, while on cardiopulmonary bypass, to the LA cavity through developed systemic-to-pulmonary collaterals. To avoid distention of the LV and to visualize the defect better, placement of a large LA vent was needed.

Intraoperative pressure measurement was done. The RA pressure increased from 9 to 15 mm Hg. The mean PA pressure did not change (13 to 14 mm Hg), and the systemic pressure and output remained adequate. The patient recovered uneventfully.

## OUTCOME

Three weeks later the patient was seen as an outpatient and generally felt well. Her oxygen saturation was 97%. An ECG showed reduced RV wall motion, no remarkable change from preoperative findings. The IVC diameter was now 14 mm, reflecting congestion of the systemic venous return and/or improved cardiac output. The PA flow pattern demonstrated that forward flow was produced by atrial contraction, indicating a stiff RV. She also had a CT showing a RVEF of 32% and an LVEF of 50%. The RA size was larger and the LA smaller, indicating a reduction of preload to the left heart.

The RV function was now a limiting factor of the overall circulation.

Increase in size of the RA is not a good sign, particularly in terms of atrial arrhythmia.

The patient performed a bicycle exercise study. Her peak HR was 146 bpm and her peak BP was 138/89. The peak $Vo_2$ was 15.0 mL/min/kg (48.0% of predicted).

Although the postoperative exercise testing result was far from ideal, the patient was satisfied with efficacy of the surgical intervention. She felt much more capable of ascending stairs than she felt before her operation.

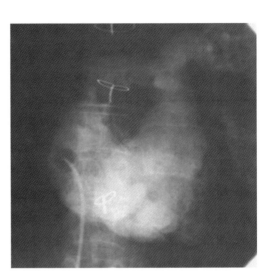

Figure 4-9 Catheterization 1 month after surgery.

### FINDINGS

At our institution, it was routine to reassess hemodynamics after surgery. The RA pressure was 10, mean PA pressure was 9, and the mean pulmonary capillary wedge pressure was 4. The cardiac output was 3.3 L/min (cardiac index 2.5 L/min/m²). Pulling back from the RV to RA showed almost no difference in the pressure tracing.

Angiography showed very poor contraction of the RV.

**Comments:** The RV does not contribute substantially to the pulmonary circulation. Although the atrial pressures are reassuring and the cardiac output has improved, the patient has a "sort of" Fontan-type physiology. It is likely that cardiac output will always be relatively low.

## Selected References

1. Celermajer DS, Deanfield JE: Hypoplasia of the apical component of the right ventricle. In Anderson RH, Baker EJ, Macartney FJ, et al (eds): Paediatric Cardiology, 2nd ed. London, Churchill Livingstone, 2002, pp 1128–1129.
2. Hanley FL, Sade RM, Blackstone EH, et al: Outcomes in neonatal pulmonary atresia with intact ventricular septum: A multiinstitutional study. J Thorac Cardiovasc Surg 105:406–423, 1993.
3. Kouchoukos NT, Blackstone EH, Doty DB, et al: Coronary arteriovenous fistula. In Kouchoukos NT, Blackstone EH, Doty DB, et al (eds): Kirklin/Barratt-Boyes Cardiac Surgery, 3rd ed. Philadelphia, Churchill Livingstone, 2003, pp 1240–1247.
4. Calder AL, Co EE, Sage MD: Coronary arterial abnormalities in pulmonary atresia with intact ventricular septum. Am J Cardiol 59:436–442, 1987.
5. Celermajer DS, Deanfield JE: Disease of the tricuspid valve: Ebstein's malformation. In Anderson RH, Baker EJ, Macartney FJ, et al (eds): Paediatric Cardiology, 2nd ed. London, Churchill Livingstone, 2002, pp 1111–1126.

6. Muster AJ, Zales VR, Ilbawi MN, et al: Biventricular repair of hypoplastic right ventricle assisted by pulsatile bidirectional cavopulmonary anastomosis. J Thorac Cardiovasc Surg 105: 112–119, 1993.

7. Kreutzer C, Mayorquim RC, Kreutzer GO, et al: Experience with one and a half ventricle repair. J Thorac Cardiovasc Surg 117: 662–668, 1999.

8. Gentles TL, Keane JF, Jonas RA, et al: Surgical alternatives to the Fontan procedure incorporating a hypoplastic right ventricle. Circulation 90(5 Pt 2):II1–6, 1994.

9. Numata S, Uemura H, Yagihara T, et al: Long-term functional results of the one and one half ventricular repair for the spectrum of patients with pulmonary atresia/stenosis with intact ventricular septum. Eur J Cardio-Thorac Surg 24:516–520, 2003.

10. Miyaji K, Shimada M, Sekiguchi A, et al: Pulmonary atresia with intact ventricular septum: Long-term results of "one and a half ventricular repair." Ann Thorac Surg 60:1762–1764, 1995.

# Partial Anomalous Pulmonary Venous Return

Masahiro Koh, Toshikatsu Yagihara, and Hideki Uemura

**Age:** 54 years old
**Gender:** Female
**Occupation:** Housewife
**Working diagnosis:** Partial anomalous pulmonary venous return

## HISTORY

The patient was well throughout her life until the age of 44 (10 years previously) when she developed paroxysmal atrial fibrillation and congestive heart failure. Her symptoms were controlled with diuretics. Workup included an ECG showing normal LV function but biatrial enlargement and a dilated RV. There were no valvular abnormalities and no pulmonary hypertension suggested by the ECG.

Further workup was pursued with cardiac catheterization, which demonstrated that the right upper pulmonary vein (RUPV) was abnormally connected to the superior caval vein. The atrial septum was intact. There was mild pulmonary hypertension (mean of 31 mm Hg), but the pulmonary vascular resistance was not elevated. The calculated Qp/Qs was 1.2. At that time, surgery was not recommended. She had been doing well on diuretics since then.

Her heart failure worsened 9 years after the initial episode. Her symptoms required hospitalization on several occasions, so that further workup was pursued.

***Comments:*** In this patient, an abnormal RUPV was found. Because the Qp/Qs ratio was believed to be close to normal (if the calculations were true, why is the RV dilated?), and because the patient's symptoms resolved easily with treatment, no intervention was felt to be necessary (see Case 6).

## CURRENT SYMPTOMS

Over the past year, the patient developed progressive dyspnea on exertion with difficulty climbing two flights of stairs, as well as intermittent ankle edema.

NYHA class: II

## CURRENT MEDICATIONS

Furosemide 40 mg daily

Spironolactone 50 mg daily

Aspirin 325 mg daily

## PHYSICAL EXAMINATION

BP 130/70 mm Hg, HR 58 bpm and irregular, oxygen saturation 97%

Height 152 cm, weight 65 kg, BSA 1.66 m$^2$

Neck veins: Severely engorged (12 cm above the sternal angle), with large V-waves present

Lungs/chest: Clear

Heart: The rhythm was irregularly irregular. There was a left parasternal lift. There was a 1/6 systolic murmur at the third left intercostal space, whereas the second heart sound had an increased pulmonary component, but was normally split.

Abdomen: Normal

Extremities: There was bilateral 2+ pitting ankle edema.

***Comments:*** The neck veins reflect tricuspid regurgitation. The clinical examination suggests that the RV dilation reported 9 years ago was still present and clinically relevant.

The second heart sound was normally split. Although this does not necessarily exclude an ASD, the absence of a fixed and wide splitting of the second heart sound is noteworthy and other causes must be explored. In this case, the only potential cause was the isolated RUPV anomaly diagnosed previously.

## LABORATORY DATA

| | |
|---|---|
| Hemoglobin | 12.3 g/dL (12.0–16.5) |
| Hematocrit/PCV | 38.0% (35.0–45.0) |
| Platelet count | **405 × 10$^9$/L** (150–350) |
| Sodium | 142 mmol/L (138–145) |
| Potassium | 3.8 mmol/L (3.4–4.9) |
| Creatinine | 0.5 mmol/dL (0.5–1.0) |
| Blood urea nitrogen | 12 mg/dL (8–20) |
| Total protein | 6.7 g/dL (6.5–8.2) |
| Albumin | 3.8 g/dL (3.6–5.5) |

***Comments:*** No specific abnormalities present.

# ELECTROCARDIOGRAM

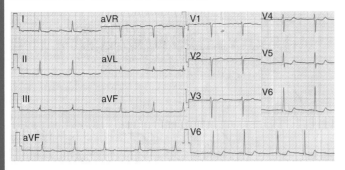

Figure 5-1 Electrocardiogram.

## FINDINGS

Heart rate: 59 bpm

QRS axis: +52°

QRS duration: 90 msec

Atypical atrial fibrillation, nonspecific ST changes

A 24-hour ECG was also performed. The heart rate ranged from 40 to 108 bpm. There were rare PVCs, and no long pauses.

***Comments:*** Atrial fibrillation reflects long-standing right atrial enlargement. What the ECG does not demonstrate here is RV hypertrophy. The QRS axis does not suggest that the RV is dilated, even though the history and physical exam point to RV overload being present.

The 24-hour ECG can be helpful in determining whether appropriate rate control is present.

# CHEST X-RAY

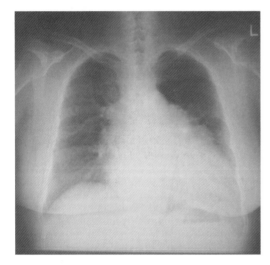

Figure 5-2 Posteroanterior projection.

## FINDINGS

Cardiothoracic ratio: 70%

Large cardiac silhouette with prominent central pulmonary arteries, and increased vascularity on the right side. The left heart border was straight, compatible with right ventricular dilation. The left main bronchus was horizontal, suggesting LA enlargement.

***Comments:*** Significant cardiomegaly here argues for long-standing volume overload from the shunt. The finding is incompatible with the previously reported Qp/Qs ratio of only 1.2:1.

# ECHOCARDIOGRAM

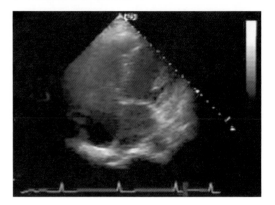

Figure 5-3 Apical four-chamber view.

## FINDINGS

The LV was normal in size with normal systolic function. The LA was mildly enlarged. The RA and RV were both enlarged, the atrial septum was intact, and no abnormal pulmonary venous drainage could be demonstrated in this study.

***Comments:*** RA and RV enlargement are signs of significant volume overload. This is not surprising here given the CXR.

What the echo does not show is an ASD. The atrial septum was well visualized and intact. In this type of setting, unexplained RV enlargement without visible shunt, the examiner should consider a TEE or a bubble study to exclude a sinus venosus ASD, and a TEE, MRI, or CT angiogram to evaluate possible anomalous pulmonary venous connections (see Case 1).

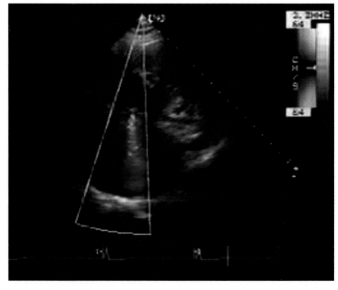

Figure 5-4 Apical four-chamber view.

## FINDINGS

There was moderate to severe tricuspid regurgitation (peak velocity mildly increased at 3.0 m/sec). The tricuspid valve appeared structurally normal.

*Comments:* The clinician may be tempted to suggest that the tricuspid regurgitation is the cause of the RV and RA enlargement, yet the valve itself was structurally normal. Because RV enlargement was described on an echocardiogram 9 years ago, it argues that the tricuspid valve regurgitation is secondary to chamber enlargement.

The patient importantly does not have pulmonary hypertension.

# MAGNETIC RESONANCE IMAGING

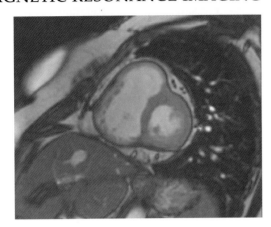

Figure 5-5  Short-axis view.

## FINDINGS

The RV was dilated with mildly reduced systolic function. The LV was normal. There was no ASD.

**Ventricular Volume Quantification**

|  | LV | (Normal range) | RV | (Normal range) |
|---|---|---|---|---|
| EDV (mL) | 91 | (52–141) | 201 | (58–154) |
| ESV (mL) | 32 | (13–51) | 92 | (12–68) |
| SV (mL) | 59 | (33–97) | 109 | (35–98) |
| EF (%) | 65 | (59–77) | 54 | (55–79) |
| EDVi (mL/m²) | 55 | (56–90) | 121 | (53–90) |
| ESVi (mL/m²) | 19 | (14–33) | 56 | (11–37) |
| SVi (mL/m²) | 36 | (37–62) | 66 | (17–37) |
| Mass index (g/m²) | 53 | (48–78) | 39 | (17–37) |

*Comments:* The Qp/Qs ratio here (comparing stroke volumes) was 1.9:1, significantly greater than what had been reported 9 years earlier by catheterization. There are potential pitfalls in such shunt calculations.

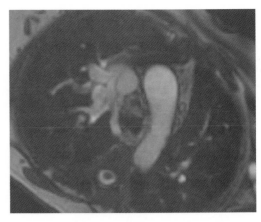

Figure 5-6  Oblique axial steady-state free precession cine.

## FINDINGS

The RUPV is connected to the upper SVC.

*Comments:* The RUPV in the upper left appears to communicate with the SVC. This location is higher than would be seen if partial anomalous veins were associated with a sinus venosus ASD (see Case 1). There are many vascular structures normally in this region, namely branches of both the right pulmonary artery and the venous tributaries, which can all seem structurally similar on MRI. Because of partial volume effects (where a thin vessel wall may not be visible if it runs parallel with the imaging plane), additional views of this area should be obtained to confirm the finding.

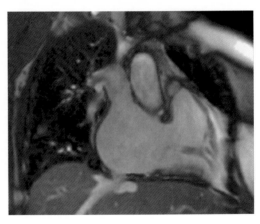

Figure 5-7  Oblique coronal steady-state free precession cine.

## FINDINGS

The RUPV drained to the upper SVC. The RA was enlarged.

*Comments:* The anomaly can be clearly appreciated in this view, as normally no structures should appear to enter the SVC at this location. It is important that anomalies are identified at the time of the MRI procedure to ensure that confirmatory views are obtained before the scan is ended. One advantage of CT is that reconstruction of any plane can be performed even after the scan has been completed.

# COMPUTED TOMOGRAPHY

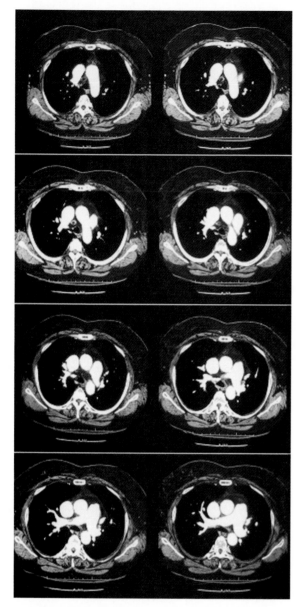

Figure 5-8 Chest computed tomography scan.

## FINDINGS

The RUPV was abnormally connected to the SVC.

***Comments:*** The fine spatial resolution of CT is extremely useful for stationary vascular structures, and is an excellent means of assessing the pulmonary venous drainage patterns, particularly if thin slices through the area of interest are used. The downside is radiation exposure and the need for contrast injection.

Partial anomalous return of the right pulmonary veins commonly coexists with ASD of the sinus venosus type (see Case 1).

## CATHETERIZATION

### HEMODYNAMICS

Heart rate    60 bpm

|  | Pressure | Saturation (%) |
|---|---|---|
| High SVC |  | 65 |
| Low SVC |  | 89 |
| IVC |  | 70 |
| RA | mean **18** | 85 |
| RV | **53/17** | 83 |
| PA | **54/29 mean 38** | 82 |
| PCWP | mean **19** |  |
| LV | 148/**16** | 98 |
| Aorta | 145/75 mean 105 | 98 |

**Calculations**

| | |
|---|---|
| Qp (L/min) | 6.20 |
| Qs (L/min) | 3.13 |
| Cardiac index (L/min/m²) | **1.89** |
| Qp/Qs | **1.98** |
| PVR (Wood units) | **3.55** |
| SVR (Wood units) | **27.84** |

***Comments:*** Catheterization was carried out to evaluate the degree of left-to-right shunt and the degree of pulmonary hypertension.

Procedurally, this is a case where the high SVC saturation is critical to determine the true mixed venous saturation. If obtained too low, the SVC saturation would contain oxygenated blood, which would be reflected in the mixed venous saturation estimate and grossly underestimate the true degree of the shunt.

The patient's pulmonary artery (PA) pressures were mildly elevated, but the pulmonary vascular resistance is not suggestive of significant pulmonary vascular disease.

The arterial pressure, left ventricular end-diastolic pressure, and wedge pressures were all high, even though the systemic cardiac index was low. If these data were correct, left ventricular dysfunction was also present.

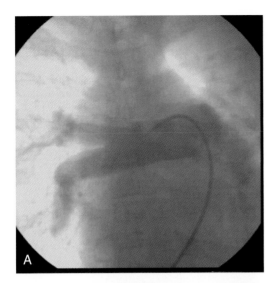

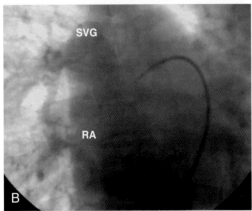

Figure 5-9 Anteroposterior projection angiogram. **A,** Early phase. **B,** Late phase.

## FINDINGS

Pulmonary angiography showed on early phase the normal branches of the pulmonary arteries (*A*), and showed on late phase (*B*) abnormal return from the RUPV to the SVC.

**Comments:** Late after an injection into the PA the blood should normally return only to the LA. In this case, there is enough contrast reaching the SVC and RA to outline these structures.

### FOCUSED CLINICAL QUESTIONS AND DISCUSSION POINTS

1. **What is the cause of this patient's congestive failure?**

*The patient has an anomalous pulmonary venous connection from the RUPV to the SVC, without an ASD. There is considerable left-to-right shunt through this defect, resulting in enlargement of the RA and RV. The LA is likely dilated as a result of the elevated left heart pressures. The treatment plan must include management of this part of her problem.*

*Why might the Qp/Qs increase over time (if it did)? With LV diastolic dysfunction, LA pressure rises relative to the RA. Indeed, the difference between the RA pressure and pulmonary capillary wedge pressure in this patient became larger over the past decade. When the RA pressure is lower than the LA pressure, the vascular bed that drains via the anomalous pulmonary vein will have lower resistance and receive more blood flow, leading to an*

increase in Qp/Qs and further right heart dilatation and symptoms.[1,2]

2. **Should this patient undergo surgical repair now?**

*There is debate about the optimal indications for surgical repair in this setting. Some argue that isolated partial anomalous pulmonary venous return without ASD, when Qp/Qs is less than 1.8:1, is not associated with adverse prognosis in terms of survival and surgery is not indicated.[3,4] Others would consider RV dilation itself to be an indication for surgery.*

*Surgical repair should be offered on the basis of right heart dilatation and symptoms. In fact, in this patient, surgical intervention would have been justified on the basis of symptoms of heart failure at initial presentation, regardless of the calculated Qp/Qs ratio. Now, with a Qp/Qs of 1.9:1 and progressive clinical symptoms, the patient should definitely undergo surgical repair.*

3. **Should her arrhythmia be addressed at the time of surgery?**

*One may choose to add a surgical ablation of the arrhythmia, elect an attempt at ablation in the electrophysiology lab, or manage the arrhythmia medically. There is some relevant surgical literature,[5,6] but largely the decision should probably favor the use of whatever local expertise and knowledge are available.*

*Regardless, this patient may come to need a pacemaker, and one or more transvenous electrodes may need to cross the surgically altered SVC-RA junction. Epicardial leads placed at the time of surgery may facilitate potential pacing in the future.*

## FINAL DIAGNOSIS

Right heart dilatation and failure with anomalous RUPV drainage and an intact atrial septum

LV diastolic dysfunction

Mild to moderate pulmonary hypertension

Chronic atrial fibrillation (intra-atrial re-entrant tachycardia)

## PLAN OF ACTION

Rerouting of the anomalous RUPV

Placement of epicardial permanent ventricular lead

## INTERVENTION

Through a median sternotomy, the suspected findings of the RUPV draining to the proximal portion of the SVC were confirmed. That part of the SVC was large in diameter. On cardiopulmonary bypass and cross-clamping of the aorta, the intact atrial septum was opened at the oval fossa, and the incision extended toward the SVC-RA junction. A 0.1-mm-thick expanded polytetrofluoroethylene patch was used to divert the right upper pulmonary venous blood into the LA. After the patient came off bypass, an epicardial pacing lead was attached to the RV.

## OUTCOME

The patient had an uneventful postoperative course. Two weeks after surgery, cardiac catheterization was carried out to evaluate the postoperative hemodynamics. The surgical channel was unobstructed. The PA pressure was 38/16 (23) mm Hg, with the pulmonary vascular resistance being calculated as 1.5.

During a 3-year follow-up the patient has been asymptomatic and doing well. She remains in chronic atrial fibrillation, with good ventricular rates, off diuretics, and on warfarin adjusted for an INR of 2 to 2.5. Her RA/RV dilatation has decreased on echo, although it has not normalized.

## Selected References

1. Alpert JS, Dexter L, Vieweg MVR, et al: Anomalous pulmonary venous return with intact atrial septum: Diagnosis and pathophysiology. Circulation 56:870–875, 1977.
2. Koh M, Uemura H, Kagisaki K: The impact, and surgical implications, of isolated anomalous connection of one pulmonary vein. Cardiol Young 17:554–556, 2007.
3. Kouchoukos NT, Blackstone EH, Doty DB, et al: Atrial septal defect and partial anomalous pulmonary venous connection. In Kirklin/Barratt-Boyes Surgery: Morphology, Diagnostic Criteria, Natural History, Techniques, Results, and Indications, 3rd ed. Philadelphia, Churchill Livingstone, 2003, pp 715–751.
4. Allen HD, Gutgesell HP, Clark EB, Driscoll DJ (eds): Moss and Adams' Heart Disease in Infants, Children and Adolescents, 6th ed. Philadelphia, Lippincott Williams & Wilkins, 2000.
5. Kobayashi J, Yamamoto F, Nakano K, et al: Maze procedure for atrial fibrillation associated with atrial septal defect. Circulation 98:II-399–402, 1998.
6. Nakajima H, Uemura H, Kobayashi J, et al: Modified cavoatriotomy for combined PAPVC repair and maze procedure. Ann Thorac Surg 77:2226–2227, 2004.

# Scimitar Syndrome

**Emmeline F. Hou, George Pantely, and Victor Menashe**

Age: 34 years
Gender: Female
Occupation: Homemaker
Working diagnosis: Partial anomalous pulmonary venous connection

## HISTORY

The patient was well at birth and throughout childhood, but had been told her heart was on the right side and that she had one pulmonary vein draining to the RA, but that this would not cause her problems. As a teenager, she had sporadic episodes of scant hemoptysis.

One year ago the patient became pregnant for the first time, and she had two episodes of cough with small amounts of bright red blood. She had no other symptoms and had no further recurrence of hemoptysis throughout the duration of her successful pregnancy.

More recently she complained of increased airway secretions and cough after exposure to second-hand smoke and described seeing bright red blood mixed with her sputum. Several days later she suddenly had another episode of hemoptysis, not precipitated by prolonged coughing, and a second similar episode later the same day. In each case, she described expectorating bright red blood with a small blood clot.

The patient was a nonsmoker and had been generally healthy in other ways.

**Comments:** Patients with isolated partial anomalous pulmonary venous connection (PAPVC) are usually asymptomatic early in life, and the anomaly can often go unrecognized. When new symptoms occur, any known congenital heart abnormality ought to be considered for its potential role in the patient's problem, as demonstrated throughout this book.

Isolated hemoptysis is an uncommon presentation of PAPVC. Because of the presence of a congenital vascular abnormality, hemoptysis may in theory also be due to rupture of a small vessel (or of a collateral) into the airway. More likely, however, abnormalities of the pulmonary veins may coexist with congenital abnormalities of the bronchial tree or bronchial arteries. These can result in small airways with limited vascular supply that are prone to recurrent infection.

Because the most common cause of hemoptysis in any patient is chronic bronchitis[1] this may be a likely scenario explaining this woman's current problem. The amount of bleeding in this patient is not life threatening, and the recurrent nature of her low-volume hemoptysis suggests bleeding from a bronchial arteriole rather than the larger pulmonary arteries.

Hemoptysis can be associated with pulmonary arterial hypertension, although this patient's history does not suggest this.

## CURRENT SYMPTOMS

Apart from hemoptysis, the patient had no other symptoms. She had not had an upper respiratory illness. She denied any chest discomfort or shortness of breath, and had a good exercise tolerance. She was able to climb three flights of stairs without difficulty. There had been no increase in abdominal girth or lower extremity edema. She denied palpitations or syncope.

**Comments:** Lack of symptoms is the rule in PAPVC. Patients who develop symptoms (dyspnea on exertion, atrial arrhythmia, or, later in life, right heart failure and pulmonary hypertension) usually have more than one anomalously connected pulmonary vein and/or associated cardiac lesions. Symptoms often relate to the magnitude of left-to-right shunt and/or the onset of atrial tachyarrhythmia.

NYHA class: I

## CURRENT MEDICATIONS

None

## PHYSICAL EXAMINATION

BP 100/68 mm Hg, HR 62 bpm, respirations 10, oxygen saturation 98% on room air

Height 142 cm, weight 64 kg, BSA 1.59 m$^2$

Oropharynx: The oropharynx was moist, nonerythematous, and without blood, postnasal drip, or exudates.

Nasal mucosa: The mucosa was slightly hyperemic without telangiectasia, blood, or polyps.

Neck veins: Her JVP was < 3 cm above the sternal angle, with a normal waveform.

Lungs/chest: Auscultation of the chest was normal.

Heart: The point of maximal impulse was in the right precordium in the fourth intercostal space just medial to the right midclavicular line. There was no RV heave. Heart sounds were regular with a normal first and second heart sound. No murmurs or gallops were heard.

Abdomen: There was normal abdominal situs. The abdomen was soft and nontender and without hepatomegaly.

Extremities: Extremities were warm and without edema, clubbing, or cyanosis.

## Pertinent Negatives

There were no petechiae, ecchymoses, or telangiectasias.

***Comments:*** The resting oxygen saturation is normal and there is no clubbing or cyanosis to suggest chronic hypoxia.

It is important to exclude oropharyngeal and nasal sources of bleeding in the setting of hemoptysis.

The cardiac impulse is rightward. A RV heave with wide splitting of S2 may be appreciated with significant PAPVC and right heart dilation. A prominent pulmonary second heart sound may also be heard if the pulmonary artery pressures are elevated.

Approximately 25% of patients presenting with PAPVC have an associated cardiac malformation, most often an ostium secundum or sinus venosus atrial septal defect. Other associated lesions include ventricular septal defect, patent ductus arteriosus, coarctation of the aorta, tetralogy of Fallot, double outlet RV, mitral stenosis or atresia, pulmonary stenosis, and aortic stenosis.

Hemoptysis and telangiectasia may be seen in hereditary hemorrhagic telangiectasia.

## LABORATORY DATA

| | |
|---|---|
| Hemoglobin | 14.6 g/dL (11.5–15.0) |
| Hematocrit | 43% (36–46) |
| MCV | 87 fL (83–99) |
| Platelet count | $198 \times 10^3$ μ/L (150–400) |
| Creatinine | 0.8 mg/dL (0.6–1.2) |
| Blood urea nitrogen | 4.9 mmol/dL (2.5–6.5) |

***Comments:*** The hemoglobin and hematocrit are normal, as would be expected for only scant hemoptysis.

## ELECTROCARDIOGRAM

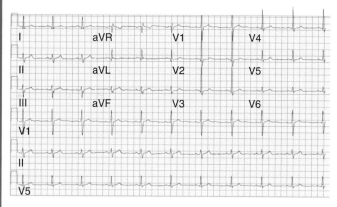

Figure 6-1 Electrocardiogram.

### FINDINGS

Heart rate: 62 bpm

QRS axis: −30°

QRS duration: 110 msec

Sinus rhythm, normal intervals, and P-wave axis. Prominent anterior forces. Leftward QRS axis.

***Comments:*** The ECG is almost entirely normal except for the high R-wave voltages in the early precordial leads. These reflect the relative position of the heart in the right chest.

The classic findings of dextrocardia, namely inverted P-wave in lead I, right axis deviation, and reversed precordial R-wave progression, are not seen. The patient more likely may have only dextroposition of the heart.

## CHEST X-RAY

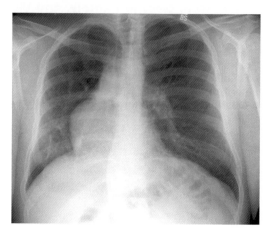

Figure 6-2 Posteroanterior projection.

### FINDINGS

Dextroposition, atrial situs solitus, and a left-sided aortic arch were seen. A large anomalous connecting vein (scimitar vein) was present in the right mid and lower lung zones. The trachea was deviated to the right. There was volume loss of the right lung and hyperinflation of the left lung.

***Comments:*** The "scimitar sign," first described in 1949, derives from the shadow of the anomalous pulmonary venous connection (scimitar vein) on posteroanterior CXR, which resembles a Turkish sword known as a scimitar.[2]

Right lung hypoplasia, a characteristic component of scimitar syndrome, causes rightward traction on the trachea and compensatory left lung hyperinflation. The heart also shifts rightward in the mediastinum.

The bronchial anatomy is normal (the left bronchus has a longer course before branching), which indicates normal atrial situs, and usually normal abdominal situs.

## EXERCISE TESTING

| | |
|---|---|
| Exercise protocol: | Modified Bruce |
| Duration (min:sec): | 13:45 |
| Reason for stopping: | Fatigue |
| ECG changes: | None |

| | Rest | Peak |
|---|---|---|
| Heart rate (bpm): | 62 | 164 |
| Percent of age-predicted max HR: | | 88 |
| $O_2$ saturation (%): | 98 | 100 |
| BP (mm Hg): | 100/68 | 184/86 |
| Double product: | | 30,176 |
| Peak $Vo_2$ (mL/kg/min): | | 38.4 |
| Percent predicted (%): | | 76 |
| Ve/$Vco_2$: | | 28 |
| Metabolic equivalents: | | 15.2 |

### FINDINGS

Normal exercise tolerance.

**Comments:** At times the patient's expression of normal exercise tolerance is worth documenting with formalized testing. Not only can this be valuable in these patients who may not note a lifelong limitation, but it will be helpful for comparison in the future.

In this case, the test confirms the patient's self-report of normal exertion capacity.

# ECHOCARDIOGRAM

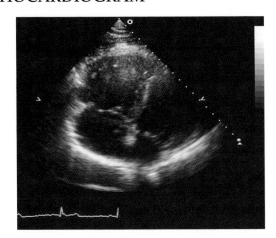

Figure 6-3 Apical four-chamber view from the right side.

## FINDINGS

There was dextroposition of the heart with normal cardiac chamber anatomy. The LV size and systolic function were normal. The RV was enlarged. The RA size was enlarged. No septal defects were identified.

**Comments:** The right heart is mildly dilated, but the RV systolic pressure and pulmonary arterial pressure are normal. Thus, the dilatation may be due to volume overloading. No valve dysfunction was present to explain the volume loading. There were no associated septal defects seen on this study (see Case 5). Thus, the findings suggest isolated PAPVC with left-to-right shunt. Hemoptysis from pulmonary hypertension or PAPVC obstruction is unlikely.

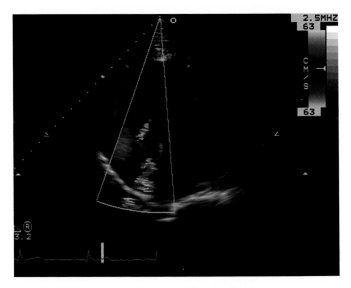

Figure 6-4 Apical four-chamber view, 2D color Doppler.

## FINDINGS

There was mild tricuspid regurgitation. The estimated RV systolic pressure was 32 mm Hg. A relatively turbulent high flow was visible in the posterior RA.

**Comments:** The high continuous flow signal seen in the posterior RA may arise from a number of sources, but suggests a possible cause of the RV enlargement, namely anomalous pulmonary venous drainage. Further planar imaging with CT or MRI would clearly demonstrate the pulmonary venous anatomy.

# MAGNETIC RESONANCE IMAGING

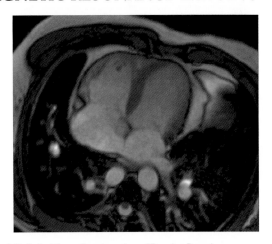

Figure 6-5 Apical four-chamber view, 2D color Doppler.

## FINDINGS

The RV was dilated with normal systolic function. The apex was deviated rightward, but still left facing. The LV had normal size and function. The Qp/Qs ratio was 1:6, based on comparison of right and left stroke volumes and confirmation from phase contrast velocity flow mapping in the pulmonary artery and aorta. Pulmonary veins from the left lung were easily seen, but not from the right lung. A large azygous vein was present.

**Comments:** The purpose of MRI in this setting is mainly to quantify the size and function of the RV, and to estimate shunt volume. The RV is clearly dilated, but its function was still normal.

The significance of the large azygos vein is possibly that it reflects an abnormally high amount of blood coming from the lower body.

### Ventricular Volume Quantification

|  | LV | (Normal range) | RV | (Normal range) |
|---|---|---|---|---|
| EDV (mL) | 124 | (52–141) | **245** | (58–154) |
| ESV (mL) | **55** | (13–51) | **121** | (12–68) |
| SV (mL) | 69 | (33–97) | **124** | (35–98) |
| EF (%) | 56 | (57–75) | 51 | (51–75) |
| EDVi (mL/m²) | 78 | (62–96) | **154** | (61–98) |
| ESVi (mL/m²) | 35 | (17–36) | **76** | (17–43) |
| SVi (mL/m²) | 43 | (40–65) | **78** | (20–40) |
| Mass index (g/m²) | 59 | (47–77) | 46 | (20–40) |

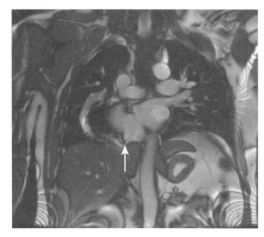

Figure 6-6  Oblique coronal steady-state free precession cine.

## FINDINGS

Flow in the scimitar vein was visible and quantifiable. The vein entered the IVC just below the RA (see arrow). The atrial septum was intact.

*Comments:* This confirmed the diagnosis of PAPVC and scimitar syndrome. This connection and continuous flow were also visible by echo, though harder to appreciate.

## COMPUTED TOMOGRAPHY

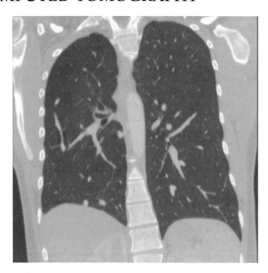

Figure 6-7  Coronal chest computed tomography scan.

## FINDINGS

The right lung was mildly hypoplastic relative to the left, with incomplete right-sided pulmonary segments. The right middle lobe was absent, as was the right upper lobe bronchus. However, both lungs had normal parenchymal attenuation without consolidation or pulmonary nodules. No bronchiectasis, architectural distortion, or pulmonary emboli were detected.

*Comments:* High resolution CT is useful to assess pulmonary parenchyma and pulmonary vasculature because of the patient's hemoptysis. This study demonstrated normal lung parenchyma, making bronchiectasis or pulmonary emboli unlikely causes for her hemoptysis.

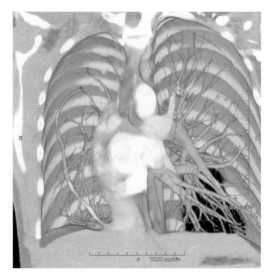

Figure 6-8  Shaded surface display, 3D reconstruction.

## FINDINGS

The anomalous pulmonary venous connection from the right upper lung was seen draining into the IVC below the diaphragm.

In addition, there were several other pulmonary venous branches draining the lower portions of the right lung demonstrating confluence with the scimitar vein at the level of the IVC.

The left-sided pulmonary venous anatomy was normal.

Bilateral SVC veins were present (not shown). The left SVC emptied into the coronary sinus.

*Comments:* Despite dextroposition of the heart (heart in the right chest but apex pointing to the left), the cardiac chamber anatomy was normal. The RV was on the right and emptied into the main pulmonary artery. The LV was on the left and emptied into a left-sided aorta.

The presence of the left SVC draining into the coronary sinus is a normal variant and not physiologically important in this case. Left SVC draining to the coronary sinus can be a source of right-to-left shunt if the coronary sinus empties to the LA, or if the coronary sinus is unroofed. It is also important when considering placement of a pacemaker.

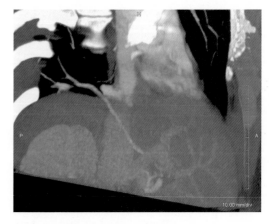

Figure 6-9  Maximal intensity projected image.

## FINDINGS

An anomalous systemic arterial supply to the right lower lobe was seen coming from an arterial branch extending from the celiac trunk and through the right hemidiaphragm.

**Comments:** The presence of arterial supply to the right lower lobe from the abdominal aorta gives the patient the more specific diagnosis of "scimitar syndrome." This specific syndrome, first described in 1836 by Chassinat and Cooper, is characterized by the presence of PAPVC of the right pulmonary vein(s) to the IVC, right lung hypoplasia, and anomalous systemic arterial supply to the right lung, usually from the underside of the aortic arch to the right upper lobe.[3,4] The syndrome was named for the scimitar vein in 1960.[5]

The abnormal arterial supply and venous drainage can be associated with recurrent pulmonary infection, hemoptysis, and lung sequestration.

## BRONCHOSCOPY

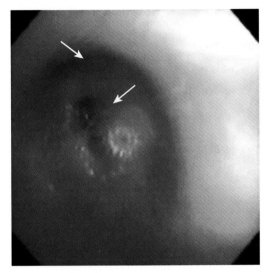

Figure 6-10 Bronchoscopy of the right main stem bronchus.

## FINDINGS

Bronchoscopy was performed to explore the etiology of hemoptysis. There was a normal right main stem bronchus, but the orifice to the right upper lobe bronchus was absent. Instead, a small indentation is seen (*top arrow*) suggesting a closed orifice. The bronchus intermedius, leading to the right middle and lower lobes, was narrowed (*bottom arrow*). Reflection of the light source off the mucosal lining is also present. The left endobronchial anatomy appeared normal.

Other findings from bronchoscopy (not shown) included hyperemic mucosa with areas of submucosal petechiae on gentle scope pressure. There were copious secretions that were clear throughout the right lung. No active bleeding was seen.

**Comments:** Bronchoscopy is used to visually inspect the airways for the source of hemoptysis and to exclude endobronchial lesions. In addition, the study demonstrated the abnormal bronchial anatomy associated with this syndrome.

### FOCUSED CLINICAL QUESTIONS AND DISCUSSION POINTS

1. What is the anatomical diagnosis?

*The patient has the classic triad of scimitar syndrome: anomalous pulmonary venous connection of the right pulmonary vein to below the diaphragm, hypoplastic right lung, and anomalous systemic arterial supply to a portion of the right lung. In addition, the patient has a large azygos venous return, and a left SVC draining to the coronary sinus.*

*The majority of patients with scimitar syndrome lead a completely asymptomatic early life and are undiagnosed in childhood. Many remain undiagnosed during adulthood as well. Those few patients who develop cardiac symptoms typically have more than one anomalously connected pulmonary vein and/or associated lesions leading to significant left-to-right shunting.*

*In a study of 122 adults with scimitar syndrome, the left-to-right shunting was less than 2:1 in 100 of the 122 patients.[6] The pulmonary arterial pressures were normal or only slightly elevated in all cases. On a follow-up study, these patients led a normal life without having surgical correction.[6]*

*A few patients with scimitar syndrome will have symptoms from lung complications such as recurrent respiratory infections and/or lung sequestration.*

2. Why does the patient have hemoptysis?

*The imaging studies demonstrated the presence of a hypoplastic right lung with incomplete pulmonary segments and anomalous vascular supply.*

*The bronchoscopy demonstrated hyperemia of the endobronchial tissue and pooling of secretions that may be related to this altered anatomy. She had incomplete pulmonary segments and abnormal distal airway anatomy. The secretions likely led to inflammation and chronic low-grade infection of the distal mucosa, causing mucosal bleeding and recurrent, low-level hemoptysis.*

*Hemoptysis can also be due to sequestered lung.[7] Sequestered lung, defined as lung parenchyma without a direct communication with the bronchial tree and pulmonary veins, receives its blood supply from the systemic arterial circulation, such as the arterial subdiaphragmatic collaterals. In this setting, it is believed to be due to abnormal development of the right lung bud during early embryogenesis. The sequestered lung parenchyma is prone to bleeding and infection, and may need to be removed surgically.[8] However, this patient did not have lung sequestration on her CT scan; her lung parenchyma was normal.*

*It is perhaps surprising and fortunate that she had not had more trouble with chronic sputum production, cough, and recurrent infections accompanying her hemoptysis. With the abnormal airway anatomy there is concern of future development of bronchiectasis.*

3. Should her PAPVC be repaired and should the anomalous small pulmonary arterial supply to the lower lobe from the celiac trunk be obliterated?

*Management of the adult patient with scimitar syndrome is dictated by the presence of associated lesions that may require intervention in their own right, the degree of right heart dilation and pulmonary hypertension due to significant left-to-right shunt, and the presence and frequency of pulmonary complications.*

*This particular patient has no other associated lesions, has a moderately enlarged right heart, and has normal pulmonary pressures. Although she has hemoptysis, this is minimal and she has not been troubled by recurrent pulmonary infections. If she had large volume hemoptysis or recurrent infection involving the hypoplastic lung, she should be considered for resection of that lung segment and ligation or catheter occlusion of the anomalous arterial blood supply.[9]*

*Indications for operative repair may be different in cases in which the atrial septum is intact, that is, where there is a pressure gradient between the left and right atria, which can affect relative resistance to different pulmonary vascular beds (see Case 5). Catheterization to measure the pulmonary to systemic flow and vascular resistance ratios would be required if and when symptoms develop. In this case, the scimitar vein is relatively small, and there is no justification for closure or redirection at present. If exercise limitations or further RV dilation occur in the future, this may warrant intervention.*

*Late after surgical repair, mortality is low, but scimitar patients have a higher propensity for pulmonary vein stenosis than patients with other types of anomalous pulmonary venous return.[10]*

## FINAL DIAGNOSIS

Scimitar syndrome with scant hemoptysis from hyperemic endobronchial mucosa

## PLAN OF ACTION

Observation and regular imaging

## INTERVENTION

None

## OUTCOME

One year later her MRI showed no change in the size or function of the RV. The patient has had no further recurrence of her hemoptysis. She has not had any serious pulmonary infections or developed signs or symptoms of bronchiectasis.

Eight years later she continues to be very well and active, chasing her growing young son.

## Selected References

1. Braunwald E: Cough and hemoptysis. In Isselbacher KJ, et al (eds): Harrison's Principles of Internal Medicine, 13th ed. New York, McGraw-Hill, 1994, p 173.
2. Dotter CT, Hardisty NM, Steinberg I: Anomalous right pulmonary vein entering the inferior vena cava; two cases diagnosed during life by angiocardiography and cardiac catheterization. Am J Med Sci 218:31–361, 1949.
3. Chassinat R: Observation d'anomalies anatomiques remarquables de l'appareil circulatoire, avec hepatocele congeniale, n'ayant donne lieu pendant la vie a aucun symptom particulier. Arch Gen Med 11:80–84, 1836.
4. Cooper G: Case of malformation of the thoracic viscera: Consisting of imperfect development of right lung and transposition of the heart. London Med Gazzette 18:600–601, 1836.
5. Neill CA, Ferencz C, Sabiston DC, Sheldon H: The familial occurrence of hypoplastic right lung with systemic arterial supply and venous drainage "scimitar syndrome." Bull Johns Hopkins Hosp 107:1–21, 1960.
6. Dupuis C, Charaf LA, Breviere GM, et al: The "adult" form of scimitar syndrome. Am J Cardiol 70:502–507, 1992.
7. Nedelcu C, Carette MF, Parrot A, et al: Hemoptysis complicating scimitar syndrome: From diagnosis to treatment. Cardiovasc Intervent Radiol (31 ) Suppl 2: S96–S98, 2008.
8. Horcher E, Helmer F: Scimitar syndrome and associated pulmonary sequestration: Report of a successfully corrected case. Prog Pediatr Surg 21:107–111, 1987.
9. Sahin S, Celebi A, Yalcin Y, et al: Embolization of the systemic arterial supply via a detachable silicon balloon in a child with scimitar syndrome. Cardiovasc Intervent Radiol 28:249–253, 2005.
10. Alsoufi B, Cai S, Van Arsdell GS, et al: Outcomes after surgical treatment of children with partial anomalous pulmonary venous connection. Ann Thorac Surg 84:2020–2026, 2007.

## Bibliography

Brody H: Drainage of the pulmonary veins into the right side of the heart. Arch Pathol 33:221–229, 1942.
Halasz NA, Halloran KH, Liebow AA: Bronchial and arterial anomalies with drainage of the right lung into the inferior vena cava. Circulation 14: 826–846, 1956.
Hickie JB, Gimlette TMD, Bacon APC: Anomalous pulmonary venous drainage. Br Heart J 18:365–377, 1956.
Khan MA, Torres AJ, Printz BF, Prakash A: Usefulness of magnetic resonance angiography for diagnosis of scimitar syndrome in early infancy. Am J Cardiol 96:1313–1316, 2005.
Mardini MK, Sakati NA, Lewall DB, et al: Scimitar syndrome. Clin Pediatr 21:350–354, 1982.
Mathey J, Galey JJ, Logeais Y, et al: Anomalous pulmonary venous return into inferior vena cava and associated bronchovascular anomalies (the scimitar syndrome): Report of three cases and review of the literature. Thorax 23:398–407, 1968.

# Part II

# Ventricular Septal Defects

# Endocarditis in a Young Man

**Emmeline F. Hou, George Pantely, and Victor Menashe**

**Age: 27 years**
**Gender: Male**
**Occupation: Graduate student**
**Working diagnosis: Residual ventricular septal defect after surgical closure**

## HISTORY

The patient was born with a perimembranous VSD. Because of severe aortic insufficiency at age 12 years, he underwent aortic valvuloplasty with plication of the noncoronary leaflet and direct suture closure of the VSD. Postoperatively there was a residual small VSD and mild to moderate aortic insufficiency. In the years following he was asymptomatic and had no activity restrictions. He participated in various sports as a student and frequently bicycled 60 to 80 miles a week. He was followed yearly in the congenital heart clinic with an echocardiogram. His VSD, aortic insufficiency, and left ventricular size and function were stable.

Six months ago, he developed fever and associated symptoms of fatigue, myalgias, shortness of breath, nonproductive cough, and wheezing. The patient was treated for a presumed bronchitis with a course of antibiotics and inhalers. His symptoms initially improved while taking antibiotics, but returned a few days after completing the antibiotic course. Over the next 6 months, he was placed on a series of antibiotics for a presumptive diagnosis of recurrent bronchitis.

The patient began to have predictable cycles of fevers up to 40° C and myalgias according to when he last took antibiotics. Approximately 5 days after completing a course of medication, he would have resumption of symptoms. The antibiotics he had been prescribed included penicillin, ampicillin, erythromycin, and tetracycline. His fevers and myalgias were relieved within 10 to 15 hours after starting the medications, except for tetracycline, which was never effective. Blood cultures were not drawn at any point.

He reported having one dental procedure for a loose dental filling a few weeks prior to his initial onset of symptoms. The patient took prophylactic antibiotics against endocarditis before dental procedures, but was not strict with the timing of the dose in relation to the procedure.

He was a nonsmoker, and had never used intravenous (IV) drugs.

**Comments:** Patients with residual VSD after early VSD repair warrant cardiology follow-up for signs of left ventricular dysfunction, aortic insufficiency, tricuspid insufficiency, pulmonary hypertension, LVOT obstruction, and infective endocarditis. Of patients who have undergone closure of their VSD, up to 5.5% needed a second operation to close residual or recurrent VSDs.[1] However, if the residual VSD is small and restrictive, surgery is not necessary.

The clinical presentation of recurrent fevers in any patient with prior surgery and/or a turbulent lesion should obviously instigate a thorough workup for infective endocarditis. The most common presenting feature is fever, although it may be absent in up to 10% of patients. In right heart endocarditis, patients may present with hemoptysis or recurrent "chest infections" due to pulmonary emboli.

In infective endocarditis, fever is initially continuous, but may become intermittent particularly when short nonbactericidal courses of antibiotics have been given.

Cleaning, filling, or extracting teeth is associated with bacteremia with positive blood cultures in 12% to 85% of dental patients. The most common organisms are alpha-hemolytic streptococcus, in particular, the viridans streptococcus group. Although most patients receive instructions for endocarditis prophylaxis consistent with older American Heart Association guidelines, a study observed that only 22% of patients who were advised by their physician to take prophylactic antibiotics actually took prophylaxis as recommended.[2]

## CURRENT SYMPTOMS

A 6-month history of intermittent fevers, myalgias, and shortness of breath after a dental procedure.

He complained of headaches and neck soreness, but no joint pain or back pain.

He denied hemoptysis and hematuria.

He had no skin lesions.

NYHA class: I

**Comments:** The incidence of infective endocarditis is 0.38 cases per 10,000 person years.[3] The major predisposing factors for the development of infective endocarditis are susceptible cardiovascular substrates and a source of bacteremia. Previously, a large proportion of patients who developed endocarditis had a history of rheumatic heart disease. Today, there is an increasing number of patients with congenital heart disease surviving into adulthood who present with infective endocarditis.

## CURRENT MEDICATIONS

Erythromycin 500 mg orally twice daily (eighth day of a 10-day course)

Amoxicillin 2 g orally before dental procedures

## PHYSICAL EXAMINATION

Temperature 36.4, BP 122/68, HR 75, oxygen saturation 96% on room air

General: Height 138 cm (63 in), weight 63 kg (137 lb), BSA 1.55 m$^2$

HEENT: There was no conjunctival hemorrhage.

Neck veins: JVP was 6 cm above the sternal angle with a normal waveform.

Lungs/chest: End-expiratory wheezes, but no rales were heard.

Heart: The precordium was hyperdynamic with a left sternal border thrill. Heart sounds were normal. A grade 4/6 holosystolic murmur was heard best along the lower left sternal border. A high-pitched long diastolic decrescendo murmur was heard best at the left lower sternal border.

Abdomen: The abdomen was soft and nontender. There was no hepatosplenomegaly.

Extremities: Extremities were warm and without edema, clubbing, or cyanosis. There were no petechiae, splinter hemorrhages, Janeway lesions, or Osler nodes.

### Pertinent Negatives

Neurologic exam was normal.

No spinal tenderness, costovertebral angle tenderness, or joint abnormalities were identified.

**Comments:** Fever will wax and wane particularly when there has been exposure to short nonbactericidal courses of antibiotics.

Conjunctival hemorrhage and Roth spots are the result of systemic septic emboli from infective endocarditis.

When present, congestive heart failure from infection-induced valvular destruction is a serious complication and portends a higher mortality.

Septic emboli to the lungs from right heart endocarditis can result in pulmonary infiltrates or pleural effusions.

Cardiac auscultation is consistent with the underlying cardiac anomaly. It is important to systematically note changes in auscultation from baseline exam as the changes may indicate valvular destruction.

Hepatomegaly is observed in many patients, and splenomegaly occurs in about 55% of patients. Splenic infarction or intraabdominal abscess should be suspected if there is left upper quadrant pain and tenderness.

Clubbing of the nails may develop with subacute endocarditis. Skin lesions are also common with subacute endocarditis.

Neurologic involvement occurs in 30% to 40% of patients.

Involvement of the large joints may occur in up to 20% to 30% of patients.

## LABORATORY DATA

| | |
|---|---|
| WBC count | $7 \times 10^3$ cells/L (4.3–10) |
| PMN | 48% (48–65) |
| Band cells | 11% (0–5) |
| Hemoglobin | 16 g/dL (13–17.0) |
| Hematocrit | 48% (41–51) |
| MCV | 90.7 fL (85–95) |
| Platelet count | $209 \times 10^3$ cells/L (150–420) |
| Sodium | 142 mg/dL (136–147) |
| Potassium | 4.2 mg/dL/dL (3.5–5.2) |
| Creatinine | 1.3 mg/dL (0.8–1.3) |
| Blood urea nitrogen | 11 mg/dL (6–23) |
| ESR | 1 mm/hr (0–5) |
| Urine analysis | No red or white blood cells, normal sediment |

**Comments:** Leukocytosis with bandemia is usually seen, although leukopenia can occur in overwhelming sepsis.

Anemia is seen in approximately 40% of patients as a manifestation of the anemia of chronic disease. Rarely is anemia due to hemolysis from large vegetations or valvular destruction.

The erythrocyte sedimentation rate (ESR) is usually elevated, but may be normal in 10% of cases, and therefore a normal result cannot exclude the diagnosis.

Microscopic hematuria is seen in more than 50% of cases.[4]

## ELECTROCARDIOGRAM

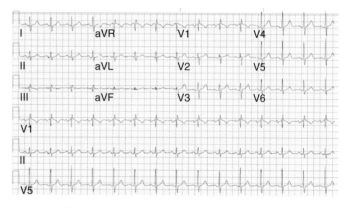

Figure 7-1 Electrocardiogram.

### FINDINGS

Heart rate: 90 bpm

QRS axis: +35°

PR interval: 162 msec

QRS duration: 96 msec

Sinus rhythm, incomplete RBBB. There was no RA overload.

**Comments:** The presenting ECG is unchanged from previous studies. The incomplete right bundle branch block is not new.

Extension of infective endocarditis into the septum may lead to atrioventricular, fascicular, or bundle branch block, so lengthening of the PR interval or QRS duration may be an important sign. Rarely, embolization to the coronary arteries can lead to myocardial infarction.

## CHEST X-RAY

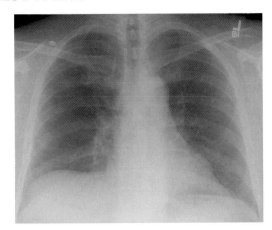

Figure 7-2 Posteroanterior projection.

### FINDINGS

Normal heart size without increased pulmonary flow or heart failure. There was no evidence of lung infiltrates, masses, or pleural effusions.

*Comments:* Septic emboli can result in pulmonary infiltrates on CXR. Pleural effusions may also be present. Acute valvular destruction can cause pulmonary vascular congestion and pulmonary edema.

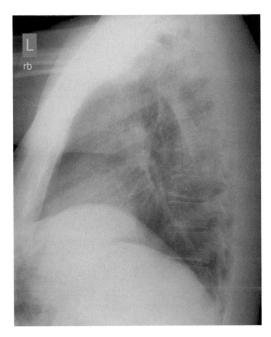

Figure 7-3 Lateral projection.

### FINDINGS

Normal examination.

## ECHOCARDIOGRAM

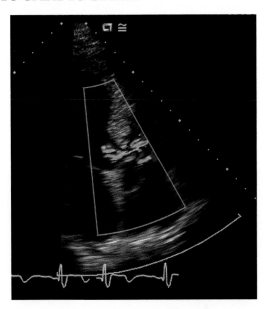

Figure 7-4 Apical four-chamber view with 2D Doppler.

### FINDINGS

The LV size and systolic function were normal. The RV size and systolic function were also normal. A small VSD (0.4 cm) was present with a peak velocity of 5.1 m/sec. The VSD jet is directed at the tricuspid valve. The aortic valve appeared normal (trileaflet) with mild regurgitation.

*Comments:* Although the patient has had prior surgical closure of his VSD, he has a residual defect. The lesion is less than one third of the aortic root size and there is a significant systolic pressure gradient between the left and right ventricles (>64 mm Hg). The residual VSD is thus restrictive.

The direction of the VSD jet toward the tricuspid valve is believed to increase the risk of developing right-sided endocarditis.

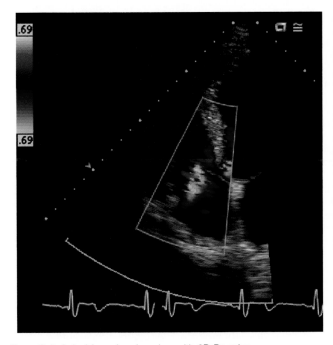

Figure 7-5 Apical four-chamber view with 2D Doppler.

## FINDINGS

No vegetations are seen on the tricuspid valve. However, the tricuspid valve is notably thicker when compared to previous studies. There is moderate tricuspid regurgitation (prior studies have demonstrated only mild tricuspid regurgitation). The peak tricuspid regurgitant velocity is 2.6 m/sec. Estimated RV systolic pressure is normal at 30 to 35 mm Hg.

**Comments:** Although a vegetation is not clearly seen, the thickened appearance of the tricuspid valve with worsened regurgitation suggests infective endocarditis involving the tricuspid valve.

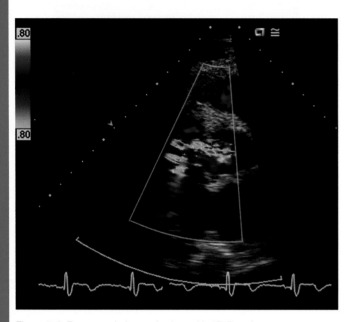

Figure 7-6 Parasternal short-axis view with 2D Doppler.

## FINDINGS

There was mild fibrocalcific sclerosis of the aortic valve. Mild central aortic insufficiency was seen with a pressure half time of 417 msec. This was unchanged compared to prior studies. No perivalvular abscess or aneurysm was identified. No vegetations were seen on the aortic valve.

**Comments:** Another potential site of infective endocarditis in this patient is the aortic valve. Aortic insufficiency is a relatively high-risk lesion for infective endocarditis. Vegetations, worsening insufficiency, and perivalvular involvement should be sought.

TTE has a high specificity (98%) but low sensitivity (<60%) for the detection of vegetations in all comers.[3] In the setting of complex congenital heart lesions, imaging can be more difficult. There should be a low threshold for transesophageal imaging in this group. However, a negative TEE still does not exclude endocarditis, and the clinical and microbiologic data should be carefully scrutinized.

### FOCUSED CLINICAL QUESTIONS AND DISCUSSION POINTS

1. **Why is this patient at risk for developing infective endocarditis?**

*Although small residual VSDs are of little hemodynamic significance, they still pose a risk for infective endocarditis.*

*The presence of additional valvular disease further increases the risk of endocarditis in the setting of VSD.*

*A recent study of 222 patients with a VSD considered too small to require surgery during childhood who were followed up for 8 years reported a 1.8% incidence of endocarditis.[4]*

*In the Second Natural History Study of Congenital Heart Defects (NHS-2), bacterial endocarditis occurred rarely in patients with small unrepaired VSDs, 1.3 per 1,000 patient-years.[1] Based on the NHS-2 data, the incidence of endocarditis was reported to be significantly less after VSD closure, provided there were no additional valvular abnormalities.[5] The risk of endocarditis, however, was not eliminated completely.*

*A 30-year postoperative follow-up study of patients with isolated VSD demonstrated a cumulative incidence of infective endocarditis of 4.1%. The risk appeared to increase 20 years after surgical closure, with all incidences of endocarditis occurring in the setting of either a residual VSD or an associated valvular abnormality. No one with complete closure of the VSD in the absence of other anomalies developed endocarditis.[6]*

*Right-sided endocarditis occurs most often in the setting of IV drug use. However, many patients with VSDs present with right-sided endocarditis without a history of IV drug use. This is presumably due to infection on the tricuspid valve from the VSD jet directed toward the valve tissue.*

2. **How does one make a diagnosis of infective endocarditis?**

*The diagnosis of endocarditis can be difficult. Attempts have been made to establish criteria, such as the Duke diagnostic criteria, to make a firm diagnosis. However, these must be adapted based on clinical experience of the congenital heart population in which complex repairs are common. The classic stigmata of endocarditis (valvulitis, peripheral emboli, and immunologic vascular findings) are often absent in this population. History, microbiologic studies, and echocardiographic imaging are essential in making a diagnosis.*

3. **What is the value of blood cultures after multiple courses of antibiotics?**

*The administration of antimicrobial agents to patients before blood cultures are obtained reduces the recovery rate of the infective organism by 35% to 40%.[7] The nature of the organism and the antimicrobial susceptibility of the organism will guide appropriate antibiotic therapy.*

*Among nontoxic, hemodynamically stable patients who have received recent antibiotics, further antibiotic therapy should be delayed to obtain blood cultures.[8] If possible, one should wait at least 3 days after prior treatment has been discontinued.[9] Blood cultures after long-term antibiotic treatment may not become positive after treatment has been discontinued for 6 to 7 days.*

*In cases complicated by sepsis, severe valvular dysfunction, conduction disturbances, or embolic events, empiric therapy should be started after three sets of blood cultures are drawn.*

4. **Once appropriate antibiotic treatment has been initiated, what is the required duration of treatment in this patient?**

*The duration of antimicrobial therapy for infective endocarditis is complex and variable. It is dependent on the infective organism, antimicrobial susceptibility of the organism, and the patient course and response to therapy. Therefore, consultation with an infectious disease specialist is recommended.*

*In this case of native valve endocarditis (i.e., no prosthetic material) with an organism suspected to be fully susceptible to penicillin, a 4-week course of IV penicillin plus 2 weeks of synergistic gentamicin is recommended. Ceftriaxone can be used instead of penicillin if there is renal dysfunction or penicillin allergy.[9]*

*A 2-week treatment regimen with penicillin and gentamycin may be considered if streptococcal isolates are fully sensitive to penicillin and the patient has a rapid (<7 days) response to antibiotic treatment. There should also be no cardiovascular com-*

*plications and no vegetations greater than 10 mm on transesoph-
ageal echocardiogram.*[10] *The efficacy and safety of this treatment
have been documented in clinical studies.*[11]

5. **Which patients with congenital defects should receive prophylactic antibiotics against infective endocarditis?**

*Antibiotic prophylaxis is recommended for the following ACHD
conditions:*
1. *Unrepaired cyanotic ACHD, including palliative shunts and
conduits*
2. *Completely repaired ACHD with prosthetic material or
device, whether placed by surgery or by catheter intervention,
during the first 6 months after the procedure*
3. *Repaired ACHD with residual defects at the site or adjacent
to the site of a prosthetic patch or prosthetic device (which
prevents endothelialization)*

## FINAL DIAGNOSIS

Subacute bacterial infective endocarditis involving the tricuspid
valve

## PLAN OF ACTION

Discontinue all antibiotics and await the recurrence of febrile
illness. Once the fever returns, obtain blood cultures and initiate
appropriate IV antibiotics.

## INTERVENTION

None

## OUTCOME

On discontinuation of his antibiotics, the patient had recurrence
of his febrile illness 7 days later. He was admitted to the hospital, and three sets of blood cultures were taken. Within 24 hours
the blood cultures were positive for gram-positive cocci in
chains. Penicillin G 3 million IU intravenously every 4 hours was
started for presumed streptococcal infection. Gentamicin 90 mg
intravenously every 12 hours was added for synergistic treatment.

The patient became afebrile 2 days after antibiotics were
started, and remained afebrile through completion of a 2-week
course of IV penicillin and gentamycin. His symptoms resolved
completely and have not returned.

The blood culture organisms were finalized as *Streptococcus
sanguis* and *Streptococcus intermedius*. Both of these organisms
are of the *S. viridans* group. They were susceptible to penicillin,
ampicillin, erythromycin, clindamycin, ciprofloxacin, and van-
comycin. They were resistant to tetracycline.

With the confirmation of uncomplicated *S. viridans* subacute
bacterial endocarditis and rapid clinical response, 2 weeks of IV
penicillin and gentamicin was felt to be sufficient for complete
treatment. A course of oral antibiotics after the IV course was
not necessary. Surveillance cultures drawn following completion of antibiotic therapy were sterile.

The patient continues to do well and is working as a speech
pathologist. He is now vigilant about his prophylactic antibiotics and the timing of his dose before procedures.

## FINAL COMMENTS

Febrile illness in such patients should prompt physicians and
other care providers to think of endocarditis. As this case illustrates, failure to consider infective endocarditis delays diagnosis and appropriate treatment and may put the patient's life at
risk.

## Selected References

1. Kidd L, Driscoll DJ, Gersony WM, et al: Second natural history
study of congenital heart defects: Results of treatment of patients
with ventricular septal defects. Circulation 87:I38–I51, 1993.
2. Van der Meer JTM, van Wijk W, Thompson J, et al: Awareness of
need and actual use of prophylaxis: Lack of patient compliance in
the prevention of bacterial endocarditis. J Antimicrob Chemother
29:187–194, 1992.
3. Durack DT: Prevention of infective endocarditis. N Engl J Med
332:38–44, 1995.
4. Pelletier LL Jr, Petersdorf RG: Infective endocarditis: A review of
125 cases from the University of Washington Hospitals, 1963–1972.
Medicine 23 (Baltimore) 56:287–313, 1977.
5. Shively BK, Gurule FT, Roldan CA, et al: Diagnostic value of
transesophageal compared with transthoracic echocardiography
in infective endocarditis. J Am Coll Cardiol 18:391–397, 1991.
6. Gabriel HM, Heger M, Innerhofer P, et al: Long-term outcome of
patients with ventricular septal defect considered not to require
surgical closure during childhood. JACC 39:1066–1071, 2002.
7. Gersony WM, Hayes CJ, Driscoll DJ, et al: Bacterial endocarditis
in patients with aortic stenosis, pulmonary stenosis, or ventricular
septal defect. Circulation 87:I52–I65, 1993.
8. Morris CD, Reller MD, Menashe VD: Thirty-year incidence of
infective endocarditis after surgery for congenital heart defect.
JAMA 279:599–603, 1998.
9. Pazin GJ, Saul S, Thompson ME: Blood culture positivity: Suppression by outpatient antibiotic therapy in patients with bacterial
endocarditis. Arch Intern Med 142:263–268, 1982.
10. Bayer AS, Bolger AS, Taubert KA, et al: Diagnosis and management of infective endocarditis and its complications, AHA scientific statement. Circulation 98:2936–2948, 1998.
11. Horstkotte D, Follath F, Gutschik E, et al: Task force on infective
endocarditis of the European Society of Cardiology: Guidelines
on prevention, diagnosis and treatment of infective endocarditis.
Eur Heart J 25:267–276, 2004.

## Bibliography

Dajani AD, Taubert KA, Wilson W, et al: Prevention of bacterial endo-
carditis: Recommendation by the American Heart Association.
Circulation 96:358–366, 1997.
Durack DT, Lukes AS, Bright DK: New criteria for diagnosis of infec-
tive endocarditis: Utilization of specific echocardiographic find-
ings. Am J Med 96:200–209, 1994.
Mylonakis E, Calderwood SB: Infective endocarditis in adults. N Engl
J Med 345:1318–1330, 2001.
Shah P, Singh WSA, Rose V, Keith JD: Incidence of bacterial endocarditis in ventricular septal defects. Circulation 34:127, 1966.
Simmons NA, Cawson RA, Eykyn SJ, et al: The antibiotic prophylaxis
of infective endocarditis: Recommendations from the Endocarditis
Working Party of the British Society for Antimicrobial Chemotherapy. Lancet 335:888–899, 1990. See update: Antibiotic prophylaxis and infective endocarditis (letter). Lancet 339:1292–1293,
1992.
Wilson W, Taubert KA, Gewitz M, et al: Prevention of infective endocarditis: Guidelines from the American Heart Association: A
guideline from the American Heart Association Rheumatic Fever,
Endocarditis, and Kawasaki Disease Committee, Council on Cardiovascular Disease in the Young, and the Council on Clinical
Cardiology, Council on Cardiovascular Surgery and Anesthesia,
and the Quality of Care and Outcomes Research Interdisciplinary
Working Group. Circulation 116:1736–1754, 2007.

# Ventricular Septal Defect and the Aortic Valve

**Hideki Uemura, Tomohiro Tsunekawa, and Toru Ishizaka**

**Age: 23 years**
**Gender: Male**
**Occupation: College student**
**Working diagnosis: Aortic regurgitation, after closure of outlet ventricular septal defect**

## HISTORY

The patient was born uneventfully at term, but at 18 months a heart murmur was noted. A cardiac workup established the diagnosis of a doubly committed VSD. The interventricular communication was small because the aortic valve leaflet covered the defect. No aortic regurgitation was noted on follow-up echos. By age 6 years, however, echo demonstrated a slight deformity of the right coronary cusp with very mild aortic valve regurgitation. At that time, a surgical procedure was not indicated on the basis of the small shunt and the mild aortic valve involvement. At 9 years old, the right coronary cusp was found prolapsing toward the LV. Soon thereafter the family moved and the patient was lost to follow-up.

The patient came back to cardiac attention when he was 16 years old, still without symptoms, but now a diastolic murmur was audible. Echo showed mild to moderate aortic valve regurgitation.

Surgical repair was carried out 4 months later, and consisted of closure of the VSD through the pulmonary trunk[1] and plasty of the aortic valve by means of the so-called Trusler method.[2] The operation was uneventful and the postoperative course was uncomplicated.

Residual aortic valve regurgitation was mild during the first several months postoperatively, but progressed later. Catheterization 1 year after surgery demonstrated an enlarged left ventricle. The patient was reluctant to undergo further surgery. On annual follow-up echos, however, left ventricular diastolic dimensions increased gradually over the ensuing years, eventually to an LV diastolic dimension of 67 mm. Therefore, the patient was discussed for further treatment.

***Comments:*** In a doubly committed and juxta-arterial VSD, the outlet septum is missing or very hypoplastic, and the aortic valve and the pulmonary valve are in fibrous continuity without an interrupting muscular bar.[3–6] There is no off-setting present between the two semilunar valves. This type of defect is more common in Asian populations.

Because of the anatomic orientation, the right coronary cusp of the aortic valve is often affected by the presence of the defect.[7] The leaflet may cover the ostium of the defect partially or completely. If this happens, interventricular shunting is diminished or even absent, and pulmonary blood flow is not excessive. Alternatively, deformity of the right coronary cusp over time tends to produce aortic valve regurgitation. Another outcome

in the natural history of such a defect is for the defect to become a sinus of Valsalva aneurysm, which may rupture.

The Trusler method[2] of surgical repair of aortic cusp prolapse/regurgitation consists of plication of the elongated edge of the right coronary cusp and suspension of the commissures.

## CURRENT SYMPTOMS

None

NYHA class: I

## CURRENT MEDICATIONS

None

## PHYSICAL EXAMINATION

BP 140/40 mm Hg, HR 58 bpm, oxygen saturation 99% on room air

Height 176 cm, weight 68 kg, BSA 1.82 m$^2$

Surgical scars: A previous median sternotomy scar was present.

Neck veins: Not distended and had a normal waveform

Lungs/chest: Normal vesicular breath sounds were heard with no rales. There was no chest deformity.

Heart: The rhythm was regular. An early 2/6 high-pitched diastolic murmur was heard at the second left intercostal space. The peripheral pulses were accentuated.

Abdomen: Flat and soft, liver and spleen were not palpable, no bruit was present.

Extremities: No edema or cyanosis was present.

***Comments:*** Unless there are other sources of arterial runoff, the patient's blood pressure (wide pulse pressure and low diastolic pressure) indicates that aortic regurgitation is clinically significant.

In severe aortic regurgitation, peripheral pulses are bounding as the pulse pressure widens (100 mm Hg, in this case). This is because the systolic arterial pressure is raised with an increased systolic volume, and diastolic pressure is low because of aortic valve regurgitation.

The high-pitched early diastolic murmur is due to aortic valve regurgitation. An Austin Flint murmur (a low-pitched apical diastolic murmur due to anterior mitral leaflet deformation by the aortic regurgitant jet) should be sought.

## LABORATORY DATA

| | |
|---|---|
| Hemoglobin | 13.9 g/dL (13.0–17.0) |
| Hematocrit/PCV | 39.2% (41–51) |
| MCV | 87.9 fL (85–100) |
| Platelet count | $239 \times 10^3$/mL (150–350) |
| Sodium | 140 mmol/L (138–145) |
| Potassium | 3.7 mmol/L (3.4–4.9) |
| Creatinine | 0.8 mg/dL (0.7–1.3) |
| Blood urea nitrogen | 15 mg/dL (8–20) |
| Uric acid | 5.3 mg/dL (3.8–8.0) |
| AST | 16 U/L (0–40) |
| ALT | 13 U/L (0–35) |
| T Bil | 1.1 mg/dL (0.2–1.2) |
| Hb A1c | **4.2%** (4.3–5.8) |
| FBS | 82 mg/dL (65–110) |

### OTHER RELEVANT LAB RESULTS
| | |
|---|---|
| HANP | **46** pg/mL (<40) |
| BNP | **25.5** pg/mL (<20) |

## ELECTROCARDIOGRAM

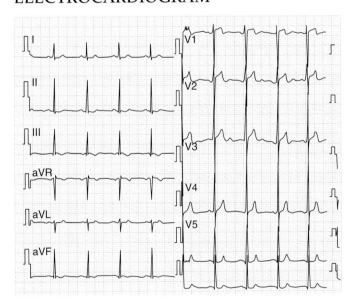

Figure 8-1 Electrocardiogram.

### FINDINGS
Heart rate: 58 bpm

QRS axis: +70°

QRS duration: 106 msec

PR interval: 0.18 sec

Normal sinus rhythm with LV hypertrophy

**Comments:** Note that the precordial leads have been taken at half standard, so the dramatic voltages in the precordial leads are understated. The ST elevation in V1–3 offers some nonspecific support for pathologic LV hypertrophy, since voltage evidence of LV hypertrophy is not very reliable in the young.

U-waves are visible in the precordial leads. These can be present in long QT syndromes or various electrolyte disturbances. In this case, they likely relate to LV hypertrophy.

## CHEST X-RAY

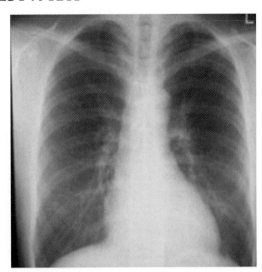

Figure 8-2 Posteroanterior projection.

### FINDINGS
Cardiothoracic ratio: 52%

The heart contour was normal with no evidence of pulmonary congestion. Sternotomy wires were seen.

**Comments:** The heart size is normal and reassuring. Apart from evidence of prior sternotomy, there is little here to suggest significant pathology.

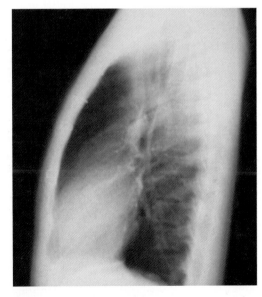

Figure 8-3 Lateral projection.

### FINDINGS
Normal apart from the sternal wires. The thoracic spine is straight.

## EXERCISE TESTING

Not performed

## ECHOCARDIOGRAM

### OVERALL FINDINGS

The LV was moderately enlarged (LVEDd 65 mm, LVESd 45 mm in parasternal long-axis view) with reasonable contraction (EF 66%). There was no LV hypertrophy. The LA size was normal. The RV was normal in appearance. There was no residual VSD. There was mild pulmonary regurgitation, trivial tricuspid regurgitation, and no mitral regurgitation. There was retrograde flow in the abdominal aorta.

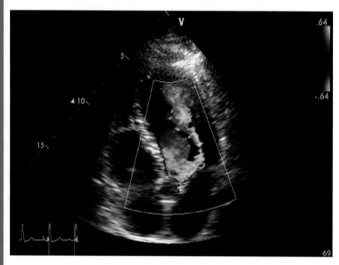

Figure 8-4 Apical five-chamber view, color Doppler.

### FINDINGS

Significant aortic regurgitation was seen in this view, with an eccentric jet directed toward the anterior leaflet of the mitral valve.

**Comments:** Holodiastolic flow reversal in the descending thoracic aorta suggests at least moderate aortic regurgitation; aortic regurgitation is probably severe when diastolic flow reversal is also present in the abdominal aorta, as with this patient.

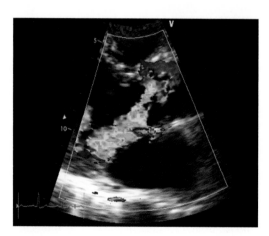

Figure 8-5 Parasternal long-axis view, 2D color Doppler.

### FINDINGS

There was severe aortic regurgitation. Leakage was mainly through a thickened and deformed right-coronary cusp with secondary malcoaptation of the cusps. The aortic root diameter was 35 mm.

**Comments:** Right aortic cusp prolapse into the defect can be best visualized with color Doppler imaging in the parasternal long-axis view, and apical five-chamber and three-chamber views. The prolapsing aortic cusp may obliterate the VSD completely; the size of the VSD can therefore be underestimated echocardiographically. Doubly committed VSDs are best seen from parasternal short-axis views, just below the pulmonary valve. This patient had previous aortic valve repair and does not have any residual VSD. The mechanism of aortic regurgitation is thus different, with probable degeneration and deformity of the previously repaired aortic cusps.

## CATHETERIZATION

### HEMODYNAMICS

Heart rate    58

|  | Pressure | Saturation (%) |
|---|---|---|
| SVC |  | 75 |
| IVC |  | 85 |
| RA | mean 6 |  |
| RV | 19/6 |  |
| PA | 18/5 mean 9 | 79 |
| PCWP | mean 6 |  |
| LA |  |  |
| LV | 137/12 |  |
| Aorta | 135/42 mean 78 | 99 |

| Calculations | |
|---|---|
| Qp (L/min) | 6.29 |
| Qs (L/min) | 5.56 |
| Cardiac index (L/min/m$^2$) | 3.05 |
| Qp/Qs | 1.13 |
| PVR (Wood units) | 0.48 |
| SVR (Wood units) | 12.94 |

### FINDINGS

Normal right-sided filling pressures with no evidence of a residual intracardiac shunt (despite the calculations shown). There was a borderline elevated LV end-diastolic pressure and no gradient across the aortic valve.

**Comments:** Many cardiologists would not have done a heart catheterization on this young man. It was the policy of our unit to do so.

Pulmonary hypertension was absent, an important consideration in patients with a previous VSD closed beyond infancy.

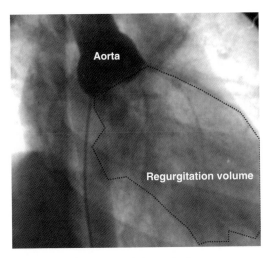

Figure 8-6 Aortogram in posteroanterior projection.

## FINDINGS

Angiographic calculations: There was severe aortic regurgitation. Aortic root diameter 34 mm (145% of anticipated normal value)

**Ventricular Volume Quantification**

|  | LV | (Normal range) | RV | (Normal range) |
|---|---|---|---|---|
| EDV (mL) | **376** | (77–195) | 181 | (88–227) |
| ESV (mL) | **138** | (19–72) | 98 | (23–103) |
| SV (mL) | **238** | (51–133) | 83 | (52–138) |
| EF (%) | 63 | (57–74) | **46** | (48–74) |
| EDVi (mL/m$^2$) | **206** | (68–103) | 99 | (68–114) |
| ESVi (mL/m$^2$) | **76** | (19–41) | **54** | (21–50) |
| SVi (mL/m$^2$) | **131** | (44–68) | 46 | (23–50) |

**Comments:** Ventriculography confirmed the LV enlargement seen by echo and preserved LV contraction.

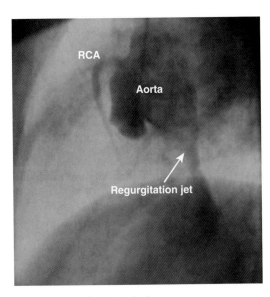

Figure 8-7 Aortogram in lateral projection.

## FINDINGS

There was an eccentric jet of aortic regurgitation toward the ventricular septum.

**Comments:** The regurgitation is produced by prolapse of the right aortic cusp toward the septal defect.

### FOCUSED CLINICAL QUESTIONS AND DISCUSSION POINTS

1. What is the significance of a juxta-arterial VSD?

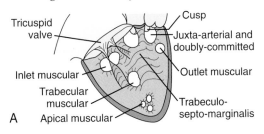

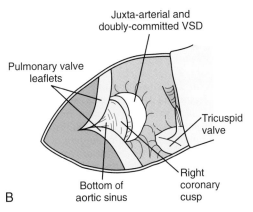

Figure 8-8 **A,** Various types of ventricular septal defect as seen from the right side of the heart. **B,** Surgical view of juxta-arterial and doubly committed ventricular septal defect through pulmonary trunk.

*Although morphologically the term VSD seems straightforward, in the setting of a doubly committed and juxta-arterial VSD there is potential for confusion. By definition, part of the border of the VSD in a juxta-arterial, doubly committed VSD is formed by fibrous continuity between the aortic and pulmonary valves. As a result, a certain proportion of the morphologic VSD orifice is provided by the right coronary cusp of the aortic valve. Prolapse of the aortic cusp into the VSD is common under these circumstances, and diminishes the actual communication between the two ventricles, even though a defect in the wall exists. Hence, the physiological communication (left-to-right shunt size) does not necessarily correlate with the true size of the morphologic defect (see Fig. 8-8A).*

*In such cases the echocardiographer may report that a VSD is small or has become smaller (in the context of aortic cusp prolapse) based on the size of the interventricular communication seen by Doppler. The surgeon sees the actual size of the VSD at the time of surgery, which can be substantial and require patch closure. This should be borne in mind when intervention is contemplated.*

*Appreciation of the anatomy of the VSD and the surrounding structures is clearly important for surgery. Through the pulmonary trunk, there often appears to be some fibrous tissue beneath the pulmonary valve attachment, which may be used for anchoring the VSD patch. This tissue is also part of the root of the aortic sinus. Some surgeons may place a stitch in this tissue, but if a* perioperative laceration occurs inadvertently, a communication between the aortic root and the right ventricle may be created (see Fig. 8-8B).

2. Should this patient have been offered surgery at an earlier age?

Our institutional policy as to when to operate on a patient with a juxta-arterial VSD with a relatively small left-to-right intracardiac shunt depends on whether the right coronary cusp of the aortic valve is deformed.[8] Patients are followed up closely, and if there is echocardiographic evidence of progressive deformation of the cusp or the development of aortic regurgitation of any degree, elective surgical closure of the VSD is recommended.

The situation may be different with adult patients, as they may be referred for surgery with a more conventional indication for surgery, namely substantial aortic regurgitation or rupture of a sinus of Valsalva. When aortic regurgitation is graded as mild or moderate, the surgeon will perform a commissural suspension and plication of the edge of elongated right coronary cusp in addition to closure of the VSD. If regurgitation is severe with obvious organic changes in the leaflets, the aortic valve will need to be replaced.

These different surgical approaches have been compared in a large surgical series performed between 1977 and 2004.[9] Of 105 patients who underwent surgery at less than 2 years of age, only 2 (2%) needed plasty of the aortic valve. Of 188 patients between 2 and 15 years, 21 (11%) needed repair or replacement of the aortic valve. In 122 adolescent and adult patients, 49 needed aortic valve repair and 21 valve replacements (57% all together). Furthermore, there was 90% freedom from reoperation at 20 years among patients who required VSD closure only (with no need for concomitant aortic valve surgery of any sort).[9] In contrast, there was a much higher rate of reoperation in those who required surgery on the aortic valve at the first operation. Whether this reflects different anatomic substrates or better preservation of the native aortic valve when patients are operated on at a young age remains speculative.

On the basis of these findings, closure of the VSD should be arranged before any additional procedure is needed to the aortic valve, even before 2 years of age. Given today's surgical techniques, VSD closure can be achieved with a very low mortality and morbidity even in early infancy.

In retrospect, it seems likely that this patient may not have developed severe aortic regurgitation if he had undergone closure of the VSD at 6 years when the aortic valve deformity was noted for the first time.

3. What surgical options should be considered in this patient?

It was felt that this particular patient would benefit from elective surgical intervention, both on the grounds of substantial aortic regurgitation and progressive dilatation of his LV. (The ACC/AHA[10] valve guidelines recommend surgery in the asymptomatic patient with severe aortic regurgitation when the LV ejection fraction is less than 50% or when the LV diastolic diameter is greater than 75 mm.

Although aortic valve repair would be attractive, it is not likely to be possible. When regurgitation is due to a perforation at one cusp, repair may be uncomplicated. More commonly, however, prior attempted repair leads to considerable organic change of the leaflets. This patient previously underwent commissural suspension together with plication of the redundant tissues of the leaflet edges. Over the ensuing 6 years the leaflets would be expected to become thickened and degenerate. Restoration of the valve geometry and optimal coaptation would be quite difficult. Therefore, replacement of the valve was thought to be more likely.

4. What type of valve replacement should be used?)

When considering aortic valve replacement, there are four choices: (1) mechanical valve, (2) bioprosthesis, (3) homograft, or (4) a pulmonary autograft (Ross procedure).

A mechanical valve is durable but requires lifelong meticulous anticoagulation, with risks of either hemorrhage or valve thrombosis. This is particularly troublesome for women of childbearing age. A xenograft bioprosthesis (made of heterogeneous tissue) does not require anticoagulation but has a limited lifespan, especially in the young, and reoperation will be required. A homograft valve is comparable to a xenograft bioprosthesis, but with time both the leaflets and the homograft wall will become calcified. Therefore, reoperation will be more challenging and somewhat more risky.

Use of the pulmonary autograft may be the least attractive option in this case. Because of the morphologic features of this type of VSD, the pulmonary valve is not easily usable. The outlet septum is either absent or very hypoplastic, in keeping with the cardinal feature of the defect, fibrous continuity between the aortic and the pulmonary valve forming part of the VSD border (as discussed previously). It is thus difficult if not impossible to harvest the pulmonary autograft, which under normal circumstances sits on a muscular "crown." Furthermore, the annular attachment of the pulmonary valve in this particular case would have previously received a few stitches for VSD closure. These surgical stitches, in turn, could have affected the geometry and competence of the pulmonary valve. An ideal Ross procedure requires a completely normal pulmonary valve; otherwise, neo-aortic valve dysfunction requiring reoperation in the ensuing years becomes likely, which negates the purpose of the Ross procedure to begin with.

In this case, the patient considered valve durability and avoidance of reoperation as a priority. Therefore, a mechanical valve prosthesis was chosen, with a commitment on his part for lifelong anticoagulation.

## FINAL DIAGNOSIS

Recurrent and progressive aortic valve regurgitation, related to doubly committed and juxta-arterial VSD

## PLAN OF ACTION

Aortic valve replacement

## INTERVENTION

Myxomatous degeneration of the aortic leaflets was evident at the time of surgery. The left coronary cusp and the right coronary cusp had been shortened, thickened, and stiffened. The noncoronary cusp was thickened and redundant. The aortic valve was replaced using a St. Jude Medical mechanical valve (size 27-mm, standard cuff). The patient made an uneventful recovery.

## OUTCOME

The patient did well and left the hospital in less than a week from surgery (on anticoagulation).

One year later the patient reported no symptoms. The blood pressure was 109/65. His echocardiogram showed an LVEDd of 45 mm and an LVESd of 28 mm. The transaortic valve velocity was 2.1 m/sec.

He had a bicycle exercise test showing a mildly reduced peak $Vo_2$ (29.6 mL/min/kg).

**Comments:** A mechanical valve usually creates a small pressure gradient. This is partly related to kinetic energy loss from opening the valve leaflets and also due to turbulence across the valve in its open position.

## Selected References

1. Kawashima Y, Fujita T, Mori T, et al: Trans-pulmonary arterial closure of ventricular septal defect. J Thorac Cardiovasc Surg 74:191–194, 1977.
2. Trusler GA, Moes CA, Kidd BS: Repair of ventricular septal defect with aortic insufficiency. J Thorac Cardiovasc Surg 66:394–403, 1973.
3. Tynan M, Anderson RH: Ventricular septal defect: Morphology and classification. In Anderson RH, Baker EJ, Macartney FJ, et al (eds): Paediatric Cardiology, 2nd ed, vol 2. Edinburgh, Harcourt, 2002, pp 983–994.
4. Ueda M, Becker AE: Classification of hearts with overriding aortic and pulmonary valves. Int J Cardiol 9:357–369, 1985.
5. Griffin ML, Sullivan ID, Anderson RH, Macartney FJ: Doubly committed subarterial ventricular septal defect: New morphological criteria with echocardiographic and angiocardiographic correlation. Br Heart J 59:474–479, 1988.
6. Schmidt KG, Cassidy SC, Silverman NH, Stanger P: Doubly committed subarterial ventricular septal defects: Echocardiographic features and surgical implications. J Am Coll Cardiol 12:1538–1546, 1988.
7. Tatsuno K, Konno S, Ando M, Sakakibara S: Pathogenetic mechanisms of prolapsing aortic valve and aortic regurgitation associated with ventricular septal defect: Anatomical, angiographic, and surgical considerations. Circulation 48:1028–1037, 1973.
8. Tomita H, Arakaki Y, Ono Y, et al: Severity indices of right coronary cusp prolapse and aortic regurgitation complicating ventricular septal defect in the outlet septum: Which defect should be closed? Jpn Circ J 68:139–143, 2004.
9. Uemura H, Kagisaki K, Adachi I, et al: Aortic valvar involvement in patients undergoing closure of ventricular septal defect via the pulmonary trunk. Int J Cardiol 129:26–31, 2008.
10. Bonow RO, Carabello BA, Chatterjee K, et al: ACC/AHA 2006 Guidelines for the Management of Patients with Valvular Heart Disease: A report of the American College of Cardiology/American Heart Association Task Force on Practice Guidelines (Writing Committee to Revise the 1998 Guidelines for the Management of Patients with Valvular Heart Disease): Developed in collaboration with the Society of Cardiovascular Anesthesiologists: Endorsed by the Society for Cardiovascular Angiography and Interventions and the Society of Thoracic Surgeons. Circulation 114:e84–e231, 2006.

# Catheter Closure of Ventricular Septal Defects

**Omar Khalid, Qi-Ling Cao, and Ziyad M. Hijazi**

**Age: 57 years**
**Gender: Female**
**Occupation: High school teacher**
**Working diagnosis: Muscular ventricular septal defect**

## HISTORY

The patient was evaluated for a heart murmur during pregnancy 20 years prior to presentation when she was 34 years old and diagnosed with a muscular VSD. She did well until 2 years prior to presentation (then 52 years old) when she started complaining of dyspnea on exertion. She occasionally complained of chest discomfort, palpitations, and dizziness that resolved spontaneously. These symptoms grew more noticeable over the ensuing years.

Past medical history was significant for a moderate degree of scoliosis.

**Comments:** One wonders why the patient has developed dyspnea at this stage. It may be that there was a component of restrictive lung disease from her scoliosis, though this would be unlikely to progress over time in the way her symptoms have. More likely, there was a change in the shunt through the VSD, secondary to aging and to a stiffer LV. This would enhance volume loading of the left heart chambers and compromise further systemic cardiac output (through a systemic "still" phenomenon), both leading to exertional dyspnea.

## CURRENT SYMPTOMS

She complained of dyspnea on exertion. The patient found herself out of breath after climbing two flights of stairs. She reported neither orthopnea nor paroxysmal nocturnal dyspnea. There was no history of cough, cyanosis, or syncope. No history of smoking or alcohol consumption.

NYHA class: II

**Comments:** Although the patient was asymptomatic for many years, she now complains of limiting dyspnea. There are many potential causes of dyspnea in a 57-year-old, one of which

is VSD. As she aged, changes in LV and RV compliance, namely increasing left ventricular end-diastolic pressures, are likely to have resulted in an increased left-to-right shunt through the defect. This in turn may have contributed to her limited exercise tolerance.

## CURRENT MEDICATIONS

None

## PHYSICAL EXAMINATION

BP 124/79 mm Hg, HR 72 bpm, oxygen saturation 97% on room air

Height 170 cm, weight 56.7 kg, BSA 1.64 m$^2$

Surgical scars: None

Neck veins: The jugular venous pressure was not elevated (0 mm above the sternal angle), and the waveform was normal.

Lungs/chest: Clear

Heart: There was a mild RV heave. First and second heart sounds were normal. There was a grade 3/6 harsh pansystolic murmur heard all across the precordium; no diastolic or ejection systolic murmurs were heard.

Abdomen: There was no hepatomegaly.

Extremities: There was no pedal edema or finger clubbing.

**Comments:** The harsh holosystolic murmur is consistent with the diagnosis of a restrictive VSD. The absence of a diastolic or ejection systolic murmur suggests that there was neither aortic regurgitation nor any significant pulmonary stenosis, respectively.

# LABORATORY DATA

| Hemoglobin | 12.0 g/dL (11.5–15.0) |
| Hematocrit/PCV | 37.5% (36–46) |
| MCV | 95.7 fL (83–99) |
| Platelet count | $183 \times 10^9/L$ (150–400) |

***Comments:*** The normal hemoglobin excludes anemia as the cause of the exertional dyspnea.

# ELECTROCARDIOGRAM

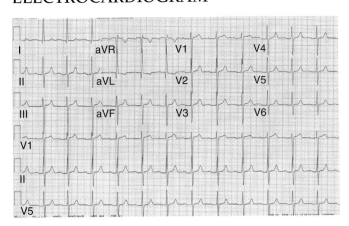

Figure 9-1 Electrocardiogram.

## FINDINGS
Heart rate: 76 bpm

QRS axis: −22°

QRS duration: 106 msec

Sinus rhythm, first-degree heart block, voltage criteria for LV hypertrophy. The P-wave duration may be increased, in keeping with LA overload associated with LV hypertrophy.

***Comments:*** This ECG supports the notion that the left-to-right shunt has been large enough to cause left heart dilation. The first-degree block is not easily explained by a muscular VSD.

# CHEST X-RAY

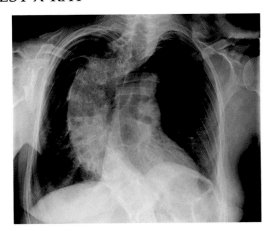

Figure 9-2 Posteroanterior projection.

## FINDINGS
Cardiothoracic ratio: Cannot be meaningfully measured

There is severe thoracolumbar scoliosis distorting the chest. There is also minimal increase in interstitial markings in the lower zones with no pleural effusion. Cardiovascular assessment is very difficult in the setting of marked scoliosis. Nevertheless, there seems to be LA enlargement (based on the horizontal appearance of the left main brochus). The pulmonary trunk and aortic arch could be seen. There was no evidence of overt heart failure.

***Comments:*** The thoracolumbar scoliosis calls into question the relative contribution of scoliosis to the patient's dyspnea. In her case, scoliosis had never limited her in the past, and it would seem unlikely to have progressed to be the sole cause of her limitations now.

The patient's scoliosis also poses a significant challenge not only for interpreting a chest radiograph, but also for maneuvering catheters and profiling the defects in the catheterization laboratory.

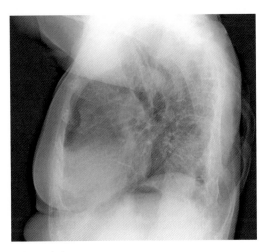

Figure 9-3 Lateral view.

## FINDINGS
There was a suggestion of LA enlargement.

***Comments:*** Scoliosis makes interpretation difficult, but the presence of LA enlargement is an important finding, as it suggests a more hemodynamically significant left-to-right shunt at the ventricular level.

# ECHOCARDIOGRAM

## OVERALL FINDINGS
By TEE, the measurements obtained were:

LVEDd (mm): 50.2

LVESd (mm): 33.9

LA (mm): 42

LVPW (mm): 9.4

Shortening fraction: 32.4%

PV (m/sec): 1.5

AV (m/sec): 1.4

VSD (m/sec): 4

Mild LV hypertrophy

Single muscular VSD with its RV opening in the area of the moderator band

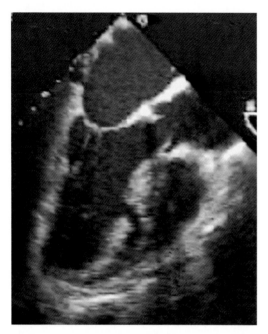

Figure 9-4  Long-axis view without color Doppler.

## FINDINGS

The echocardiogram showed normal LV function with mild LV hypertrophy, a left-to-right shunt at the midseptal level, mild LA dilatation, mild to moderate tricuspid regurgitation, and mild pulmonary hypertension.

The 2D four-chamber view by TEE showed two separate openings into the right ventricular side separated by the moderator band. Color Doppler showed left-to-right shunt through the defect. The Doppler gradient across the ventricular septum was 4 m/sec (suggesting an RV systolic pressure of 124 – 64 = 60 mm Hg).

**Comments:** Imaging adults with muscular VSDs can be difficult, especially in the presence of significant scoliosis. In this patient, the VSD was well seen in the longitudinal plane.

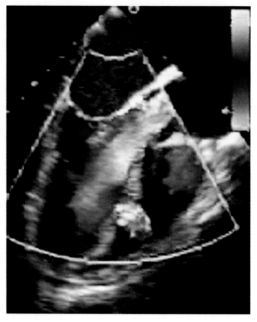

Figure 9-5  The same view as Figure 9-4, with Color Doppler transesophageal echocardiography demonstrating the effect.

## FINDINGS

Color Doppler showed left-to-right shunt through the defect. The Doppler gradient across the valve was 4 m/sec.

**Comments:** Color Doppler adds sensitivity to identifying muscular septal defects. The Doppler velocity through the defect should reflect the pressure gradient between the RV and LV. Flow is almost all during systole. If diastolic flow were present, this would indicate a significant elevation of LV end-diastolic pressure (not seen in this patient).

## CATHETERIZATION

### HEMODYNAMICS (FIG. 9-6)

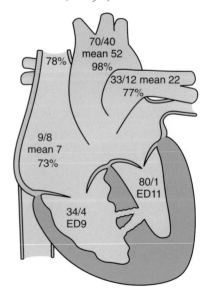

Figure 9-6  Hemodynamic values obtained at cardiac catheterization.

Heart rate    72 bpm

**Calculations**

| | |
|---|---|
| Qp (L/min) | 7.44 |
| Qs (L/min) | 5.23 |
| Cardiac index (L/min/m$^2$) | 3.19 |
| Qp/Qs | 1.42 |
| PVR (Wood units) | 1.48 |
| SVR (Wood units) | 8.61 |

## Findings

Cardiac catheterization was done under general anesthesia and transesophageal guidance to facilitate closure of the defect, if appropriate. Low blood pressures relate to anesthesia. The patient was breathing 25% inspired oxygen (see Case 2), though the calculations used here do not account for supplemental oxygen.

There was a significant systolic pressure gradient across the VSD. Left ventricular end-diastolic pressure was not raised.

**Comments:** It is well known that under general anesthesia, oximetry data are altered such that routine shunt calculations of flow and shunt volume are potentially flawed. Specifically, lowered metabolism may raise the mixed venous saturation and underestimate the shunt, and positive pressure ventilation may change the pulmonary vascular resistance and limit shunting. Therefore, the calculated Qp/Qs ratio does not necessarily reflect the true magnitude of the shunt. These authors mainly rely on echocardiographic data (chamber size and shunt gradients) and symptoms to make clinical decisions.

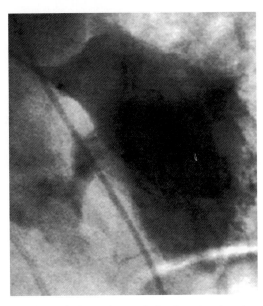

Figure 9-7 Left ventricular angiogram in the four-chamber view demonstrating the left-to-right shunt.

## Findings

The midseptal muscular VSD is clearly visible, with shunted blood from the LV to the RV. It appears that the RV side has two openings.

**Comments:** Due to the presence of significant scoliosis, the traditional views may not profile the septum in this patient. Therefore, the angulation must change to allow good profiling of the ventricular septum.

This angiogram was performed to delineate the exact location of the VSD and its relationship to other structures. The view also serves to facilitate crossing the VSD from the left ventricle to the RV at the time of intervention.

## Focused Clinical Questions and Discussion Points

1. When should a VSD be closed?

*Closure of a VSD in general is considered in patients with attributable symptoms, left heart dilatation, and/or a Qp/Qs greater than 1.5:1 in the absence of advanced pulmonary vascular disease. A careful clinical evaluation for signs and symptoms of congestive heart failure is important. It is also important to assess the hemodynamic effects of a VSD such as the degree of LA and LV dilatation and the presence and extent of PAH.*

*Anatomical considerations also weigh in the decision whether to close a defect. An echocardiogram, transesophageal if necessary, is essential to define the size and location of the defect, and to look for other coexisting septal defects, as more than one muscular defect may coexist. The lesion in this patient could be easily closed transcutaneously, thus avoiding the potential risks and hazards of cardiopulmonary bypass surgery.*

*The goals of closure are to prevent clinical deterioration, prevent further enlargement of the LA and LV, and lower the risk of atrial and/or ventricular dysrhythmia.*

*In this patient, the decision to proceed with catheter closure was based on left heart dilatation (suggestive of a significant left-to-right shunt, despite the low shunt calculation from oxygen saturations) and on the patient's symptoms. An additional consideration was the technical feasibility of transcutaneous closure. Once other causes of symptoms including dyspnea are excluded, a strong argument can be made for closure. In this case, after consideration of these issues and following prior discussions with the patient, the operators proceeded with defect closure.*

2. Should muscular VSDs be closed surgically or transcutaneously using a closure device?

*Muscular VSDs pose a significant challenge to the surgeon. Midmuscular or apical VSDs cannot be reached via the tricuspid valve, and thus for optimal visualization of the VSD a right ventriculotomy may be required. Even with a right ventriculotomy, due to the presence of large trabeculations, the view may not be optimal for successful closure. Left ventriculotomy is the best approach to see the VSD; however, such a procedure may lead to cardiac dysfunction and arrhythmogenesis. Alternatively, device closure of a muscular VSD in experienced hands is successful in 93% to 100% with a reported mortality of 0% to 2.7% and a morbidity of 3% to 10% including device embolization and postprocedural conduction abnormalities. Therefore, the authors submit that device closure is the best option for patients with a muscular VSD.*

3. What kind of device is most suitable for such a lesion?

*Device VSD closure has been used since the late 1980s. The ideal device should be user friendly. The operator should have full control of the device with the ability to reposition or recapture it prior to its final release. It should have a small delivery system, and the device should achieve complete or near complete closure with no adverse effects. The immediate and mid-term results of the Amplatzer muscular VSD device (see Holzer et al) seem to be promising.*

*The Amplatzer muscular VSD occluder (AGA Medical Corp.) is made of nitinol wire. It is a self-expandable device consisting of two flat disks that are linked via a central connecting waist, the diameter of which determines the size of the device.*

*The two disks are 4 mm larger than the connecting waist. Dacron fabric is incorporated into each disk to enhance thrombosis and prevent shunting through the device. The device has now been approved by the U.S. Food and Drug Administration for VSD closure (since September 2007).*

## FINAL DIAGNOSIS

Single muscular VSD

## PLAN OF ACTION

Transcutaneous closure of VSD

## INTERVENTION

The defect was closed in the catheterization laboratory under TEE guidance. To be able to close a midseptal VSD, it must be approached from the jugular vein. An arteriovenous loop was performed to facilitate passage of the delivery sheath from the jugular vein to the mid-LV cavity. The defect was crossed initially from the LV side using a Judkins left catheter. A wire was snared into the right jugular vein, then a 9 French Mullins sheath was placed over the wire from the right internal jugular vein through the RA and RV, crossing the VSD to the ascending aorta. Then a 12 mm Amplatzer muscular VSD occluder was positioned appropriately.

During deployment of the LV disk, the patient's blood pressure suddenly dropped to 50/30. Immediate attention to the mitral valve revealed that the anterior leaflet was caught between the disk and the septum resulting in wide-open mitral regurgitation. The disk was recaptured immediately and the mitral valve leaflet was freed. The regurgitation disappeared and the blood pressure returned to normal.

The length of the Amplatzer muscular VSD device was not sufficient to extend onto both sides of the septum. The ventricular septum in an adult is about 10 mm in thickness, yet the length of the waist in the Amplatzer muscular VSD device is only about 7 to 8 mm; hence, it may not completely straddle the septum. Significant constriction of the waist of the device after deployment confirmed the suspicion that the VSD had two openings on the RV side. The presence of two exits on the RV side makes closure more challenging, as the operator needs to position the device away from the moderator band to avoid inducing tricuspid regurgitation.

On final left ventriculography, a small residual shunt was seen near the inferior border of the VSD. The patient recovered quickly and without complication.

The changes in the QRS complexes compared to the previous ECG are due to new left anterior fascicular block. There is a low incidence of permanent and transient cardiac conduction disturbances with catheter-based closure of a muscular VSD.

## INTRAOPERATIVE ECHOCARDIOGRAM

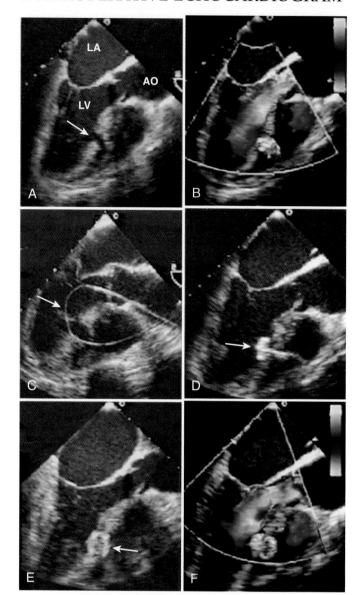

Figure 9-8 Transesophageal images in the long-axis view demonstrating the steps of closure.

### FINDINGS

**A,** Large VSD on the LV side *(arrow)*, opening into two separate defects into the RV side separated by the moderator band. **B,** Color Doppler confirming a left-to-right shunt through the VSD. **C,** A wire loop *(arrow)* passing from the ascending aorta to the LV through the VSD to the RV and out the right internal jugular vein. **D,** The left disk *(arrow)* deployed in the LV. **E,** The Amplatzer muscular VSD device *(arrow)* deployed in optimal position, straddling the ventricular septum. **F,** Color Doppler showing no significant flow through the defect or device.

***Comments:*** This figure composite outlines the procedure as seen echocardiographically. TEE guidance during the procedure helps to position the device and assess for any dysfunction of the mitral or aortic valves after deployment.

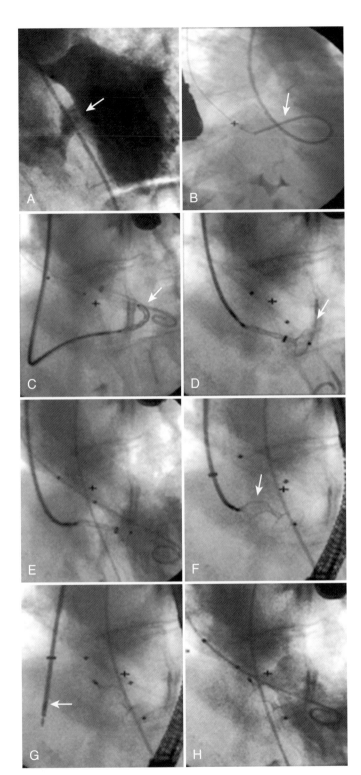

loop from the femoral artery through the VSD (*arrow*) and out the right internal jugular vein. **C**, Amplatzer device within Mullins sheath passing from the right internal jugular vein to the RA to the RV through the VSD (*arrow*) into the LV. **D**, LV disk was deployed (*arrow*). Note the pigtail in the LV for angiography. **E**, An angiogram in the LV while the LV disk (*arrow*) and the connecting waist were positioned in place. **F**, Cine image showing the deployment of the right disk. **G**, Cine image immediately after the device was released from the cable (*arrow*). **H**, Repeat LV angiogram demonstrating the device straddling the ventricular septum with trivial residual shunt through the posterior-inferior part of the device.

## OUTCOME IMAGING

Images were unavailable.

### FINDINGS

The anatomic features are identical to the preprocedure film except for the addition of the Amplatzer device seen in the midcardiac silhouette.

   ***Comments:*** A simple posteroanterior and lateral CXR can be a reassuring confirmation of position after the procedure.

## OUTCOME

The patient was discharged home in sinus rhythm the following day. She was told to take 75 mg of aspirin daily and antibiotic prophylaxis when needed for 6 months.
   During her follow-up visits, she expressed significant improvement in her dyspnea. Transthoracic echocardiography revealed good ventricular function and a trivial residual shunt from the inferior border of the device. This small residual shunt had completely resolved at her 6-month follow-up echocardiogram.

## Bibliography

Hijazi ZM: Device closure of ventricular septal defects. Cathet Cardiovasc Interven 60:107–114, 2003.

Hijazi ZM, Hakim F, Al-Fadley F, et al: Transcatheter closure of single muscular ventricular septal defects with the Amplatzer muscular VSD occluder: Initial results and technical consideration. Cathet Cardiovasc Intervent 49:167–172, 2000.

Holzer R, Balzer D, Cao QL, et al: Amplatzer muscular ventricular septal defect investigators. Device closure of muscular ventricular septal defects using the Amplatzer muscular ventricular septal defect occluder: Immediate and mid-term results of a US registry. J Am Coll Cardiol 43:1257–1263, 2004.

Minette MS, Sahn DJ: Ventricular septal defects. Circulation 114:2190–2197, 2006.

Robinson JDC, Zimmerman FJ, De Loera O, Hijazi ZM: Cardiac conduction disturbances seen after transcatheter device closure of muscular ventricular septal defects with the Amplatzer MVSD occluder. Am J Cardiol 97:558–560, 2006.

Serraf A, Lacour-Gayet F, Bruniaux J, et al: Surgical management of isolated multiple ventricular septal defects. J Thorac Cardiovasc Surg 103:437–443, 1992.

Thanopoulos BD, Rigby ML: Outcome of transcatheter closure of muscular ventricular septal defects with the Amplatzer ventricular septal defect occluder. Heart 91:513–516, 2005.

Thanopoulos BD, Tsaousis GS, Konstadopoulou GN, Zarayelyan AG: Transcatheter closure of muscular ventricular septal defects with the Amplatzer ventricular septal defect occluder: Initial clinical applications in children. J Am Coll Cardiol 33:1395–1399, 1999.

Figure 9-9 Cine fluoroscopic images demonstrating the steps of closure.

## FINDINGS

The same interventional sequence is shown angiographically:
   **A**, LV angiogram in the four-chamber view demonstrating a midseptal muscular VSD (*arrow*) measuring 16 mm on the LV side. **B**, Cine image demonstrating the arteriovenous wire

# Straddling of the Tricuspid Valve: Long-Term Outcome

**Craig S. Broberg**

**Age: 36**
**Gender: Female**
**Occupation: Office clerk**
**Working diagnosis: Severe tricuspid valve regurgitation**

## HISTORY

The patient presented in early infancy with dyspnea and failure to thrive. Cardiac catheterization and angiography showed a very large VSD with left-to-right shunting, and she underwent pulmonary artery (PA) banding at the age of 8 weeks. During her early childhood, the patient gradually became cyanotic but otherwise remained asymptomatic, and the decision to close the defect was postponed several times.

At age 14 she underwent surgical closure of the VSD with a Dacron patch and release of the PA band. Several of the chordae tendinae supporting the tricuspid valve ran through the defect and inserted on the LV side of the septum. The surgeon placed the patch around these insertions so as to minimize any tricuspid valve insufficiency.

Postoperatively, however, an echocardiogram showed severe tricuspid regurgitation, severe pulmonary stenosis, and a persistent VSD. Furthermore, the patient developed postoperative complete heart block. Endocardial pacing wires failed to capture, so an epicardial pacing system was placed. She also had postoperative paralysis of the right hemidiaphragm and a recurrent right pleural effusion, which eventually required a right pleurodesis.

In the ensuing years, the patient remained cyanotic. Her clinicians debated about the merits of further surgery. Her outpatient workup continued to show severe tricuspid regurgitation, pulmonary stenosis, and a VSD. A diagnostic catheterization was done to measure the PA pressures and was complicated by a right femoral venous thrombosis. She was started on warfarin.

The patient remained free of overt symptoms, and so surgery was avoided as long as possible. However, two isolated episodes of infective endocarditis in her late adolescent years, both treated successfully with antibiotics, made the tricuspid regurgitation even worse.

At age 25, she finally underwent repeat surgery. There was contraction and thickening of the septal leaflet of the tricuspid valve. A 10-mm VSD was closed, and a patch placed in the RVOT to widen the outflow. A tricuspid valve annuloplasty was also performed. Her epicardial pacemaker was replaced with an endovascular system, but the ventricular lead had to be placed in the RVOT for reliable capture.

The patient recovered from surgery without complications. A postoperative echocardiogram showed moderate tricuspid regurgitation with moderate RV dysfunction.

Medical management of her "failing RV" and tricuspid regurgitation continued, and the patient remained asymptomatic and able to work full time. Several years later she had an episode of sustained ventricular tachycardia (VT) requiring urgent cardioversion. An electrophysiologic study showed VT arising from a focus near the pacing wire in the RVOT. After catheter ablation, VT could no longer be induced.

At age 27 she again developed sustained VT in the setting of hyperkalemia and acute renal failure. This was likely related to overdiuresis. With fluid balance and correction of her electrolytes her renal function returned to normal. The patient was considered for tricuspid valve replacement (TVR) and RA maze, and admitted to the hospital for surgery. However, on further review the night before the procedure, and considering her relative lack of symptoms, the procedure was cancelled.

After 2 more years of follow-up, the patient began to note more marked exercise intolerance. A repeat workup included a nuclear angiogram; her RVEF was 27%. After group discussion, it was felt her TR was secondary to her RV failure, and a conservative approach was again elected.

Over the next 2 years the patient continued to deteriorate clinically. She had several hospital admissions for right-sided heart failure and/or renal dysfunction.

Eventually, she had to stop working as a bank clerk. Because of her worsening clinical status, her case was again reviewed with consideration of repeat surgery.

*Comments:* PA banding has been used to protect infants with large or multiple VSDs or otherwise complex anatomy to reduce pulmonary blood flow and pressures and thus prevent pulmonary vascular disease.

Chordal insertion from an AV valve through a VSD to the contralateral septum or free wall, as was later found here, is known as valve "straddling." Valve straddling poses a major challenge to the surgeon, in that it makes closure of the VSD difficult, if not impossible, without affecting the function of the AV valve. It is unclear as to whether the straddling was fully appreciated before surgery. Nevertheless, VSD closure was associated with severe dysfunction of the tricuspid valve immediately after surgery. In addition, sutures placed near the conduction system can result in heart block, as occurred in this patient. Removal of the PA band may leave residual obstruction; the RVOT obstruction was fortuitous in her case, as a residual, moderate-sized VSD was present at the end of the operation.

In a patient in whom the first operation was complicated and unsuccessful, further surgery is daunting both for the patient and family as well as the surgeon. The pulmonary stenosis was preventing pulmonary vascular disease from developing as a result of her persistent VSD. Yet pulmonary stenosis also worsened the tricuspid valve regurgitation by causing elevated RV pressures. The delay and difficult decision making in this case are easy to understand.

The venous thrombosis, endocarditis, and problems with pacing are complications that arise both as a result of inherent congenital abnormalities and as iatrogenic complications, both seen in this patient.

Contraction and shrinking of the leaflets were felt to be related both to prior endocarditis and to previous repair. The chordal structures that initially straddled the VSD were no longer intact.

The patient is now no longer cyanotic, but still has tricuspid valve insufficiency and impaired RV function.

Sustained arrhythmias in patients with ACHD often reflect or coexist with severe hemodynamic problems, as in this patient. It is a good rule of thumb to consider each arrhythmia as a reminder to look for correctable hemodynamic problems.

The decision not to operate reflected the patient's lack of symptoms and concern that the high risks of further tricuspid surgery might not be rewarded by clinical improvement.

It can be difficult to determine whether tricuspid insufficiency is entirely due to RV dilation and dysfunction, or vice versa.

This patient had continued to work despite several years of medical problems for which disability would have been an easy option. She is a good example of many congenital heart patients who continue to live their lives as fully as possible despite worsening problems and physical disability. It is a testament to their stamina and stoicism. Furthermore, the fact that she now feels incapable of continuing to do so is a sign of how much worse she has become.

## CURRENT SYMPTOMS

The patient had a very limited exercise capacity, approximately 80 m on flat ground, limited by fatigue.

She denied palpitations, lightheadedness, or near-syncope. She had moderate bilateral lower extremity edema.

NYHA class: IV

## CURRENT MEDICATIONS

Enalapril 10 mg twice daily

Furosemide 80 mg mornings, 40 mg evenings

Spironolactone 50 mg twice daily

Amiodarone 200 mg daily

Warfarin adjusted dose to maintain an INR of 2.0–3.0

**Comments:** Her medical regimen was being adjusted according to her symptoms, weight, neck veins, and creatinine levels.

Amiodarone had been given after the patient's episode of VT, although, arguably, her risk for VT was probably low after successful ablation, due because her second episode of VT was metabolic in origin.

## PHYSICAL EXAMINATION

BP 100/60, HR 80 (paced), oxygen saturation 94%

Height 156 cm, weight 63 kg, BSA 1.63 m²

Surgical scars: Median sternotomy scar

Neck veins: The JVP was seen at 7 cm above sternal angle, with large V waves.

Lungs/chest: Clear to auscultation, but breath sounds were absent at the right base.

Heart: Regular rhythm with a persistently split second heart sound. There was a grade 2/6 holosystolic murmur at the left lower sternal border, increasing in inspiration. A right ventricular lift was not appreciated. The left ventricular apex beat was normal.

Abdomen: The liver was palpable just 1 cm beyond the costal margin. No ascites was present.

Extremities: There was 3+ bilateral pitting edema to above the knees.

**Comments:** Signs of right heart failure are present despite medical therapy.

The murmur is consistent with tricuspid regurgitation, which may become less audible as it becomes more severe. Such a murmur will increase on inspiration in about half of patients with substantial tricuspid regurgitation.

## LABORATORY DATA

| | |
|---|---|
| Hemoglobin | 13.2 g/dL (11.5–15.0) |
| Hematocrit/PCV | 39% (36–46) |
| MCV | 92 fL (83–99) |
| Platelet count | 234 × 10⁹/L (150–400) |
| Sodium | 134 mmol/L (134–145) |
| Potassium | 3.6 mmol/L (3.5–5.2) |
| Creatinine | 0.94 mg/dL (0.6–1.2) |
| Blood urea nitrogen | 4.2 mmol/L (2.5–6.5) |

### OTHER RELEVANT LAB RESULTS
Prior creatinine had been as high as 3.2 mg/dL. Liver function tests were normal.

**Comments:** Her renal function at this time is normal, although she has had labile creatinine levels dependent on intravascular volume status.

## ELECTROCARDIOGRAM

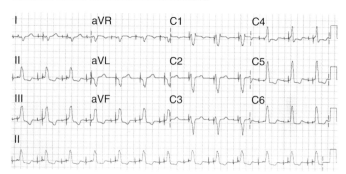

Figure 10-1 Electrocardiogram.

### FINDINGS
Heart rate: 75 bpm (paced)

AV sequential pacing

**Comments:** The patient had no reliable escape rhythm when the pacemaker was turned off. She was, therefore, pacemaker dependent.

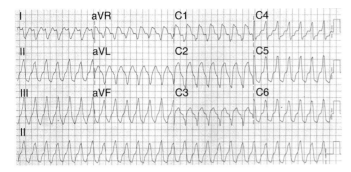

Figure 10-2 Electrocardiogram.

## FINDINGS

Regular, wide QRS complex tachycardia at a rate of 160

LBBB conduction pattern, suggesting an RV origin.

**Comments:** This ECG was obtained at the time of a prior hospitalization. The rhythm is VT. An electrophysiologic study showed a similar rhythm inducible in the RVOT near the existing pacing wire (see Fig. 10-3). Following successful catheter ablation, the VT could no longer be induced.

## CHEST X-RAY

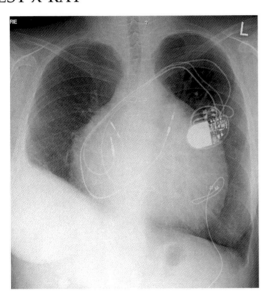

Figure 10-3 Posteroanterior projection.

## FINDINGS

Cardiothoracic ratio: 70%

There was a prior sternotomy. There was also gross cardiomegaly with marked RA enlargement. An epicardial pacing lead near the LV apex was seen. A transvenous pacing system was present with two leads in the RA and one in the RVOT. The pulmonary arteries were normal, and the lung fields had a normal vascular pattern. There was no LA enlargement. There was an opacity at the right lung base, seen on prior films.

**Comments:** The aftermath of complications from her first surgery are visible, namely the elevated right hemidiaphragm from a phrenic nerve palsy and epicardial pacing wires. The ventricular lead in the RVOT was the site of prior VT (see the

section "History"). Cardiomegaly here is largely secondary to RA enlargement.

## EXERCISE TESTING

| Exercise protocol: | Modified Bruce |
|---|---|
| Duration (min:sec): | 6:27 |
| Reason for stopping: | Dyspnea |
| ECG changes: | Paced |

|  | Rest | Peak |
|---|---|---|
| Heart rate (bpm): | 80 | 100 |
| $O_2$ saturation (%): | 94 | 98 |
| BP (mm Hg): | 100/60 | 142/78 |
| Double product: |  | 14,200 |
| Peak $V_{O_2}$ (mL/kg/min): |  | 11.1 |
| Percent predicted (%): |  | 38 |
| $Ve/V_{CO_2}$: |  | 78 |
| Metabolic equivalents: |  | 2 |

### Comparison Values

| Time before presentation | 3 yr | 1 yr | Current |
|---|---|---|---|
| Peak $V_{O_2}$ | 19.0 | 10.7 | 11.1 |
| Percent predicted (%) | 65 | 38 | 38 |
| $Ve/V_{CO_2}$ slope | 34 | 82 | 78 |

**Comments:** Formal exercise testing is a good way to evaluate exercise capacity. In this case, the patient was severely limited, and comparison with the results of previous tests illustrates her functional decline.

Both the low peak $V_{O_2}$[1] and the rise in her $Ve/V_{CO_2}$ slope are poor prognostic markers for survival.[2]

## ECHOCARDIOGRAM

### OVERALL FINDINGS

The RV was dilated and showed severe systolic dysfunction. The LV was mildly dilated with mild systolic dysfunction. There was moderate mitral regurgitation. The RA and LA were both severely dilated. There was no residual VSD and no obstruction of the RVOT tract or pulmonary valve.

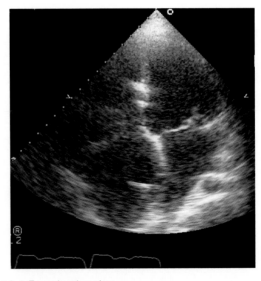

Figure 10-4 Four-chamber view.

## FINDINGS

The RV was severely dilated and dysfunctional. The LV was also dilated and mildly dysfunctional. The RA was severely enlarged, the LA was moderately enlarged.

**Comments:** Tricuspid regurgitation causes RV dilatation, which in turn perpetuates tricuspid regurgitation. The patient had faced tricuspid regurgitation since her first surgical repair and is now at the end stage of this vicious cycle.

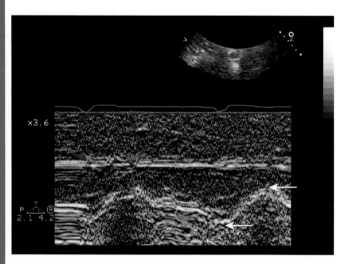

Figure 10-5 Apical M-mode of the right ventricle free wall near the tricuspid annulus.

## FINDINGS

This M-mode of the RV free wall demonstrated severely reduced longitudinal function of the ventricle. The tricuspid annulus moves only 6 mm toward the apex during systole (see Fig. 10-5; vertical distance between arrows).

**Comments:** Although longitudinal motion of the RV free wall in a patient with prior sternotomy and pericardiotomy may not necessarily reflect true RV function, in this case the finding seems consistent with the subjective appreciation of RV dysfunction. Generally, less than 10 mm displacement of the tricuspid annulus is considered to indicate severe RV dysfunction.

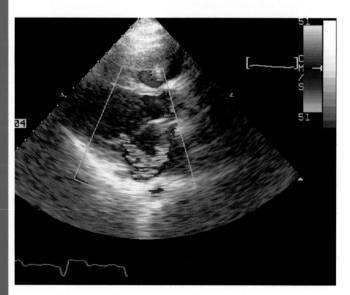

Figure 10-6 Parasternal long-axis view.

## FINDINGS

The ventricle was mildly dilated. Systolic function was mildly impaired. The mitral valve was moderately regurgitant, and the LA was moderately enlarged.

**Comments:** Since the mitral valve is structurally normal, regurgitation is likely due to an enlarged LV, which is likely due to the failing RV (ventricular interaction).

### Echo Summary

|  | 11 yr ago | 7 yr ago | 4 yr ago | 2 yr ago | Current |
|---|---|---|---|---|---|
| LVEDd | Normal | 5.5 | 5.8 | 5.6 | **6.4** |
| LVESd | Normal | 4.1 | 3.9 | **4.1** | 4.2 |
| MR | None | None | None | None | Mod |
| TR | Mod | Mod | Sev | Sev | Sev |
| RV dysfunction | Mod | Mod | Mod | Sev | Sev |

Mod, moderate; Sev, severe.

## FINDINGS

Echocardiographic findings over last decade are compared.

**Comments:** Although assessment of tricuspid regurgitation and RV function is often done by subjective visualization, the trend demonstrates that severe tricuspid regurgitation most likely preceded the deterioration of RV function. In addition, the dilatation of the LV is a more recent concern (see bold in the table, "Echo Summary").

# MAGNETIC RESONANCE IMAGING

Not performed

# CATHETERIZATION

## HEMODYNAMICS

Heart rate    80 bpm

|  | **Pressure** | **Saturation** (%) |
|---|---|---|
| SVC | mean 12 | 59 |
| IVC | mean 12 | 69 |
| RA | mean 12, v waves to 18 | |
| RV | 29/12 | |
| PA | 31/12 mean 17 | 62 |
| PCWP | mean 12 | |
| LV | 95/10 | 98 |
| Aorta | 107/50 mean 71 | 96 |

### Calculations

| | |
|---|---|
| Qp (L/min) | 2.74 |
| Qs (L/min) | 2.86 |
| Cardiac index (L/min/m²) | 1.73 |
| Qp/Qs | 0.96 |
| PVR (Wood units) | 2.55 |
| SVR (Wood units) | 20.62 |

## FINDINGS

PA pressures were normal, as was pulmonary vascular resistance. The RA pressure was elevated and rose further with RV systole due to the significant tricuspid regurgitation. The cardiac index was low.

**Comments:** The catheterization was done primarily to assess PA pressures in the setting of the long-standing left-to-right shunt through the VSD. The initial PA banding, and subsequent RVOT obstruction, however, have successfully protected the patient from developing pulmonary arterial hypertension.

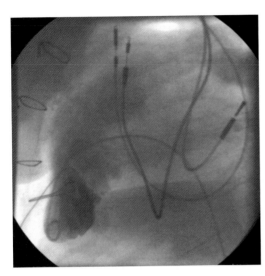

Figure 10-7 Lateral projection RVgram.

## FINDINGS

The RV was severely dysfunctional. There was severe TR.

**Comments:** The multiple pacing catheters are seen, including one in the RVOT, the site of prior VT ablation (compare with Fig. 10-3). Contrast is seen flowing backward from the RV (appreciable on cine) into the dilated RA. Function of the RV is difficult to assess, but qualitatively it appears enlarged and severely dysfunctional. The RA is severely enlarged, which is one reason it does not completely fill with contrast despite severe tricuspid regurgitation.

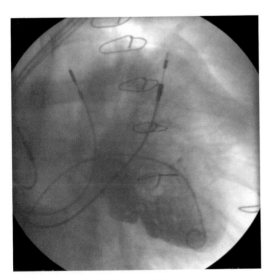

Figure 10-8 Anteroposterior projection RVgram.

## FINDINGS

The RV was severely dysfunctional.

**Comments:** The RAO and AP projections are more favorable for determining the degree of contrast regurgitation into the RA.

## FOCUSED CLINICAL QUESTIONS AND DISCUSSION POINTS

1. Should a patient with significant tricuspid valve straddling undergo surgical closure?

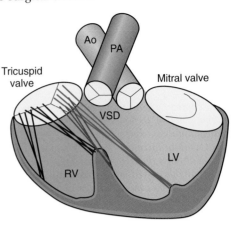

Type A ———
Septal attachment at the VSD

Type B ———
Septal attachment in the contralateral ventricle

Type C ———
Attachment on the contralateral free wall

Figure 10-9 Schematic representation of various types of atrioventricular valve straddling, based on the insertion site of the chordal structures (see text).

*Straddling, defined as AV valve chordal insertion to the contralateral ventricular septum or free wall, such that the chordae travel through the VSD, was first described by Rastelli and colleagues.[3] It is usually associated with other congenital abnormalities, including double-outlet RV, TGA, or AVSD.[4-6] Insertion on the septum may be within the AVSD itself (type A), on the septum but within the contralateral ventricle (type B), or on the contralateral free wall (type C, see Fig. 10-9).[4] Straddling in some instances may result in obstruction of either the LVOT or the infundibulum.*

*The surgeon's challenge is to close the septal defect without disrupting the integrity of the affected AV valve. In patients with type C, palliative procedures are usually offered as the defect cannot be closed without major sacrifice of atrioventricular valve function.*

*Like any surgery involving a VSD, in the setting of straddling there is a risk of disruption of the conduction system resulting in AV block, as occurred in this patient. Pacemaker insertion was required in 3 of 5 patients after correction of tricuspid valve straddling.[7] However, others have stated that the presence of straddling does not increase this risk, which was only 3.8% in one series.[4]*

*This case exemplifies both of these complications, namely valve dysfunction and AV block, and the long-term outcome from attempted correction of the straddling defect are evident.*

2. What is the best therapeutic approach to this patient?

*Three options are available to this patient. The first is to continue with medical management. This would effectively be a palliative approach, with little improvement over her current state and likely continued progression of symptoms and a high mortality rate over the next several years. Her recurrent hospitalizations are evidence of failing medical therapy.*

*The second option is to replace the tricuspid valve in the hope of relieving RV volume loading and stabilizing or perhaps* even improving RV function. In turn, AV valve replacement in the setting of impaired ventricular function is known to be problematic, whereas repair may be better tolerated.[8] Repair was not felt to be feasible here, however. Given the prior operations and complications in this patient, any reoperation would carry considerable risks, and a failing RV would hamper recovery from bypass. Even if surgery were successful at alleviating heart failure, there would still be a risk of recurrent VT or even sudden death. Further, decisions about which replacement valve to use were difficult. A mechanical valve would present difficulties for pacing, on which she is dependent. A bioprosthetic valve might require replacement in the future.

The third option is heart transplantation. Prior pleurodesis and diaphragmatic palsy, though troubling, would not disqualify her from transplantation. Suitability would depend on a complete transplant workup including the measurement of her creatinine clearance. Although the option would potentially require a long wait for a suitable organ, and a significant operative risk, this would offer her the best chance of meaningful functional improvement long term.

These issues were discussed at length at a multidisciplinary conference on two separate occasions, as well as with the patient and her family. Pursuit of transplantation was initially felt to be the best course.

3. If TVR were considered, what plans should be made for her pacemaking system and/or potential for VT?

One reason the second therapeutic option (i.e., TVR) was felt to be more difficult was because of the need to ensure adequate pacing. Her current pacing system is problematic. Initially, endocardial capture had not been possible and epicardial leads were placed. After her second surgery endocardial capture was successful in the RVOT, which eventually led to VT from the pacing site. Somewhat surprisingly, the patient had not had atrial arrhythmias to this point. A new endocardial system would need to be placed through the newly inserted bioprosthetic valve, or placed epicardially.

The other consideration was whether to place an implantable cardioverter/defibrillator. She had two episodes of VT but both were secondary to correctable causes. Overall, it was not felt that there was a strong enough indication to warrant implantable cardioverter/defibrillator placement.

4. What is the most accurate method for determining RV function?

Assessment of RV function, a recurring challenge in this book and in clinical practice, is critically important in cases such as this in which clinical decisions are based on interpretations of function. The methods currently available, namely echocardiography, nuclear imaging, angiography, MRI, and CT, all have limitations. MRI and CT are believed to be most accurate and reproducible in terms of assessment of systolic function[9,10] though variability in methodology still exists.

Since MRI was not an option in this patient due to the pacemaker, and gated CT scanning was not available at the time, the clinicians relied on older methods. These all showed RV dysfunction, although with some disagreement as to its degree. Whatever imaging method used, serial measurements are often of value in making clinical decisions, as with this case, and are best when the same modality is compared over time. Certain echo Doppler tools add sophistication to RV functional assessment, as is discussed elsewhere (see Case 56).

It should also be mentioned that RV dysfunction may be masked by unloading in the setting of severe TR (reduced afterload), just as with LV function in the setting of severe mitral regurgitation. Issues about the feasibility of AV valve replacement in the setting of severe ventricular dysfunction are also equally applicable to the RV and the LV. It is often tempting to assume that valve replacement will solve the patient's problems in these circumstances, but caution is advised.

## FINAL DIAGNOSIS

Severe tricuspid regurgitation

Severe RV systolic dysfunction

Mild LV dilatation and systolic dysfunction

Complete AV block, pacemaker dependent

Prior VT

Mild chronic renal dysfunction

## PLAN OF ACTION

Pursue workup for cardiac transplantation

## OUTCOME

The patient underwent her pretransplantation workup. Her creatinine clearance was 64 mL/min (normal range 80–120) and her 24-hour urine protein was 0.11 g/day (normal range 0–0.1). A repeat echocardiogram showed left ventricular dimensions to have returned to normal range (54 mm at end-diastole and 37 mm at end-systole) with normal LV function. There was severe tricuspid regurgitation, but the overall RV function was thought to be mildly to moderately reduced. These latest data were compared to previous echocardiograms. A repeat exercise test was performed; the exercise duration and peak $Vo_2$ (11.1 mL/kg/min, 38% of predicted) were unchanged.

In light of the more optimistic echocardiographic picture (regarding both RV and LV function) and low creatinine clearance, her plans were again reviewed at a multidisciplinary meeting. The various risks and benefits were discussed at length, and it was felt that an attempt at TVR would be worthwhile, especially considering the anticipated wait for a suitable organ for transplantation and borderline renal function.

A few weeks later, while waiting for elective surgery, the patient was admitted because of worsening heart failure symptoms and a rising creatinine. After heart failure symptoms improved with intravenous diuresis, the patient was taken to the operating room for TVR. It had been 11 years since her last operation, with tricuspid regurgitation and RV dysfunction present ever since then.

In the operating room, vascular access was problematic from both the right and left femoral regions. The left femoral artery thrombosed during a cannulation attempt, leaving the leg ischemic and requiring fasciotomy. Through very dense adhesions the heart was finally freed and limited bypass was obtained. After much effort, the tricuspid valve was replaced with a St. Jude prosthetic valve. The endocardial pacing system was completely removed and epicardial atrioventricular pacing was ensured before closure.

Postoperatively in the intensive care unit the patient experienced a prolonged period of systemic hypotension and low cardiac output. Though there was no evidence of hemopericardium or hemothorax by echo, a surgical reexploration was performed to exclude pericardial bleeding or thrombus. The patient required vasoconstrictors to maintain an arterial blood pressure of 75 mm Hg systolic. The patient's renal function deteriorated, and she required hemofiltration to remove fluid and accumulating lactate.

She developed sustained atrial arrhythmia on the second postoperative day, further compromising her hemodynamics, and recurrent atrial fibrillation after cardioversion. Unfortunately, the epicardial atrial pacing wire failed to capture and a transvenous atrial pacing wire was placed transjugularly. With atrial pacing, no further atrial tachycardia occurred.

During the following weeks she remained in critical condition on assisted ventilation with low cardiac output and tenuous blood pressure felt to be secondary to RV dysfunction. She developed further deterioration and evidence of sepsis during her fourth postoperative week. An echocardiogram showed vegetations on the atrial pacing wire. She was taken back to the operating room where the pacing wire was completely removed and her thorax reexplored. Eventually *Candida albicans* was grown from the removed wire. Postoperatively, blood pressure could not be maintained despite maximal pressors. Oxygenation diminished and severe metabolic acidosis could not be controlled. After discussing the situation with the family, care was withdrawn.

***Comments:*** The unfortunate outcome from redo/redo surgery highlights the major challenges faced in this situation. These include technical challenges in establishing cardiopulmonary bypass but also multiple postoperative problems such as systemic hypotension, renal failure, and sepsis/endocarditis, which all related to pacing, RV dysfunction, and low cardiac output status. All these ultimately led to the patient's eventual demise.

Optimally, when a decision to undergo surgery is made in a tenuous patient such as this, it is crucial that a clear backup plan is available if and when the RV fails to meet the hemodynamic demands. One lesson learned from this case in retrospect was that a preemptive decision as to whether an RV assist device as a bridge to transplantation would be an option might have helped the care team address the difficult postoperative period. In addition, more clearly defined plans about pacing might have avoided the transcutaneous pacing wire that was placed and subsequently became a nidus for infection. Yet even in the best of circumstances, it is important to recognize the fragility

of this particular patient going to surgery and that perioperative mortality was high. In retrospect, and purely speculatively, heart transplantation may have been a better option for this patient.

## Selected References

1. Diller GP, Dimopoulos K, Okonko D, et al: Exercise intolerance in adult congenital heart disease: Comparative severity, correlates, and prognostic implication. Circulation 112:828–835, 2005.
2. Dimopoulos K, Okonko DO, Diller GP, et al: Abnormal ventilatory response to exercise in adults with congenital heart disease relates to cyanosis and predicts survival. Circulation 113:2796–2802, 2006.
3. Rastelli GC, Ongley PA, Titus JL: Ventricular septal defect of atrioventricular canal type with straddling right atrioventricular valve and mitral valve deformity. Circulation 37:816–825, 1968.
4. Serraf A, Nakamura T, Lacour-Gayet F, et al: Surgical approaches for double-outlet right ventricle or transposition of the great arteries associated with straddling AV valves. J Thorac Cardiovasc Surg 111:527–535, 1996.
5. Bharati S, McAllister HA Jr, Lev M: Straddling and displaced atrioventricular orifices and valves. Circulation 60:673–684, 1979.
6. Freedom RM, Bini R, Dische R, Rowe RD: The straddling mitral valve: morphological observations and clinical implications. Eur J Cardiol 8:27–50, 1978.
7. Pacifico AD, Soto B, Bargeron LM: Surgical treatment of straddling tricuspid valves. Circulation 60:655–664, 1979.
8. Bolling SF, Pagani FD, Deeb GM, Bach DS: Intermediate-term outcome of mitral reconstruction in cardiomyopathy. J Thorac Cardiovasc Surg 115:381–386; discussion 387–388, 1998.
9. Jauhiainen T, Järvinen VM, Hekali PE: Evaluation of methods for MR imaging of human right ventricular heart volumes and mass. Acta Radiol 43:587–592, 2002.
10. Babu-Narayan SV, Goktekin O, Moon JC, et al: Late gadolinium enhancement cardiovascular magnetic resonance of the systemic right ventricle in adults with previous atrial redirection surgery for transposition of the great arteries. Circulation 111:2091–2098, 2005.

# Atrioventricular Septal Defects

# Long-Term Follow-Up of Atrioventricular Septal Defect

**Per Lunde and Craig S. Broberg**

**Age: 58**
**Gender: Female**
**Occupation: Professional gardener**
**Working diagnosis: Repaired partial atrioventricular septal defect**

## HISTORY

The patient was well until her mid-20s, when she noted progressive shortness of breath. Workup led to the diagnosis of a large primum ASD with left AV valve regurgitation (LAVVR).

She underwent surgery to close the defect and address the regurgitation. To repair the valve, the surgeon placed sutures between the mural and superior bridging leaflets that formed the left AV valve. When tested intraoperatively, this repair left a small residual leak, but it was felt that further suturing would create valvular stenosis.

The patient did well during the next 20 years, enjoying a full, active life including having and raising her three children.

Ten years ago she developed atrial fibrillation, which was converted to sinus rhythm with direct current (DC) cardioversion. Digoxin was started. She had several further episodes of atrial fibrillation in the next 4 years, each treated successfully with DC cardioversion. Multiple antiarrhythmic medications were tried, but each failed to prevent recurrent atrial fibrillation. Five years ago the patient had a few spells of lightheadedness. Sinus pauses up to 5 seconds long were noted on 24-hour ECG monitoring. Therefore a VVI pacemaker was inserted.

Apart from hypertension treated medically, she had no other medical problems. However, the patient noted gradual deterioration in her exertional tolerance and was seen again in clinic for review.

**Comments:** Not uncommonly the presence of a large primum ASD will not be found until adulthood. Partial AVSD implies that there are two discrete valvular orifices although there is a common AV "annular" ring (junction).

The left valve has three leaflets; therefore, technically, it is not a "mitral" valve, as the latter implies two leaflets. Instead, the proper terminology used is "left AV valve."

The surgeon's drawing of the intraoperative findings is shown (Fig. 11-1), drawn from the perspective of an open right atrium, looking through the ASD toward the right and left AV valves. The surgeon may face the dilemma of relieving completely the regurgitation at the expense of inducing valve stenosis. Most surgeons would restore competence of the trileaflet

AV valve by placing sutures between the superior and inferior bridging leaflets (and not between the mural and one of the bridging leaflets, as in this patient).

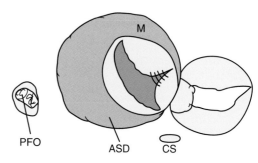

Figure 11-1 Surgeon's drawing of the anatomic features of the left atrioventricular valve with a cleft between the inferior and superior bridging leaflets that have been sutured together to restore valve competence.

In today's practice, left AV valve competence is assessed intraoperatively by TEE while weaning from cardiopulmonary bypass. This method assists optimal surgical repair and could potentially improve the long-term outcome following repair of the left AV valve.[1]

**Comments:** In this patient, recurrent episodes of atrial fibrillation over 2 decades may suggest the development of significant LAVVR and LA enlargement. Recurrent atrial fibrillation per se may, in turn, worsen valvular regurgitation.

Even with optimal valvar repair, long-term LAVVR is not uncommon; reported reoperation rates for LAVVR vary from 6% to 18% between adult and pediatric series.[2]

AVSD is associated with inherent abnormalities of the conduction system, relating to the abnormal common AV junction. Thus, AV block is not uncommon. Sinus node dysfunction is less common, but known to occur even before surgery[3]; it may relate to long-standing RA dilatation and stretch, as per any type of large ASD in the older patient.[4] Furthermore, because of the surgical approach to repair through the RA, sinus node injury may also occur (less common in contemporary cohorts).

## CURRENT SYMPTOMS

The patient has a markedly reduced exertional tolerance. Although she can walk slowly on flat ground, she has trouble with one flight of stairs. She sleeps with three pillows to avoid dyspnea when recumbent.

NYHA class: III

## CURRENT MEDICATIONS

Digoxin 0.25 mg daily

Sotalol 80 mg twice daily

Losartan 50 mg twice daily

Amlodipine 5 mg daily

Warfarin adjusted for an INR of 2.0–3.0

**Comments:** The combination of digoxin and sotalol should provide optimal rate control for atrial fibrillation, and the doses could be increased if needed without the risk of bradycardia because of the indwelling pacemaker. Losartan and amlodipine were added for hypertension.

## PHYSICAL EXAMINATION

BP 145/70, HR 70 bpm (paced), oxygen saturation 98%

Height 148 cm, weight 47 kg, BSA 1.39 m²

Surgical scars: Median sternotomy

Neck veins: The JVP was mildly elevated, but a normal waveform was seen.

Lungs/chest: Clear to auscultation

Heart: The heart rhythm was regular. There was a widened and somewhat displaced apical impulse. The first and second heart sounds were normal, including a normal A2 and P2. There was a grade 3/6 holosystolic murmur at the apex, but no basal murmur or diastolic murmur.

Abdomen: Normal without organomegaly

Extremities: Mild lower extremity edema

**Comments:** BP control may not be optimal despite therapy.
The nature and location of the murmur clearly indicate LAVVR. The fact that neither a third heart sound nor a diastolic heart murmur was heard may indicate that the regurgitation is not severe. There is no evidence for concomitant AV valve stenosis.

## LABORATORY DATA

| Hemoglobin | 13.6 g/dL (11.5–15.0) |
|---|---|
| Hematocrit/PCV | **47%** (36–46) |
| MCV | 87 fL (83–99) |
| Platelet count | 210 × 10⁹/L (150–400) |
| Sodium | 143 mmol/L (134–145) |
| Potassium | 4.0 mmol/L (3.5–5.2) |
| Creatinine | 0.8 mg/dL (0.6–1.2) |
| Blood urea nitrogen | 3.1 mmol/L (2.5–6.5) |

## ELECTROCARDIOGRAM

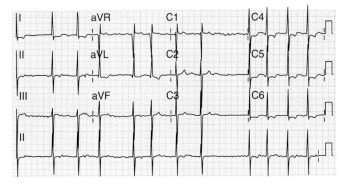

Figure 11-2 Electrocardiogram (prior to pacemaker implantation).

### FINDINGS
Heart rate: 72 bpm

QRS axis: −60°

QRS duration: 100 msec

Atrial fibrillation with leftward axis, LV hypertrophy, and nonspecific ST segment depression with T-wave inversion. No pacemaker function seen.

**Comments:** LV hypertrophy is not a typical finding in AVSD patients but was present here prior to insertion of her pacemaker, indicating that systemic hypertension or outflow tract obstruction may have been long-standing.
Patients with AVSD typically have a leftward or extreme right QRS axis (superior axis) from inherent differences in their AV conduction. The ST changes could be related to digoxin or to LV hypertrophy.

## CHEST X-RAY

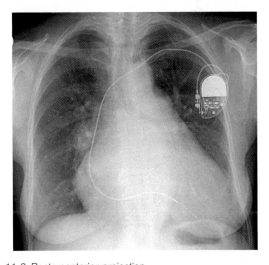

Figure 11-3 Posteroanterior projection.

### FINDINGS
Cardiothoracic ratio: 71%

The cardiac silhouette was grossly enlarged. The prominent bulging at the right cardiac border indicates RA enlargement. The LA was also enlarged as indicated by the wide tracheal bifurcation angle and the relatively horizontal left main bronchus. The central pulmonary arteries were prominent. The patient had a transvenous pacing system with a single electrode placed in the RV apex.

**Comments:** The CXR suggests both RA and LA enlargement, in this case almost certainly reflecting long-standing atrial fibrillation and AV valve regurgitation (although a significant left-to-right shunt at the atrial level needs to be excluded).

## EXERCISE TESTING

| Exercise protocol: | Modified Bruce |
| Duration (min:sec): | 6:23 |
| Reason for stopping: | Dyspnea |
| ECG changes: | None |

| | Rest | Peak |
|---|---|---|
| Heart rate (bpm): | 70 | 117 |
| Percent of age-predicted max HR: | | 72 |
| O₂ saturation (%): | 98 | 99 |
| Blood pressure (mm Hg): | 145/70 | 160/85 |
| Double product: | | 18,720 |
| | | |
| Peak Vo₂ (mL/kg/min): | | 11.9 |
| Percent predicted (%): | | 50 |

**Comments:** The test confirmed the patient's self-reported exercise limitation. She was only able to complete just over 6 minutes of the protocol and obtained a peak Vo₂ of only 50% of predicted. Additional information gained from the study was the absence of oxygen desaturation with exercise, and that she has a limited chronotropic response because of her underlying atrial fibrillation and medication.

## ECHOCARDIOGRAM

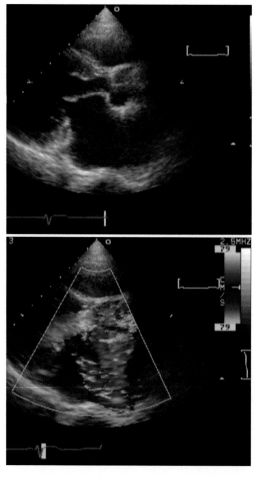

Figure 11-4 Parasternal long-axis view, with and without 2D color Doppler.

### FINDINGS

Normal LV systolic function present with moderate concentric LV hypertrophy. The LVOT was narrow but the peak velocity was only 1.8 m/sec at rest. The left AV valve was thickened, and there was severe mitral regurgitation. The LA was severely dilated.

**Comments:** The major finding is the severe LAVVR, seen in Figure 11-4, extending to the far end of the enlarged LA. In addition to inherent structural abnormalities of the left AV valve, the valve leaflets are chronically thickened, which contributes further to the valve dysfunction.

The relatively long LVOT can also be seen. Severe concentric LV hypertrophy cannot be explained by moderate/severe AV valve regurgitation.

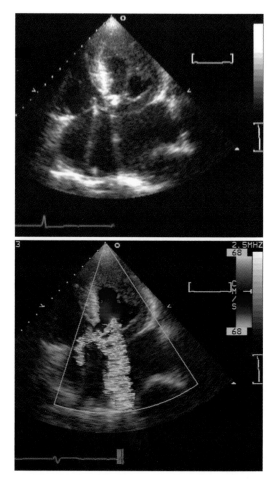

Figure 11-5 Apical four-chamber view, with and without 2D color Doppler.

### FINDINGS

Normal LV and RV size and systolic function were seen. There was severe LA and RA enlargement. The tricuspid regurgitation velocity was 3.2 m/sec, giving an estimated RV systolic pressure of 51 mm Hg.

Severe LAVVR seen with two discrete regurgitant jets was visualized with color Doppler.

**Comments:** Two regurgitant jets are not an uncommon finding following AV valve repair. One jet is secondary to annular dilatation and thickening of the leaflets. The other jet is through the septal commissure ("cleft").

Enlargement of the right atrium is likely due to the patient's long-standing atrial fibrillation, right AV valve regurgitation, and mild pulmonary hypertension.

## STRESS ECHOCARDIOGRAPHY

Stress echocardiography was performed.

|  | Rest | Dobutamine (40 µg/kg/min) |
|---|---|---|
| HR | 54 | 82 (paced) |
| BP | 115/50 | 132/61 then fell to 107/43 |
| LVOT | 1.8 m/sec | 4.2 m/sec (70 mm Hg) |
| TR velocity | 3.2 m/sec | 4 m/sec |

***Comments:*** The purpose of the study was to determine if significant LVOT obstruction occurred during stress.

The patient is in atrial fibrillation, and the rise in heart rate is due to increased conduction across her AV node.

The patient's BP rose then fell. Dobutamine can cause vasodilatation and hypotension, but one questions whether this drop is due to dynamic LVOT obstruction causing significant impairment of LV emptying. The gradient through the LVOT rose significantly during the procedure, which probably supports this concept. However, the result of this test should be interpreted with caution as a dobutamine stress test may provoke high gradients even in normal individuals, especially in the setting of LV hypertrophy.[5]

Thus, the test may not be a reliable means to provoke latent LVOT gradients. The more physiologic alternative of provoking a latent LVOT gradient is to measure the pressure gradient during dynamic exercise testing.[6]

# MAGNETIC RESONANCE IMAGING

Not performed, as the patient has a pacemaker

# CATHETERIZATION

## HEMODYNAMICS

Heart rate 70 bpm

|  | Pressure | Saturation (%) |
|---|---|---|
| SVC |  | 59 |
| IVC |  | 66 |
| RA | mean 7 | 61 |
| RV | **58/9** |  |
| PA | **62/15 mean 31** | 61 |
| PCWP | **mean 25 (v waves to 43)** |  |
| LA |  |  |
| LV | 141/**19** |  |
| Aorta | 141/78 mean 105 | 94 |

**Calculations**

| Qp (L/min) | 1.94 |
|---|---|
| Qs (L/min) | 2.16 |
| Cardiac index (L/min/m²) | **1.55** |
| Qp/Qs | 0.90 |
| PVR (Wood units) | 6.19 |
| SVR (Wood units) | 45.46 |

## FINDINGS

Oximetry showed no evidence of a left-to-right shunt. RV function was preserved. There was moderate pulmonary hypertension secondary to severe left AV "mitral" valve regurgitation as demonstrated by large v-waves and a mean capillary wedge pressure of 25 mm Hg. There was some elevation of LV diastolic pressures, having an adverse effect on both LAVVR and PAH. There was no pullback gradient between the LV and aorta at rest.

***Comments:*** Catheterization was performed to exclude coronary artery disease as a factor in her symptoms, to clarify whether an LVOT gradient was contributing to her LV hypertrophy, and to assess the severity of LAVVR.

Overall cardiac output was low and systemic vascular resistance relatively high. As a consequence oxygen extraction was high and mixed venous oxygen saturation was low, further emphasizing how compromised her circulation really was.

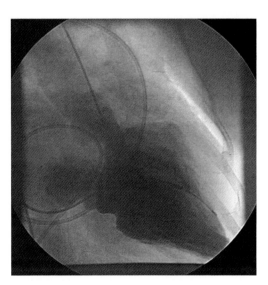

Figure 11-6 Right anterior oblique view ventriculogram.

## FINDINGS

The RAO ventriculogram showed normal LV systolic function with seemingly moderate LAVVR.

***Comments:*** Although affected by PVCs and the irregular heart rate, the LAVVR by this ventriculogram seemed less significant than anticipated by the echocardiogram and hemodynamic data. The regurgitation by ventriculography can be underestimated if there is insufficient contrast injection or if the left atrium is not framed properly during the injection. Still, the data question whether AV valve regurgitation is significant enough to warrant reoperation.

The RAO ventriculogram also demonstrates the relatively long LVOT, sometimes referred to as a "goose neck" deformity, which contributes to the development of LVOT obstruction.

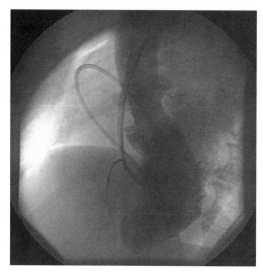

Figure 11-7 Left anterior oblique view ventriculogram.

## FINDINGS
Moderate LAVVR.

**Comments:** Again, this left ventriculogram in this LAO view showed moderate LAVVR and normal LV function. Significant dynamic LVOT obstruction does not seem present during systole.

### FOCUSED CLINICAL QUESTIONS AND DISCUSSION POINTS

1. What is the cause of this patient's symptoms and low exercise capacity?

*Several cardiopulmonary factors are likely to contribute to her poor exercise capacity, including mild PAH,[7] severe LAVVR, loss of left atrial contraction, chronotropic incompetence,[8] restrictive filling of the thickened left ventricle, and perhaps dynamic LVOT obstruction. Furthermore, the patient has marked cardiomegaly, which has an adverse effect on lung volume and is likely to have impaired ventilatory response to exercise, although not formally tested here.[9] Although speculative, most if not all of these factors would have a detrimental effect on cardiac output and thus lead to exercise intolerance.*

2. Which of the above factors is expected in a patient with an AVSD?

*This patient exhibits several of the long-term complications of an AVSD. First, LAVVR is very common, as the valve is inherently abnormal and valve repair does not always convey a perfect result. Regurgitation is not usually severe, but some patients will require a second operation to replace (or less often repair) the left AV valve.[10]*

*Second, due to the nature of the AV junction, the aortic valve and annulus are "unwedged," that is, somewhat distal from the superior leaflet of the left AV valve (see Case 15), unlike the normal arrangement, where the aortic and mitral valve annuli are in fibrous continuity. On ventriculography a "goose neck" deformity is seen (and had been a pathognomonic feature for establishing the diagnosis before the advent of echocardiography) and reflects the disproportion between the longer outlet versus the shorter inlet portion of the left ventricle. Because of the former (longer LVOT) and the frequent presence of tissue tags in the region, LVOT obstruction (dynamic or fixed) is not uncommon and may develop many years after repair.[11]*

*Third, AVSD affects the AV conduction system, and some patients will require permanent pacing for complete heart block over their lifetime. This patient is slightly unusual in that her pacemaker was placed because of sinus pauses rather than AV block.*

*All these potential complications reiterate the need for lifelong follow-up and for tertiary input for patients with AVSDs, even after successful repair.*

3. What is the cause of the patient's LV hypertrophy?

*The LV hypertrophy in this patient is striking, and more than one would expect from the dynamic LVOT obstruction provoked during the dobutamine stress test. There is nothing obviously inherent about an AVSD that should lead to a thickened myocardium other than significant obstruction. The patient's hypertension, though aggressively treated, likely contributed to LV hypertrophy.*

4. Should the patient be offered an intervention?

*There is certainly a rationale to replace the left AV valve. The surgeons could also consider an atrial maze procedure and possibly a septal myectomy to relieve any dynamic obstruction. This would be a long procedure, with considerable risk of morbidity and mortality for the patient. Recovery would be long.*

*Much of the argument for or against valve surgery hinges on the severity of the mitral regurgitation. There was disagreement between echocardiography and catheterization in this patient, as sometimes is encountered in clinical practice.*

*After a long multidisciplinary discussion about this patient's findings, the comorbid problems of LV hypertrophy, diastolic dysfunction, and permanent atrial fibrillation were also considered as possible factors limiting her exercise capacity. In addition, the patient's view that she did not wish to undergo further surgery swayed the decision toward medical therapy. Accepting the relatively high risks of surgery, however, one should expect a reduction in cardiothoracic ratio, improvement in systemic cardiac output, and as a result improved exercise capacity and probably quality of life.*

## FINAL DIAGNOSIS
Partial AVSD

Left AV valve regurgitation

Chronic atrial fibrillation

Severe LV hypertrophy

## PLAN OF ACTION
Improve medical management of heart failure and low output state

## INTERVENTION
None at present

## OUTCOME
Several adjustments were made to the patient's medical regimen. Diuretic therapy was increased given the peripheral edema and likely diastolic dysfunction. The addition of an aldosterone antagonist was also made. To improve the chronotropic response during exercise, digitalis was stopped, and the pacemaker rate responsive function was altered to better respond to activity.

Two years later the patient remains clinically stable, if not slightly improved, normotensive with no peripheral edema. Her LAVVR remains unchanged, and she has maintained LV and RV systolic function.

## Selected References

1. Freeman WK, Schaff HV, Khandheria BK, et al: Intraoperative evaluation of mitral valve regurgitation and repair by transesophageal echocardiography: Incidence and significance of systolic anterior motion. J Am Coll Cardiol 20:599–609, 1992.
2. Gatzoulis MA, Hechter S, Webb GD, et al: Surgery for partial atrioventricular septal defect in the adult. Ann Thorac Surg 67:504–510, 1999.
3. Clark EB, Kugler JD: Preoperative secundum atrial defect with coexisting sinus node and atrioventricular node dysfunction. Circulation 65:976–980, 1982.
4. Webb GD, Gatzoulis MA: Atrial septal defects in the adult: Recent progress and overview. Circulation 114:1645–1653, 2006.
5. Wagner S, Mohr-Kahaly S, Nixdorff U, et al: Intraventricular obstructions in dobutamine stress echocardiography: Determinants of their development and clinical sequelae. Z Kardiol 87:327–335, 1997.
6. Meimoun P, Benali T, Saya S, et al: Significance of systolic anterior motion of the mitral valve during dobutamine stress echocardiography. J Am Soc Echocardiogr 18:49–56, 2005.
7. Engelfriet PM, Duffels MGJ, Møller T, et al: Pulmonary arterial hypertension in adults born with a heart septal defect. The Euro Heart Survey on Adult Congenital Heart Disease. Heart 93: 682–687, 2007.
8. Diller G-P, Dimopoulos K, Okonko D, et al: Heart-rate response during exercise predicts survival in adults with congenital heart disease. J Am Coll Cardiol 48:1250–1256, 2006.
9. Dimopoulos K, Okonko DO, Diller G, et al: Abnormal ventilatory response to exercise in adults with congenital heart disease relates to cyanosis and predicts survival. Circulation 113:2796–2802, 2006.
10. Amira AA, Lincoln CR, Shore DF, et al: The left atrioventricular valve in partial atrioventricular septal defect: Management strategy and surgical outcome. Eur J Cardio Thorac Surg 26:754–761, 2004.
11. Van Arsdell GS, Williams W, Boutin C, et al: Subaortic stenosis in the spectrum of atrioventricular septal defects. J Thorac Cardiovasc Surg 110:1534–1542, 1995.

# Outflow Tract Obstruction after Atrioventricular Septal Defect Repair

**Thomas K. Kaltsas, Elena Nikiphorou, and Panayiotis Zarvos**

**Age: 35**
**Gender: Female**
**Occupation: Hairdresser**
**Working diagnosis: Repaired atrioventricular septal defect**

## HISTORY

The patient was diagnosed at birth with an intermediate AVSD. At age 3 she underwent repair of the defect with a large Dacron patch and suture repair of the "cleft" in the left AV valve. The surgery was successful, and her follow-up was unremarkable.

At age 17 she was readmitted for cardiac catheterization due to repeated episodes of syncope and left arm pain. The results revealed a gooseneck deformity of the LVOT, mild left AV valve regurgitation (LAVVR), and a 38 mm Hg gradient across her LVOT. No abnormality of the aortic arch vessels was demonstrated. The gradient was not felt to be hemodynamically significant, and the episodes were attributed to vasovagal attacks.

The patient had thereafter remained completely asymptomatic for an additional 18 years. Recent outpatient review revealed a long ejection systolic murmur over the left sternal edge, and further arrangements were made for investigation.

**Comments:** The term "intermediate AVSD" describes a variant of AVSD in which there is a large atrial communication with a common AV junction (which is a unifying feature of all AVSDs), yet there are two separate AV valves. In addition, there is a small, restrictive interventricular communication between the chordal attachments of the bridging leaflets.[1]

In patients with partial or intermediate AVSDs, elective repair of the left AV valve at the time of ASD closure has been recommended to improve outcome, although reoperation may be needed in a certain percentage of patients. Obviously, repair of AVSD before pulmonary vascular disease develops is essential, although the latter is unlikely to develop early in life unless there is additional pathology (such as upper airway obstruction in a patient with Down syndrome). Early repair improves long-term survival prospects and functional class and reduces the risk of subsequent AV valve degeneration.[2]

The development of subaortic stenosis is usually progressive, and patients may be asymptomatic (symptoms may be absent or mild). The reported interval from repair to the development of subaortic obstruction in partial or intermediate AVSDs ranges from months to many years after repair,[3] hence the need for indefinite follow-up.

## CURRENT SYMPTOMS

The patient denied any cardiovascular symptoms, including chest pain, breathlessness, or further episodes of loss of consciousness.

NYHA class: I

**Comments:** No further symptoms in this patient confirm that her previous symptoms had not been due to the subaortic stenosis.

## CURRENT MEDICATIONS

None

## PHYSICAL EXAMINATION

BP 135/90, HR 90 bpm, oxygen saturation on room air 98%

Height 168 cm, weight 105 kg, BSA 2.21 m$^2$

Surgical scars: Median sternotomy scar

Neck veins: A normal JVP was seen.

Lungs/chest: The chest was clear.

Heart: There was a regular heart rhythm with occasional ectopic beats. No thrills or heaves were palpable. The heart sounds were normal with a 3/6 ejection systolic murmur heard best at the left sternal edge.

Abdomen: No abnormality detected

Extremities: No abnormality detected. Peripheral pulses were all present. There was no edema.

**Comments:** In this setting of an intermediate AVSD, an ejection systolic heart murmur over the left sternal edge suggests LVOT obstruction. A pansystolic murmur near the apex would, in turn, suggest LAVVR.

## LABORATORY DATA

| | |
|---|---|
| Hemoglobin | 15.0 g/dL (11.5–15.0) |
| Hematocrit/PCV | 46% (36–46) |
| MCV | 91 fL (83–99) |
| Platelet count | 250 × 10$^9$/L (150–400) |
| Sodium | 139 mmol/L (134–145) |
| Potassium | 4.3 mmol/L (3.5–5.2) |
| Creatinine | 0.76 mg/dL (0.6–1.2) |
| Blood urea nitrogen | 3.5 mmol/L (2.5–6.5) |

Liver function tests: Normal

Thyroid function tests: Normal

# ELECTROCARDIOGRAM

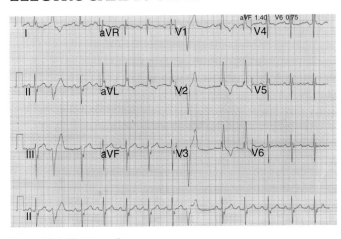

Figure 12-1 Electrocardiogram.

## FINDINGS
Heart rate: 96 bpm

QRS axis: −30°

QRS duration: 120 msec

PR duration: 220 msec

Sinus rhythm, frequent PVCs. Left axis deviation, and a very atypical RBBB. LA overload is likely.

**Comments:** The hallmark finding of AVSDs on ECG is a superior (leftward or extreme right) QRS axis, seen in 95% of patients. This is a result of the abnormal AV junction and inferior displacement of the conduction system. RV volume overload, when present, is reflected by an rsR pattern in the right precordial leads or, less commonly, by a qR pattern. The PR interval may be prolonged. This finding is thought to be due to increased intra-atrial conduction time, and, in general, these patients are at risk of complete heart block.[4]

# CHEST X-RAY

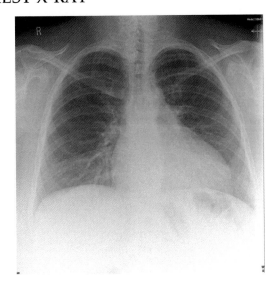

Figure 12-2 Posteroanterior projection.

## FINDINGS
Cardiothoracic ratio: 57%

Situs solitus, levocardia with a left aortic arch. Increased cardiothoracic ratio with a relatively small pedicle of the heart and a small aortic knuckle. Mild dilatation of the pulmonary trunk.

**Comments:** Apart from cardiomegaly, the CXR is normal. A small aortic knuckle is common in patients with congenital heart disease, in keeping with long-standing low systemic cardiac output.

# EXERCISE TESTING

| Exercise protocol: | Modified Bruce |
| Duration (min:sec): | 9:31 |
| Reason for stopping: | Fatigue |
| ECG changes: | LAD, RBBB |

| | Rest | Peak |
| --- | --- | --- |
| Heart rate (bpm): | 90 | 171 |
| Percent of age-predicted max HR: | | 92 |
| O₂ saturation (%): | 98 | 99 |
| Blood pressure (mm Hg): | 135/90 | 184/80 |

| | |
| --- | --- |
| Peak Vo₂ (mL/kg/min): | 24.1 |
| Percent predicted (%): | 53 |
| Ve/Vco₂: | 37 |
| Metabolic equivalents: | 7.2 |

**Comments:** The patient's peak $Vo_2$ is below normal for her age and gender, but is fairly representative of many asymptomatic adult congenital heart disease patients.

Exercise intolerance is prevalent in adult congenital heart diseases, even among asymptomatic patients, and is as severe as in patients with noncongenital heart failure. Lack of heart rate response to exercise, pulmonary arterial hypertension, and impaired pulmonary function can all be important covariates for impaired exercise performance, as are underlying cardiac anatomy and physiology. Poor exercise capacity carries prognostic information in these patients and is associated with an increased risk of hospitalization or death independent of symptom status.[5]

# ECHOCARDIOGRAM

## OVERALL FINDINGS
The LV was hypertrophied with hyperdynamic function (EF 75%).

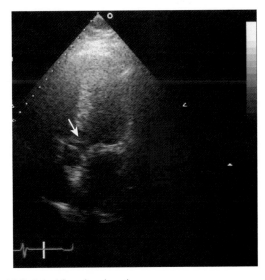

Figure 12-3 Apical five-chamber view.

## FINDINGS

A thin ridge *(arrow)*—probably fibromuscular—seems to narrow the LVOT. The aortic valve was competent; the obstruction point was clearly subaortic. Doppler interrogation across the LVOT revealed a peak pressure gradient of 74 mm Hg. There may also be a slight systolic anterior motion of the tip of the anterior leaflet of the mitral valve, although this does not seem to be causing any significant stenosis at rest.

**Comments:** Clinically significant subaortic obstruction after partial AVSD repair has been reported in up to 11% of patients.[6] Previous repair of the left AV valve has been implicated as a possible mechanism for the development of subaortic stenosis by some authors. Mobility of the AV valve may be decreased considerably by closing the "cleft" such that the leaflets may be tethered to the ventricular septum. This, in turn, limits the normal systolic displacement of the valve leaflets away from the septum and can precipitate obstruction in what is already an elongated and "narrowed" subaortic area. The only long-term follow-up[7] reported a 90% freedom from subaortic obstruction 14 years after AV septal repair in 180 patients.

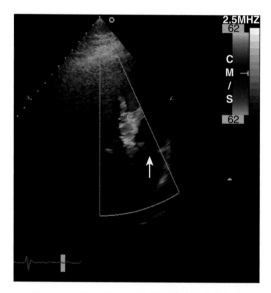

Figure 12-4 Four-chamber view during diastole.

## FINDINGS

The posterior leaflet of the left AV valve is relatively immobile *(arrow)*. The diastolic filling jet is slightly turbulent. The mean gradient across the valve was 4.5 mm Hg. There was only mild left AV valve regurgitation as estimated from multiple views.

**Comments:** LAVVR is the main indication for reoperation in patients after repair of either partial or complete AVSD. Up to 20% of patients with partial or complete AVSD repair were observed to have severe LAVVR during follow-up. While 25% of patients who had severe LAVVR immediately after

AVSD repair showed some spontaneous improvement with follow-up, 50% of patients with moderate to severe LAVVR ultimately required reoperation.[8] In our patient, the left AV valve is only mildly regurgitant and slightly stenotic 33 years after her original operation.

# MAGNETIC RESONANCE IMAGING

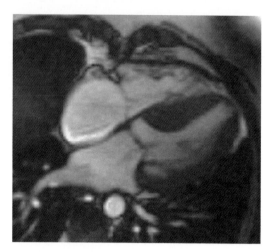

Figure 12-5 Oblique axial plane steady-state free precession cine (four-chamber view, diastolic frame).

## FINDINGS

There is concentric LV hypertrophy. The basal part of the septum is 19 mm thick at end diastole.

**Comments:** Guidelines are sometimes not explicit regarding the right timing of intervention in patients with subaortic stenosis.

Operating on this patient would be a sensible approach as her significant gradient has increased over the years (see also Fig. 12-6), and important LV hypertrophy is now present. Surgery produces relief of obstruction and frees the valve leaflets with long-term adequate relief of LVOT obstruction.[9] Adult patients with stable gradients of less than 50 mm Hg (on Doppler) without significant LV hypertrophy must also be followed closely, as some of them will eventually require surgery.[10]

### Ventricular Volume Quantification

|  | LV | (Normal range) | RV | (Normal range) |
|---|---|---|---|---|
| EDV (mL) | 140 | (52–141) | 132 | (58–154) |
| ESV (mL) | 51 | (13–51) | 49 | (12–68) |
| SV (mL) | 89 | (33–97) | 83 | (35–98) |
| EF (%) | 64 | (57–75) | 63 | (51–75) |
| EDVi (mL/m²) | 63 | (62–96) | **60** | (61–98) |
| ESVi (mL/m²) | 23 | (17–36) | 22 | (17–43) |
| SVi (mL/m²) | 40 | (40–65) | 37 | (20–40) |
| Mass index (g/m²) | **84** | (47–77) | 31 | (20–40) |

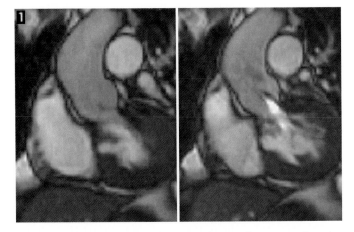

Figure 12-6 Oblique coronal plane steady-state free precession cine (aortic valve view), in diastole and systole.

## FINDINGS

Two images in both diastole and systole (from left to right) showed moderate to severe subaortic stenosis (white-colored jet in systole). The peak recorded velocity was 4.1 m/sec. The stenosis was shown, on another view, to be due to narrowing between the hypertrophied basal septum and fibromuscular bands or ridges just anterior to the septal leaflet of the repaired mitral valve, close to its "hinge" region. There was also slight systolic anterior motion of the septal leaflet of the mitral valve explained by a Venturi effect associated with the subaortic jet.

**Comments:** Despite an improvement in surgical mortality over time, there are some patients who appear to be at higher risk of early death[11] and late complications after AVSD repair. Abnormalities of the LVOT and left AV valve are two major risk factors for the aforementioned patients.[11,12] Freedom from reoperation is only 70% at 10 years. The majority of reoperations are for left AV valve dysfunction or LVOT obstruction, which are more prevalent in patients with a partitioned orifice (partial or intermediate AVSD).[12]

## CATHETERIZATION

### HEMODYNAMICS
Heart rate 85 bpm

| | Pressure | Saturation (%) |
|---|---|---|
| SVC | | 73 |
| IVC | | 77 |
| RA | 3 mean | 74 |
| RV | 25/2 end diastolic pressure 10 | 75 |
| PA | 20/4 mean 11 | 75 |
| PCWP | 11 mean | |
| LA | 9 mean | 98 |
| LV | **200/8** | 98 |
| Aorta | 140/80 mean 100 | 99 |

### Calculations

| | |
|---|---|
| Qp (L/min) | 5.09 |
| Qs (L/min) | 4.68 |
| Cardiac index (L/min/m²) | **2.12** |
| Qp/Qs | 1.09 |
| PVR (Wood units) | 0.39 |
| SVR (Wood units) | 20.70 |

## FINDINGS

The catheter revealed a gooseneck deformity of the LVOT,[13] mild, and a 60 mm Hg pullback gradient across the LVOT. The LV was hypertrophied and hyperdynamic. The aortic valve was trileaflet and nonobstructive, and no other abnormalities were demonstrated.

**Comments:** The patient had poor echo images, and in such a case the "real" gradient may be over- or underestimated. The catheter would confirm the resting gradient and give information on the structure of the distorted LVOT. If there is suspicion of coronary artery disease, the catheter study could address that point at the same time.

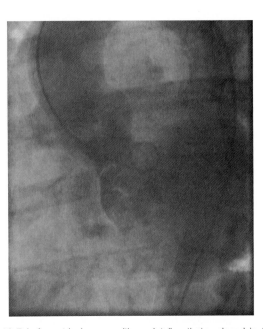

Figure 12-7 Left ventriculogram with a pigtail catheter placed in the left ventricular outflow tract.

## FINDINGS

The aortic valve was trileaflet. Within the LVOT, subaortic tissue was visualized, contributing to obstruction.

**Comments:** Note the abnormal configuration of the LVOT (elongated, with tissue tags contributing to the obstruction.

### FOCUSED CLINICAL QUESTIONS AND DISCUSSION POINTS

1. **What is the underlying pathophysiological mechanism for the development of discrete subaortic stenosis (DSS)?**

   *The mechanisms of DSS development and progression have been studied in children.[14] Minor morphologic changes in the LVOT can produce marked modifications in dynamic forces and septal shear stress, which in turn can induce a cellular proliferative response. It is likely that if septal shear stress is increased earlier in life, then this response will be more rapid and foster the progression of LVOT obstruction. Progression of DSS can be very rapid in infants and small children at vulnerable periods of development, whereas the obstruction progresses much more slowly during adult life.[15]*

   *There are other considerations in understanding the pathogenesis of DSS in the context of an AVSD. The distance from the left AV valve annulus to the LV apex is appreciably less than that from the apex to the aortic annulus, whereas normally the two distances are equal. This inlet-to-outlet disproportion creates the characteristic gooseneck deformity that used to be a major diagnostic feature on left ventriculography. Furthermore, this elongation of the LVOT, in combination with the fact that there are chordal attachments of the left AV valve to the ventricular septum in these patients, forms the basis for the development of discrete subaortic obstruction, which may occur even late after successful repair of the defect.*[16]

2. **What other complications are seen in patients with AVSD, irrespective of surgery?**

*Patients with AVSDs are prone to a number of complications irrespective of surgery: LVOT obstruction, LAVVR or stenosis (see Case 13), and residual shunts are the most common among them. Furthermore, complete AV block and atrial arrhythmia are relatively common and infective endocarditis, which in turn contributes to morbidity and mortality.*[17]

3. **What are the criteria for surgical resection of DSS in AVSD?**

*There are only a few published reports on the evolution of DSS in adult patients with AVSDs. One study demonstrated that the severity of the LVOT obstruction (peak gradient by echo) and the age of the patient are the major factors determining whether surgery should be undertaken.*[15] *In patients older than 50 years of age the severity of obstruction increased significantly at follow-up (over a period of 4.8 years). In addition, in the overall group, 50% of patients with peak gradients higher than 50 mm Hg showed significant increase in the severity of obstruction, whereas only one sixth of patients with initial gradients lower than 50 mm Hg showed significant progression of the subaortic obstruction. Another important remark from the same study was that "prevention" of aortic regurgitation should not be a criterion for surgery in patients with mild obstruction. Aortic regurgitation was more prominent in patients after surgical reintervention than in unoperated patients. Also, aortic regurgitation, although common, was rarely hemodynamically significant in this patient group.*

## FINAL DIAGNOSIS

LVOT obstruction after intermediate AVSD repair

## PLAN OF ACTION

Surgical subaortic resection

## INTERVENTION

The patient underwent successful and uneventful relief of subaortic stenosis. The surgeon described multiple tissue tags obstructing the LVOT. He was able to resect them without interfering with the function and competence of the left AV valve, nor did he need to operate on or replace the aortic valve (which in itself was somewhat small but trileaflet, nonobstructive, and placed some distance from the LVOT).

***Comment:*** In the setting of an AVSD, the tensors or fibrous tissues supporting the left AV valve are much closer in proximity to the subaortic region than in the normal heart. At the same time, the AV conduction bundles are more posteroin-

feriorly displaced than normal. Therefore, the conduction axis is more remote from the subaortic area, and thus ventricular septal musculature can be excised extensively without fear of causing complete surgical heart block.

## OUTCOME

The patient was discharged home on the sixth postoperative day in sinus rhythm and reported improved functional capacity at her 6-month follow-up appointment.

She continued to have first degree heart block and was reminded that she may require permanent pacing over her lifetime for "acquired" heart block.

## Selected References

1. Shinebourne EA, Ho SY: In Gatzoulis MA, Webb GD, Daubeney PE (eds): Diagnosis and Management of Adult Congenital Heart Disease. London, Churchill Livingstone, 2003.
2. Boening A, Scheeve J, Heine K, et al: Long term results after surgical correction of atrioventricular septal defects. Eur J Cardiothoracic Surg 22:167–173, 2002.
3. Gurbuz TA, Novick WM, Pierce CA, Watson DC: Left ventricular outflow tract obstruction after atrioventricular septal defect repair. Ann Thorac Surg 68:1723–1726, 1999.
4. Fournier A, Young M, Garcia OL, et al: Electrophysiologic cardiac function before and after surgery in children with atrioventricular canal. Am J Cardiol 57:1137–1141, 1986.
5. Diller GP, Dimopoulos K, Okonko D, et al: Exercise intolerance in adult congenital heart disease. Comparative severity correlates, and prognostic implication. Circulation 112:828–835, 2005.
6. El-Najdawi EK, Driscoll DJ, Puga FJ, et al: Operation for partial atrioventricular septal defect: A forty-year review. J Thorac Cardiovasc Surg 119:880–889, 2000.
7. Najm HK, Williams WG, Churatanaphong S, et al: Primum atrial septal defect in children: Early results, risk factors and freedom from reoperation. Ann Thorac Surg 66:829–835, 1998.
8. Jan Ten Harkel DA, Cromme-Dijkhuis AH, Heinerman BC, et al: Development of left atrioventricular valve regurgitation after correction of atrioventricular septal defect. Ann Thorac Surg 79:607–612, 2005.
9. Erentrug V, Bozburga N, Kirali K, et al: Surgical treatment of subaortic obstruction in adolescents and adults: Long-term follow-up. J Card Surg 20(1):16–21, 2005.
10. Gersony WM: Natural history of discrete subaortic stenosis: Management implications. JACC 38:843–845, 2001.
11. Baufreton C, Jaurnois D, Leca F, et al: Ten-year experience with surgical treatment of partial AVSD: Risk factors in the early postoperative period. J Thorac Cardiovasc Surg 112:4–20, 1996.
12. Sittiwangkul R, Ma RY, McCrindle BW, et al: Echocardiographic assessment of obstructive lesions in atrioventricular septal defects. JACC 38:253–261, 2001.
13. Blieden LC, Randall PA, Castaneda AR, et al: The "goose-neck" of the endocardial cushion defect: Anatomical basis. Chest 65:13–17, 1974.
14. Cape EG, Vanauker MD, Sigfusson G, et al: Potential role of mechanical stress in the etiology of pediatric heart disease: Septal shear stress in subaortic stenosis. J Am Coll Cardiol 30:247–254, 1997.
15. Oliver JM, Gonzalez A, Gallego P, et al: Discrete subaortic stenosis in adults: Increased prevalence and slow rate of progression of the obstruction and aortic regurgitation. JACC 38:835–842, 2001.
16. Taylor NC, Somerville J: Fixed subaortic stenosis after repair of ostium primum defects. Br Heart J 45:689–697, 1981.
17. Gatzoulis MA, Hechter S, Webb G, Williams W: Surgery for partial atrioventricular septal defect in the adult. Ann Thorac Surg 67:504–510, 1999.

# Left Atrioventricular Valve Regurgitation: Criteria for Intervention

**Jonathon B. Ryan, Elisabeth Bédard, and Hideki Uemura**

**Age: 30 years**
**Gender: Female**
**Occupation: Mother**
**Working diagnosis: Atrioventricular septal defect**

## HISTORY

As a child, the patient was diagnosed with a partial AVSD (ostium primum ASD). Corrective surgery was performed at the age of 8 years. The left AV valve was repaired and the interatrial communication was closed with autologous pericardium. She was followed up intermittently and remained well.

At the age of 27, the patient underwent a successful pregnancy. Following the pregnancy, however, she became aware of increasing shortness of breath on exertion and occasional palpitations. She was first seen in a specialist cardiology clinic 10 months postpartum. At that time she had become increasingly breathless with moderate exertion. She lived in a first-floor apartment and struggled with the stairs, especially when carrying her son.

A transthoracic echocardiogram showed moderate left atrioventricular valve regurgitation (LAVVR) through the commissure between the superior and inferior bridging leaflets. There was dilatation of the LA and LV. Transesophageal echocardiography confirmed the anatomic findings but also showed that the superior bridging leaflet of the left AV valve was thickened and had a rolled edge. The degree of LAVVR was judged as moderate to severe.

The patient noted increasing difficulty keeping up with her new motherhood role. The initial view was that she should be considered for surgical intervention. The patient expressed a desire to have additional children but was advised not to consider a further pregnancy until after her LAVVR had been re-repaired.

When the patient's case was discussed at a multidisciplinary care conference, concerns were raised that the valve may not be repairable. It was suggested that intensive medical management through a second planned pregnancy may be a better alternative to risking either a bioprosthetic mitral valve replacement (with inevitable re-replacement) or a mechanical prosthesis requiring anticoagulation.

To help confirm the indications for surgery and safety of pregnancy, the group recommended a cardiopulmonary exercise test, a cardiac MR study to reassess the severity of regurgitation and its impact on the LV, and 24-hour ECG monitoring as it was unclear from her standard 12 lead electrocardiogram whether her rhythm was sinus or junctional. In the interim, she was started on an ACE inhibitor (not to be taken when attempting to become pregnant) and a diuretic.

A few months later, the patient had an unplanned pregnancy, despite being on the oral contraceptive pill. This created a great deal of anxiety, as her recollection of the pregnancy advice was that she would place herself at considerable risks with pregnancy. The patient chose to have the pregnancy terminated.

The patient was not seen for 18 months, having missed several appointments. When she returned to the clinic at age 30 years, she reported a further deterioration in her symptoms.

*Comments:* Failure to address clefts in the left AV valve at the time of closure of a partial AVSD is an important cause of late AV valve regurgitation. In the past, it was believed that the left AV valve in AVSD should be operated in a trifoliate fashion.[1,2] It appears, however, that most surgeons today would close the apposition between the bridging leaflets of the left AV valve, thus leading to improving overall results.[3] This argument, however, is not universally accepted.[4]

Although many women may complain of fatigue or breathlessness through pregnancy and in caring for a newborn, such complaints in patients with congenital heart disease should prompt a careful cardiovascular assessment and workup.

The pathogenesis of valve dysfunction must be carefully studied to determine the etiology, as the etiology influences the decision to recommend surgery. Regurgitation may be due to acquired pathology rather than the original congenital abnormality.[4] If the regurgitation relates to a persisting cleft in the valve, it is also important to assess the size of the mural leaflet and the size of the left AV valve orifice (which may have been restricted by the previous repair or dilated by the volume loading of the ventricle). These factors help determine whether valve repair is feasible and influence the choice of the method of repair. In the literature, late reoperation for LAVVR was around 10%[5] or even higher.[4]

Primary repair of a cleft left AV valve is almost always successful, particularly if there is a well-formed mural leaflet. The results of re-repair, however, are less predictable and the possibility of iatrogenic left AV valve stenosis is greater.

Further testing could be seen as simply a stalling tactic for a difficult clinical situation, but coupled with additional time, it can help clarify what the optimal management should be. The appropriate medical management of LAVVR is unclear. Afterload reduction may reduce the regurgitant fraction, and ACE inhibition has been shown to improve the functional class of patients with mitral regurgitation. However, this patient was normotensive and almost certainly had a normal systemic vascular resistance. The consequences of inducing abnormally low afterload have not been established. Similarly, in the absence of physical signs of congestive heart failure, the potential benefit of diuretics is likely to be limited.

The implications of congenital heart disease for pregnancy and thus contraception are critically important for all female adult congenital heart disease (CHD) patients of childbearing age, as shown repeatedly in this book. The cardiologist should not disregard the responsibility of discussing pregnancy and contraception clearly and openly with female patients, nor assume that such discussions have taken place with other health care providers.

## CURRENT SYMPTOMS

The patient's main complaint was shortness of breath on exertion. She was now able to manage only 10 steps on stairs. She also described occasional palpitations, which were associated with dizziness. However, she denied orthopnea, nocturnal dyspnea, ankle swelling, and chest pain.

NYHA class: II

## CURRENT MEDICATIONS

Lisinopril 10 mg daily

Furosemide 40 mg daily

## PHYSICAL EXAMINATION

BP 130/80 mm Hg, HR 74 bpm, oxygen saturation 98%

Height 183 cm, weight 89.0 kg, BSA 2.13 m²

Surgical scars: Previous median sternotomy

Neck veins: Jugular venous pressure was not elevated.

Lungs/chest: Lungs were clear to auscultation.

Heart: The rhythm was regular. The first heart sound was normal. There was an accentuated pulmonary component of the second heart sound. There was a third heart sound. A loud pan-systolic murmur was present at the apex, radiating to the back and axilla. There was no diastolic rumble.

Abdomen: The abdomen was soft, and the liver was not enlarged.

Extremities: No peripheral edema was present.

***Comments:*** LV enlargement on echocardiography cannot always be demonstrated clinically. Accentuation of the pulmonary component of the second heart sound suggests a degree of pulmonary hypertension, which would be consistent with chronic, severe LAVVR. This is a clinically important sign, especially if accompanied by a prominent a-wave in the JVP, an RV heave, or signs of tricuspid regurgitation. The patient does not show any signs of congestive heart failure at present.

## LABORATORY DATA

| | | |
|---|---|---|
| Hemoglobin | 12.6 g/dL | (11.5–15.0) |
| Hematocrit/PCV | 37% | (36–46) |
| MCV | 83 fL | (83–99) |
| Platelet count | 246 × 10⁹/L | (150–400) |
| Sodium | 139 mmol/L | (134–145) |
| Potassium | 4.0 mmol/L | (3.5–5.2) |
| Creatinine | 0.62 mg/dL | (0.6–1.2) |
| Blood urea nitrogen | 3.6 mmol/L | (2.5–6.5) |

***Comments:*** No significant abnormalities apart from possible borderline iron deficiency (borderline microcytosis).

## ELECTROCARDIOGRAM

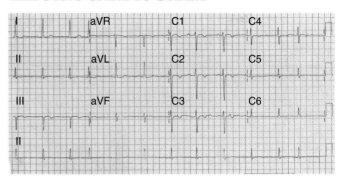

Figure 13-1 Electrocardiogram.

### FINDINGS

Heart rate: 73 bpm

QRS axis: −7°

QRS duration: 96 msec

Sinus rhythm, atrial premature beats, and a superior (leftward) axis as expected.

***Comments:*** Nonspecific T-wave inversions are seen.

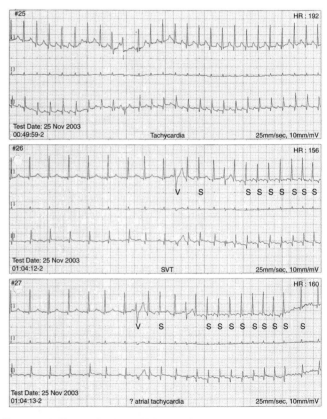

Figure 13-2 Twenty-four-hour Holter monitor.

## FINDINGS

Overall sinus rhythm. Episodes of ectopic atrial rhythm with atrial reentry and also fibrillation. Occasional episodes of accelerated junctional rhythm. Ventricular rates between 78 and 189 bpm.

## CHEST X-RAY

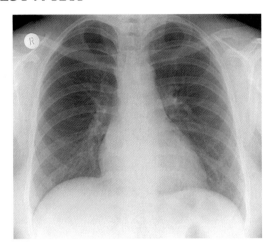

Figure 13-3 Posteranterior projection.

## FINDINGS

Cardiothoracic ratio: 50%

No overt left heart chamber enlargement or evidence of congestive cardiac failure seen. Mild cardiomegaly.

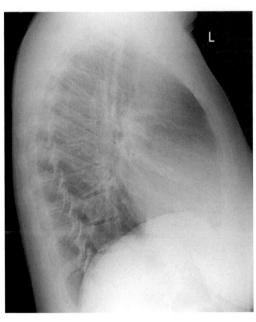

Figure 13-4 Lateral view.

## FINDINGS

No overt left heart chamber enlargement or congestive cardiac failure as per posteroanterior film.

## EXERCISE TESTING

| | | |
|---|---|---|
| Exercise protocol: | Modified Bruce | |
| Duration (min:sec): | 10:20 | |
| Reason for stopping: | Dyspnea | |
| ECG changes: | None | |

| | Rest | Peak |
|---|---|---|
| Heart rate (bpm): | 74 | 179 |
| Percent of age-predicted max HR: | | 94 |
| $O_2$ saturation (%): | 98 | 100 |
| Blood pressure (mm Hg): | 130/80 | 160/72 |
| Double product: | | 28,640 |
| Peak $Vo_2$ (mL/kg/min): | | 23.2 |
| Percent predicted (%): | | 73 |
| $Ve/Vco_2$: | | 39.1 |
| Metabolic equivalents: | | 9.0 |

***Comments:*** The results are somewhat better than anticipated from the patient's subjective report on exercise capacity.

## ECHOCARDIOGRAM

### OVERALL FINDINGS

There was LV enlargement (LVEDd 66 mm, LVESd 42 mm) with maintained LV systolic function. The LA was dilated (51 mm).

Severe LAVVR was present, with a posteriorly directed jet arising at the commissure between the superior and inferior bridging leaflets and reaching the rear wall of the LA.

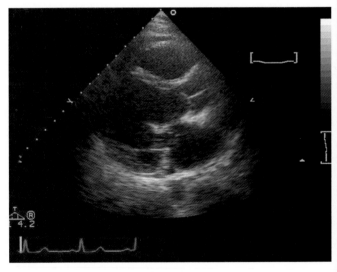

Figure 13-5 Parasternal long-axis view.

***Comments:*** There was significant progression in both the severity of the LAVVR and the degree of left heart chamber enlargement since the initial transthoracic echocardiogram 18 months earlier.

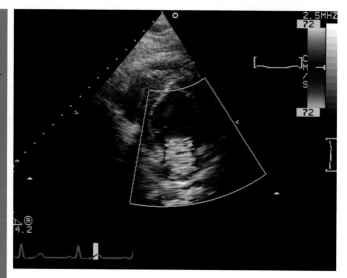

Figure 13-6 Parasternal short-axis view.

## FINDINGS

The parasternal short-axis view revealed severe LAVVR, with a posteriorly directed jet arising at the repaired commissure between the superior and inferior bridging leaflets and reaching the rear wall of the LA.

**Comments:** In short axis, one can appreciate both the trajectory of the jet posteriorly and its width.

## MAGNETIC RESONANCE IMAGING

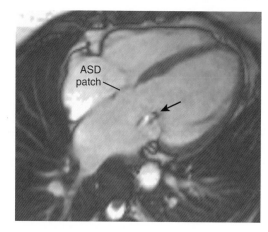

ASD patch

Figure 13-7 Magnetic resonance image.

## FINDINGS

In the left AV valve there was severe regurgitation due to central lack of coaptation of the leaflets resulting in an eccentric jet of regurgitation *(arrow)* directed toward the base of the posterior wall of the LA. The regurgitant fraction by stroke volume difference was 50%. The LA was moderately dilated (LA volume index 56 mL/m²).

## Ventricular Volume Quantification

| | LV | (Normal range) | RV | (Normal range) |
|---|---|---|---|---|
| EDV (mL) | **267** | (52–141) | 142 | (58–154) |
| ESV (mL) | **111** | (13–51) | 51 | (12–68) |
| SV (mL) | **156** | (33–97) | 91 | (35–98) |
| EF (%) | 58 | (57–75) | 64 | (51–75) |
| EDVi (mL/m²) | **126** | (62–96) | 67 | (61–98) |
| ESVi (mL/m²) | **52** | (17–36) | 24 | (17–43) |
| SVi (mL/m²) | **73** | (40–65) | **43** | (20–40) |
| Mass index (g/m²) | 49 | (47–77) | 26 | (20–40) |

**Comments:** The nature of the regurgitant jet is consistent with regurgitation through the repaired commissure between the superior and inferior bridging leaflets. Separation of the superior and inferior bridging leaflets at the cleft may be interpreted as a central lack of coaptation.

Overall, this MRI demonstrates severe LAVVR, significant left heart chamber enlargement, and mild LV systolic impairment.

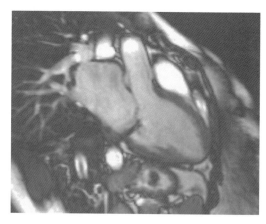

Figure 13-8 Oblique sagittal view steady-state free precession cine (three-chamber view).

## FINDINGS

A discrete posteriorly directed jet of LAVVR was seen. The LA was enlarged.

**Comments:** In this view, one can appreciate that the jet is very narrow and hugs the wall of the atrium as it wraps around to the posterior wall. Also note the unwedged position of the aorta (not engaged in the usual way between the ventricular septum and the anterior leaflet of the mitral valve), one of the hallmarks of AVSDs.

### FOCUSED CLINICAL QUESTIONS AND DISCUSSION POINTS

1. **What is the cause of LAVVR in patients with AVSD?**

   *Both partial and complete AVSDs result from a failure of fusion of the septum primum, the ventral and dorsal endocardial cushions, and the interventricular septum. The consequence of this is a common AV junction. The AV valve can arise only from the subendocardial tissue around the periphery of the valve orifice and thus arises as a common five-leaflet valve.*

   *In the "ostium primum" ASD form of partial AVSD, the common AV valve is fused with the muscular interventricular septum. The superior and inferior bridging leaflets of the valve are also fused together as they pass over the muscular interven-*

tricular septum. This limits shunting across the defect at the atrial level and produces separate left and right AV valvular orifices. The gaps between the superior and inferior bridging leaflets are what form the so-called clefts. Because the clefts lack chordal support, and the overall quantity of valvular tissue is relatively deficient, these valves are typically regurgitant.

2. What is the natural history of residual LAVVR following surgical repair of the cleft?

Some degree of LAVVR is common following appropriate surgical repair of partial or complete AVSD. Severity is largely determined by the adequacy of the valve leaflets, particularly the mural leaflet, but is usually mild unless there were significant abnormalities of the leaflets preoperatively. Patients with an AVSD and no interventricular communication are more liable to have residual or progressive regurgitation, because the flow across the left-sided AV valve increases after closure of the interatrial communication. The orifice of the left-sided valve tends to become larger in this setting, causing failure of coaptation. In contrast, in patients with a common AV valve, a surgeon can choose a line to place a proper amount of the bridging leaflets for the more important left-sided component. The size of the annular attachment of the AV valve can become smaller by reduction of a left-to-right shunt particularly through the interventricular communication.

Unlike acquired mitral valve regurgitation, where the underlying pathological process is progressive, LAVVR following complete or partial AVSD repair is often stable over time because the defect is anatomical. However, the effect of the original repair on the geometry of the annulus alters as the patient grows, particularly following repair of the complete form of AVSD in which the use of a synthetic patch to septate the ventricular component of the defect markedly restricts the natural growth of the annulus at one part. This may promote growth of the opposite side—that is, the lateral attachment for the mural leaflet that is a key for better valvar function. If the surgeon does not use any synthetic material that might restrict the anteroposterior distance in repairing the defect initially, the "septal" aspect of the valvar attachment would dilate, but growth compensation of the other parts would not occur. Thus, the mural leaflet could potentially remain relatively hypoplastic.

Regardless of the initial cause, if the degree of regurgitation is sufficient to produce volume loading, the severity of the LAVVR will be progressive (i.e., generally mitral regurgitation leads to more mitral regurgitation). In this case, it is possible that the hypervolumic circulatory state associated with pregnancy influenced the natural history.

3. What are the indications for reoperation in this patient?

The indications for redo left AV valve surgery (repair or replacement) late after repair of partial AVSD are essentially the same as for acquired mitral valve regurgitation. In general, patients with severe regurgitation who are either symptomatic (NYHA II–IV) or who have evidence of early LV dysfunction (defined as LVESd > 40 mm or EF < 60%) should undergo surgery.

In the present case, the degree of LAVVR was initially assessed as moderate and her subjective assessment was somewhat inconsistent with her performance on MVo$_2$ testing. However, over time further imaging showed clear evidence of worsening severity of regurgitation and LV enlargement, such that she reached the thresholds defined in the ACC/AHA guidelines.[6]

4. What influence should the patient's expressed desire to have a second child have on clinical decision making?

Potential pregnancy is a very significant factor. A decision on the timing of surgery relative to a planned pregnancy in patients with significant LAVVR is dependent on the likelihood of repair and the likelihood of LV decompensation. This highlights the importance of communication between the cardiologist and surgeon and obstetrician, which is best achieved in a multidisciplinary environment.

The initial intent was perhaps to get the patient through her second pregnancy first, then replace the valve. This plan would place the patient at risk of congestive cardiac failure during the pregnancy. Furthermore, it is unknown as to whether further volume loading due to pregnancy has an adverse long-term effect on patients with dilated ventricles and severe valvular lesions. The alternative plan, likely valve replacement, would have required anticoagulation through a successive pregnancy. The MRI and subsequent clinical course showed that the former option was not favorable and that surgery had become necessary.

## FINAL DIAGNOSIS

Severe LAVVR late after repair of partial AVSD

## PLAN OF ACTION

Left AV valve surgery

## INTERVENTION

The patient was admitted 4 months later for elective surgery. The repeat sternotomy was uneventful. The LA was approached through Waterson's groove (i.e., the prominent groove between the right pulmonary veins and the RA). On inspection of the left AV valve, the superior and inferior bridging leaflets were thickened and there was a persistent cleft at the commissure between them. This was closed with 5-0 prolene. The annulus was markedly dilated. Thus suture annuloplasty at the superior bridging leaflet (mural leaflet commissure 35 mm) and the inferior bridging leaflet (mural leaflet commissure 20 mm) was performed using 2-0 Ethibond.

Intraoperative transesophageal echocardiography and postoperative transthoracic echocardiography confirmed an adequate repair, with only a trace of central LAVVR.

**Comments:** Despite the preoperative imaging, the surgeon here felt that a repair was achievable, hence avoiding the pitfalls associated with replacement. Some surgeons would advocate the use of an annuloplasty band or ring to support the suture annuloplasty, with the expectation that this will improve the durability of the repair. While there is evidence to support this approach for routine mitral valve repair, there are important differences in AVSD that affect the appropriateness of these devices in this setting (see Fig. 13-8). In these patients, the natural shape of the annulus is different from a normal mitral annulus. This is particularly true in complete AVSD in which the use of a synthetic patch to septate the ventricular defect during the original operation markedly restricts the natural growth of the annulus and further alters its shape (see Fig. 13-8). The role of the anterior leaflet of a normal mitral valve is usually played by the mural leaflet in AVSD. Plication of the circumferential length at this part is less than ideal (see Fig. 13-8), particularly when the mural leaflet width is small. Also, the abnormal location of the AV node makes placement of a ring more difficult.

## OUTCOME

The patient's postoperative stay was uneventful, and she was discharged home on the sixth postoperative day. She was, however, readmitted 9 days later in atrial flutter with variable block. She underwent successful direct current cardioversion and was discharged home on a trial of beta-blockers and warfarin therapy for 6 months.

Two years later the patient was free of sustained arrhythmia, with much improved functional capacity, 3 months pregnant (off beta-blockers and warfarin for 18 months, on low-dose aspirin only).

**Comments:** Atrial arrhythmias are very common following cardiac procedures. In view of this episode and the nonsustained atrial flutter observed on the 24-hour Holter monitor 18 months earlier, it may have been appropriate to have performed a bi-atrial maze procedure at the time of left AV valve repair.[7] The exact origin of her atrial arrhythmia was uncertain. Preoperatively, the patient had not experienced sustained arrhythmias. She had undergone previous repair at the age of 8 years; hence the risk of late sustained arrhythmia would be small. In addition, a maze procedure during a reoperation is more difficult due to adhesions, which increases the risks associated with the procedure. Furthermore, hemodynamic improvement by surgical correction of the LAVVR may decrease her arrhythmic risk.

In LAVVR, one possible focus of atrial arrhythmia is the sleeve muscles of the pulmonary veins. During a proper maze, the surgeon needs to isolate the pulmonary venous ostia.[8] Alternatively, re-entry tachyarrhythmias may arise from slow conduction circuits around the abnormally large common AV junction, the right atriotomy scar,[9] or, rarely, around the fossa ovalis (particularly if the muscle bar between a patent foramen ovalis or incidental secundum ASD and the AVSD has not been divided at the original operation). If this patient continues to experience palpitations, she should undergo electrophysiological studies to look for such pathways, which may be amenable to percutaneous catheter ablation.

## Selected References

1. Carpentier A: Surgical anatomy and management of the mitral component of atrioventricular canal defects. In Anderson RH, Shinebourne EA (eds): Paediatric Cardiology. Edinburgh, Churchill Livingstone, 1977, pp 477–486.

2. Pacifico AD: Atrio-ventricular septal defect. In Stark J, de Leval M (eds): Surgery for Congenital Heart Defects. Philadelphia, WB Saunders, 1994, pp 373–388.

3. Kouchoukos NT, Blackstone EH, Doty DB, et al: Atrioventricular septal defect: Technique of operation. In Kouchoukos NT, Blackstone EH, Doty DB, et al (eds): Kirklin/Barratt-Boyes Cardiac Surgery, 3rd ed. Philadelphia, Churchill Livingstone, 2003, pp 824–835.

4. Ebels T, Anderson RH: Atrioventricular septal defects: Treatment. In Anderson RH, Baker EJ, Macartney FJ, et al (eds): Paediatric Cardiology, 2nd ed. London, Churchill Livingstone, 2002, pp 968–975.

5. Najm HK, Coles JG, Endo M, et al: Complete atrioventricular septal defects: Results of repair, risk factors, and freedom from reoperation. Circulation 96:II311–II315, 1997.

6. Bonow RO, Carabello BA, Kanu C, et al: ACC/AHA 2006 guidelines for the management of patients with valvular heart disease: A report of the American College of Cardiology/American Heart Association Task Force on Practice Guidelines (Writing Committee to Revise the 1998 Guidelines for the Management of Patients with Valvular Heart Disease): Developed in collaboration with the Society of Cardiovascular Anesthesiologists: Endorsed by the Society for Cardiovascular Angiography and Interventions and the Society of Thoracic Surgeons. Circulation 114:84–231, 2006.

7. Bando K, Kasegawa H, Okada Y, et al: Impact of preoperative and postoperative atrial fibrillation on outcome after mitral valvuloplasty for nonischemic mitral regurgitation. J Thorac Cardiovasc Surg 129:1032–1040, 2005.

8. Cox JL, Jaquiss RD, Schuessler RB, Boineau JP: Modification of the maze procedure for atrial flutter and atrial fibrillation. II. Surgical technique of the maze III procedure. J Thorac Cardiovasc Surg 110:485–495, 1995.

9. Kalman JM, VanHare GF, Olgin JE, et al: Ablation of "incisional" reentrant atrial tachycardia complicating surgery for congenital heart disease: Use of entrainment to define a critical isthmus of conduction. Circulation 93:502–512, 1996.

# Anticoagulation in a Pregnant Patient with a Mechanical Valve

**Eapen Thomas and Sara Thorne**

Age: 31 years
Gender: Female
Occupation: Nurse
Working diagnosis: Repaired atrioventricular septal defect

## HISTORY

The patient had an AVSD diagnosed in infancy and repaired in childhood. By age 6, however, she needed left AV valve repair. However, AV valve regurgitation persisted. One year later she underwent left AV valve replacement with a Bjork Shiley (single disc mechanical) valve.

She developed paroxysmal, then chronic atrial fibrillation at 21 years. This required medical management with amiodarone initially, followed by bisoprolol. She was also on warfarin. In addition she was started on losartan for elevated blood pressure.

At 23 years she experienced sudden chest pain and shortness of breath and suffered a large anterior myocardial infarction. She was found to have an occlusion of the left anterior descending coronary artery, felt to be embolic in origin. Eventually, a large LV aneurysm formed.

Three years later she had worsening ventricular dilatation and dysfunction, and symptoms of severe heart failure. It was decided that she should undergo LV aneurysmectomy with further left AV valve replacement using a bileaflet Carbomedics 27-mm valve. The procedure went well, and she made an excellent recovery, though remained in permanent atrial fibrillation.

At age 30 she and her partner were considering having their first child. She was referred for prepregnancy counseling to a multidisciplinary pregnancy cardiac clinic.

The patient had no family history of congenital heart disease and had no chromosomal anomaly.

**Comments:** AVSD denotes a deficiency of AV muscular and membranous septa. A prevalence of 0.19 per 100 live births, accounting for 2.9% of congenital cardiac malformations, has been quoted.[1]

Primary repair of AVSD in the first 3 to 6 months of age has been the preferred surgical management since the early 1980s. This patient had her surgical repair in an earlier era. Because the left AV valve is not a normal mitral valve, postoperative AV valve function is as important to assess as the septal closure itself. Failure of adequate left AV valve repair occurs in up to one fifth of procedures. The need for valve replacement occurs in about 5%.[2]

Chronic atrial fibrillation occurs in 18% of patients long term after repair of incomplete AVSD[3] and in up to 50% of adult patients who undergo valve surgery. The combination of these factors in this case makes atrial fibrillation seem unsurprising even at this young age.

The cause of the embolus was not clear, but felt most likely related to the presence of a prothrombotic valve. There was no residual ASDs, and she has always been compliant with warfarin. The LA was not huge.

Aneurysmectomy can at times restore some LV geometry and more favorable LV mechanics. The Bjork Shiley valve was functioning normally at the time of surgery, but was replaced both to offer a more appropriately sized valve now that the patient was an adult, and because it had been implicated in the coronary embolus.

## CURRENT SYMPTOMS

The patient was asymptomatic. She felt able to carry on all her typical activities of daily living, including shopping, walking, and climbing stairs. She denied palpitations, orthopnea, or chest pain.

NYHA class: I

**Comments:** Despite her remarkable history of LV dysfunction, she has no self-reported symptoms.

## CURRENT MEDICATIONS

Bisoprolol 1.25 mg daily

Digoxin 125 µg daily

Warfarin 10 mg (target INR 2.5–3.5)

## PHYSICAL EXAMINATION

BP 110/70 mm Hg, HR 82 bpm, oxygen saturation 99%

Height 161 cm, weight 63 kg, BSA 1.68 m²

Surgical scars: There was a midline sternotomy scar.

Neck veins: Seen 2 cm above the sternal angle with a normal waveform

Lungs/chest: Clear to auscultation

Heart: The pulse was regular. There was a prosthetic first heart sound. No murmurs were audible. The apical impulse was not palpable.

Abdomen: No abnormalities were seen.

Extremities: Peripheral pulses were normal, there was no edema.

***Comments:*** The findings are fairly nondescript and as expected for a patient with a prior valve replacement. She was not in atrial fibrillation at the time of the exam.

## LABORATORY DATA

| | |
|---|---|
| Hemoglobin | 13.2 g/dL (11.5–15.0) |
| Hematocrit/PCV | 41% (36–46) |
| MCV | 85 fL (83–99) |
| Platelet count | $260 \times 10^9$/L (150–400) |
| Sodium | 136 mmol/L (134–145) |
| Potassium | 4.2 mmol/L (3.5–5.2) |
| Creatinine | 0.88 mg/dL (0.6–1.2) |
| Blood urea nitrogen | 6 mmol/L (2.5–6.5) |

***Comments:*** All within normal/desirable limits.

## ELECTROCARDIOGRAM

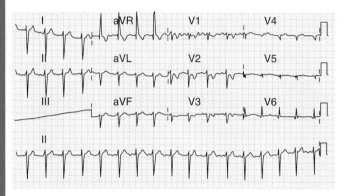

Figure 14-1 Electrocardiogram.

### FINDINGS
Heart rate: 105 bpm

QRS axis: −160°

QRS duration: 100 msec

Sinus tachycardia

Extreme axis deviation

There are precordial Q-waves and mild ST elevation from the prior anterior infarction.

***Comments:*** The axis deviation reflects her prior LV aneurysmectomy surgery and her AVSD.

Because of the intermittent atrial fibrillation, a 24-hour ECG was performed, which showed several episodes of atrial fibrillation, all with appropriate ventricular rate control.

## CHEST X-RAY

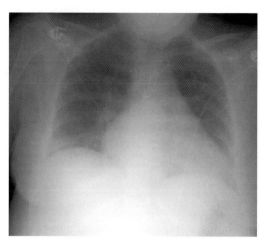

Figure 14-2 Anteroposterior projection.

### FINDINGS
Cardiothoracic ratio: 64%

***Comments:*** Even for an AP projection, the heart size seems enlarged with a prominent RA, but there is no frank evidence of heart failure.

## EXERCISE TESTING

| | | |
|---|---|---|
| Exercise protocol: | Modified Bruce | |
| Duration (min:sec): | 10:28 | |
| Reason for stopping: | Dyspnea | |
| ECG changes: | Atrial fibrillation | |

| | Rest | Peak |
|---|---|---|
| Heart rate (bpm): | 82 | 154 |
| Percent of age-predicted max HR: | | 81 |
| O$_2$ saturation (%): | 99 | 100 |
| Blood pressure (mm Hg): | 110/70 | 174/82 |
| Peak Vo$_2$ (mL/kg/min): | | 26.9 |
| Percent predicted (%): | | 68 |
| Ve/Vco$_2$: | | 37 |
| Metabolic equivalents: | | 9.1 |

***Comments:*** Cardiopulmonary exercise testing can be useful prior to pregnancy. A "normal" test is reassuring. However, the interpretation of an abnormal test is more difficult: There are no data at present to correlate a particular maximum oxygen consumption with adverse outcome, or suggest a cut-off value for a safe pregnancy.

Here the results were fairly reassuring considering her background of severe LV dysfunction requiring aneurysmectomy surgery. She went into atrial fibrillation during the test but had an appropriate ventricular rate throughout, including recovery.

# ECHOCARDIOGRAM

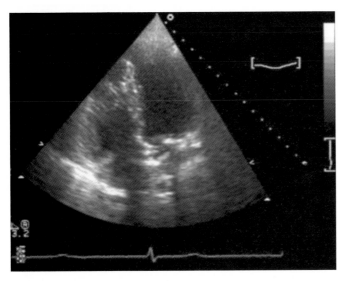

Figure 14-3 Apical four-chamber view.

## FINDINGS

There was mildly reduced LV systolic function with an ejection fraction of 48% with a normal functioning prosthetic left AV valve.

The RV was normal, as was the right AV valve. Normal estimated pulmonary artery pressure was noted. There was no evidence of LVOT obstruction or LV aneurysm.

***Comments:*** The echo demonstrates an excellent result from her prior aneurysmectomy. In a patient with prior AVSD, it is also important to look for evidence of LVOT obstruction or regurgitation of the right AV valve, though the latter is less common.

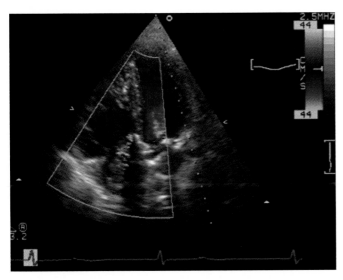

Figure 14-4 Apical four-chamber view, 2D color Doppler.

## FINDINGS

There was moderate right AV valve regurgitation. There is no residual intracardiac shunt detected.

***Comments:*** It is important to document normal function of a mechanical valve in the "mitral" position prior to preg-

nancy, given the issues surrounding proper anticoagulation for such a valve.

## FOCUSED CLINICAL QUESTIONS AND DISCUSSION POINTS

1. **What is this patient's most significant risk from pregnancy?**

*Currently the patient has no residual shunt, a competent left AV valve, and good LV function. However, she has a prosthetic left AV valve and has paroxysmal atrial fibrillation, with a history of significant thromboembolism while on anticoagulation. The greatest risk to her and the fetus is therefore related to anticoagulation. All mechanical valve prostheses carry a significant risk of thromboembolism during pregnancy. The risk is greatest for small, single-leaflet tilting disc prostheses and least for large, aortic-bileaflet tilting disc valves.*

*There is no universally safe anticoagulant regime for pregnant women with mechanical valve prostheses. The interests of the mother and fetus are in conflict—warfarin is safer for the mother while heparin safer for the fetus.*

*Warfarin is the most effective anticoagulant at preventing valve thrombosis. Unfortunately, it crosses the placenta and can cause warfarin embryopathy in the first trimester, affecting 4% to 8% of live births.[4] The risk of fetal complication is greatest at daily doses greater than 5 mg.[5] In addition, there is a risk of fetal hemorrhage throughout gestation. Warfarin also increases the risk of peripartum maternal hemorrhage.*

*In contrast, heparin does not cross the placenta and is therefore safer for the fetus. However, the risk of valve thrombosis in pregnant patients with mechanical valves is higher on heparin (4.92%) than warfarin (0.33%).[6] This risk can be reduced by administering low molecular weight heparin (LMWH) at twice daily doses and monitoring anti-Xa levels regularly (>1 unit/mL in the blood sample taken 4 to 6 hours after the last dose).*

2. **What are the current recommendations for proper anticoagulation during pregnancy in women with prosthetic heart valves?**

*There are three basic anticoagulant regime options: (1) Warfarin throughout pregnancy, (2) LWMH (twice daily, with anti-Xa monitoring) and 75 mg aspirin throughout pregnancy, and (3) LMWH (twice daily, with anti-Xa monitoring) plus 75 mg aspirin for the first trimester, switching to warfarin after 12 weeks, then back to LMWH after 36 weeks.*

*The choice of anticoagulation regime should be tailored to each individual. For example, a patient with a small thrombogenic valve in the mitral position who is adequately anticoagulated on less than 5 mg warfarin (i.e., highest risk of thrombosis and relatively low risk of warfarin-associated fetal complications) may be best advised to continue warfarin. However, a patient with an aortic bileaflet tilting disc valve requiring more than 5 mg warfarin may choose to be managed on LMWH.*

*Women should be fully informed of risks and benefits of all options and should participate in the choice of anticoagulation. Meticulous antenatal care and attention to anticoagulation monitoring are crucial whichever regime is chosen, especially during changes between warfarin and heparin and in the first few postpartum days. Detailed and serial fetal scans should be performed.*

*LMWH is now the preferred option for thromboprophylaxis in Europe.[7,8] The advantages of LMWH over unfractionated heparin include an enhanced anti-Xa:anti-IIa ratio, resulting in a reduced risk of bleeding. It has stable and predictable pharmacokinetics with increased bioavailability and half-life, allowing less frequent fixed or weight-based dosing without the need for monitoring for most patients (however, anti-Xa monitoring is mandatory for patients with mechanical valves).[9,10]*

3. How should anticoagulation be handled through labor and delivery?

*If warfarin has been used throughout pregnancy, then this should ideally be stopped at least 10 days before delivery to allow the fetus to metabolize the drug and reduce the risk of neonatal hemorrhage during delivery. LMWH should be used as a bridging therapy.*

*Careful planning is needed if the patient is to receive epidural anesthesia. Guidelines from the Royal College of Obstetrics and Gynecology for the use of an epidural in fully anticoagulated patients state that 24 hours should elapse between the last dose of LMWH and the insertion of an epidural. If a further dose of LMWH is given, there should be a 4-hour delay before removal of the epidural catheter.*

*In practice, one may have to accept that epidural anesthesia may not be possible. However, options for a safe epidural can be implemented with proper planning in situations where timing may be more predictable. For vaginal delivery LMWH should be stopped 24 hours before a planned epidural, with the recognition that if labor is prolonged, the woman may be left without anticoagulation for several hours. For elective cesarean section, a thromboprophylactic dose of LMWH should be used on the day prior to the procedure but omitted on the morning of planned delivery, a thromboprophylactic dose of LMWH should be given 3 hours postop, and a treatment dose should be recommenced that evening. If the epidural catheter has to be left in place for analgesia overnight, a dose of LMWH should be administered once hemostasis is achieved.*

*Heparin should be resumed 6 to 12 hours after a vaginal delivery.*

*Warfarin can be restarted 2 to 3 days postpartum assuming no postpartum hemorrhage has occurred. Anticoagulation should be maintained with LMWH until an appropriate INR is reached.*

4. What are the considerations for the choice of contraception in women with a mechanical heart valve?

*Estrogen is thrombogenic and is contraindicated even though patients are on warfarin because of the risk of valve thrombosis. Progesterone is not thrombogenic. The progestogen-only or minipill is safe but not very effective. The newer progestogen-only pill, Cerazette, is safe and as effective as the combined oral contraceptive pill. Depo Provera is safe and effective but hematomas may occur from deep intramuscular injections (every 3 months) and secondary to anticoagulation.*

*The progestogen-eluting Mirena coil is safe and as effective as sterilization. In addition, most women become amenorrhoeic, which is beneficial as menorrhagia is common in anticoagulated women. Implanon is a single-rod, nonbiodegradable implantable contraceptive that contains progestogen. This is inserted subdermally and is as effective as sterilization with no cardiac contraindications.*

## FINAL DIAGNOSIS

AVSD repair

Mechanical left AV valve

Permanent atrial fibrillation

## PLAN OF ACTION

Thorough planning of anticoagulation strategy before conception

## INTERVENTION

None

## OUTCOME

The patient and her partner had the opportunity to discuss a potential pregnancy with the cardiologist, obstetrician, cardiac clinical nurse specialist, and the midwife before planning conception. Emphasis in these discussions was on choice of anticoagulants during pregnancy, labor, and postdelivery. A specific plan was outlined with the patient and all her providers. She opted for LMWH twice daily throughout pregnancy.

The patient conceived and discontinued warfarin immediately, starting LMWH, for which she had already been trained. She attended a joint cardiac and obstetrics clinic monthly. She was monitored with transthoracic echocardiography and anti-Xa levels regularly.

Her other medications including digoxin, bisoprolol, and aspirin were continued.

Pregnancy was uneventful until 34 weeks gestation when absent end-diastolic flow was demonstrated on antenatal scan. At that point she underwent an uneventful cesarean section. The baby was immediately assessed by a neonatal team and was healthy.

At the time of the decision to deliver the fetus, the patient was 12 hours post LMWH dose and due for another dose. This dose was omitted and replaced with intravenous unfractionated heparin. The intravenous heparin was stopped 1 hour prior to cesarean section, which was performed with regional (epidural) analgesia 24 hours after the last treatment dose of LMWH.[11] Four hours after removal of the epidural catheter, she was given one half of her usual dose of LMWH. Twelve hours later she resumed her twice-daily LMWH regime.

On the second post–cesarean section day she became tachycardic and dyspneic. Her hemoglobin fell to 7 g/dL. Transesophageal examination revealed a normal mitral valve prosthesis with no evidence of thrombus. She therefore underwent surgery under general anesthesia for removal of thrombus from the uterovesical pouch. Warfarin was restarted on day 4. Dalteparin sodium (LMWH) was continued until her INR was above 2.5.

Later, contraception was offered using a single-rod, nonbiodegradable implantable contraceptive (Implanon) that contains the progestogen etonogestrel.

**Comments:** Absent end-diastolic flow in the umbilical arteries is a specific indicator of serious fetal compromise and is an indication for immediate delivery.

Even with careful planning, catastrophic bleeding and/or thromboses may occur. The most risky period is the immediate postpartum when clotting mechanisms are activated and bleeding risk is high. Skilled and vigilant attention must be paid during this fragile period.

The Implanon device is not associated with any prothrombotic effects, and there are no cardiac contraindications to its use. It is at least as effective as sterilization and there is a rapid return to normal fertility after removal of the implant.[12]

## Selected References

1. Samanek M, Benesova D, Geotzova J, Hycejova I: Distribution of age at death in children with congenital heart disease who died before the age of 15. Br Heart J 59:581–585, 1988.
2. Suzuki K, Tatsumu K, Kikuchi T, Mimori S: Predisposing factors of valve regurgitation in complete atrioventricular septal defect. J Am Coll Cardiol 32:1449–1453, 1998.
3. Goldfaden DM, Jones M, Morrow AG: Long-term results of repair of incomplete atrioventricular canal. J Thorac Cardiovasc Surg 82:69–73, 1981.
4. Chan WS, Anand S, Ginsberg JS: Anticoagulation of pregnant women with mechanical heart valves: A systematic review of literature. Arch Intern Med 160:191–196, 2000.
5. Oakley CM: Valvular disease in pregnancy. Curr Opin Cardiol 11:155–159, 1996.

6. Meschengieser SS, Fondevila CG, Santerelli MT, Lazzari MA: Anticoagulation of pregnant women with mechanical heart valve prostheses. Heart 82:23–26, 1999.

7. Scottish Intercollegiate Guidelines Network (SIGN): Guideline 62: Prophylaxis of Venous Thromboembolism. Edinburgh, SIGN, 2002.

8. Scottish Intercollegiate Guidelines Network (SIGN): Guideline 36: Antithrombotic Therapy. Edinburgh, SIGN, 1999.

9. Nelson-Piercy C: Hazards of heparin allergy, heprin induced thrombocytopenia and osteoporosis. Baillieres Clin Obst Gynaecol 11:489–509, 1997.

10. Warkentin TE, Levine MN, Hirsh J, et al: Heparin-induced thrombocytopenia in patients treated with low-molecular weight heparin or unfractionated heparin. N Engl J Med 332:1330–1335, 1995.

11. Thromboembolic disease in pregnancy and the puerperium. Green-top Guideline No 28. London, RCOG, 2007.

12. Funk S, Miller MM, Mishell DR Jr, et al: The Implanon™ US Study Group: Safety and efficacy of Implanon™, a single-rod implantable contraceptive containing etonogestrel. Contraception 11: 319–326, 2005.

# Atrial Septal Defect Associated with Pulmonary Hypertension—Cause and Effect

**Gerhard-Paul Diller**

**Age: 32 years**
**Gender: Female**
**Occupation: Nurse's assistant**
**Working diagnosis: Atrial septal defect with pulmonary arterial hypertension**

## HISTORY

The patient was well until 10 years ago (22 years old) when she had a successful pregnancy but developed a deep vein thrombosis 1 week postpartum. She was treated with warfarin for 6 months.

She was then well until 2 years ago (30 years old) when she developed pneumonia and was admitted to her local hospital. CXR showed a large heart, and an echocardiogram showed a large ASD.

Three months later, she presented with a swollen leg and sudden shortness of breath. For the first time, a bluish discoloration of her lips and fingertips was noted. An echocardiogram demonstrated elevated right ventricular systolic pressure. She was felt to have had a pulmonary embolus and was again started on warfarin. She was also started on nocturnal oxygen with continuous positive airway pressure therapy.

She is a nonsmoker.

**Comments:** Patients with an isolated ASD are usually asymptomatic even well into adult life. Early symptoms may include exertional dyspnea or fatigue, atrial flutter, or occasionally thromboembolic events.

The patient has developed cyanosis. In a patient with an ASD, cyanosis is worrisome as it implies new right-to-left shunting through the defect. This suggests the presence of elevated RV filling pressures and PAH, which was confirmed by echo.

Causes to consider here include recurrent deep venous thrombosis; primary PAH, which can sometimes affect young women; and pulmonary vascular disease from chronic volume overload (i.e., Eisenmenger syndrome). However, only very large ASDs, especially in patients living at high altitude, can easily explain the development of Eisenmenger syndrome.[1] Otherwise, other causes should be sought.

## CURRENT SYMPTOMS

Currently she can walk slowly about 200 m on level ground. Sometimes she is pushed in a wheelchair while shopping. She has experienced lightheadedness on exertion. She denies chest pain, palpitations, or syncope but at the end of each day notes ankle swelling. She sleeps well but apparently snored until her continuous positive airway pressure therapy was started.

NYHA class: III

**Comments:** Snoring should not be ignored, since sleep apnea can be a cause of or contribute to PAH, heart failure, and stroke risk.

## CURRENT MEDICATIONS

Warfarin 4 mg orally at bedtime (target INR 2–3)

Digoxin 250 µg daily by mouth

Nifedipine 60 mg twice daily by mouth (as pulmonary hypotensive therapy)

**Comments:** Anticoagulation is indicated because of the history of presumed deep venous thrombosis as well as suspected pulmonary embolism. In general, anticoagulation is recommended in patients with primary PAH.[2] In patients with Eisenmenger syndrome, the use of anticoagulants is controversial and can be dangerous if the INR is not carefully controlled.

## IMMUNIZATION STATUS

She is immunized against influenza but not against pneumococcal pneumonia.

**Comments:** Pneumonia accounts for 7% of deaths in patients with PAH. Immunization against influenza and pneumococcal infections is accordingly recommended.[3]

## PHYSICAL EXAMINATION

BP 110/70 mm Hg, HR 90 bpm, oxygen saturation 78% on room air measured in the right hand and 76% in the left foot

Height 162 cm, weight 91 kg, BSA 2.02 m$^2$

Surgical scars: None

Neck veins: JVP was elevated to 8 cm above the sternal angle with a prominent CV-wave.

Lungs/chest: Chest was clear.

Heart: There was a RV lift. There was wide fixed splitting of the second heart sound with a loud pulmonary component. A third heart sound was heard at the left lower sternal border. There was a grade 2 pansystolic murmur medial to the apex.

Abdomen: There was mild hepatomegaly.

Extremities: There was moderate symmetric pitting edema of both ankles. Clubbing was seen in both fingers and toes.

## PERTINENT NEGATIVES
There were no findings of scleroderma or rheumatoid arthritis.

*Comments:* Cyanosis is clearly present as the history suggested, and the workup must try to clarify the etiology.

A CV-wave is indicative of tricuspid regurgitation.

A wide and fixed split second heart sound is a cardinal clinical sign in patients with a significant ASD. It reflects delayed pulmonary valve closure and a relatively fixed and increased right ventricular stroke volume. In fact, fixed splitting is not always seen in typical ASDs, especially in a case like this in which the left-to-right shunt has lessened in the face of pulmonary hypertension, which is suggested by the loud pulmonary component of the second heart sound.

The pansystolic murmur indicates mitral or tricuspid regurgitation or a VSD. There are various clinical ways of making the distinction. If this were felt to be of mitral origin, one should consider whether this is a primum ASD with a regurgitant left AV valve.

The presence of clubbing suggests that right-to-left shunting has been more chronic than the history indicates.

## LABORATORY DATA

| | | |
|---|---|---|
| Hemoglobin | **16.9 g/dL** | (11.5–15.0) |
| Hematocrit | **50%** | (36–46) |
| MCV | **81 fL** | (83–99) |
| MCH | **26 pg** | (27–32.5) |
| Sodium | 135 mmol/L | (134–145) |
| Potassium | 4.3 mmol/L | (3.5–5.2) |
| Creatinine | 0.8 mg/dL | (0.6–1.2) |
| Blood urea nitrogen | 4.2 mmol/L | (2.5–6.5) |
| Iron | **5.7 μg/L** | (12.6–26.0) |
| Ferritin | **8 ng/mL** | (20–186) |
| TIBC | **88 μmol/L** | (50–80) |
| Transferrin saturation | **7%** | (20–45) |

*Comments:* The elevated hemoglobin concentration in this patient represents secondary erythrocytosis. Secondary erythrocytosis is seen in chronically cyanotic patients and should be proportional to the severity of the hypoxemia. The term "secondary erythrocytosis" refers to an isolated increase in red blood cells (as opposed to polycythemia in which all cell lines proliferate) and is a physiologic adaptation to chronic hypoxemia.

If the oxygen saturation is 78%, one should expect the hemoglobin to be as high as 20 to 23 g/dL.[4] Thus, this patient is relatively anemic despite her raised hemoglobin. This is because she is iron deficient. There are several potential etiologies for this (see Case 72). Iron deficiency is associated with an increased risk for stroke in cyanotic heart disease.[5] This should be treated with oral iron supplementation or intravenous iron if the oral form is not tolerated. Her exercise capacity may improve with a higher hemoglobin.

The expected pattern of microcytosis and hypochromia seen here may be found in as few as 16% of cyanotic patients with iron deficiency. Instead, patients often present with hyperchromia and/or macrocytosis.[6]

## ELECTROCARDIOGRAM

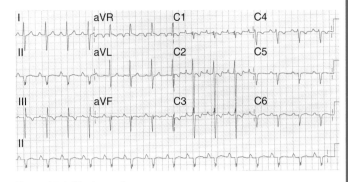

Figure 15-1 Electrocardiogram.

## FINDINGS
Heart rate: 89 bpm

PR int: 220 msec

QRS axis: +246°

QRS duration: 109 msec

Sinus rhythm with borderline first-degree block

P-wave forces compatible with dextrocardia

Some peaking of P-waves in V1–3, indicating RA overload

Marked deviation of the QRS axis

Inferior Q-waves unlikely to reflect prior infarction. Poor R-wave progression in the left chest leads. T-wave inversion in leads V1–4.

*Comments:* In a patient with dextrocardia, one needs to know where the limb and precordial leads were placed. This tracing suggests reversed limb lead placement. Inverted T-waves in V1–4, together with a prominent S-wave in V6 may indicate right ventricular hypertrophy.

Extreme axis deviation is strongly suggestive of pulmonary hypertension in this context.

First-degree AV block is also common in adults with ostium primum ASD, but may be seen in "older" patients with a large secundum ASD.

Thus the ECG suggests that the patient may indeed have an ostium primum ASD, that is, an AVSD, rather than a secundum ASD.

## CHEST X-RAY

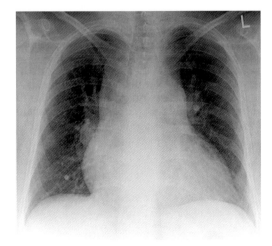

Figure 15-2 Posteroanterior projection.

## FINDINGS

Cardiothoracic ratio: 67%

The cardiac silhouette was grossly enlarged. Dilatation of the central pulmonary arteries was suspected, although this was not well seen. The SVC was dilated. The prominent bulging at the right cardiac border indicated RA enlargement.

**Comments:** Abnormal findings in patients with PAH usually include prominent central pulmonary arteries and attenuation of peripheral vascular markings (pruning). Signs of RA and RV enlargement may also be present. Enlargement of the RA is expected, given the findings on the physical examination and ECG. If LA enlargement were also present (not seen here in Fig. 15-2), one should consider left AV valve regurgitation as a cause.

## EXERCISE TESTING

A cardiopulmonary test was not performed.

Distance walked: 185 m

Pretest $O_2$ saturation: 78% (room air)

Posttest $O_2$ saturation: 65% (room air)

Posttest heart rate: 119 bpm

**Comments:** The 6-minute walk test (6MWT) is commonly used as an "objective" measure of exercise capacity in patients with PAH.[7] It has been demonstrated that, in patients with idiopathic PAH, the distance walked in 6 minutes is related to functional class and is predictive of mortality.[8] For example, 185 m is a very low distance for this test, even in cyanotic patients.

Also, a 6MWT distance of less than 300 m with a reduction in oxygen saturation of more than 10% is associated with an increased mortality in patients with idiopathic PAH.[8] But in a cyanotic patient with PAH due to congenital heart disease, this amount of exertional desaturation is expected, and has no known prognostic implications.

## ECHOCARDIOGRAM

### OVERALL FINDINGS

The LV was normal in size and function. The RV was moderately dilated and hypertrophied due to pressure overload, but RV systolic function was preserved. The LA and RA were mildly dilated. There was mild left AV valve and moderate right AV valve regurgitation. The peak velocity through the right AV valve was 4.0 m/sec, suggesting an estimated right ventricular pressure of approximately 80 mm Hg.

There was a large defect in the lower part of the atrial septum. The insertion of the left AV valve and tricuspid valve were at the same level (loss of the normal apical offset with the septal tricuspid leaflet normally being closer to the apex, characteristic of AVSDs).

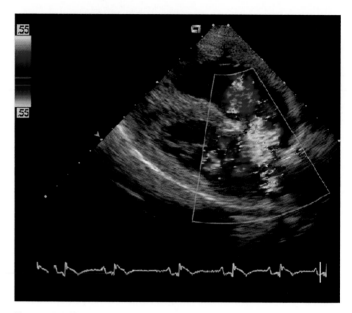

Figure 15-3 Parasternal long-axis view, 2D color Doppler.

**Comments:** Echo confirms the presence of an AVSD, as well as elevated pulmonary arterial pressure. In AVSD, because the AV valves have a different structure, the terms "mitral" and "tricuspid" are replaced by "left" and "right" AV.

Left-sided AV valve regurgitation is common in patients with primum ASD or partial AVSD. In this case, there is only mild left AV valve regurgitation.

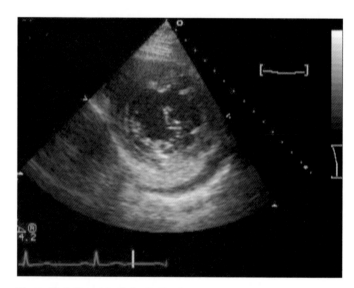

Figure 15-4 Parasternal short-axis view.

## FINDINGS

A common AV junction. The left AV valve had three leaflets, sometimes described as a "cleft mitral valve."

**Comments:** Again, the diagnosis of AVSD is made. The "mitral" valve is actually made up of two bridging leaflets and a mural leaflet, which gives the appearance of having a "cleft."

In this case, there is a known large atrial septal communication (primum ASD), but no ventricular septal communication was seen. Although there is a common AV valve ring, there are two separate valve orifices. Hence, this should be called a partial

AVSD, as opposed to a complete AVSD, where only one undivided AV orifice is present.

## MAGNETIC RESONANCE IMAGING

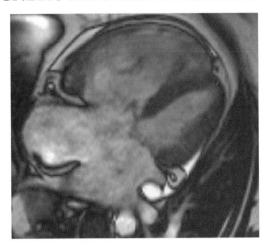

Figure 15-5 Oblique transaxial plane, four-chamber view, early systole.

### Ventricular Volume Quantification

|  | LV | (Normal range) | RV | (Normal range) |
|---|---|---|---|---|
| EDV (mL) | 138 | (52–141) | 184 | (58–154) |
| ESV (mL) | 50 | (13–51) | 101 | (12–68) |
| SV (mL) | 88 | (33–97) | 83 | (35–98) |
| EF (%) | 64 | (57–75) | 45 | (51–75) |
| EDVi (mL/m$^2$) | 68 | (62–96) | 91 | (61–98) |
| ESVi (mL/m$^2$) | 25 | (17–36) | 50 | (17–43) |
| SVi (mL/m$^2$) | 43 | (40–65) | 41 | (20–40) |

### FINDINGS

There was a large atrial septal communication (common atrium) but no signal loss to suggest substantial flow across the defect. The atria were both enlarged. The left and right AV valves shared a common insertion point on the septum. The RV was mildly dilated and hypertrophied, with mildly reduced function. LV function was normal. There was no ventricular septal communication. The study also showed moderate right AV valve regurgitation and mild left AV valve regurgitation. The Qp/Qs ratio was 0.94.

*Comments:* Because the right and left AV valves share a common ring, they meet at the septum. That is, the usual deviation of the septal leaflet of the tricuspid valve toward the apex is not present in AVSD patients.

The hypertrophy of the RV reflects pulmonary hypertension. RV volumes are greater than LV volumes because of the tricuspid regurgitation, since the previous left-to-right shunt has disappeared. The lack of visible flow across the defect is not surprising given both its size (flow will be laminar rather than turbulent, and signal loss will not occur) and the equalization of atrial pressures.

The additional findings support the diagnosis of PAH. The Qp/Qs ratio does not mean that little or no shunting occurs, only that the net shunt is very small (i.e., left-to-right shunt volume is approximately equal to right-to-left shunt volume). MRI can estimate flow, and *net* right-to-left shunt and flow ratio, but not the actual amount of shunt.

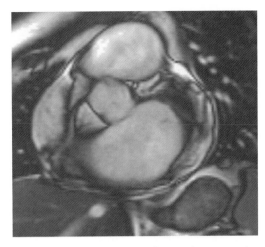

Figure 15-6 Oblique sagittal plane, steady-state free precession cine.

### FINDINGS

The aortic valve is in the center of the image. Below it the large oval is the common atrium. No atrial septum is seen, and the "defect" measures 50 mm in diameter.

*Comments:* The size of this defect is large enough to result in pulmonary vascular disease and pulmonary hypertension.[1]

This again confirms the presence of a common AV valve ring. The valve itself is made up of two bridging leaflets (superior and inferior), a mural leaflet on the left, and usually an anterior and mural leaflet on the right. The left AV valve is made up of portions of the two bridging leaflets and the left mural leaflet.

## COMPUTED TOMOGRAPHY

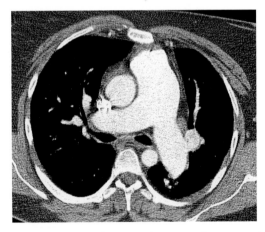

Figure 15-7 Chest computed tomography scan, pulmonary angiogram.

### FINDINGS

There was dilatation of the main pulmonary artery (50 mm, normally less than 27 mm) and branches (30 mm on the right and 25 mm on the left). No pulmonary arterial thrombus was found.

*Comments:* High resolution CT is especially useful to assess pulmonary arterial thrombi and to exclude intrapulmonary hemorrhage or infarction in patients with PAH. It is also the test of choice for assessing the lung parenchyma. In this case, it is important to identify whether thrombi are present given the known PAH and history of possible pulmonary embolus.

# CATHETERIZATION

## HEMODYNAMICS

Hemodynamic findings are shown on the drawing below.

| Calculations | Room Air | Oxygen |
|---|---|---|
| Qp (L/min) | 3.43 | 3.83 |
| Qs (L/min) | 4.47 | 4.11 |
| Cardiac index (L/min/m²) | 2.21 | 2.03 |
| Qp/Qs | 0.77 | 0.93 |
| PVR (Wood units) | 13.69 | 7.05 |
| SVR (Wood units) | 20.34 | 22.17 |

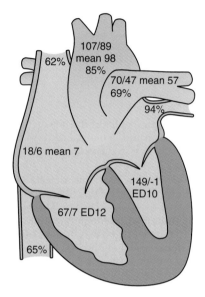

Figure 15-8 Hemodynamic findings.

## FINDINGS

Cardiac catheterization was performed to assess pulmonary arterial pressures and vascular resistance, and to determine vasoreactivity.

The study demonstrated moderate PAH with pulmonary artery pressures two thirds of systemic level. There was a positive vasoreactivity study. With oxygen and nitric oxide inhalation, mean pulmonary artery pressure fell from 57 to 37 mm Hg, and pulmonary vascular resistance fell from 13.7 to 7.0 Wood units.

**Comments:** The data confirm that pulmonary vascular resistance is high, meaning that elevated pulmonary artery pressures are not merely secondary to high flow or left atrial hypertension. RV hypertrophy will restrict filling and favor right-to-left shunting.

In addition, vasodilator testing (using inhaled nitric oxide) showed an acute vasoreactive response with a marked reduction in pulmonary vascular resistance. This finding is an important prognostic sign, as responsiveness to inhaled nitric oxide (NO) is associated with a better outcome.[9] However, in this case, even after NO inhalation, the pulmonary vascular resistance is too high to recommend closure of the ASD.

Ventriculography was not performed.

### FOCUSED CLINICAL QUESTIONS AND DISCUSSION POINTS

1. What is the anatomical diagnosis?

*The patient has a partial AVSD, or ostium primum ASD. This is different from a secundum ASD in that it cannot be closed by a device (though not relevant in this case). Left AV valve regurgitation may be or become important (see Case 13), and subaortic stenosis may develop (see Case 12) in patients with AVSD.*

2. Why is the patient cyanotic?

*This patient clearly shunts a large volume of venous blood right to left through her large atrial septal communication due to increased pulmonary vascular resistance. But what is the cause of PAH? Normally patients with even large atrial defects do not develop Eisenmenger physiology even later in life.[1] In this patient the defect is very large, so this is still definitely a possibility. But are there other potential mechanisms for her cyanosis?*

*Alternatively, PAH may be idiopathic or secondary to chronic thromboembolic disease or sleep apnea, both potentially relevant in this case (for a more in-depth discussion of etiologies, see Case 81). Regardless of why PAH develops, RV hypertrophy will occur and will lower RV compliance, favoring right-to-left shunting at the atrial level.*

*Catheterization was undertaken here to measure pulmonary vascular resistance and vasoreactivity. The results demonstrated pulmonary vascular disease. Distinguishing primary pulmonary hypertension from secondary or Eisenmenger syndrome may be clinically irrelevant. This patient should be treated as having Eisenmenger syndrome.*

3. Should the ASD be closed? What are the potential risks of closing the ASD?

*Closure of an atrial communication should be considered if the patient has a substantial left-to-right shunt. She does not, as evidenced by her pulmonary artery saturation of only 69% (rather than the 80% or more expected with a large left-to-right shunt). Were the pulmonary flow rates high, ASD closure could reduce pulmonary arterial pressures, but this is not true for this patient. The patient is not a candidate for ASD closure under these circumstances.*

4. Is the patient a candidate for other therapy for PAH?

*The patient has been on a calcium-channel blocker (nifedipine) for some time. Use of high-dose calcium-channel blockers has been found to improve clinical condition and prognosis in vasoreactive idiopathic pulmonary hypertension patients—that is, patients with a positive vasoreactive response to nitric oxide (see Case 81).[10] Whether calcium-channel blocker treatment is equally beneficial for patients with PAH as part of Eisenmenger syndrome is unknown.*

*Other therapeutic options include prostacyclin in various forms, phosphodiesterase inhibitors such as sildenafil, and endothelin-receptor antagonists such as bosentan. A recent randomized, blind placebo control study showed that bosentan, an oral dual-receptor endothelin antagonist, was safe and led to improved pulmonary hemodynamics and improved 6MWT and functional class in patients with Eisenmenger syndrome.[3] Therefore, bosentan may represent a therapeutic option for class III patients, and other treatment options may be considered when the evidence base widens.[11]*

## FINAL DIAGNOSIS

Partial AVSD (primum ASD) with PAH and Eisenmenger syndrome

Iron deficiency

## PLAN OF ACTION

Medical therapy

## INTERVENTION

None

# OUTCOME

The first goal of medical therapy was to replace the patient's iron stores. This was done with oral ferrous sulfate, which she tolerated well. After 3 months, her laboratory results were as follows:

| | | |
|---|---|---|
| Hemoglobin | **23.5 g/dL** | (11.5–15.0) |
| MCV | 94 fL | (83–99) |
| MCH | 32.4 pg | (27–32.5) |
| Hematocrit | **68%** | (36%–46%) |
| Ferritin | 121 ng/mL | (20–186) |

These results show a marked elevation in her hemoglobin due to restoration of normal iron stores. The patient noted improvement in her symptoms. A repeat 6MWT distance was 350 m, a marked improvement, although still within the range of therapeutic indications for advanced therapies (150 to 450 m).

The patient was maintained on warfarin because of her documented PAH and her previous history of deep venous thrombosis with presumed pulmonary embolism. Warfarin requires special monitoring in the setting of cyanosis (see Case 41).

The patient was then started on oral bosentan therapy, which she tolerated well. At 6 months she was feeling better and her 6MWT had improved further to 470 meters.

## Selected References

1. Wood P: The Eisenmenger syndrome or pulmonary hypertension with reversed central shunt. Br Med J 2:701–709, 755–762, 1958.
2. Archer S, Rich S: Primary pulmonary hypertension: A vascular biology and translational research "work in progress." Circulation 102:2781–2791, 2000.
3. Galie N, Torbicki A, Barst R, et al: Guidelines on diagnosis and treatment of pulmonary arterial hypertension. The Task Force on Diagnosis and Treatment of Pulmonary Arterial Hypertension of the European Society of Cardiology. Eur Heart J 25:2243–2278, 2004.
4. Broberg C, Jayaweera R, Diller G, et al: The optimal relationship between oxygen saturation and hemoglobin in adult patients with cyanotic congenital heart disease can be determined and correlates with exercise capacity [abstract]. Circulation 114:11–503, 2006.
5. Ammash N, Warnes CA: Cerebrovascular events in adult patients with cyanotic congenital heart disease. J Am Coll Cardiol 28: 768–772, 1996.
6. Kaemmerer H, Fratz S, Braun SL, et al: Erythrocyte indexes, iron metabolism, and hyperhomocysteinemia in adults with cyanotic congenital cardiac disease. Am J Cardiol 94:825–828, 2004.
7. Hoeper MM, Rubin LJ: Update in pulmonary hypertension 2005. Am J Respir Crit Care Med 173:499–505, 2006.
8. Miyamoto S, Nagaya N, Satoh T, et al: Clinical correlates and prognostic significance of six-minute walk test in patients with primary pulmonary hypertension: Comparison with cardiopulmonary exercise testing. Am J Respir Crit Care Med 161:487–492, 2000.
9. Post MC, Janssens S, Van de Werf F, Budts W: Responsiveness to inhaled nitric oxide is a predictor for mid-term survival in adult patients with congenital heart defects and pulmonary arterial hypertension. Eur Heart J 25:1651–1656, 2004.
10. Rich S, Kaufmann E, Levy PS: The effect of high doses of calcium-channel blockers on survival in primary pulmonary hypertension. N Engl J Med 327:76–81, 1992.
11. Diller G-P, Gatzoulis MA: Pulmonary vascular disease in adults with congenital heart disease. Circulation 115:1039–1050, 2007.

## Bibliography

Galiè N, Beghetti M, Gatzoulis MA, et al, on behalf of the BREATHE-5 Investigators: Bosentan therapy in patients with Eisenmenger syndrome: A multi-centre, double-blind randomised placebo-controlled study. Circulation 114:48–54, 2006.

Humbert M, Sitbon O, Simonneau G: Treatment of pulmonary arterial hypertension. N Engl J Med 351:1425–1436, 2004.

Schwerzmann M, Zafar M, McLaughlin PR, et al: Atrial septal defect closure in a patient with "irreversible" pulmonary hypertensive arteriopathy. Int J Cardiol 110:104–107, 2006.

# Patent Ductus Arteriosus

# Catheter Closure of a Patent Ductus Arteriosus

**Vaikom S. Mahadevan, Eric M. Horlick, and Peter R. McLaughlin**

**Age: 68**
**Gender: Female**
**Occupation: Housewife**
**Working diagnosis: Patent ductus arteriosus**

## HISTORY

The patient had a normal birth and upbringing but was told a cardiac murmur was present.

Within the previous year she had two episodes of pneumonia. The workup that ensued included an echocardiogram, which suggested a PDA.

## CURRENT SYMPTOMS

She is generally healthy and asymptomatic. She experiences shortness of breath after climbing three flights of stairs. She denies palpitations, unexplained fevers, or hemoptysis.

NYHA class: I

**Comments:** Patients with a small PDA often remain asymptomatic throughout a normal lifespan.

## CURRENT MEDICATIONS

None

## PHYSICAL EXAMINATION

General: Moderate build. Pink.

BP (right upper limb) 140/50 mm Hg, HR 65 bpm, oxygen saturation 98% in both fingers and toes

Height 163 cm, weight 56 kg, BSA 1.59 m²

Neck veins: Venous pulse was not elevated and the waveform was normal.

Lungs/chest: Clear

Heart: Normal precordial examination. There were normal first and second heart sounds, with a grade 2/6 continuous murmur at the upper left sternal edge and the infraclavicular area.

Abdomen: Normal

Extremities: No cyanosis or clubbing of fingers or toes

**Comments:** The wide pulse pressure and low diastolic pressure suggest a moderately large PDA (most commonly seen in aortic regurgitation, but common in high to low pressure communications involving the aorta).

In patients with a PDA and severe pulmonary hypertension there may be differential cyanosis and clubbing seen only in the toes and not in the fingers (see Case 17). This is due to the right-to-left shunt being distal to the upper limb circulation.

The continuous murmur is typical of a PDA, and is classically described as machinelike due to its "rough" quality. There are a number of other lesions producing continuous murmurs, including ruptured sinus of Valsalva aneurysm and coronary AV fistulas.

## LABORATORY DATA

| | |
|---|---|
| Hemoglobin | 12.9 g/dL (11.5–15.0) |
| Hematocrit/PCV | 38% (36–46) |
| Platelet count | 193 × 10⁹/L (150–400) |
| Sodium | 141 mmol/L (134–145) |
| Potassium | 3.7 mmol/L (3.5–5.2) |
| Creatinine | 0.64 mmol/dL (0.6–1.2) |

**Comments:** These results are all normal, as expected.

## ELECTROCARDIOGRAM

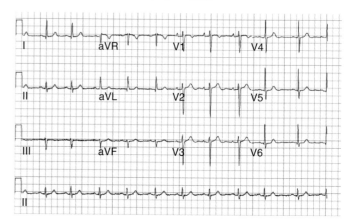

Figure 16-1 Electrocardiogram.

## FINDINGS

Heart rate: 65 bpm

QRS axis: −10°

QRS duration: 106 msec

Sinus rhythm with normal axis, intervals, and segments. Normal ECG.

**Comments:** There is no evidence of LV or LA overload in this ECG, which would suggest a substantial left-to-right shunt. Likewise, there is no evidence of right ventricular hypertrophy, which would be expected in a patient with a large PDA that has caused pulmonary arterial hypertension (see Case 17).

## CHEST X-RAY

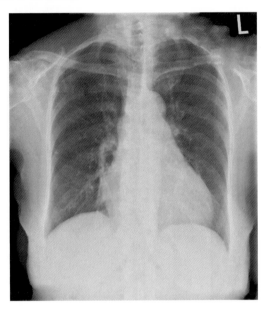

Figure 16-2 Posteroanterior projection.

## FINDINGS

Cardiothoracic ratio: 62%

The cardiac silhouette is enlarged. There is mild prominence of the main pulmonary artery segment.

**Comments:** Cardiomegaly can occur in older patients even with relatively small shunts due to long-standing volume overloading of the heart. For patients with a PDA, the left-to-right shunt involves the LA and LV as well as the proximal aorta and pulmonary arteries. If the PDA was very large, the left-to-right shunt would have reversed early in childhood, due to the development of severe PAH. This clearly does not apply in this patient.

Ductal calcification can be seen superimposed on the aortic knuckle.

## ECHOCARDIOGRAM

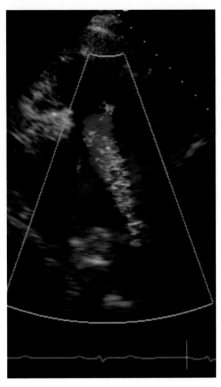

Figure 16-3 Color Doppler imaging in the parasternal short-axis view.

## FINDINGS

Normal LV size and systolic function. The LVEDD was 4.9 cm. The LA dimension was 3.8 cm. RV chamber sizes were normal. The main pulmonary artery was dilated and measured 40 mm. There was mild tricuspid regurgitation with a calculated RV systolic pressure of 42 mm Hg.

This revealed turbulent flow from the aorta (seen in cross section) toward the pulmonary trunk (toward the transducer, top of the image).

**Comments:** Color flow from the aorta into the pulmonary artery, especially the left pulmonary artery, as in this case, confirms the diagnosis of a PDA. Rarely, a native, small aorto-pulmonary window can present with a somewhat similar color flow pattern in an adult patient. The communication in such a case is much more proximal in the main pulmonary artery and not at the level of bifurcation as with PDA. Mild pulmonary hypertension is seen in this patient as a result of a long-standing left-to-right shunt, but pulmonary vascular resistance is not likely to be significantly elevated.

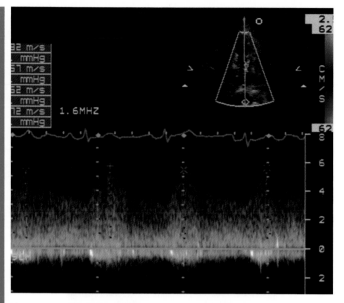

Figure 16-4 Continuous Doppler examination of ductus flow.

## FINDINGS

Continuous Doppler examination reveals high-velocity continuous flow in the pulmonary artery with a peak systolic gradient of 135 mm Hg.

***Comments:*** With a patent ductus there is continuous flow from the aorta to the pulmonary artery during systole and diastole, often described as a "machinery" murmur. When significant pulmonary hypertension develops, flow may be only systolic or bidirectional. In patients with severe pulmonary hypertension there may be reversal of flow from the pulmonary artery into the aorta, leading to differential (lower body) cyanosis and toe clubbing.

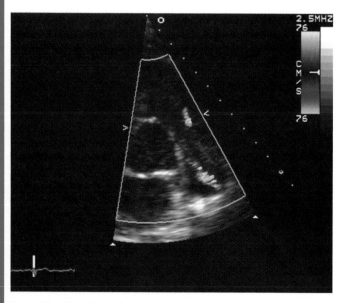

Figure 16-5 Two-dimensional color Doppler examination of the pulmonary artery.

## FINDINGS

There was trace pulmonary valve regurgitation. In addition, left-to-right flow from the PDA was visible.

***Comments:*** In this view, angled slightly differently from the first, the Doppler data show both PR and PDA flow in diastole. The two jets demonstrate the relative anatomical relationship of these two structures. The aortic valve in cross section is visible to the left.

# MAGNETIC RESONANCE IMAGING

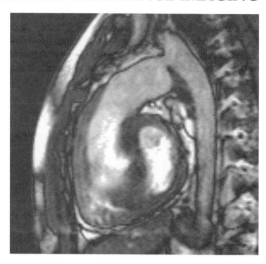

Figure 16-6 Sagittal steady-state free precession cine (right ventricular outflow tract view).

### Ventricular Volume Quantification

|  | LV | (Normal range) | RV | (Normal range) |
|---|---|---|---|---|
| EDV (mL) | 152 | (52–141) | 111 | (58–154) |
| ESV (mL) | 42 | (13–51) | 43 | (12–68) |
| SV (mL) | 110 | (33–97) | 68 | (35–98) |
| EF (%) | 72 | (60–78) | 61 | (57–81) |
| EDVi (mL/m²) | 95 | (53–87) | 70 | (49–86) |
| ESVi (mL/m²) | 26 | (13–31) | 27 | (8–34) |
| SVi (mL/m²) | 69 | (36–60) | 43 | (16–36) |
| Mass index (g/m²) | 84 | (48–78) | 65 | (16–36) |

## FINDINGS

A patent ductus was visible with flow from the descending intrathoracic aorta (to the right in Fig. 16-6) to the main pulmonary artery (on the left). Phase contrast velocity flow mapping showed output through the proximal main pulmonary artery and through the aorta was consistent with the ventricular stroke volumes measured. Function of both ventricles was normal. The LV was mildly enlarged.

***Comments:*** Though not necessary to make the diagnosis, the MRI study confirmed the predominant left-to-right shunt, and normal function of the RV and LV. All this is reassuring information in relation to plans to close the defect.

It should be pointed out that velocity flow mapping of the proximal great vessels quantifies flow before the shunt, and therefore does not give information about the volume flowing to each capillary bed. In other words, the RV and LV stroke volumes here, or comparable aortic and pulmonary artery flow mapping data, would give a Qp/Qs ratio of 0.6, implying significant right-to-left shunt, which is erroneous. Since PDA flow volume loads the left heart chambers, and not the right, the LV stroke volume reflects Qp, and thus the true Qp/Qs is actually the inverse of the RV and LV stroke volumes. The LV and RV stroke volumes here of 110 and 68 mL, respectively, when properly considered, give an approximate shunt of 1.6. It is important that these concepts are understood for proper interpretation of the data obtained.

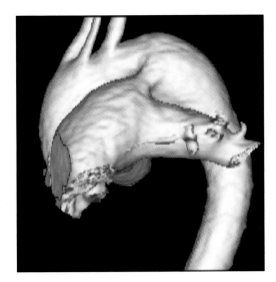

Figure 16-7 Three-dimensional volume reconstruction of cardiac magnetic resonance image showing duct anatomy.

## FINDINGS

The PDA and its relationship to surrounding structures was clearly evident.

**Comments:** Reconstructed images such as these can assist the interventionalist in planning closure.

## CATHETERIZATION

### HEMODYNAMICS

| | Pressure | Saturation (%) |
|---|---|---|
| SVC | | 79 |
| IVC | | 74 |
| RA | 6 | |
| RV | 39/5 | |
| PA | 38/12 mean 22 | 87 |
| PCWP | 8 | 98 |
| LA | | |
| LV | 138/7 | |
| Aorta | 136/52 mean 82 | 98 |

| Calculations | |
|---|---|
| Qp (L/min) | 7.49 |
| Qs (L/min) | 4.07 |
| Cardiac index (L/min/m²) | 2.55 |
| Qp/Qs | 1.84 |
| PVR (Wood units) | 2.00 |
| SVR (Wood units) | 18.68 |

**Comments:** Hemodynamic measurements are not essential unless there is a question about increased pulmonary vascular resistance. In this case, the findings were confirmatory of the suspected shunt estimated by MRI.

The measured saturation in the pulmonary artery will differ among the main, right, and left branches because of "streaming." Estimates of pulmonary flow and the Qp/Qs ratio based on oximetry data may not be accurate as a result. The MRI data, if properly done and interpreted, may give a more reliable measurement of shunt fraction. In this case, the two modalities agree fairly well.

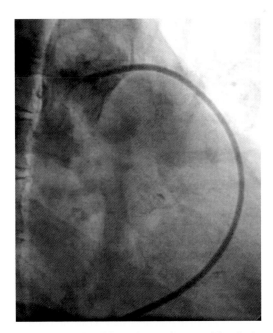

Figure 16-8 Right anterior oblique view angiogram of the duct.

## FINDINGS

Image obtained as part of the interventional therapeutic procedure.

**Comments:** The catheter has been introduced into the right heart and through the PDA into the descending aorta, and there is calcification seen at the aortic ampulla of the ductus.

### FOCUSED CLINICAL QUESTIONS AND DISCUSSION POINTS

1. **Is the patent ductus responsible for any of the symptoms in this patient?**

   *Mild exercise intolerance could be attributed to this amount of shunting. Left-to-right shunts are said be associated with more frequent lower respiratory infections, but it is difficult to be sure about the causal relationship between her pneumonia and the PDA.*

2. **Should a PDA in an asymptomatic adult be closed?**

   *In view of the risk of endocarditis, any ductus with an audible murmur should be considered for closure even in the absence of symptoms.[1] While many practitioners would agree, others would feel the risk of endocarditis is very small, and would not recommend proceeding to PDA closure.*

3. **What technical considerations or limitations must be considered for closure?**

   *Almost any PDA found today will be closed via catheter rather than surgery. In children, this is usually done with coils, since these can be delivered through smaller sheaths. In adults, sheath size is not a major issue and defects are usually larger; hence, coil embolization is not the best method, as it is more likely to lead to incomplete closure. In contrast, the Amplatzer PDA occluder device is particularly suited for the older child or adult with a PDA. This particular device has been shown to have excellent initial and 1-year outcomes for closure of moderate to large ducts.[2] Calcified ducts may be difficult to cannulate from the pulmonary end. If so, these can be entered from the aortic side with a JL4 catheter, and the wire snared from the pulmonary side. Furthermore, small, calcified ducts may require a smaller size sheath (e.g., 7 Fr), since larger sheaths may not be able to traverse the ductus.*

## FINAL DIAGNOSIS

Incidental PDA

## PLAN OF ACTION

Transcatheter device closure of the defect

## INTERVENTION

Access was obtained via the right femoral vein and an 8 Fr sheath was inserted. A Gensini catheter was used to enter the pulmonary artery, and a straight-tipped wire was used to traverse the ductus into the descending aorta. The catheter was maneuvered over the wire into the descending aorta, and an angiogram was obtained in the right oblique projection. The duct measured 2 mm in diameter with a calcified ampulla. Subsequently, a long 10 Fr Amplatzer delivery system sheath was exchanged for the Gensini catheter, and an 8 × 6 mm Amplatzer duct occluder was deployed under fluoroscopic guidance.

## OUTCOME

The patient underwent successful device closure of a calcified patent ductus. There were no complications. The continuous murmur disappeared after the procedure. She was advised to practice antibiotic prophylaxis for dental and other potentially infective procedures for a further 6-month period.

At follow-up she had no audible murmur. By echocardiography no flow was seen across the closed duct. She was told that endocarditis prophylaxis was no longer necessary.

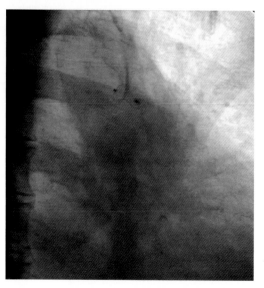

Figure 16-9   Angiogram.

### FINDINGS

RAO imaging showing the Amplatzer ductal occluder in position.

**Comments:** Device embolization is less likely with the Amplatzer ductal occluder, which is the preferred method for a patent ductus in adults as compared to coils. The newer Amplatzer Duct Occluder II can also be deployed for duct closure from the aortic end.

## Selected References

1. Rao PS: Transcatheter occlusion of patent ductus arteriosus: Which method to use and which ductus to close. Am Heart J 132:905–909, 1996.
2. Pass RH, Hijazi Z, Hsu DT, et al: Multicentre USA Amplatzer patent ductus arteriosus device trial: Initial and one-year results. J Am Coll Cardiol 44:513–519, 2004.

# Erythrocytosis with Normal Oxygen Saturation

**Gerhard-Paul Diller**

**Age: 27 years**
**Gender: Female**
**Working diagnosis: Down syndrome**

## HISTORY

The patient has Down syndrome and was suspected to have cardiac disease shortly after birth. Echocardiography, however, showed only a subaortic membrane with a peak gradient of 43 mm Hg across the LVOT. The atrial and ventricular septa were intact, and no other lesions were seen.

She was assessed again at the age of 18. She had a good exercise capacity (498 m walked in 6 minutes) without significant desaturation during exercise. Echocardiography showed an unchanged gradient across the LVOT, as well as normal LV and RV dimensions and function. The patient was subsequently lost to follow-up.

A blood count arranged by her local general practitioner 1 year before presentation showed an elevated hematocrit and hemoglobin. There was a normal white cell and platelet count. She was seen by a hematologist, who found no other abnormality.

She began to experience increasing dyspnea on exertion and was referred for further workup.

***Comments:*** Down syndrome, or trisomy of chromosome 21, is present in approximately 0.7 out of 1000 live births[1] and accounts for 95% of all syndromic congenital malformations. The various types of congenital heart defects seen include ventricular septal defect, PDA, atrioventricular septal defect, and atrial septal defect.[1,2]

The hematologic finding of increased hemoglobin/hematocrit with a normal white cell and platelet count is consistent with erythrocytosis, rather than polycythemia (in which all cell lines are increased). This finding therefore should alert the physician to look for evidence of hypoxemia due to a right-to-left shunt.

## CURRENT SYMPTOMS

The patient notes dyspnea after walking 200 m on level ground and becomes breathless when climbing stairs. The patient denies chest pain, palpitations, or syncope. She sleeps well and does not snore.

NYHA class: III

***Comments:*** Snoring may be important, since sleep apnea, common in patients with Down syndrome, can contribute to PAH, heart failure, and stroke risk.

## CURRENT MEDICATIONS

None

## PHYSICAL EXAMINATION

BP 110/60, HR 86 bpm, oxygen saturation 96% on room air (right hand) and 83% in left foot

Height 152 cm, weight 87 kg, BSA 1.92 m$^2$

Surgical scars: None

Neck veins: JVP was not elevated, and there was a normal waveform.

Lungs/chest: Clear

Heart: An RV impulse was palpable. There was variable splitting of the second heart sound with a loud pulmonary component. There was a grade 3 systolic ejection murmur loudest at the upper right sternal edge.

Abdomen: No hepatomegaly

Extremities: Peripheral pulses were all easily palpable. Clubbing was seen in the toes, but not the fingers.

***Comments:*** In any patient such as this it is imperative to look for evidence of differential cyanosis. Lower body cyanosis was present in this patient. If the oximetry data and physical findings are correct, the diagnosis must be a pulmonary hypertensive PDA.

A loud second heart sound is a cardinal clinical sign in patients with pulmonary hypertension.

In this patient the systolic murmur was best heard in the aortic area and it is most likely related to the subaortic ridge described in previous echocardiograms.

## LABORATORY DATA

| | |
|---|---|
| Hemoglobin | **20.2 g/dL** (11.5–15.0) |
| Hematocrit | **58%** (36–46) |
| MCV | **104 fL** (83–99) |
| MCH | **36 pg** (27–32.5) |
| Platelets | 157 × 10$^9$/L (150–400) |
| WBC | 6.7 × 10$^9$/L (3.5–10.8) |
| Sodium | 138 mmol/L (134–145) |
| Potassium | 4.2 mmol/L (3.5–5.2) |
| Creatinine | 0.9 mg/dL (0.6–1.2) |
| Blood urea nitrogen | 4.4 mmol/L (2.5–6.5) |
| Iron | 21 µg/L (12.6–26.0) |
| Ferritin | 37 ng/mL (20–186) |
| TIBC | 73 µmol/L (50–80) |
| Transferrin saturation | 29% (20–45) |
| Vitamin B$_{12}$ | 449 ng/L (180–914) |
| Folate | >20 (>20) |

***Comments:*** The elevated hemoglobin concentration in this patient represents secondary erythrocytosis. Secondary erythrocytosis is seen in chronically cyanotic patients. The term *secondary erythrocytosis* refers to an isolated increase in red blood cells (as opposed to polycythemia, in which all cell lines proliferate) and is a physiologic adaptation to chronic hypoxemia.

The oxygen saturation on room air is 96% in the upper extremity and does not explain a hemoglobin value as high as 20 g/dL. However, there is clinical evidence of lower body cyanosis. Therefore, low renal saturations may account for elevated erythropoietin levels leading to her raised hemoglobin.

There is no evidence of iron, vitamin $B_{12}$, or folate deficiency in this patient. Macrocytosis is common in patients with Down syndrome and is not necessarily related to other deficiencies.[3]

# ELECTROCARDIOGRAM

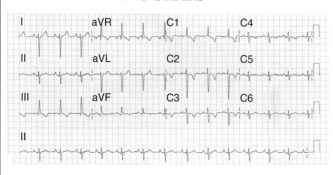

Figure 17-1 Electrocardiogram.

## FINDINGS

Heart rate: 84 bpm

PR int: 170 msec

QRS axis: +160°

QRS duration: 99 msec

Sinus rhythm. Marked right axis deviation. RV hypertrophy with strain pattern in V1–4.

Some peaking of P-waves in I and II

***Comments:*** There is voltage evidence of RV hypertrophy (R/S $V_1$ > 1; R $V_1$ > 7 mm, R/S $V_6$ < 1). There is also right axis deviation and T-wave inversion anteroseptally, consistent with RV "strain."

# CHEST X-RAY

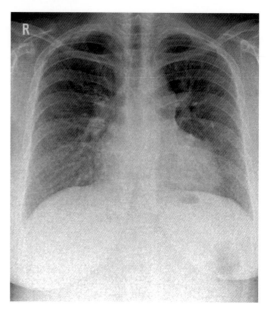

Figure 17-2 Posteroanterior projection.

## FINDINGS

Cardiothoracic ratio: 54%

Mild cardiomegaly, predominantly due to enlargement of the RA. Mildly prominent central pulmonary arteries.

***Comments:*** From what is known so far in this case, the provider should look for evidence of pulmonary hypertension. Abnormal findings in patients with PAH usually include prominent central pulmonary arteries and attenuation of peripheral vascular markings (pruning). Signs of RA and RV enlargement may also be present. Calcification of the PDA should also be sought.

# EXERCISE TESTING

Sinus rhythm throughout

| Exercise protocol: | Modified Bruce |
| --- | --- |
| Duration (min:sec): | 5:48 |
| Reason for stopping: | Dyspnea |
| ECG changes: | None |

|  | Rest | Peak |
| --- | --- | --- |
| Heart rate (bpm): | 86 | 164 |
| Percent of age-predicted max HR: |  | 85 |
| $O_2$ saturation (%): | 96 (83 in foot) | 92 (36 in foot) |
| Blood pressure (mm Hg): | 110/60 | 150/80 |
| Double product: |  | 24,600 |
| Peak $V_{O_2}$ (mL/kg/min): |  | 11.3 |
| Percent predicted (%): |  | 58 |
| $Ve/V_{CO_2}$: |  | 60 |
| Metabolic equivalents: |  | 4.5 |

***Comments:*** Cardiopulmonary exercise testing is used as an objective measure of exercise capacity in patients with adult congenital heart disease. Peak oxygen consumption is related to functional class and is predictive of morbidity in this cohort.[4]

The patient's exercise tolerance is severely reduced.

There is only a mild drop in oxygen saturation in the fingers. A common mistake in these cases is to fail to measure lower body oxygen saturation with exercise, which in this case is markedly reduced. This is consistent with her erythrocytosis. This confirms the presence of a substantial right-to-left shunt with preferential streaming of unoxygenated blood into the lower body during exercise. This finding is diagnostic of a PDA with PAH (Eisenmenger syndrome).

## ECHOCARDIOGRAM

### OVERALL FINDINGS
The LV was normal. The RV was enlarged and hypertrophied with preserved RV systolic function. A flattened interventricular septum throughout the cardiac cycle was seen. The RA was severely enlarged. There was no intracardiac shunt. There was trace tricuspid regurgitation. The mitral valve was normal.

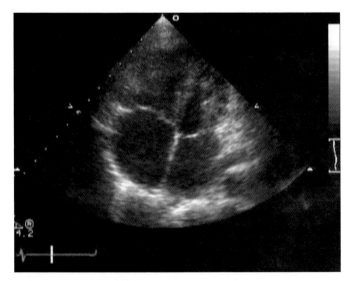

Figure 17-3  Echocardiogram.

***Comments:*** Although no shunt was seen on these images, there is evidence of RV pressure overload from the flattened septum throughout the cycle. In contrast, a volume load, which could be a cause of chamber enlargement, may still allow the septum to bulge toward the RV during systole. There is no significant tricuspid regurgitation or visible shunt to explain RA enlargement, thus this finding more likely reflects elevated RV filling pressures, consistent with the noted RV hypertrophy and expected pressure overload.

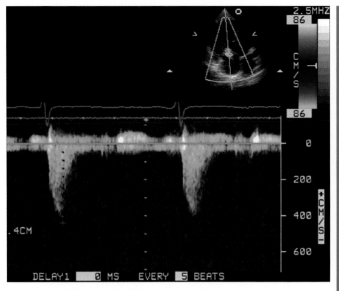

Figure 17-4  Echocardiogram.

### FINDINGS
There was trace tricuspid regurgitation. The peak tricuspid regurgitation velocity was 4.4 m/sec, giving an estimated RV systolic pressure of 88 mm Hg (based on an assumed central venous pressure of 10 mm Hg).

***Comments:*** The tricuspid regurgitation velocity confirms the finding of pulmonary hypertension suggested by the abnormal septal motion, RV hypertrophy, and RA enlargement. Although raised pulmonary artery pressure is almost certain (since no RVOT obstruction is present), Doppler-based predictions of pressure measured in the catheterization laboratory in the setting of PAH are not as accurate.[5]

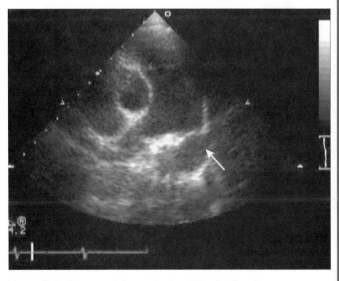

Figure 17-5  Parasternal short-axis view, 2D color Doppler.

### FINDINGS
A PDA measuring 10 mm was seen between the left pulmonary artery and the descending aorta (*arrow*). There was little bidirectional shunt on color Doppler, suggestive of equalized pressures in the main pulmonary artery and the aorta.

**Comments:** This confirms the presence of a large PDA. The lack of visible flow across the defect is explained by the equalization of pressures between the aorta and the main pulmonary artery. This also explains why no typical continuous heart murmur was audible.

# MAGNETIC RESONANCE IMAGING

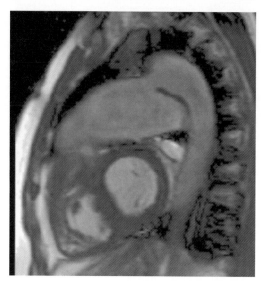

Figure 17-6 Magnetic resonance image.

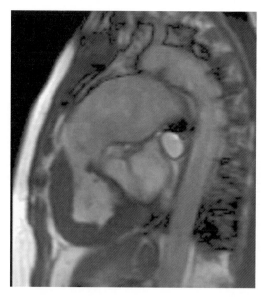

Figure 17-7 Magnetic resonance image.

## FINDINGS

The MRI showed a PDA with no net flow across the defect at rest. The Qp/Qs ratio was 1. The pulmonary artery was dilated, reflecting increased pressure rather than flow in this instance. The RV was hypertrophied but functioned normally. In addition, there was mild LVOT.

**Comments:** A PDA can be easily seen by MRI if specifically sought, but is often missed if the diagnosis is not questioned (see Fig. 17-7). The additional estimates of flow and ventricular size and function can be helpful in determining the physiological significance of the lesion. The quality of imaging is suboptimal, perhaps because of limited patient coordination.

This is the same patient with a slightly different imaging plane, where the PDA is not readily apparent.

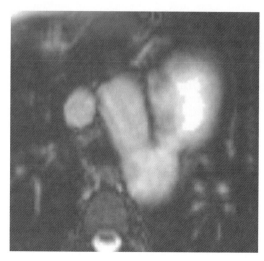

Figure 17-8 Oblique axial steady-state free precession cine of the aortic arch.

**Ventricular Volume Quantification**

| | LV | (Normal range) | RV | (Normal range) |
|---|---|---|---|---|
| EDV (mL) | 96 | (52–141) | 133 | (58–154) |
| ESV (mL) | 34 | (13–51) | 61 | (12–68) |
| SV (mL) | 62 | (33–97) | 72 | (35–98) |
| EF (%) | 65 | (56–75) | 54 | (49–73) |
| EDVi (mL/m$^2$) | **50** | (65–99) | 69 | (65–102) |
| ESVi (mL/m$^2$) | **18** | (19–37) | 32 | (20–45) |
| SVi (mL/m$^2$) | **32** | (42–66) | 38 | (22–42) |
| Mass index (g/m$^2$) | 55 | (47–77) | **50** | (22–42) |

## FINDINGS

A PDA is visible between the descending aorta and the enlarged main pulmonary artery.

**Comments:** Enlargement of the pulmonary artery is typical when pulmonary hypertension is present. It appears more dilated than it actually is in this view (see Fig. 17-8) because of the obliquity of the viewing plane. Just below this level, the right and left pulmonary arteries branch to either side of the ductus.

# COMPUTED TOMOGRAPHY

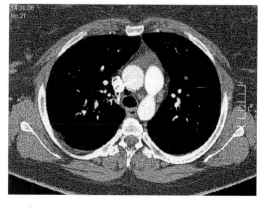

Figure 17-9 Chest computed tomography scan, high resolution.

## FINDINGS

There was a patent duct. The main pulmonary artery was mildly dilated compatible with raised pulmonary artery pressure.

Elsewhere, throughout both lungs there was a mosaic pattern typical of PAH.

There was no evidence of thrombus within the pulmonary arteries, as may be seen in approximately 20% of Eisenmenger patients.[6]

***Comments:*** High-resolution CT is especially useful to assess pulmonary arterial thrombi and to exclude intrapulmonary hemorrhage or infarction in patients with PAH. It is also the test of choice for assessing lung parenchyma. In this case, it also confirms the presence of a PDA.

## CATHETERIZATION

### HEMODYNAMICS

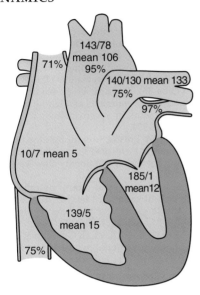

Figure 17-10 Hemodynamic findings.

Saturation descending aorta: 84%

**Calculations**

| | |
|---|---|
| Qp (L/min) | 3.63 |
| Qs (L/min) | 3.47 |
| Cardiac index (L/min/m²) | 1.81 |
| Qp/Qs | 1.05 |
| PVR (Wood units) | 33.34 |
| SVR (Wood units) | 29.09 |

### FINDINGS

Cardiac catheterization was performed to confirm the diagnoses and to assess pulmonary arterial pressures. In retrospect, this was not necessary.

The study demonstrated severe PAH with pulmonary artery pressures at systemic level. A large PDA with bidirectional shunting was found.

***Comments:*** The data confirm that the patient has a large PDA with Eisenmenger physiology.

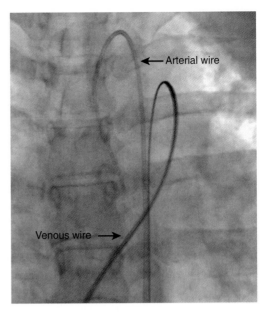

Figure 17-11 Anteroposterior projection angiogram.

***Comments:*** AP projection with one wire placed in the ascending aorta and a second wire introduced into the descending aorta from the venous side via the persistent duct.

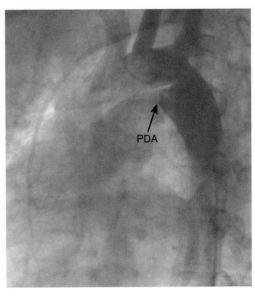

Figure 17-12 Lateral aortogram showing the persistent arterial duct.

### FOCUSED CLINICAL QUESTIONS AND DISCUSSION POINTS

1. **What is the diagnosis?**

   *The patient has a PDA with Eisenmenger physiology. The case is a reminder that in any patient with an elevated hemoglobin and normal right arm oxygen saturation, a pulmonary hypertensive patent ductus should be considered.*

2. **Why does the patient have erythrocytosis despite having "normal" oxygen saturations?**

   *This patient clearly shunts venous blood right to left through her PDA into the descending aorta. The oxygen saturations in the descending aorta are substantially lower than those in the ascend-*

*ing aorta, especially during heart catheterization and at peak exercise. Therefore, the renal parenchyma receives hypoxic blood leading to an increased erythropoietin production with subsequent secondary erythrocytosis. Again, abnormal oxygen saturations may be missed if oxygen saturation is measured only in the upper extremities. Therefore, if a pulmonary hypertensive PDA is suspected, oxygen saturations should also be determined in the lower extremities and digital clubbing should be sought in both upper and lower limbs.*

### 3. What is the cause of pulmonary hypertension?

*The fact that a large nonrestrictive arterial communication between the systemic and pulmonary circulation can lead to pulmonary vascular disease with subsequent shunt reversal is well recognized.[7] Therefore, the presence of a large PDA—as in this patient—explains the presence of Eisenmenger physiology. It is noteworthy, however, that patients with Down syndrome are more susceptible to the development of pulmonary hypertension even in the absence of structural heart disease.[8] This may be in part because of upper airway obstruction and a sleep apnea type of mechanism, although there was no suggestion of that for our patient from the history. Whether routine sleep studies should be performed in such patients is unclear.*

### 4. Is the patient a candidate for drug therapy?

*Different therapeutic options including prostacyclin in various forms, phosphodiesterase inhibitors such as sildenafil, calcium antagonists, and endothelin-receptor antagonists such as bosentan may be beneficial in patients with idiopathic pulmonary hypertension.[9] A recent randomized placebo-controlled trial has demonstrated that oral bosentan (a dual-receptor endothelin antagonist) therapy is effective in improving functional capacity and pulmonary hemodynamics in patients with Eisenmenger syndrome.[10] Therefore, bosentan may be a therapeutic option for this patient even though currently experience with bosentan in patients with Down syndrome is limited.*

## FINAL DIAGNOSIS

Persistent ductus arteriosus with PAH and Eisenmenger syndrome

## PLAN OF ACTION

Conservative management, with advice against therapeutic phlebotomies and for avoidance of dehydration

## INTERVENTION

None

## OUTCOME

Two years after her diagnosis, the patient is doing well. Though she still experiences dyspnea on exertion, she is able to cope with this limitation and still participates in daily activities at her school, including walks to local shops, dances, and theater. She has regular follow-up with measurement of oxygen saturation, hemoglobin, and a 6-minute walk test.

## Selected References

1. Grech V, Gatt M: Syndromes and malformations associated with congenital heart disease in a population-based study. Int J Cardiol 68:151–156, 1999.
2. Figueroa JR, Magana BP, Hach JLP, et al: Heart malformations in children with Down syndrome. Rev Esp Cardiol 56:894–899, 2003.
3. Roizen NJ, Amarose AP: Hematologic abnormalities in children with Down syndrome. Am J Med Genet 46:510–512, 1993.
4. Diller GP, Dimopoulos K, Okonko D, et al: Exercise intolerance in adult congenital heart disease: Comparative severity, correlates, and prognostic implication. Circulation 112:828–835, 2005.
5. Brecker SJ, Gibbs JS, Fox KM, et al: Comparison of Doppler derived haemodynamic variables and simultaneous high fidelity pressure measurements in severe pulmonary hypertension. Br Heart J 72:384–389, 1994.
6. Broberg CS, Ujita M, Prasad S, et al: Pulmonary arterial thrombosis in Eisenmenger syndrome is associated with biventricular dysfunction and decreased pulmonary flow velocity. J Am Coll Cardiol 50:634–642, 2007.
7. Wood P: The Eisenmenger syndrome or pulmonary hypertension with reversed central shunt. Br Med J 2:701–709, 755–762, 1958.
8. Cooney TP, Thurlbeck WM: Pulmonary hypoplasia in Down's syndrome. N Engl J Med 307:1170–1173, 1982.
9. Galie N, Torbicki A, Barst R, et al: Guidelines on diagnosis and treatment of pulmonary arterial hypertension: The Task Force on Diagnosis and Treatment of Pulmonary Arterial Hypertension of the European Society of Cardiology. Eur Heart J 25:2243–2278, 2004.
10. Galie N, Beghetti M, Gatzoulis MA, et al: Bosentan Randomized Trial of Endothelin Antagonist Therapy-5 (BREATHE-5) Investigators. Bosentan therapy in patients with Eisenmenger syndrome: A multicenter, double-blind, randomized, placebo-controlled study. Circulation 114:48–54, 2006.

# Left-Sided Lesions

# Part I

# Left Ventricular Inflow

# Cor Triatriatum

**Candice K. Silversides and Andrew Crean**

**Age: 31**
**Gender: Female**
**Occupation: Salesperson**
**Working diagnosis: Palpitations**

## HISTORY

The patient was first noted to have a murmur at age 6 years. The murmur was felt to be a "functional murmur," and no echocardiogram was performed.

She was active in sports during adolescence and had no functional limitations.

She came to medical attention at age 31 because of two episodes of tachycardia. Each episode lasted for 15 seconds and was not associated with syncope. She did not feel overly stressed, had no symptoms of heat or cold intolerance, and did not drink more than one caffeinated beverage a day.

***Comments:*** A young woman presenting with palpitations is common in any adult cardiology clinic. Some associations such as mitral valve prolapse are common, but in many cases, no cardiac abnormalities are found. The subsequent workup should look for clues of structural heart malformations, such as evidence of atrial enlargement or valvular abnormalities. Although the history of a childhood murmur is suspicious, innocent murmurs in children are common.

## CURRENT SYMPTOMS

The patient had no functional limitations. She engaged in aerobics three times weekly without experiencing dizziness, light-headedness, or palpitations.

NYHA class: I

## CURRENT MEDICATIONS

None

## PHYSICAL EXAMINATION

BP 102/68 (in the right arm), HR 80 bpm (regular), oxygen saturations 99% on room air

Height 163 cm, weight 48 kg, BSA 1.5 m$^2$

Surgical scars: None

Neck veins: The JVP was normal with a normal venous waveform.

Lungs/chest: Clear to auscultation

Heart: There were no heaves or thrills. The first heart sound was normal. There was a fixed split second heart sound. The pulmonary component of the second heart sound was normal. At the apex, there was a midsystolic click followed by a grade 2/6 mid-to-late systolic murmur. There were no diastolic murmurs.

Abdomen: There was no evidence of hepatosplenomegaly.

Extremities: There was no pedal edema.

***Comments:*** The midsystolic click followed by the mid-late systolic murmur is diagnostic of mitral valve prolapse. A fixed split second heart sound strongly suggests an ASD.

Notably absent findings in this case include a loud pulmonary component of the second heart sound suggestive of idiopathic pulmonary hypertension, which can affect younger women and lead to RA enlargement and arrhythmia. The right heart was not palpable, making a significant left-to-right shunt less likely. There was no evidence of left heart failure.

## LABORATORY DATA

| | |
|---|---|
| Hemoglobin | 12.7 g/dL (11.5–15.0) |
| MCV | 88 fL (83–99) |
| Platelet count | 233 × 10$^9$/L (150–400) |
| Sodium | 140 mmol/L (134–145) |
| Potassium | 3.8 mmol/L (3.5–5.2) |
| Creatinine | 0.6 mg/dL (0.6–1.2) |

***Comments:*** Normal laboratory findings.

# ELECTROCARDIOGRAM

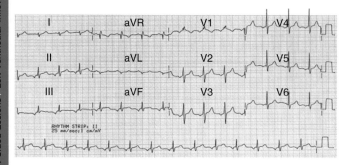

Figure 18-1 Electrocardiogram.

## FINDINGS

Heart rate: 95 bpm

QRS axis: +95°

QRS duration: 104 msec

Coronary sinus or low atrial rhythm with inverted P-waves in the inferior leads, and an RSR' pattern was in lead V1 with a modest persistent S-wave to V6

24-hour Holter monitor: Predominantly "atrial" rhythm with an average heart rate of 78 bpm. Rare isolated premature supraventricular complexes.

**_Comments:_** Inverted P-waves in the inferior leads can indicate lead misplacement or an ectopic atrial pacemaker. In the setting of an ASD, such P-waves suggest a sinus venosus defect. The P-wave axis makes interpretations about atrial size from this ECG difficult. The incomplete RBBB and rightward axis are suspicious for RV hypertrophy. The borderline right axis deviation and 3-mm R-wave suggest RV volume (rather than pressure) overload.

In this patient, the abnormal P-wave forces turned out to be a red herring.

# CHEST X-RAY

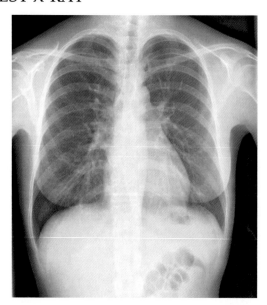

Figure 18-2 Posteroanterior projection.

## FINDINGS

Cardiothoracic ratio: 43%

**_Comments:_** The normal CXR offers strong evidence against pulmonary hypertension. RV hypertrophy is not confirmed, but cannot be excluded.

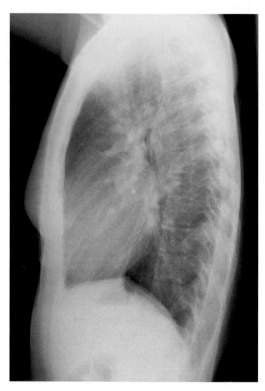

Figure 18-3 Lateral view.

# EXERCISE TESTING

Not performed

# ECHOCARDIOGRAM

## OVERALL FINDINGS

There was normal LV size and function. The RV was mildly enlarged. RV function was normal. The RV systolic pressure was 28 mm Hg. The RA was normal in size. There was mild tricuspid regurgitation. There were myxomatous mitral valve leaflets with mild bileaflet mitral valve prolapse and mild mitral regurgitation.

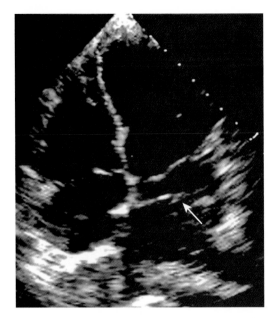

Figure 18-4 Transthoracic echocardiogram, apical four-chamber view.

## FINDINGS

An ASD (secundum type) was present. In addition, the LA was divided by a membranous structure at the midlevel of the LA (*arrow*), which divided the atrium into a pulmonary venous chamber and the true functional atrium communicating with the mitral valve. There was a small orifice in the membrane with turbulent flow across it (peak gradient at rest of 13 mm Hg, mean gradient 4 mm Hg).

**Comments:** This patient has cor triatriatum. Associated anomalies are common and found in 70% of patients. These include ASD (as with this patient), patent foramen ovale, ventricular septal defect, persistent left SVC, partial anomalous pulmonary venous return, patent ductus arteriosus, and aortic coarctation.[1–3]

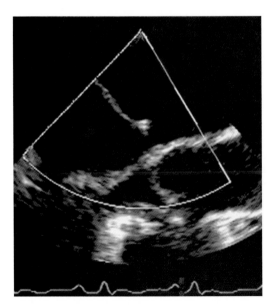

Figure 18-5 Transesophageal echocardiogram.

## FINDINGS

A thin membrane is stretched across the LA. The membrane lay between the left atrial appendage/mitral valve and the common

pulmonary venous chamber. There was an opening in the membrane measuring 7 × 5 mm. All four pulmonary veins drained normally into the common venous chamber. The ASD communicated with the common venous chamber rather than the true LA.

**Comments:** TEE can help to define the location of the membrane or fibromuscular diaphragm and the size and number of fenestrations. There are three anatomic types of cor triatriatum: (1) diaphragmatic, (2) hourglass, and (3) tubular.[4] This is an example of the diaphragmatic type. Cor triatriatum can also be classified according to the size of the opening across the membrane: Group 1, no opening; Group II, one or more openings; and Group III, a wide opening.[5] The size and number of fenestrations in the membrane are variable.

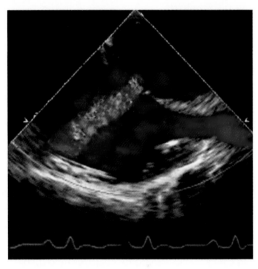

Figure 18-6 Transesophageal echocardiogram of the intra-atrial septum.

## FINDINGS

A small, 0.8-cm secundum ASD was seen between the RA and the pulmonary venous compartment.

**Comments:** Turbulent color flow suggests obstruction. Pulsed Doppler is used to measure the gradient across the opening in the membrane. Three-dimensional echocardiography may provide additional information.[6]

The presence of the ASD allows runoff into the RA. Thus the velocity through the LA membrane may underestimate the true amount of obstruction.

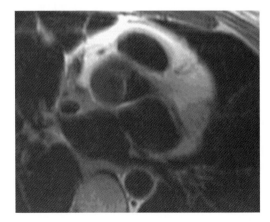

Figure 18-7 Axial double inversion recovery.

## FINDINGS

A membrane or fibromuscular diaphragm separated the pulmonary vein confluence and the true LA.

**Comments:** Cor triatriatum can also be diagnosed by cardiac MRI or CT.[7,8] MRI flow velocities can give estimates of the degree of obstruction and the amount of left-to-right shunting.

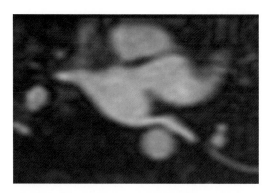

Figure 18-8 Axial reconstruction of a 3D magnetic resonance angiogram.

## FINDINGS

Again, the diaphragm dividing the LA into two components was easily visible. In this view, the right upper pulmonary vein and the left lower pulmonary vein were seen draining into the common pulmonary venous chamber. The common pulmonary venous chamber was separated from the true LA chamber by a membrane. The left atrial appendage is seen in the true LA chamber. The RA and RV, not seen on this view, are mildly dilated. RV systolic function was normal.

**Comments:** These anatomic features help distinguish cor triatriatum from other congenital anomalies such as a supravalvular mitral ring.

### FOCUSED CLINICAL QUESTIONS AND DISCUSSION POINTS

1. **What is the differential diagnosis for the finding of a membrane in the LA?**

   *The differential diagnosis includes prominent folds in the atrial wall, supravalvular mitral rings, and persistent left SVC. Further, the membrane may occasionally appear as an artifact. In cor triatriatum, the distinguishing feature of this type is that the membrane or fibromuscular diaphragm typically originates from the LA wall and lies between the left atrial appendage and the common pulmonary venous chamber.*

   *In patients with cor triatriatum, there may be no defining features on the physical exam. Patients may have nonspecific murmurs. An RV lift or a loud pulmonary component of the second sound would suggest pulmonary hypertension.*

2. **Are the patient's palpitations related to the defect?**

   *The finding of cor triatriatum was fortuitous in this woman with mild mitral valve prolapse and brief episodes of presumed supraventricular tachycardia.*

   *Clinical manifestations of cor triatriatum depend on the size of the orifice(s) in the left atrial diaphragm and the presence of*

associated anomalies. In its most severe form, symptoms begin in infancy. In less severe cases, cor triatriatum may not be detected until adulthood. Symptoms are those of pulmonary venous congestion, with dyspnea and orthopnea being the most common.[9] The development of symptoms may be due to fibrosis of the orifice, the development of mitral regurgitation, or the occurrence of atrial fibrillation.

*If symptoms seem out of proportion to the measured gradient by echocardiography, provocative tests such as exercise echocardiography, exercise cardiac catheterization, or volume challenges may help to assess the functional significance of the gradient. In this case, the gradient across the membrane was not severe, and provocative tests were not performed.*

3. **What is the significance of an ASD in patients with cor triatriatum?**

   *ASDs may mask the hemodynamic effects of the pulmonary venous obstruction. Since flow is preferentially redirected across the ASD into the RA, the gradient across the membrane orifice will be lower than anticipated. Depending on the severity of the left-to-right shunt, subsequent RV dilation and/or systolic dysfunction may develop.*

4. **What are the indications for surgical intervention and what are the outcomes after surgery?**

   *The patient with an unobstructed form of cor triatriatum does not require intervention. For patients with significant obstruction, surgery is the treatment of choice.[9,10] In this case, the presence of the ASD and the dilated right ventricle were felt to be appropriate indications for surgery.*

   *Surgery consists of removal of the membrane or fibromuscular diaphragm and repair of the associated cardiac defects. With long-standing severe obstruction, pulmonary pressure may not revert to normal levels even after the removal of the membrane, as can be seen after repair of mitral stenosis.*

## FINAL DIAGNOSIS

Cor triatriatum

Small secundum ASD

## PLAN OF ACTION

Surgical resection of the membrane and closure of the secundum ASD

## INTERVENTION

Through a median sternotomy and after establishing bypass, the RA was opened. The LA membrane was clearly seen, and its fenestration was close to the atrial septum and measured 8 mm in diameter. The pulmonary veins were markedly dilated. The membrane was resected and the secundum ASD was closed. There were no postoperative complications.

## OUTCOME

Since her operation, the patient has remained asymptomatic. She has had further episodes of palpitations. She still has mild mitral regurgitation. Her myxomatous mitral valve disease is being monitored with periodic clinical exams and echocardiograms.

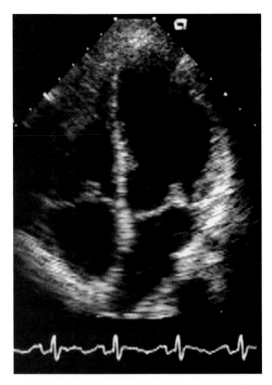

Figure 18-9 Transthoracic echocardiogram, four-chamber view.

## FINDINGS

The echocardiogram showed a small lateral ridge at the midatrial level. There was no residual gradient or ASD. The mitral valve leaflets were myxomatous with mild mitral valve prolapse and mild mitral regurgitation.

***Comments:*** Operative results were good in this adult patient.

## Selected References

1. Van Praagh R, Corsini I: Cor triatriatum: Pathologic anatomy and a consideration of morphogenesis based on 13 postmortem cases and a study of normal development of the pulmonary vein and atrial septum in 83 human embryos. Am Heart J 78:379–405, 1969.
2. Van Son JA, Danielson GK, Schaff HV, et al: Cor triatriatum: Diagnosis, operative approach, and late results. Mayo Clin Proc 68:854–859, 1993.
3. Oglietti J, Cooley DA, Izquierdo JP, et al: Cor triatriatum: Operative results in 25 patients. Ann Thorac Surg 35:415–420, 1983.
4. Marin-Garcia J, Tandon R, Lucas RV, Jr, Edwards JE: Cor triatriatum: Study of 20 cases. Am J Cardiol 35:59–66, 1975.
5. Loeffler E: Unusual malformation of the left atrium: Pulmonary sinus. Arch Pathol 48:371–376, 1949.
6. Bartel T, Muller S, Geibel A: Preoperative assessment of cor triatriatum in an adult by dynamic three dimensional echocardiography was more informative than transoesophageal echocardiography or magnetic resonance imaging. Br Heart J 72:498–499, 1994.
7. Ibrahim T, Schreiber K, Dennig K, et al: Images in cardiovascular medicine: Assessment of cor triatriatum sinistrum by magnetic resonance imaging. Circulation 108:e107, 2003.
8. Tanaka F, Itoh M, Esaki H, et al: Asymptomatic cor triatriatum incidentally revealed by computed tomography. Chest 100: 272–274, 1991.
9. McGuire LB, Nolan TB, Reeve R, Dammann JF, Jr: Cor triatriatum as a problem of adult heart disease. Circulation 31:263–272, 1965.
10. Chen Q, Guhathakurta S, Vadalapali G, et al: Cor triatriatum in adults: Three new cases and a brief review. Tex Heart Inst J 26:206–210, 1999.

# Part II

# Left Ventricular Outflow

# Considerations for the Ross Procedure

**David B. Meyer and Thomas L. Spray**

**Age: 26 years**
**Gender: Female**
**Lifestyle information: Active athlete and traveler, engaged to be married**
**Working diagnosis: Aortic insufficiency and neoaortic root dilatation**

## HISTORY

The patient was born with a tricuspid aortic valve, but as a child she developed aortic valve endocarditis resulting in perforation of the noncoronary cusp. Aortic insufficiency worsened, and at age 9 she required surgery to repair the insufficiency. The procedure was unsuccessful, however, and again at age 10 she underwent repeat surgical repair aortic valvuloplasty, with better results. She was started on lisinopril.

At age 18, aortic insufficiency had progressed and she required further surgery. She underwent a Ross procedure, which was uncomplicated. In early follow-up both her neoaortic root and pulmonary homograft were functioning well.

Eight years after the Ross procedure, she reported a significant decline in her exercise tolerance, growing steadily worse over the past year.

*Comments:* Endocarditis in the young is uncommon but does occur, with risk factors similar to those in adults. It is more common in patients with a bicuspid aortic valve, or any source of turbulent flow around the valve. Sometimes a tricuspid aortic valve can be "functionally bicuspid" if there is considerable fusion along one of the commissures.

Often valvuloplasty is performed in children or adolescents, even if results are less than optimal, to delay valve replacement until growth is complete.

The Ross procedure reduces the need for future aortic valve surgery (although pulmonary valve redo surgery may be required, see Case 23), and avoids the need for long-term warfarin, especially important in a woman of childbearing age.

## CURRENT SYMPTOMS

The patient complained of exercise intolerance. She was no longer able to carry out her usual daily workout routine, and found herself breathless after climbing two flights of stairs. She denied dizziness or light-headedness, palpitations, fever, chills, or shakes.

NYHA class: II

## CURRENT MEDICATIONS

Lisinopril 10 mg daily

## PHYSICAL EXAMINATION

BP 100/42 mm Hg, HR 100 bpm, oxygen saturation 100%

Height 178 cm, weight 67 kg, BSA 1.82 m²

Surgical scars: Median sternotomy

Neck veins: The venous waveform was normal.

Lungs/chest: Clear to auscultation

Heart: The precordium was active. There was a 2/6 blowing diastolic murmur heard along the left sternal border. Peripheral pulses were bounding. There was a diastolic flow murmur at the femoral artery.

Abdomen: Soft with no organomegaly or masses

Extremities: Warm and well perfused

*Comments:* The physical exam suggests worsening aortic insufficiency, from the wide pulse pressure, the early diastolic murmur, the bounding peripheral pulses, and possible flow reversal in the femoral artery.

## LABORATORY DATA

| | |
|---|---|
| Hemoglobin | 14.8 g/dL (11.5–15.0) |
| Hematocrit | 43% (36–46) |
| MCV | 83 fL (83–99) |
| Platelet count | 225 × 10³ μ/L (150–400) |
| Creatinine | 1.1 mg/dL (0.6–1.2) |
| Blood urea nitrogen | 12 mg/dL (6–24) |

*Comments:* No abnormalities were found.

# ELECTROCARDIOGRAM

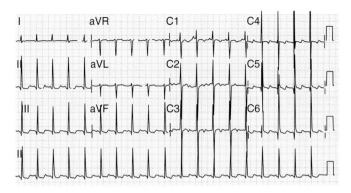

Figure 19-1 Electrocardiogram.

## FINDINGS

Heart rate: 110 bpm

QRS axis: Between +30° and +60°

PR interval: 120 msec

QRS duration: 100 msec

Sinus tachycardia. Presence of LV hypertrophy and diffuse ST-T abnormalities.

**Comments:** This ECG (see Fig. 19-1) shows some of the typical characteristics of LV hypertrophy (voltage criteria) as can be found in patients with significant chronic aortic regurgitation. Left precordial Q-waves can reflect chronic volume overload. However, the diffuse ST-T abnormalities are nonspecific and could also be related to myocardial injury from previous cardiac surgery.

## CHEST X-RAY

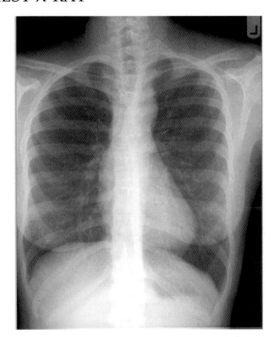

Figure 19-2 Posteroanterior projection.

## FINDINGS

Cardiothoracic ratio: 51%

The cardiac silhouette is normal in size, with normal appearance of the pulmonary arteries and aorta. There is no pulmonary edema. The aortic knuckle is somewhat prominent for a young woman, and the ascending aorta also seems prominent. Sternotomy wires are present.

**Comments:** The absence of cardiomegaly in a patient with potential aortic insufficiency is a reassuring sign. Pulmonary outflow tract obstruction can occur after a Ross procedure, sometimes resulting in right heart enlargement. The apex on this CXR points upward slightly, which can be seen if the RV is enlarged, but there is no RA enlargement, and the pulmonary arteries do not appear dilated.

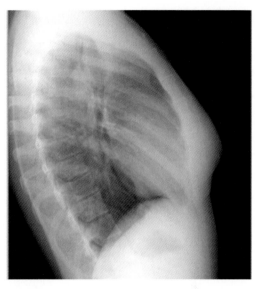

Figure 19-3 Lateral projection.

## FINDINGS

The retrosternal space is full, compatible with RV dilation, ascending aortic dilation, or possibly the placement of the homograft in the pulmonary position.

**Comments:** Again, one would look for evidence of an enlarged LV or RV to highlight problems related to a prior Ross procedure. No abnormalities were seen here.

## EXERCISE TESTING

Not performed

## ECHOCARDIOGRAM

### OVERALL FINDINGS

The LV was dilated, with an LVEDd of 62 mm and an LVESd of 45 mm, giving a shortening fraction of 29%.

The leaflets of the neoaortic valve appear normal, but there is aortic root dilatation (diameter 55 mm). There was no obstruction or significant regurgitation in the pulmonary homograft valve/conduit.

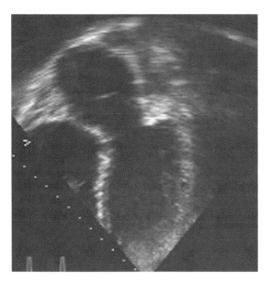

Figure 19-4 Apical view of the left ventricular outflow tract.

**Comments:** The etiology of the aortic dilatation is not well understood, though there is some evidence suggesting that molecular abnormalities of the tunica media that may be related to aortic root dilatation in bicuspid valve patients may also be present in the pulmonary artery.[1]

There is no obstruction of RV outflow. When it occurs, obstruction can be subvalvular, valvular, or supravalvular.

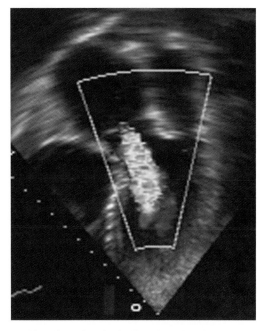

Figure 19-5 Two-dimensional color Doppler apical view.

## FINDINGS

There was severe neoaortic valve regurgitation, with a jet diameter of 6 mm.

**Comments:** Any dilatation of the aortic root will compromise neoaortic valve function. Figure 19-5 shows there is aneurysmal degeneration of the autograft root, with normal appearing autograft leaflets. Thus the mechanism of regurgitation is likely dilatation and distortion of the valve due to the aneurysm of the root.

## FOCUSED CLINICAL QUESTIONS AND DISCUSSION POINTS

1. **What was the cause of neoaortic valve dysfunction in this patient?**

   *The neoaortic valve, previously the patient's own pulmonary valve, is checked carefully for abnormalities and size compatibility before being harvested originally, so there should be no inherent leaflet dysfunction of the valve to explain its dysfunction. Endocarditis of the valve can occur and compromise function. Another common cause of regurgitation soon after surgery is distortion of the valve ring at the time of implant, which leads to failure of appropriate coaptation. This problem is not always appreciated immediately after surgery, but can develop slowly as healing and scarring occur. The other potential cause of dysfunction is dilatation of the aortic root. The Ross procedure as originally described left the coronary arteries in place, whereas newer adaptations involve a neoaortic root with reimplantation of the coronary ostia, as in this patient's case. In either case, dilatation of the aortic root can occur and eventually lead to dilatation of the valve ring and regurgitation, which was the mechanism in this patient.[2-4]*

2. **When is the optimal time to reintervene for either aortic root dilatation or neoaortic valve insufficiency late after a Ross procedure?**

   *For this size patient, in the absence of Marfan's disease, we consider a diameter greater than 50 mm to be an indication for surgery. In addition, the aortic insufficiency related to the dilatation of the aorta is a motivation toward repair, since at this point the leaflets themselves appear nondiseased and may be able to be spared, with restoration of aortic valve competence.*

   *Even without the coexistence of aortic root dilatation, traditional criteria for deciding to intervene for severe aortic insufficiency also apply, including LV dilatation and systolic dysfunction, as well as attributable symptoms.*

3. **What is the optimal type of valve replacement/repair to use for neoaortic regurgitation and root dilatation following a Ross operation?**

   *The classical operation for this set of problems is a modified Bentall procedure (composite mechanical aortic valve and root replacement). However, this is suboptimal for this patient because it would require permanent anticoagulation, and the patient, soon to be married, is hoping to start a family in the near future.*

   *There are numerous reports of the success of valve-sparing root replacement with remodeling of the dilated annulus as an alternative to the Bentall procedure. The valve-sparing procedure involves the replacement of the aortic wall with a graft, into which the native valve is resuspended. This alternative allows preservation of the autograft valve with no requirement for anticoagulation.[5-7]*

   *In either case, the patient is still at risk of pulmonary homograft dysfunction in the future, and requires lifelong follow-up both for her aortic and pulmonary valves.*

## FINAL DIAGNOSIS

Neoaortic root aneurysm

Neoaortic valve insufficiency

## PLAN OF ACTION

Valve-sparing neoaortic root replacement

## INTERVENTION

The patient was taken to surgery. Findings at operation, as expected, included significant dilatation of the autograft to the suture line of the native aorta. The valve leaflets themselves appeared normal, and the annulus was less dilated than the sinuses themselves. The aorta was replaced with a David technique, sewing a 26-mm Dacron graft (with a preformed sinus) down to the annulus, with the valve resuspended within the graft. The coronary arteries were reimplanted into the sinus portion of the graft as in a Bentall procedure. Hence, the graft itself provides an obligate downsize annuloplasty if a size is chosen that is smaller than the annulus itself, as it was in this case.

## OUTCOME

The operation was performed without complication. Postoperative imaging showed no neoaortic regurgitation. The patient underwent a catheterization on postoperative day 2 because of abnormalities on the ECG suspicious for new ischemia, but there was normal coronary flow. She was discharged approximately 1 week after surgery.

The patient was married as planned and remains asymptomatic. She and her husband are contemplating having their first child.

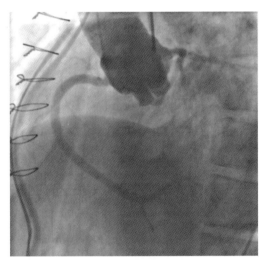

Figure 19-6 Postoperative aortogram.

## FINDINGS

There was no obstruction to flow in the coronary arteries. Aortography showed no regurgitation of the neoaortic valve and a normal-sized aortic root.

***Comments:*** This aortogram was done to examine the coronary flow, which was normal, but demonstrates the remodeled valve annulus and the absence of neoaortic regurgitation.

## Selected References

1. Fedak PW, de Sa MP, Verma S, et al: Vascular matrix remodeling in patients with bicuspid aortic valve malformations: Implications for aortic dilatation. J Thorac Cardiovasc Surg, 126:797–806, 2003.
2. David TE, Omran A, Ivanov J, et al: Dilation of the pulmonary autograft after the Ross procedure. J Thorac Cardiovasc Surg 119:10–20, 2000.
3. Pasquali SK, Cohen MS, Shera D, et al: The relationship between neo-aortic root dilation, insufficiency, and reintervention following the Ross procedure in infants, children, and young adults. J Am Coll Cardiol 49:806–812, 2007.
4. Luciani GB, Mazzucco A: Aortic root disease after the Ross procedure. Curr Opin Cardiol 21:55–60, 2006.
5. Yacoub MH, Gehle P, Chandrasekaran V, et al: Late results of a valve-preserving operation in patients with aneurysms of the ascending aorta and root. J Thorac Cardiovasc Surg 115:80–90, 1998.
6. Feindel CM, David TE: Aortic valve sparing operations: Basic concepts. Int J Cardiol 97(Suppl 1):61–66, 2004.
7. David TE, Ivanov J, Armstrong S, et al: Aortic valve-sparing operations in patients with aneurysms of the aortic root or ascending aorta. Ann Thorac Surg 74:1758–1761; discussion S92–S99, 2002.

# Aortic Stenosis and Endocarditis during Pregnancy

**Sofian Johar and Michael A. Gatzoulis**

**Age: 33**
**Gender: Female**
**Occupation: Housewife**
**Working diagnosis: Subaortic stenosis**

## HISTORY

The patient had been diagnosed with mild subaortic stenosis in early childhood but did not require intervention. She had been discharged from pediatric cardiology follow-up at age 13.

She remained asymptomatic throughout her adult life and led an unrestricted lifestyle. She had no complications or events, but was not receiving regular medical care or cardiology follow-up.

The patient became pregnant at the age of 33. At 23 weeks gestation she developed fevers, sweats, headaches, and general lethargy for 3 days. Blood cultures were positive, and she was referred with a provisional diagnosis of bacterial endocarditis. Hospital admission was arranged.

**Comments:** Subaortic stenosis is an uncommon lesion and accounts for approximately 1% of congenital heart defects. It is usually caused by a fixed lesion in the LVOT and consists of a fibrous ridge in the LVOT proximal to the aortic valve. Less commonly the obstruction can take the form of a less discrete, tunnellike narrowing. It is often associated with other forms of congenital heart disease such as ventricular septal defect, patent ductus arteriosus, coarctation of the aorta, bicuspid aortic valve, abnormal left ventricular papillary muscle, and atrioventricular septal defect.

It is uncommon for subaortic stenosis to present with symptoms in infancy or early childhood unless there is other, concomitant congenital heart disease. It is usually diagnosed after evaluation of a childhood murmur. Symptoms are related to the degree of LVOT obstruction and may include exertional dyspnea, effort syncope, angina, congestive cardiac failure, and sudden death.

Once diagnosed, progression can be anticipated, although in childhood this is variable and many patients remain stable and asymptomatic for a long period of time. Occasionally, subaortic stenosis can be rapidly progressive. Once adulthood is reached patients may remain stable for years, though some do eventually require surgery to relieve the obstruction.[1] Patients with subaortic stenosis are at risk of developing aortic regurgitation, usually related to the eccentric jet from the membrane striking and adversely affecting the aortic valve (which in itself is usually morphologically normal to start). The risk of bacterial endocarditis is substantial. It is more common in patients with a damaged aortic valve and can lead to significant aortic regurgitation and congestive heart failure.

## CURRENT SYMPTOMS

She was well throughout pregnancy until the 23rd week, and reported fevers, sweats, headaches, and general lethargy that began 3 days prior to presentation. In particular she denied any exertional dyspnea, syncope, palpitations, or chest discomfort.

NYHA class: I

**Comments:** The risk to the pregnant woman with subaortic stenosis depends on the degree of LV outflow obstruction, LV function, and the presence of any associated congenital heart defects.

Ideally, patients would have been assessed prior to conception with in-depth counseling, and patients with severe obstruction and/or symptoms would have been repaired prior to pregnancy.[2]

The hemodynamic changes during pregnancy result in a predictable increase in the gradient across the LVOT as the stroke volume rises during the second trimester and the systemic blood pressure falls.

Unfortunately, the patient was discharged from tertiary care in her early teens even though she had a commonly progressive lesion. Furthermore, and regrettably, the patient received no information on pregnancy risks to herself or her infant, or information on the risks of recurrence of congenital heart disease (estimated at up to 10% for left-sided obstructive lesions). Paradoxically, this case represents the rule rather than the exception for most of the developed world, emphasizing the need for raising awareness of pregnancy and heart disease among professionals and patients alike.

## CURRENT MEDICATIONS

None

## PHYSICAL EXAMINATION

BP 125/80 (right arm), HR 90 bpm, oxygen saturation 99% on room air

Height 165 cm, weight 73 kg, BSA 1.83 m$^2$

Surgical scars: None

Neck veins: Her JVP was not elevated.

Lungs/chest: Clear

Heart: The heart rate was regular. The cardiac impulse was slightly increased but not displaced. She had a palpable thrill with a normal first heart sound, split second, and a 3–4/6 harsh ejection systolic murmur throughout her precordium together with an early soft diastolic murmur at the left sternal edge.

Abdomen: Normal

Extremities: There was no peripheral edema and no radio-femoral delay. The patient was not clubbed and there were no splinter hemorrhages or other stigmata of infective endocarditis.

***Comments:*** Peripheral pulses are generally of normal volume unless the LVOT obstruction is severe.

A forceful apex beat is usually present in most patients with more than mild subaortic stenosis. The presence of an increased cardiac impulse suggests significant LV hypertrophy.

The second heart sound can be narrowly split or single because of prolonged LV systole.

An ejection systolic murmur is typically heard with the length of the murmur being proportional to the degree of obstruction when LV function is preserved.

The high-pitched early diastolic murmur indicates coexisting aortic regurgitation, which may be present in 50% of patients with fixed subaortic stenosis.

## LABORATORY DATA

| | |
|---|---|
| Hemoglobin | **10.7 g/dL** (11.5–15.0) |
| Platelet count | $198 \times 10^9/L$ (150–400) |
| Total white cell count | **$9.2 \times 10^6/L$** (1.0–7.6) |
| Sodium | **133 mmol/L** (134–145) |
| Potassium | 4.0 mmol/L (3.5–5.2) |
| Creatinine | 0.6 mg/dL (0.6–1.2) |
| Blood urea nitrogen | 3.9 mmol/L (2.5–6.5) |
| CRP | **58 mg/dL** (0.0–5.0) |

Blood cultures grew *Streptococcus mitis* sensitive to penicillin.

***Comments:*** The raised white cell count, elevated C-reactive protein (CRP) concentration levels, and positive blood cultures with a typical organism strongly suggest the diagnosis of infective endocarditis. Echocardiography would be indicated to look for vegetations.

Renal function is normal, which is important as aminoglycosides, normally given in conjunction with another antibiotic for the treatment of infective endocarditis, are nephrotoxic. Furthermore, renal dysfunction can result from hemodynamic compromise secondary to acute endocarditis. The latter constitutes an indication for surgery when medical treatment is failing.[3]

## ELECTROCARDIOGRAM

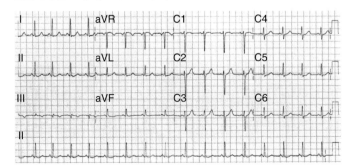

Figure 20-1 Electrocardiogram.

### FINDINGS

Heart rate: 98 bpm

QRS axis: +32°

QRS duration: 86 msec

***Comments:*** There was sinus rhythm with normal AV conduction. The QRS axis was normal with normal QRS progression and a normal PR interval.

No ECG evidence of LV hypertrophy.

The normal PR interval is important. PR prolongation may suggest the development of an aortic root abscess in patients with aortic valve endocarditis. An aortic root abscess in this case was excluded with a transesophageal echocardiogram.

## CHEST X-RAY

Not performed because of pregnancy

## EXERCISE TESTING

Not performed

## ECHOCARDIOGRAM

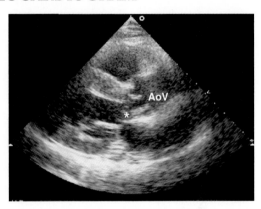

Figure 20-2 Parasternal long-axis view.

### FINDINGS

There was subaortic stenosis caused by a subaortic ridge (*asterisk*). The aortic valve (AoV) was slightly thickened. LV size was normal with mild concentric LV hypertrophy and good LV function.

***Comments:*** The echo confirmed the anatomical diagnosis of subaortic stenosis. The LV hypertrophy suggests significant outflow tract obstruction.

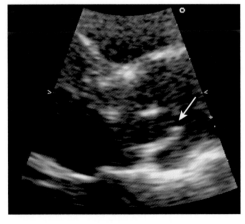

Figure 20-3 Parasternal long-axis view.

## FINDINGS

Close-up of the aortic valve showed a small vegetation (*arrow*) on the nonceronary cusp, confirming the diagnosis of bacterial endocarditis.

***Comments:*** The vegetation on the aortic valve is fairly small. However, even small vegetations can give rise to significant embolic events. Systemic embolization occurs in 22% to 50% of cases with infective endocarditis.[3] Common sites are major arterial beds, including the lungs, coronary arteries, spleen, bowel, and extremities. Up to 65% of embolic events involve the central nervous system.[4] The individual patient risk of embolization is difficult to predict. However, there is a trend toward higher embolic rates with left-sided vegetations above 10 mm in diameter.[5] This constitutes an indication for surgery particularly if there is already evidence of systemic embolization.[3]

There is a high maternal and fetal mortality rate associated with surgery during pregnancy (22.1% and 14.7%, respectively).[6]

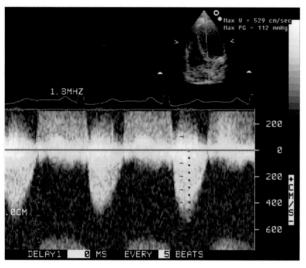

Figure 20-4 Continuous-wave Doppler through the aortic valve in five-chamber view.

## FINDINGS

Doppler through the LVOT in the five-chamber view demonstrates a peak velocity of 5.3 m/sec, giving a peak gradient of 112 mm Hg. There was also mild aortic regurgitation.

***Comments:*** The gradient across the LVOT demonstrates important obstruction, although the gradient is higher than it would have been before pregnancy because of increased cardiac output related to pregnancy (up to a 50% increase of the Doppler gradient is common).

### FOCUSED CLINICAL QUESTIONS AND DISCUSSION POINTS

1. **What are the risks for the patient with subaortic stenosis during pregnancy?**

*The patient has moderate to severe LVOT obstruction with only mild aortic regurgitation and preserved LV systolic function. Predictors of adverse maternal cardiac or neonatal events applicable here are a high-pressure gradient across the LVOT and a previous cardiac event. Therefore, the patient's "baseline" risk is significantly elevated.[7] Her aortic regurgitation is likely to be well toler-*

*ated unless there is acute failure of her aortic valve due to endocarditis. Cesarean section may be considered for patients with significant subaortic stenosis; however, vaginal delivery with an epidural is generally safe.[8]*

2. **What is the optimal management of pregnancy in a patient with acute bacterial endocarditis?**

*Infective endocarditis is rare during pregnancy and occurs in 1 in 8000 pregnant women with or without heart disease. It is obviously a serious complication. When it occurs, maternal and fetal mortality rates have been reported as 22.1% and 14.7%, respectively.[6]*

3. **How should this patient be managed?**

*This patient was hemodynamically stable despite evidence of severe subaortic stenosis and acute bacterial endocarditis. There was only mild aortic regurgitation, and renal function was normal. In addition, the fetus, assessed by ultrasound, was alive and thriving.*

*Such a complex case clearly merits multispecialty consideration. Thus, she was reviewed by obstetrics and cardiothoracic surgery, and discussed at a joint clinical conference.*

*If the patient had a good response to antimicrobial therapy, it was decided to delay delivery to maximize the survival chances of the fetus. If uncontrolled sepsis or complications such as aortic root abscess or severe aortic regurgitation developed, corrective surgery could be undertaken. Cardiopulmonary bypass prior to the 24th week of gestation carries significant risk to the fetus. However, the patient was advised that she should remain hospitalized, both for intravenous antibiotics and for observation, for the remainder of her gestation. Detailed plans for delivery should be made ahead of time in cases such as this, and the need for a multidisciplinary approach cannot be overemphasized.[8]*

## FINAL DIAGNOSIS

Severe subaortic stenosis

Acute bacterial endocarditis of the aortic valve

Pregnancy

## PLAN OF ACTION

Hospitalization and intravenous antibiotic therapy for 6 weeks and monitoring until completion of gestation

## OUTCOME

Treatment with intravenous benzylpenicillin and gentamycin continued for 6 weeks. The patient stayed as an inpatient at the cardiac center until the 29th week of pregnancy. On completion of her intravenous course of antibiotics she was transferred to the neighboring high-risk obstetric unit (due to concerns about possible atrial fibrillation secondary to LV hypertrophy, mild LV dilatation, and mild to moderate LA dilatation).

She had a good response to antimicrobial therapy and remained well throughout her pregnancy. Her aortic regurgitation did not deteriorate.

She had a fetal echocardiogram showing no cardiac abnormalities.

She became clinically depressed toward the end of the third trimester, being totally unprepared for such a prolonged hospital stay. The couple had moved into their new house when the patient was admitted with acute endocarditis and hospitalized, and she was anxious to return home to prepare for the baby's arrival.

Eventually, at 41 weeks, labor was induced, and the team proceeded with vaginal delivery with epidural anesthesia, according to predetermined plans. Forceps were required during delivery. She did very well and was discharged home after 24 hours. She had a healthy baby boy.

She was seen in clinic 6 weeks postpartum with her son; the patient was free of cardiac symptoms. Follow-up echocardiography demonstrated a peak gradient across the LVOT of 72 mm Hg.

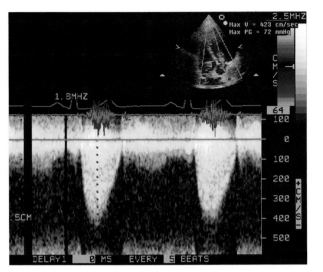

Figure 20-5 Continuous-wave Doppler through the aortic valve in five-chamber view.

## FINDINGS

Continuous-wave Doppler 6 months postpartum through the LVOT in the five-chamber view demonstrates a peak gradient of 72 mm Hg. There is mild aortic regurgitation only and mild LV hypertrophy with maintained systolic function.

***Comments:*** The gradient across the LVOT has decreased following delivery, which was expected due to a return to normal plasma volume and cardiac output following pregnancy. There was still a significant gradient, however, and there was mild LV hypertrophy. Further investigations were therefore undertaken to determine the need/timing and suitability for reparative surgery.

Cardiac catheterization showed a peak-to-peak pullback gradient across the LVOT of 52 mm Hg. LV end-diastolic pressure was 17 mm Hg, and the patient had normal coronary arteries. Her exercise capacity was impaired with an $MVo_2$ reduced at 45% of predicted. The patient and her husband wished to have

more children. She was, therefore, referred for surgical relief of her subaortic stenosis.

Surgery was carried out uneventfully 12 months after the birth of her first child. It consisted of surgical excision of a circumferential fibromuscular ridge. The aortic valve was inspected; it was a trileaflet valve, with normal excursion and evidence of mild aortic regurgitation only, and thus required no surgery. The patient returned from theater in sinus rhythm and made a timely recovery, leaving the hospital on the sixth postoperative day.

Six months later she felt very well, free of dyspnea and/or fatigue and coping very well with her 18-month-old son. A repeat echocardiogram showed a Doppler gradient of 25 mm Hg, mild aortic regurgitation, and maintained LV systolic function. She was advised of the need for lifelong follow-up and endocarditis prophylaxis and of the possible risk of developing heart block. She was also felt to have moved to a low-risk category if she was to become pregnant again, albeit she was advised to remain under close joint cardiac and obstetric care for any future pregnancies.

## Selected References

1. Oliver JM, Gonzalez A, Gallego P, et al: Discrete subaortic stenosis in adults: Increased prevalence and slow rate of progression of the obstruction and aortic regurgitation. J Am Coll Cardiol 38:835–842, 2001.
2. Steer PJ: Pregnancy and contraception. In Gatzoulis MA, Swan LS, Therrien J, Pantely G (eds): Adult Congenital Heart Disease: A Practical Guide. Oxford, Blackwell, 2005, pp 16–35.
3. Baddour LM, Wilson WR, Bayer AS, et al: Infective endocarditis: Diagnosis, antimicrobial therapy, and management of complications: A statement for healthcare professionals from the Committee on Rheumatic Fever, Endocarditis, and Kawasaki Disease, Council on Cardiovascular Disease in the Young, and the Councils on Clinical Cardiology, Stroke, and Cardiovascular Surgery and Anesthesia, American Heart Association: Endorsed by the Infectious Diseases Society of America. Circulation 111:e394–e434, 2005.
4. Heiro M, Nikoskelainen J, Engblom E, et al: Neurologic manifestations of infective endocarditis: A 17-year experience in a teaching hospital in Finland. Arch Intern Med 160:2781–2787, 2000.
5. Sanfilippo AJ, Picard MH, Newell JB, et al: Echocardiographic assessment of patients with infectious endocarditis: Prediction of risk for complications. J Am Coll Cardiol 18:1191–1199, 1991.
6. Campuzano K, Roque H, Bolnick A, et al: Bacterial endocarditis complicating pregnancy: Case report and systematic review of the literature. Arch Gynecol Obstet 268:251–255, 2003.
7. Siu SC, Sermer M, Colman JM, et al: Prospective multicenter study of pregnancy outcomes in women with heart disease. Circulation 104:515–521, 2001.
8. Uebing A, Steer PJ, Yentis SM, Gatzoulis MA: Pregnancy and congenital heart disease. BMJ 332:401–406, 2006.

# Subaortic Stenosis: Indications for Surgery

**Naser M. Ammash and Joseph A. Dearani**

**Age: 47 years**
**Gender: Female**
**Occupation: Elementary school teacher**
**Working diagnosis: Subaortic stenosis**

## HISTORY

The patient was noted to have a heart murmur at age 5. She was referred to a cardiologist at age 26 when she was contemplating pregnancy. The diagnosis of bicuspid aortic valve was made, based on the cardiac examination. She had two successful uneventful pregnancies at age 28 and age 32. She did well until a year ago (46 years old) when she started noticing dyspnea on exertion and exercise intolerance. At that time an echocardiogram revealed severe subaortic stenosis with LV hypertrophy, a tricuspid aortic valve associated with moderate aortic regurgitation, and a possible small ASD with left-to-right shunt. Based on these findings she was referred to the adult congenital heart disease clinic.

**Comments:** Fibromuscular subvalvular aortic stenosis accounts for 15% to 20% of all types of congenital LVOT obstruction, and commonly presents in adulthood.[1] The fibromuscular obstruction typically is localized and extends in the shape of a ring around the outflow tract while inserting into the anterior mitral valve leaflet and the anteroseptum. It is more common than the tunnel-like subaortic stenosis that extends over several centimeters in the outflow tract. Although congenital aortic valve stenosis is much more common in males, this male prevalence is less in fixed subaortic stenosis. Familial occurrence of subaortic stenosis has been reported.[1,2]

Subaortic stenosis is thought to be an acquired anomaly caused by altered shear stress in the LVOT. The alterations in shear stress are created by a combination of congenital abnormalities of LVOT morphometry including a steeper aortoseptal angle, a longer mitral-aortic separation, and an exaggerated aortic override.[3,4] These abnormalities could alter the angle of ejection of blood and cause abnormal in utero accumulation of embryonic cells that eventually differentiate into fibroelastic tissue and a membrane that is often not noted at birth. Therefore, in contrast to a bicuspid aortic valve, a systolic murmur is rarely present at birth but appears later in life.

The associated symptoms depend on the severity of the stenosis. They may be entirely absent until physical stress results in an inadequate increment in cardiac output and an increase in the left ventricular diastolic pressure, initially causing exertional dyspnea, lightheadedness, and/or easy fatigability. Chest pain, exertional syncope, and congestive heart failure occur later as the left ventricular obstruction worsens, similar to a patient with valvular aortic stenosis.

## CURRENT SYMPTOMS

The patient complained of exertional dyspnea and fatigue not allowing her to perform as well on her treadmill. Prior to the onset of her symptoms, she used to exercise regularly on a treadmill at a speed of 3 miles an hour, 5 to 7 days a week for a period of 1 hour.

She had no dyspnea, orthopnea, or paroxysmal nocturnal dyspnea. She complained of nonpleuritic, nonradiating chest pain occurring at rest, lasting for few seconds to a few minutes and resolving spontaneously. She also reported short episodes of rapid palpitations without dizziness or syncope.

NYHA class: II

**Comments:** Dyspnea on exertion occurs as a result of an inadequate incremental rise in cardiac output due to the fixed LV outflow obstruction. This leads to an increase in LV diastolic pressure and pulmonary congestion. As with aortic valve stenosis, the risk of developing congestive heart failure increases as the severity of the obstruction increases.

Angina pectoris can occur either as a result of acquired coronary atherosclerosis in the adult age group or secondary to the LV hypertrophy leading to subendocardial ischemia.

Exertional syncope can occur in patients with severe subaortic stenosis possibly because of an exaggerated fall in systemic vascular resistance during exercise, and a reflex bradycardia mediated by LV baroreceptors.[2] Sudden death has been reported in patients with this condition.

## CURRENT MEDICATIONS

Premarin (conjugated estrogen) 0.9 mg by mouth daily

Zyrtec (cetirizine, for allergy) 10 mg by mouth daily

Ditropan XL (oxybutynin, for bladder spasm) 5 mg by mouth daily

## PHYSICAL EXAMINATION

BP 120/65 mm Hg (right arm), 125/65 (left arm), 124 systolic (right leg); HR 84 bpm, oxygen saturation 99% on room air

Height 170 cm, weight 97.9 kg, BSA 2.18 m$^2$

Neck veins: The neck veins were normal, with a mildly diminished and delayed carotid pulse.

Lungs/chest: The lungs were clear to auscultation with no wheezes, rales, or rhonchi.

Heart: There was a right upper sternal thrill, but no parasternal lift. The rhythm was regular. The first and second heart sounds were soft. No extra heart sounds or clicks were appreciated. There was a grade 4/6 late-peaking systolic murmur noted at the left sternal border radiating to the base of the neck and into the carotids. There was also a grade 2/6 diastolic blowing murmur appreciated best at the mid-left sternal border.

Abdomen: Soft and nontender, with no hepatomegaly or splenomegaly, and no masses felt. There was no abdominal bruit.

Extremities: The peripheral pulses were normal with no brachial-femoral delay. There was no edema, cyanosis, or clubbing.

***Comments:*** The JVP can be normal in the absence of secondary pulmonary hypertension. However, significant septal hypertrophy may result in reduced distensibility of the RV, causing the RA to contract with greater force and resulting in a higher amplitude jugular venous A-wave.

As with aortic valve stenosis, the carotid pulse is often reduced and delayed as the severity of LV obstruction increases. The pulse volume, however, can be elevated in the presence of significant aortic regurgitation.

A sustained and strong LV impulse or heave can be found in patients with severe obstruction and ventricular hypertrophy. The first heart sound is often normal whereas the aortic component of the second heart sound can be normal, delayed, diminished, or even absent, depending on the severity of the subaortic stenosis. Ejection clicks are not a feature of fixed subaortic stenosis.

A systolic crescendo-decrescendo murmur and associated thrill, if severe stenosis, can be noted at the left sternal border and apex. This radiates into the second right intercostal space, and often into the suprasternal notch, and both carotid and subclavian arteries.

The configuration, length, and loudness of the murmur are similar to that of aortic valve stenosis.

A blowing decrescendo murmur of aortic regurgitation is heard in 50% of patients with fixed subaortic stenosis.[2] A fourth heart sound is a sign of hemodynamically significant stenosis causing an increase in atrial contraction and contribution to ventricular filling.

# LABORATORY DATA

| | |
|---|---|
| Hemoglobin | 12.6 g/dL (11.5–15.0) |
| Hematocrit/PCV | 37.1% (36–46) |
| MCV | 89.5 fL (83–99) |
| Platelet count | $224 \times 10^9$/L (150–400) |
| Sodium | 139 mmol/L (134–145) |
| Potassium | 4.3 mmol/L (3.5–5.2) |
| Creatinine | 1.0 mg/dL (0.6–1.2) |
| Blood urea nitrogen | **16 mmol/L** (2.5–6.5) |

## OTHER RELEVANT LAB RESULTS

| | |
|---|---|
| TSH | 3.3 mIU/L (0.30–5.0) |
| Cholesterol | 157 mg/dL (<200) |
| Triglyceride | 102 mg/dL (<150) |
| HDL | 71 mg/dL (>40) |
| LDL | 66 mg/dL (<130) |

***Comments:*** Laboratory tests are usually normal in patients with subaortic stenosis.

# ELECTROCARDIOGRAM

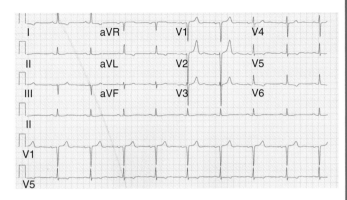

Figure 21-1 Electrocardiogram.

## FINDINGS

Heart rate: 55 bpm

PR interval: 204 msec

QRS axis: −4°

QRS duration: 92 msec

Sinus bradycardia with borderline first-degree AV block, poor R-wave progression, and nonspecific lateral ST-T abnormalities

***Comments:*** Electrocardiographic criteria do not distinguish valvular from subvalvular or supravalvular stenosis, nor do they reliably reflect the severity of aortic stenosis.

Left-axis deviation occurs more in adults than in children with severe stenosis; however, the QRS axis can be normal even in the presence of severe stenosis. Signs of LVH with and without ST-T abnormalities may be seen in 60% to 85% of patients, including 50% of patients with mild stenosis, and therefore cannot predict the severity of subaortic stenosis.[1] On the other hand, severe subaortic stenosis has been associated at times with a normal ECG.[2,5]

# CHEST X-RAY

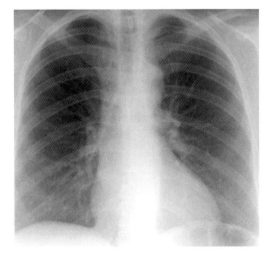

Figure 21-2 Posteroanterior projection.

## FINDINGS

Cardiothoracic ratio: 50%

The cardiac silhouette was normal with no rib notching. There was no pulmonary venous congestion. The CXR was normal.

***Comments:*** The cardiac silhouette in patients with subaortic stenosis can be normal or show signs of left ventricular enlargement leading to downward and posterior displacement of the heart. These can be evident by the appearance of an elongated heart on the posteroanterior view and a more convex ventricular shadow on the lateral view. Significant LV enlargement often suggests significant aortic regurgitation.

There may be LA enlargement related to chronically increased LA pressure. Pulmonary venous congestion occurs only in the presence of severe stenosis leading to elevated filling pressure and at times pulmonary hypertension.

Dilatation of the aorta is not a feature of subaortic stenosis, which helps distinguish it from congenital bicuspid or unicuspid aortic valvular stenosis.

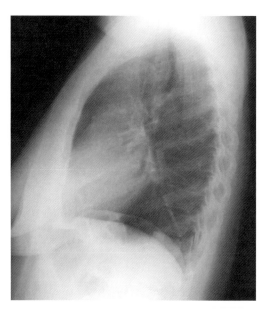

Figure 21-3 Lateral view.

## FINDINGS

Normal lateral CXR.

## ECHOCARDIOGRAM

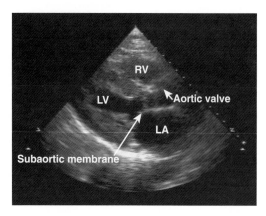

Figure 21-4 Parasternal long-axis 2D view.

## FINDINGS

There was a discrete subaortic stenosis caused by a fibromuscular membrane. The aortic valve annulus was normal in size, and the valve opens normally. The LV was normal in size and function. The LA was enlarged. The RV was normal in size.

***Comments:*** A transthoracic echocardiogram is the preferred technique for the diagnosis and serial assessment of discrete fibromuscular stenosis and delineation of associated lesions. The membrane can be noted in several locations, including within the elongated and narrow outflow tract, or extending across the anterior portion of the LVOT in a crescentic shape, or circumferential, extending onto the anterior mitral valve leaflet. It can also vary in thickness and in its proximity to the aortic valve. Rarely does the fibromuscular membrane attach to the aortic valve cusps.

The aortic valve cusps may be either normal or thickened but do not show systolic doming. The leaflets may flutter with early valve closure as a result of the proximal outflow obstruction.

The aortic valve annulus is normal in size in patients with discrete membranous aortic stenosis in comparison to the tunnellike stenosis that is often associated with small aortic annulus.[6]

The distance between the aortic annulus and mitral annulus is increased. The LV is usually normal in size, but can be hypertrophied.

LA enlargement is a sign of chronic elevation in LA pressure that occurs in severe subaortic stenosis.

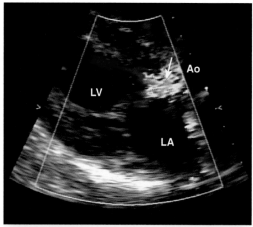

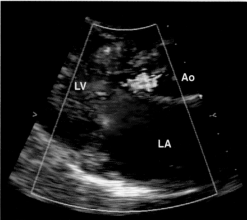

Figure 21-5 Parasternal long-axis 2D color Doppler.

# Findings

The top image demonstrates systolic color flow turbulence (*arrow*) caused by the stenosis in the LVOT (LV) and not at the level of the aortic valve. The bottom picture is a diastolic frame showing the abnormal diastolic flow caused by the aortic valve regurgitation. The latter was felt to be moderate in severity.

**Comments:** Color flow Doppler is helpful in identifying the level of aortic stenosis. The turbulence caused by the subaortic membrane should originate from the LVOT rather than either the aortic valve annulus (valvular stenosis) or above the aortic valve (supravalvular stenosis).

Aortic regurgitation is seen in 40% to 60% of cases and is most often caused by leaflet trauma from the high-velocity subaortic jet. Aortic valve deformation could also result from extension of the fibromuscular membrane onto the aortic valve itself.[5] The severity of the aortic regurgitation can also be assessed by the relative width of the color flow signal in the LVOT. A width of more then 50% is suggestive of grade III or IV/V aortic regurgitation.

If the anterior mitral valve is significantly distorted by the subaortic membrane, mitral regurgitation ensues.[1] This was not present as demonstrated on the echocardiogram shown in Figure 21-5.

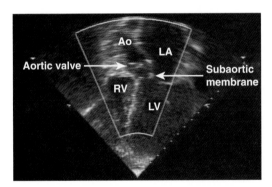

Figure 21-6 Apical four-chamber 2D view.

# Findings

The subaortic membrane was seen just underneath the aortic valve. The LV was normal in size with mild hypertrophy and normal function. The ejection fraction was 72%. The LA was mildly enlarged with a volume of 36.1 mL/m$^2$ (normal < 32 mL/m$^2$). The RA and RV were normal in size. The RV systolic pressure estimated by the tricuspid regurgitation velocity was 39 mm Hg (right atrial pressure = 5 mm Hg).

**Comments:** This view again can show the level of LV outflow obstruction (valvular, subvalvular, supravalvular), and its type, that is, discrete membranous or tubular subaortic stenosis. It is also important to assess the size of the LA and LV, as well as evaluate the degree and the distribution of LV hypertrophy.

In older patients with suboptimal transthoracic image quality, transesophageal echocardiography may be needed to confirm the diagnosis, assess its severity, and exclude associated septal defects.

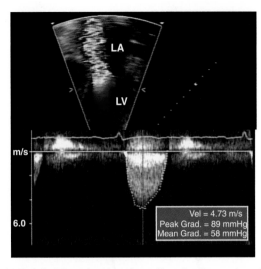

Figure 21-7 Apical four-chamber view with color flow and continuous-wave Doppler.

# Findings

The level and severity of subaortic stenosis on Doppler were again noted (top picture). The color flow turbulence originated in the LVOT. The continuous wave Doppler interrogation (bottom picture) showed a peak velocity of 4.7 m/sec, a mean gradient of 58 mm Hg, and a peak gradient of 89 mm Hg.

**Comments:** The severity of subaortic stenosis is estimated by the peak instantaneous gradient using the simplified Bernoulli equation (peak gradient = 4V$^2$). The peak Doppler gradient tends to be greater than the peak-to-peak gradient obtained at catheterization by as much as 30% to 40%.[7] On the other hand, the mean Doppler gradient, which takes an average of all instantaneous gradients throughout systole, is also useful in assessing the severity of aortic stenosis and correlates better with the mean gradient recorded at cardiac catheterization. A peak Doppler gradient of at least 50 mm Hg or mean Doppler gradient of at least 30 mm Hg is suggestive of severe stenosis.[2]

Doppler gradient estimation is less accurate with subaortic tunnel stenosis because it neglects the pressure drop caused by the viscous friction along its flow path.[1] Simultaneous pressure recordings in the LV and the aorta during catheterization are the preferred method for assessing the severity of subaortic tunnel stenosis. Three-dimensional echocardiogram and MRI have also been used to assess the anatomic and functional severity of subaortic stenosis.

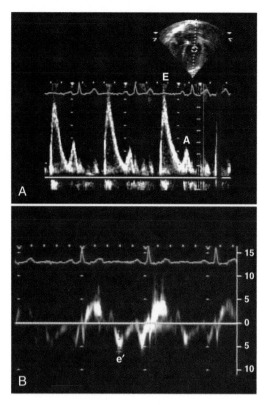

Figure 21-8 Apical four-chamber pulse wave spectral Doppler assessment of the mitral valve inflow (**A**). Doppler tissue imaging of the mitral annulus (**B**).

## FINDINGS

The mitral Doppler pattern showed increased, early LV filling (E = 1.3 m/sec) and reduced late filling (A = 0.4 m/sec), suggestive of elevated LV filling pressure. This can lead to LA enlargement and exertional dyspnea. Doppler tissue imaging of the mitral annulus (bottom) showed an e' velocity of 0.06 m/sec. The E/e' was 22, consistent with elevated LV filling pressure.

***Comments:*** Pulsed-wave spectral Doppler assessment of the mitral valve inflow, with and without Valsalva, as well as interrogation of the pulmonary venous flow, and Doppler tissue imaging of the mitral valve annulus, together with measurement of LA volume, is a reliable, noninvasive technique used for the evaluation of diastolic function of the LV. The latter plays an important role in the development of elevated LV filling pressure and dyspnea. This pattern of abnormal diastolic LV filling can persist even after surgical relief of the LV outflow obstruction.

## CATHETERIZATION

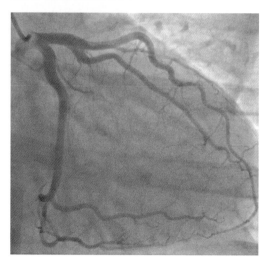

Figure 21-9 Left main coronary angiogram.

## FINDINGS

The epicardial coronary arteries were normal with no significant coronary disease.

***Comments:*** Coronary angiography was performed because of the patient's chest pain. There was no epicardial coronary disease. Today, this could also be done using CT coronary angiography.

No hemodynamic assessment of the severity of subaortic stenosis was performed at the time of cardiac catheterization because the echocardiogram had demonstrated unequivocal findings of severe subaortic stenosis caused by a fibromuscular membrane and the associated moderate aortic regurgitation. Therefore, it was determined that right and left heart catheterization would not influence the decision as to whether to proceed with surgical repair.

A combination of noninvasive and invasive investigative techniques might, however, be needed in certain cases to define the morphology and to assess the functional severity of the subaortic stenosis. Simultaneous pressure recording in the LV and aorta or careful withdrawal of an end-hole catheter from the body of the LV to the ascending aorta can provide us with a direct measurement of the peak-to-peak gradient, as well as the mean gradient created by the subaortic membrane. Biplane left ventriculography with cranial angulation in a left anterior oblique or lateral projection can be performed to visualize the LV outflow obstruction.[5] The severity of the aortic regurgitation can also be assessed by aortic root angiography if echocardiographic images were suboptimal.

### FOCUSED CLINICAL QUESTIONS AND DISCUSSION POINTS

1. What is the anatomic diagnosis?

   *This patient has a discrete subaortic stenosis caused by a fibromuscular membrane that is produced by the accumulation of fibroelastic tissue. It is four times more common than the tunnel-like subaortic stenosis that involves the whole length of the LVOT.[1] It is anatomically different from other types of subaortic stenosis such as that created by redundant accessory anterior mitral valve tissue or by the systolic anterior motion of the mitral valve in the presence of hypertrophic obstructive cardiomyopathy.*

2. **What congenital anomalies are associated with subaortic stenosis?**

*Discrete subaortic stenosis caused by a fibromuscular membrane is an isolated defect in 40% of cases.[2,3] In the remaining 60%, the stenosis is more often associated with left-sided obstructive defect as including aortic valve stenosis, coarctation of the aorta, or part of Shone syndrome, which typically includes a supravalvular mitral ring and parachute mitral valve. Simple defects such as septal defects, and complex defects such as double outlet RV, single ventricles, and tetralogy of Fallot have also been noted in association with this condition.*

3. **What is the natural history of subaortic stenosis?**

*Subaortic stenosis is often a progressive lesion that leads to LV hypertrophy and distortion of the aortic valve (jet lesion) resulting in aortic regurgitation.[8,9] This progression is variable and can be due to further narrowing, elongation, or thickening of the membrane, or from septal hypertrophy. A longitudinal study by Oliver and colleagues[9] has shown that the outflow obstruction increased at a rate of 2.25 ± 4.7 mm Hg/year. Data from the presurgical era have shown an increased risk of death, either sudden or with congestive heart failure, when subaortic stenosis is severe.[5] The degree of aortic regurgitation appears to increase with age and with the severity of stenosis,[5,10,11] at times requiring valve replacement at initial surgery. Endocarditis has been reported at a rate of 19.3/1000 patient-years.[5] The risk of endocarditis is related to the severity of the gradient and aortic regurgitation.*

4. **What are the indications for intervention?**

*Although surgical repair is clearly indicated in symptomatic patients for relief of the obstruction, the timing of surgical repair remains controversial in asymptomatic patients. Since many believe that operative resection slows progression of aortic regurgitation, surgery is generally considered in the presence of a stenosis with a peak Doppler gradient of more than 50 mm Hg, or a mean Doppler gradient or peak-to-peak catheter gradient more than 30 mm Hg.[7,11–14] At our institution we would also consider an operation with less severe stenosis in the presence of electrocardiographic signs of LV strain (at rest or postexercise), or progressive LV hypertrophy or dilatation. In addition, surgery may be considered in the presence of mild aortic regurgitation with lesser degrees of obstruction to preserve the valve.*

5. **Is percutaneous balloon dilatation an option?**

*Transluminal balloon dilatation of a discrete subaortic membrane, with resultant tear of the fibrous tissue and stretching of the stenotic orifice, has been performed in a limited number of patients with good immediate results.[15] A 70% overall reduction in the gradient has been reported without worsening of the aortic regurgitation. Better results were noted in the patients with a smaller baseline gradient, a larger aortic annulus, and a longer valve-to-membrane distance. However, although this technique may be a promising and safe alternative to surgery in patients with thin discrete stenosis, the experience is limited and the long-term benefit is unknown.*

6. **What is the long-term outcome following surgical repair?**

*Both surgical repair and balloon dilatation are only palliative procedures that may not cure the disease. They both reduce the pressure gradient but do not eliminate the underlying morphological and rheologic factors that relate to the formation of the membrane. Therefore, it is not surprising that the event-free survival following surgery is about 65% at 10 years. Reoperation for recurrent subaortic stenosis or progressive aortic regurgitation has been reported in up to 25% of patients at a mean follow-up of 5 years.[5]*

*Long-term follow-up studies have shown a mean peak residual gradient of 20 to 30 mm Hg.[15] The recurrence rate was sevenfold lower in the patients who had early surgical repair, and in those whose peak gradient prior to the operation was less the 40 mm Hg.[7] The addition of septal myectomy to membrane enucleation at the time of repair has also been shown to reduce the incidence of recurrent LV outflow obstruction on follow-up.[16,17]*

*Aortic regurgitation following operation has been reported in up to 25% to 40% of patients and can progress even after relief of the obstruction. The strongest predictors of late regurgitation are the degree of preoperative regurgitation and, to a lesser extent, the preoperative peak gradient. A preoperative peak gradient of more than 40 mm Hg is associated with late progressive aortic regurgitation. Therefore, early operation may decrease the incidence of late aortic regurgitation.[5,13,14] The combined approach of membranectomy and septal myectomy has also been shown to reduce the risk of late important aortic regurgitation to less than 10%.[16]*

*Late sudden death and endocarditis have also been reported, but subaortic resection does appear to reduce the risk of endocarditis.[5,11]*

*Although LV systolic function remains well preserved after operation, Chan and colleagues have demonstrated with echocardiography a persistent restrictive LV pattern suggestive of elevated LV filling pressure; this should be carefully monitored.[18]*

## FINAL DIAGNOSIS

Discrete subaortic stenosis caused by a fibromuscular band, associated with aortic regurgitation

### SURGICAL FINDINGS

Tricuspid aortic valve with marked attenuation of the right coronary cusp

Circumferential subaortic membrane with extension of the fibrous membrane onto the ventricular aspect of the aortic valve cusps and onto the anterior leaflet of the mitral valve

## PLAN OF ACTION

Excision of subaortic band, left ventricular septal myectomy, posterior aortic root enlargement with autologous pericardium

Aortic valve replacement with a 23-CarboMedics mechanical prosthesis[3]

Suture closure of PFO

**Comments:** Fixed subaortic stenosis is responsible for up to 20% of LV outflow obstruction requiring intervention. Operative techniques include excision of the membrane with or without septal myectomy.

Concomitant aortic valve repair has been reported in one third of patients, and more often in patients with a preoperative peak gradient of more than 40 mm Hg (49% vs. 20%).[7] Alternatively, aortic valve replacement is needed in 6% to 29% of patients at the time of initial repair.[11,19] The biggest risk factor for valve replacement was older age at the time of operation.[20] In addition, when the aortic valve annulus is small and aortic valve replacement is required, additional maneuvers to enlarge the outflow tract and/or annulus may be required so that a properly sized prosthesis can be inserted.

The operative risk is reported to be as low as 0% and as high as 3.8%.[16,19] The risk of complete heart block is less than 2%.[16] The operative risk is higher if aortic valve replacement is needed.[11]

The addition of surgical septal myectomy is thought to reduce the risk of proliferation of residual tissue. In a study published by the Mayo Clinic, the rate of recurrent stenosis and aortic regurgitation was significantly lower in patients who had membrane removal and concomitant myectomy.[16] Because the ventricular septum is often not markedly hypertrophied with discrete subaortic stenosis, a more limited left ventricular septal myectomy is performed.[17] Such myectomy carries a low risk of complete heart block, VSD,[16] or injury to the anterior mitral valve leaflet.[21] Intraoperative transesophageal echo is used routinely for assessment of satisfactory relief of obstruction and to exclude aortic or mitral valve dysfunction, or VSD.

## OUTCOME

The patient did well after the operation with an initial excellent improvement in her functional capacity, such that she is now exercising regularly.

Four years after the operation, she continues to report no effort-induced dyspnea. Her only cardiac medication is warfarin.

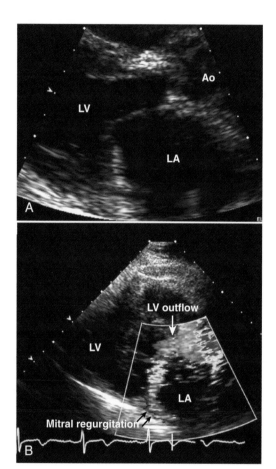

Figure 21-10 Parasternal long-axis view.

Her echocardiogram demonstrated no evidence of any residual subaortic membrane (A), and the flow in the LVOT is unobstructed (B). However, color-flow Doppler does demonstrate an eccentric jet of mitral regurgitation, which was felt to be moderate to severe (grade II–III/IV). The regurgitant volume was 54 mL. The mitral regurgitation, not present on preoperative echocardiogram, was felt to be related to a small, unsupported segment involving the anterior mitral valve leaflet, a potential complication of surgical repair.

The mechanical aortic valve prosthesis is seen and had normal function. The mitral regurgitation has potential to cause progressive volume overload with associated dyspnea and might need surgical repair in the future.

## Selected References

1. Walker F: Subvalvular and supravalvular aortic stenosis. In Gatzoulis MA, Webb GD, Daubeney PEF (eds): Diagnosis and Management of Adult Congenital Heart Disease. Philadelphia, Churchill Livingstone, 2003, pp 223–230.
2. Perloff JK: Congenital aortic stenosis: Congenital aortic regurgitation. In Perloff JK (ed): The Clinical Recognition of Congenital Heart Disease, 4th ed. Philadelphia, WB Saunders, 1994, pp 91–131.
3. Kleinert S, Geva T: Echocardiographic morphometry and geometry of the left ventricular outflow tract in fixed subaortic stenosis. J Am Coll Cardiol 22:1501–1508, 1993.
4. Gewillig M, Daenen WIM, Dumoulin M, Van Der Hauwaert L: Rheologic genesis of discrete subvalvular aortic stenosis: A Doppler echocardiographic study. J Am Coll Cardiol 19:818–824, 1992.
5. Neutze JM, Calder AL, Gentles TL, Wilson NJ: Aortic stenosis. In Moller JH, Hoffman JIE (eds): Pediatric Cardiovascular Medicine, 1st ed. Philadelphia, Churchill Livingstone, 2000, pp 511–551.
6. Kitchiner D, Jackson M, Malaiya R, et al: Morphology of left ventricular outflow tract structures in patients with subaortic stenosis and a ventricular septal defect. Br Heart J 72:251, 1994.
7. Brauner R, Laks H, Drinkwater DC, et al: Benefits of early surgical repair in fixed subaortic stenosis. J Am Coll Cardiol 30:1835–1842, 1997.
8. Freedom RM, Pelech A, Brand A, et al. The progressive nature of subaortic stenosis in congenital heart disease. Int J Cardiol 8:137–143, 1958.
9. Oliver JM, Gonzalez A, Gallego P, et al. Discrete subaortic stenosis in adults: Increased prevalence and slow rate of progression of the obstruction and aortic regurgitation. J Am Coll Cardiol 38:35–42, 2001.
10. De Vries AG, Hess J, Witsenburg M, et al: Management of fixed subaortic stenosis: A retrospective study of 57 cases. J Am Coll Cardiol 19:1013–1017, 1992.
11. Douville EC, Sade RM, Crawford FA, Wiles HB: Subvalvular aortic stenosis: Timing of operation. Ann Thorac Surg 50:29–34, 1990.
12. Frommelt MA, Snider AR, Bove EL, Lupinetti FM: Echocardiographic assessment of subvalvular aortic stenosis before and after operation. J Am Coll Cardiol 19:1018–1023, 1992.
13. Somerville J, Stone S, Ross D: Fate of patients with fixed subaortic stenosis after surgical removal. Br Heart J 43:629–647, 1980.
14. Stellin G, Mazzucco A, Bortolotti U, et al: Late results after resection of discrete and tunnel subaortic stenosis. Eur J Cardio-Thorac Surg 3:235–240, 1989.
15. Suarez de Lezo J, Pan M, Medina A, et al: Immediate and follow-up results of transluminal balloon dilatation for discrete subaortic stenosis. J Am Coll Cardiol 18:1309–1315, 1991.
16. Van Son JAM, Schaff HV, Danielson GK, et al: Surgical treatment of discrete and tunnel subaortic stenosis: Late survival and risk of reoperation. Circulation 88(5 Pt 2):I159–169, 1993.
17. Dearani JA, Danielson GK: Septal myectomy for obstructive hypertrophic cardiomyopathy: Operative techniques. J Thorac Cardiovasc Surg 9:278–292, 2004.
18. Chan KY, Redington AN, Rigby ML, Gibson DG: Cardiac function after surgery for subaortic stenosis: Non-invasive assessment of left ventricular performance. Br Heart J 66:161–165, 1991.
19. Stassano P, Di Tommaso L, Contaldo A, et al: Discrete subaortic stenosis: Long-term prognosis on the progression of the obstruction and of the aortic insufficiency. J Thorac Cardiovasc Surg 53:23–27, 2005.
20. Hazekamp MG, Frank M, Hardjowijono R, et al: Surgery for membranous subaortic stenosis. Eur J Cardio-Thorac Surg 7:356–359, 1993.
21. Wright GB, Keane JF, Nadas AS, et al: Fixed subaortic stenosis in the young: Medical and surgical course in 83 patients. Am J Cardiol 52:830–835, 1983.

# Pericardial Constriction after Relief of Subaortic Stenosis

**Nilesh Sutaria, Derek G. Gibson, and Mary N. Sheppard**

**Age: 17 years**
**Gender: Male**
**Occupation: Student**
**Working diagnosis: Subaortic stenosis**

## HISTORY

Neurofibromatosis type 1 (NF1) was diagnosed soon after birth. No other health issues were identified, however, and the patient grew up normally.

One year ago at a routine clinic visit he was noted to have a systolic murmur. An echocardiogram confirmed significant fibromuscular subaortic stenosis. He was asymptomatic.

He underwent resection of the subaortic obstruction and longitudinal myectomy via a median sternotomy and longitudinal pericardiotomy. The pericardium was completely closed at the end of the procedure. Postoperative recovery was uneventful apart from a persistent 8-mm pericardial effusion without hemodynamic compromise, treated with aspirin.

Two months later he was readmitted to the hospital with dyspnea. Echocardiography showed a minimal pericardial effusion, good LV function, no LVOT obstruction, and mild aortic regurgitation. However, he was very breathless with large bilateral pleural effusions of uncertain etiology. Bilateral chest drains were inserted. The pleural fluid was a transudate. There was continuous drainage from both sides of the chest. Various means were tried in an attempt to reduce the drainage, including albumin replacement, somatostatin infusions, and even total parenteral nutrition and a fat-free diet in case this was a chylothorax. He was also developing a large ascites. Despite these empiric remedies, recurrent pleural effusions remained a problem. Therefore, 5 months later, the patient underwent open thoracotomy, pleural biopsy, and right talc pleurodesis. Repeat echocardiography demonstrated a thickened pericardium, confirmed on CT scanning. He was transferred for further assessment.

**Comments:** NF1 is an autosomal dominant disease affecting 1 in 4000 births. The involvement of neurofibromin in cardiac development is strongly supported by NF1 "knockout" mouse models; thus there is a higher-than-expected frequency of congenital heart disease among NF1 patients, ranging from 0.4% to 6.4% in published series. Of congenital heart defects seen, valvular pulmonary stenosis predominates and is a recognized feature of three uncommon clinical subtypes: (1) NF1, Watson syndrome; (2) NF1, Noonan syndrome; and (3) individuals with large deletions of the NF1 gene.[1]

Subvalvular aortic stenosis spans a spectrum of anomalies from a simple fibrous membrane to a tunnellike fibromuscular band. A small proportion present de novo and are often referred for investigation of an asymptomatic heart murmur as in this case, although others may have a recurrence of a previously resected subvalvular membrane. Subaortic stenosis tends to be progressive, and surgery is recommended for symptomatic patients. The management of asymptomatic individuals is not well defined. In the young adult, a resting LVOT peak pressure gradient of 50 mm Hg or higher has been used as a criterion for intervention. Surgical resection should also be considered in patients with lower gradients if there is LV systolic dysfunction, moderate/severe aortic regurgitation, or a VSD.[2]

## CURRENT SYMPTOMS

The patient had mild exercise limitation, although he was able to walk around the hospital ward. He had no specific complaints.

NYHA class: II

## CURRENT MEDICATIONS

Spironolactone 25 mg daily

Furosemide 40 mg twice daily

## PHYSICAL EXAMINATION

BP 114/77 mm Hg, HR 110 bpm, oxygen saturation 98% on room air

Height 170 cm, weight 66.3 kg, BSA 1.77 m$^2$

Surgical scars: Median sternotomy, right thoracotomy

Neck veins: The neck veins were markedly distended. Examiners were unable to identify the top of the venous pulsation even with the patient upright. There were prominent X and Y descents.

Lungs/chest: There was dullness to percussion and reduced breath sounds at the right lung base.

Heart: The rhythm was regular. There were normal heart sounds, no murmurs heard, and no third heart sound or friction rub.

Abdomen: Significant ascites and hepatomegaly were appreciated.

Extremities: Mild ankle edema was present.

**Comments:** The patient has obvious elevation of the central venous pressure (CVP). Elevated JVP is the hallmark of constrictive pericarditis. The X and Y descents in systole and early diastole, respectively, are prominent.

Kussmaul's sign (not noted in this patient) was first described in patients with constrictive pericarditis and denotes the abnormal inspiratory increase in venous pressure when the heart is unable to accept the increase in systemic venous return without a marked increase in the filling pressure.

## LABORATORY DATA

| | |
|---|---|
| Hemoglobin | **11.2 g/dL** (13.0–17.0) |
| Hematocrit/PCV | 44% (41–51) |
| MCV | 92 fL (83–99) |
| Platelet count | $362 \times 10^9$/L (150–400) |
| Sodium | 140 mmol/L (134–145) |
| Potassium | 4.3 mmol/L (3.5–5.2) |
| Creatinine | 0.95 mg/dL (0.6–1.2) |
| Blood urea nitrogen | 4.8 mmol/L (2.5–6.5) |

## ELECTROCARDIOGRAM

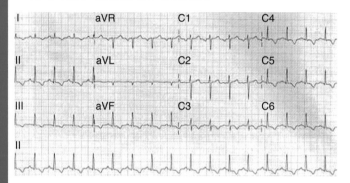

Figure 22-1 Electrocardiogram.

### FINDINGS

Heart rate: 102 bpm

QRS axis: +74°

QRS duration: 76 msec

Sinus tachycardia, normal axis, widespread T-wave inversion

**Comments:** Voltage criteria for LV hypertrophy, although absent in this case, would be expected in 65% to 85% of patients with subaortic stenosis.

Generalized T-wave inversion is a common finding in constrictive pericarditis. Other recognized changes include low QRS voltage and LA abnormalities suggestive of "p mitrale."

## CHEST X-RAY

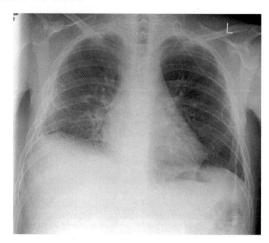

Figure 22-2 Posteroanterior projection.

### FINDINGS

Cardiothoracic ratio: 47%

Situs solitus, levocardia, left aortic arch.

Median sternotomy clips were present. The heart size was at the upper limit of normal. An elevated right hemidiaphragm was seen with a possible right pleural effusion.

**Comments:** There was no evidence of pericardial calcification, which would be suggestive of tuberculous or idiopathic constrictive pericarditis (see also Case 72).

## EXERCISE TESTING

Not performed

## ECHOCARDIOGRAM

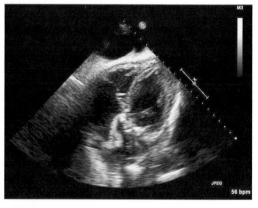

Figure 22-3 Apical four-chamber view.

### FINDINGS

The ventricular chambers were normal in size. There was normal LV systolic function (LVEDd 45 mm, LVESd 35 mm). Peak LVOT velocity was 1.0 m/sec. The atria were dilated.

**Comments:** The systolic function is not impaired, but on cine imaging, limited diastolic expansion could be appreciated as a result of pericardial constriction. It is difficult to assess the pericardial thickness with echocardiography, but it appears thickened and bright in this window.

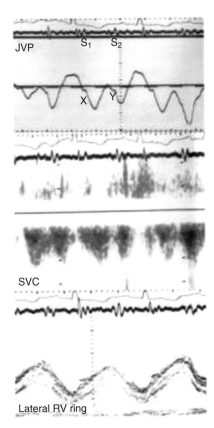

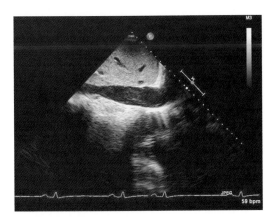

Figure 22-4 *Top,* Jugular venous pressure (JVP) recording with ECG and phonocardiogram. *Middle,* Pulsed Doppler flow in the superior vena cava (SVC). *Bottom,* RV long-axis function from M-mode through the lateral RV ring (lateral tricuspid annulus).

***Comments:*** The jugular venous waveform has a steep systolic X descent occurring before the second heart sound (S$_2$), which is associated with predominant systolic flow in the SVC. This is a very reliable finding for pericardial constriction. A stiff fibrous pericardium adherent to the epicardial layer of the myocardium limits its normal minor axis movement through the cardiac cycle. It cannot, however, affect long-axis shortening and lengthening associated with motion of the two atrioventricular rings. The downward displacement of the RV free wall in systole results in increased RA capacity that may be greater than the volume of venous return. Hence, RA pressure falls. This causes the characteristic X descent. The lateral RV ring moves normally toward the apex in systole (bottom panel), indicating that long-axis function is well maintained.

Figure 22-5 Subcostal view.

## FINDINGS

The IVC was dilated and did not collapse normally during inspiration.

***Comments:*** The IVC size can reflect the CVP. In this case, its appearance is consistent with elevated RA pressure.

# MAGNETIC RESONANCE IMAGING

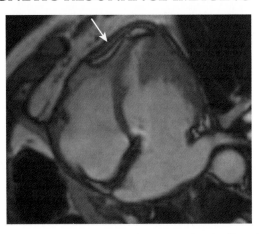

Figure 22-6 Oblique axial steady-state free precession cine (four-chamber view).

## FINDINGS

Relatively small RV and LV volumes but normal LV and RV systolic function. The pericardium was thickened (*arrow*) and adherent in some areas to the myocardium.

***Comments:*** The indexed volumes were low, reflecting limited filling of the ventricles from external constriction.

### Ventricular Volume Quantification

|  | LV | (Normal range) | RV | (Normal range) |
|---|---|---|---|---|
| EDV (mL) | 104 | (77–195) | 90 | (88–227) |
| ESV (mL) | 46 | (19–72) | 32 | (23–103) |
| SV (mL) | 58 | (51–133) | 58 | (52–138) |
| EF (%) | **56** | (57–74) | 64 | (48–74) |
| EDVi (mL/m$^2$) | **59** | (68–103) | **51** | (68–114) |
| ESVi (mL/m$^2$) | 26 | (19–41) | **18** | (21–50) |
| SVi (mL/m$^2$) | **33** | (44–68) | 33 | (23–50) |
| Mass index (g/m$^2$) | 80 | (59–93) | 38 | (23–50) |

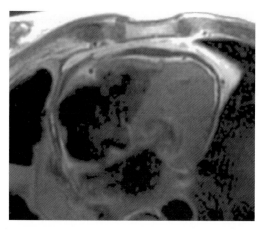

Figure 22-7 Axial turbo spin echo sequence.

## FINDINGS

The pericardial thickening is visualized.

**Comments:** Turbo spin (black blood) imaging demonstrates low signal from the dense pericardium, particularly well seen at the apex (black). The white material on either side is epicardial or extrapericardial fat.

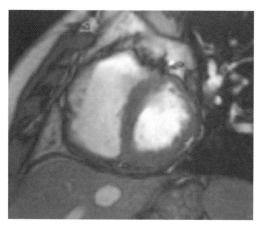

Figure 22-8 Oblique sagittal steady-state free precession cine (short-axis view).

## FINDINGS

There was significant shift of the septum during the cardiac cycle. The pericardial thickening was again seen, particularly along the inferior border of the heart.

**Comments:** There are several ways to assess for pericardial constriction by MRI. The most sophisticated are to use tagging to show that the myocardium and pericardium move together during contraction rather than slide past each other, or to use real-time imaging to demonstrate ventricular interdependence to differentiate restriction from constriction. In this cine image, one can see the free movement of the septum from the relative differences in filling between RV and LV. This finding confirms that the restrictive physiology seen on physical exam and echo is not due to changes in the myocardium.

Note also on the cine image some artifacts (darker discoloration near the RVOT and within the septum) from prior surgery.

## CATHETERIZATION

### HEMODYNAMICS
Heart rate    110 bpm

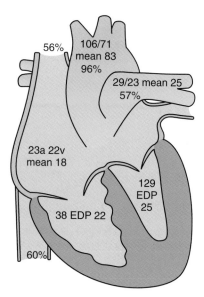

Figure 22-9 Hemodynamic data obtained at catheterization.

**Calculations**

| | |
|---|---|
| Qp (L/min) | 4.17 |
| Qs (L/min) | 4.38 |
| Cardiac index (L/min/m$^2$) | 2.48 |
| Qp/Qs | 0.95 |
| PVR (Wood units) | 0.00 |
| SVR (Wood units) | 14.83 |

### FINDINGS
Severely elevated diastolic pressures were present in all chambers. There was a mild pullback gradient from the aorta to the LV. There was no intracardiac shunt.

**Comments:** Cardiac catheterization was performed to confirm the hemodynamic changes of pericardial constriction. The equalization of pressures in diastole is consistent with the restrictive filling due to constrictive pericarditis. The calculated pulmonary vascular resistance is zero because the main pulmonary artery pressure is the same as the LV end-diastolic pressure, though physiologically speaking there is still resistance.

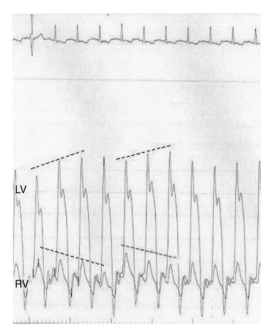

Figure 22-10 Simultaneous left ventricular and right ventricular pressures traces obtained at cardiac catheterization.

## FINDINGS

The LV trace has a "dip and plateau" waveform, and there is equalization of end-diastolic pressures in the LV and RV—the hallmark of the restrictive physiology in constrictive pericarditis.

**Comments:** The rigid pericardium in constrictive pericarditis shields the intracardiac chambers from respiration-related changes in intrathoracic pressure. There is increased ventricular interdependence (*dotted lines*) as assessed by respiratory discordance of LV and RV pressures (upsloping for the LV but downsloping for the RV), consistent increase in RV pressure during peak inspiration, and a time when LV pressure is at its lowest.

This has been shown to be the most reliable hemodynamic finding for distinguishing patients with constrictive pericarditis from those with other disease entities, in particular restrictive cardiomyopathy in which one would expect both right and left peak systolic ventricular pressures to fall with inspiration and rise with expiration, parallel with the changes in intrathoracic pressures.[3]

### FOCUSED CLINICAL QUESTIONS AND DISCUSSION POINTS

1. **What is the cause of the bilateral pleural effusions and ascites in this patient?**

*The patient has constrictive pericarditis secondary to his previous cardiac surgery for subaortic stenosis.*

*Constrictive pericarditis is a syndrome defined as chronic fibrous thickening of the wall of the pericardial sac, such that normal diastolic filling of the heart is hindered.[4] This causes symptoms and signs of right-sided heart failure with systemic venous congestion. Typically, the disease is slowly progressive, and the diagnosis, as in this case, may often be delayed for months.*

*It is crucial to differentiate between constrictive pericarditis, which is often treatable by pericardiectomy, and restrictive cardiomyopathy, which is not. Both have similar clinical presentations. Proper differentiation requires demonstration of (1) dissociation between intrathoracic and intracardiac pressures and (2) exaggerated ventricular interdependence in diastolic filling. Echo Doppler data and dynamic respiratory changes in simultaneous LV and RV pressure shown at cardiac catheterization are invaluable techniques for establishing the diagnosis.*

*Prior pericarditis, cardiac surgery, and chest irradiation now account for 50% of cases, although one third are idiopathic. Of more than 5000 adults who underwent cardiac surgery, postoperative constrictive pericarditis was recognized in only 11 patients (0.2%) despite the pericardium being left open in all cases. The average interval between surgery and presentation of pericardial constriction was 82 days, in a range of 14 to 186.[5] Tuberculous pericarditis causing constriction has become rare in developed countries.*

2. **How should this patient be treated?**

*Although medical treatment with diuretics and salt restriction may temporarily alleviate symptoms, patients do poorly without surgical pericardiectomy, which is the only definitive treatment for constrictive pericarditis. The perioperative mortality rate ranges from 5% in recent reports to nearly 15% in older series. Symptomatic improvement is reported in more than 90% of patients with 5-year survival rates of 75% to 85%.*

3. **What is the patient's long-term prognosis?**

*Older age at diagnosis and a history of chest irradiation are associated with poorer outcome. Furthermore, long-term survival is worse for patients with poorer NYHA class at operation, underscoring the need for early recognition and treatment of this frequently overlooked condition.[6]*

*The patient will require further assessment of body weight, liver enlargement, CVP, and ascites to guide the dosage of diuretics over time. Even with successful surgery, CVP and ventricular filling in many instances will not return to normal.*

*It is important to note that following repair for subaortic stenosis, recurrence of LVOT obstruction is common (15%–27%) with an average time to recurrence of 3.6 and 4.7 years.[7] Progressive aortic regurgitation is reported in 25% to 40% of patients during long-term follow-up. All patients therefore require surveillance.*

## FINAL DIAGNOSIS

Repair of subaortic stenosis

Postoperative constrictive pericarditis

## PLAN OF ACTION

Pericardiectomy

## INTERVENTION

The patient underwent pericardiectomy 6 months after his initial surgery for subaortic stenosis. At operation, the pericardium was extremely thick, although the fibrotic process did not appear to infiltrate the myocardium. The pericardial layer was relatively easily stripped with a clear line of cleavage. The CVP dropped from 25 mm Hg to 17 mm Hg immediately.

## OUTCOME

The patient made an uncomplicated recovery. JVP remained elevated postoperatively. However, at a 2-month follow-up visit, his JVP was normal. He felt well without exertional limitation, and no longer required diuretics.

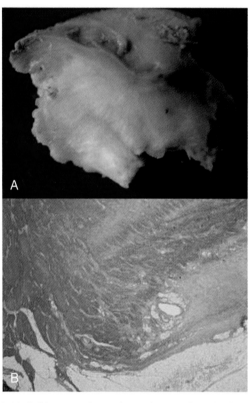

Figure 22-11 **A**, Macroscopic specimen of pericardium obtained at operation shows grossly thickened pericardium (15 mm). Beneath a layer of fibrous pericardium, one can see collagen infiltrating the pericardial fat (white). **B**, Microscopic histology of pericardium, collagen stained with Elastin von Geisen. Dense fibrosis with collagen (stained red) infiltrating pericardial fat (white).

***Comments:*** The pathologic findings are consistent with constriction due to a thickened, noncompliant pericardium.

BEFORE PERICARDIECTOMY     AFTER PERICARDIECTOMY

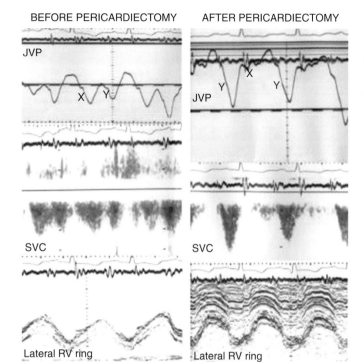

Figure 22-12 *Top*, Jugular venous pressure (JVP) recording with electrocardiogram and phonocardiogram. *Middle*, Pulsed-Doppler flow in the superior vena cava (SVC). *Bottom*, RV long-axis function from M-mode through the lateral right ventricle ring (lateral tricuspid annulus).

## FINDINGS

Neck vein, Doppler, and M-mode examination was performed following his pericardiectomy.

After pericardiectomy, the JVP trace changed to show a dominant diastolic Y descent indicating a shift from pericardial to myocardial disease. This is accompanied by predominant diastolic flow in the superior vena cava. RV long-axis function, assessed by excursion of the lateral tricuspid annulus, remains preserved.

***Comments:*** The venous pressure and waveform had returned to normal in 1 to 2 months.

## Selected References

1. Lin AE, Birch PH, Korf BR, et al: Cardiovascular malformations and other cardiac abnormalities in neurofibromatosis 1 (NF1). Am J Med Genet 95:108–117, 2000.
2. Aboulhosn J, Child J: Left ventricular outflow obstruction: Subaortic stenosis, bicuspid aortic valve, supravalvar aortic stenosis, and coarctation of the aorta. Circulation 114:2412–2422, 2006.
3. Hurrell DG, Nishimura RA, Higano ST, et al: Value of dynamic respiratory changes in left and right ventricular pressures for the diagnosis of constrictive pericarditis. Circulation 93:2007–2013, 1996.
4. White P: Chronic constrictive pericarditis (Pick's disease): Treated by pericardial resection. Lancet 2:539–548, 597–603, 1935.
5. Kutcher MA, King SB, III, Alimurung BN, et al: Constrictive pericarditis as a complication of cardiac surgery: Recognition of an entity. Am J Cardiol 50:742–748, 1982.
6. Ling LH, Oh JK, Schaff HV, et al: Constrictive pericarditis in the modern era: Evolving clinical spectrum and impact on outcome after pericardiectomy. Circulation 100:1380–1386, 1999.
7. Brauner R, Laks H, Drinkwater DCJ, et al: Benefits of early surgical repair in fixed subaortic stenosis. J Am Coll Cardiol 30:1835–1842, 1997.

# Ventricular Arrhythmia Following a Ross Procedure

**Jonathan Lyne and Tom Wong**

Age: 57 years
Gender: Male
Occupation: Logistics planner
Working diagnosis: Pulmonary stenosis with prior Ross repair

## HISTORY

Aortic regurgitation was diagnosed when the patient was 23 years old. The patient underwent a Ross procedure 6 months later. He recovered uneventfully.

Ten years postoperatively he developed symptoms of rapid palpitation. No arrhythmias were documented. Coronary angiography revealed a normal neoaortic valve with mild aortic regurgitation. The pulmonary homograft was calcified, and there were normal coronary arteries. The patient was prescribed digoxin 250 μg daily with some symptomatic improvement.

A presyncopal episode occurred 6 years later and was associated with further palpitation. On 24-hour ECG recording, nonsustained ventricular tachycardia (VT) was present. Atenolol was prescribed, but the patient continued to experience intermittent palpitations without further presyncope.

The patient was reviewed on an annual basis and remained asymptomatic apart from occasional palpitations. During the last consultation he complained of a mild reduction in exercise tolerance.

*Comments:* In August 1967 Donald Ross in London performed the first successful procedure to replace a diseased aortic valve with a pulmonary autograft (the patient's own harvested pulmonary valve), while placing a human homograft valve in the pulmonary position. The pulmonary autograft has been shown to be resistant to long-term degeneration, showing high and stable survival rates.[1]

It is important that any congenital heart disease patient with palpitations and/or documented arrhythmia undergo a thorough hemodynamic assessment. Often arrhythmia can be the first sign of underlying hemodynamic abnormalities that need to be addressed. Hence, the angiographic study performed initially was done bearing this in mind.

## CURRENT SYMPTOMS

The patient is able to walk up one flight of stairs but finds more than this difficult and slows due to dyspnea. He is able to walk his dog on flat ground at a measured pace.

NYHA class: II

*Comments:* Although subjective assessment of symptoms can often be difficult in patients with congenital heart disease, this patient had previously been extremely fit as a soldier, and was hence more aware of his own exertional limitation and concerned about his recent physical decline.

## CURRENT MEDICATIONS

Atenolol 25 mg daily

## PHYSICAL EXAMINATION

BP 155/75 mm Hg, HR 72 bpm, oxygen saturation 97%

Height 180 cm, weight 102 kg, BSA 2.26 m²

Surgical scars: Median sternotomy

Neck veins: JVP was not elevated, with normal waveform.

Lungs/chest: Chest was clear.

Heart: The patient was in sinus rhythm. There was a right ventricular heave and a soft pulmonary second sound. There was a grade 2 ejection systolic murmur in the pulmonary area.

Abdomen: Unremarkable

Extremities: There was no pitting edema or clubbing.

## LABORATORY DATA

| | |
|---|---|
| Hemoglobin | 15.9 g/dL (13.0–17.0) |
| Hematocrit/PCV | 46% (41–51) |
| MCV | 90 fL (83–99) |
| Platelet count | 262 × 10⁹/L (150–400) |
| Sodium | 137 mmol/L (134–145) |
| Potassium | 3.9 mmol/L (3.5–5.2) |
| Creatinine | 0.97 mg/dL (0.6–1.2) |
| Blood urea nitrogen | 5.8 mg/dL (6–24) |

### OTHER RELEVANT LAB RESULTS

| | |
|---|---|
| Corrected calcium | 2.24 mmol/L (2.20–2.62) |
| Magnesium | 0.8 mmol/L (0.7–1.0) |

*Comments:* The serum potassium and magnesium are within the normal range. Electrolyte imbalance is an important cause of VT and needs to be excluded.

# ELECTROCARDIOGRAM

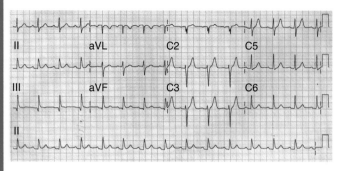

Figure 23-1 Electrocardiogram.

## FINDINGS

Heart rate: 72 bpm

PR interval: 205 msec

QRS axis: +74°

QRS duration: 106 msec

QTC duration: 410 msec

Normal sinus rhythm with normal axis and PR/QT intervals. Normal ECG.

***Comments:*** There is no evidence of a long QT syndrome or pre-excitation to explain the palpitation. Atrial arrhythmias in the setting of pre-excitation may lead to broad complex tachycardia.

## CHEST X-RAY

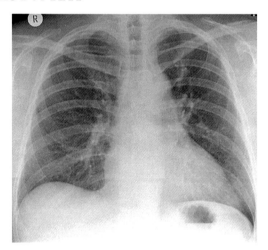

Figure 23-2 Posteroanterior projection.

## FINDINGS

Cardiothoracic ratio: 58%

The cardiac silhouette was enlarged. There was mild dilatation of the main pulmonary trunk.

***Comments:*** No obvious calcification of the pulmonary homograft is seen (30 years after its original implantation). When severe RVOT obstruction is present, RA and RV enlargement are common. The latter is better seen on a lateral film, not available for this patient.

Also note the lack of dilatation of the ascending aorta.

# EXERCISE TESTING

| | | Rest | Peak |
|---|---|---|---|
| Exercise protocol: | Modified Bruce | | |
| Duration (min:sec): | 9:50 | | |
| Reason for stopping: | Dizziness | | |
| ECG changes: | Ventricular tachycardia | | |

| | Rest | Peak |
|---|---|---|
| Heart rate (bpm): | 72 | 190 |
| O2 saturation (%): | 97 | 97 |
| Blood pressure (mm Hg): | 155/75 | 210/80 |
| Peak Vo2 (mL/kg/min): | | 21.5 |
| Percent predicted (%): | | 74 |
| Ve/Vco2: | | 23 |
| Metabolic equivalents: | | 8.2 |

The test was stopped due to clinical tachyarrhythmia, which terminated abruptly approximately 1 minute after cessation of exercise, with spontaneous restoration of sinus tachycardia.

***Comments:*** Exercise testing can be very helpful in the assessment of valvular lesions, providing information on the hemodynamic responses to exercise and the effect of exercise stress on symptoms and/or arrhythmia. In turn, this information may guide timing of necessary intervention(s).

The patient in this case was able to attain an acceptable level of exertion (>85% maximum predicted HR) but developed what seemed like VT. This was unexpected, as the patient was thought to have a history of supraventricular tachycardia.

# ELECTROCARDIOGRAM

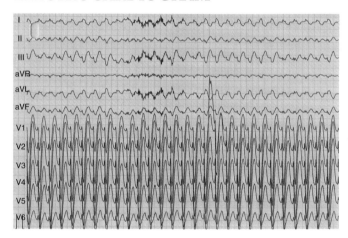

Figure 23-3 Electrocardiogram during exercise.

## FINDINGS

Regular, wide complex tachycardia, heart rate 190 bpm, with LBBB conduction.

***Comments:*** The significance of this ECG is that it is likely to reflect RV pressure overload exacerbated by exertion, thereby causing RV strain and resulting in the induction of sustained VT.

However, there is also the possibility that this represents aberrant conduction of a supraventricular arrhythmia. It may represent an atypical atrial flutter circuit with 1:1 conduction. This could be possibly related to the atriotomy performed at the initial operation, or this could be another type of atrial tachycardia with aberrant conduction.

Overall, the rhythm here was felt to be most consistent with VT.

# ECHOCARDIOGRAM

## Overall Findings

Mild to moderate pulmonary stenosis with a peak velocity of just over 3 m/sec (i.e., Doppler pressure gradient approximately 36 mm Hg). Note the A-wave (forward flow under the curve, coinciding with the P-wave and preceding systole) suggestive of RV restriction.[2]

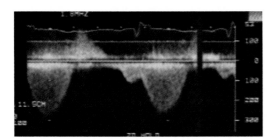

Figure 23-4 Continuous-wave Doppler recording from transthoracic echocardiogram.

***Comments:*** Echocardiography using continuous wave Doppler imaging allows determination of the transvalvular gradient. For pulmonary stenosis (unlike aortic stenosis) there is a good correlation between the Doppler-derived peak gradient and the catheter-derived peak-to-peak gradient. This is because the pressures are lower in amplitude in the pulmonary artery than in the aorta and the dP/dt is slightly different from the right side.[3]

The presence of an A-wave throughout the respiratory cycle suggests that the RV is somewhat stiff, thus counteracting the effects of any pulmonary regurgitation and limiting the extent of RV dilatation.

# MAGNETIC RESONANCE IMAGING

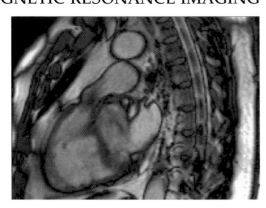

Figure 23-5 Oblique sagittal trueFISP cine image, right ventricular outflow tract view.

## Findings

There was obstruction of the pulmonary homograft.

***Comments:*** MRI provides the most accurate, available assessment of RV function and is very useful in visualizing the exact level of the RV outlet obstruction. The pulmonary valve is usually identifiable by visualizing the valve cusps as they close at the onset of diastole. Identifying the level of obstruction is important, as the obstruction may not only be valvular but also sub- and/or supravalvular following a Ross procedure. In a follow-up study of 144 patients following a Ross procedure, in 14 of 15 patients with RVOT gradients above 30 mm Hg, MRI showed evidence of narrowing of the whole homograft or distal suture line, with obvious excess surrounding tissue in 11 patients.[4]

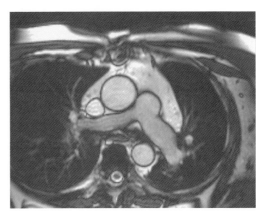

Figure 23-6 Oblique transverse plane, aligned to image the main, left, and right pulmonary arteries.

***Comments:*** There was disproportionate dilatation of the left pulmonary artery as seen on the CXR, the poststenotic jet being directed mainly into the left pulmonary artery.

# CATHETERIZATION

## Hemodynamics

Heart rate    72 bpm

| | Pressure | Saturation (%) |
|---|---|---|
| SVC | | 70 |
| IVC | | 74 |
| RA | mean 7 | |
| RV | 72/9 | |
| PA | 34/10 mean 20 | 71 |
| PCWP | mean 12 | |
| LV | 161/**15** | |
| Aorta | 156/75 mean 107 | 97 |

**Calculations**

| | |
|---|---|
| Qp (L/min) | 4.60 |
| Qs (L/min) | 4.77 |
| Cardiac index (L/min/m²) | 2.11 |
| Qp/Qs | 0.96 |
| PVR (Wood units) | 1.74 |
| SVR (Wood units) | 1.68 |

## Findings

There was a 38 mm Hg gradient (peak to peak) across the pulmonary outflow tract. The aortic pulse pressure was wide, compatible with aortic regurgitation or inelastic arteries. The left ventricular end-diastolic pressure was mildly elevated, with the wedge pressure at the upper limit of normal.

***Comments:*** The procedure was done primarily to measure the gradient across the pulmonary homograft and to look for coronary artery disease. Given both the VT with exercise and the possible need for pulmonary valve replacement surgery, excluding significant coronary disease was imperative.

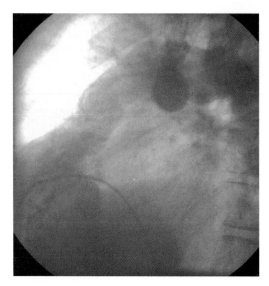

Figure 23-7 X-ray contrast right ventriculography, lateral projection.

## FINDINGS

The pulmonary homograft was heavily calcified and restricted. There was only minor atheroma in the left coronary artery.

***Comments:*** The findings are consistent with both the echocardiogram and the MRI.

### FOCUSED CLINICAL QUESTIONS AND DISCUSSION POINTS

1. What is the cause of exercise-induced VT in this patient?

*This patient had long episodic arrhythmias following a Ross procedure. There are a number of possible mechanisms for the induction and maintenance of arrhythmia. Scar tissue from the procedure itself may partially isolate areas of myocardium permitting reentry circuits to be generated and sustained.*

*A previous follow-up study has described both atrial and ventricular exercise-induced arrhythmias in this population.[5] Arrhythmias were more common in those with higher transpulmonary gradients, indicating a possible relation to RV pressure overload. It is not known whether these arrhythmias are related to preoperative, surgical, or postoperative factors. Interestingly, most patients with arrhythmia as in this case had a preoperative diagnosis of aortic regurgitation, suggesting that preoperative LV enlargement may also be a risk factor for developing later arrhythmia.*

*Increased LV mass has been associated with an increased frequency and complexity of ventricular arrhythmia and was also noted in this study.*

2. What is the expected long-term outcome after the Ross procedure?

*The pulmonary autograft procedure offers low rates of degeneration, endocarditis, and thromboembolism for a period lasting more than 20 years, particularly in the young. Freedom from reoperation to the autograft is approximately 75% at 20 years postoperatively.[1] In the early postoperative period, malposition of the autograft cusps is the most common reason for reoperation. Over the long term, a degree of mild to moderate aortic regurgitation is common.*

*Pulmonary homograft stenosis and insufficiency have been well recognized, and require reoperation in approximately 20% of patients within 20 years.[1] Stenosis may be present at any level of the RVOT including subvalvular, valvular, or supravalvular stenoses. It has been hypothesized that the immune response mounted against the donor homograft may result in dysfunction.*

*There may also be a degree of postoperative inflammation leading to shrinkage and/or compression of the pulmonary homograft.*

3. What therapy, if any, should be offered to this patient?

*Overall, the data in this patient suggest there is only a moderate degree of homograft stenosis at the most, which in isolation would not constitute an indication for pulmonary homograft replacement. Despite his complaints of exercise deterioration, his exercise capacity remains quite good. In fact, it seemed that his exercise test was limited by the tachycardia. However, the question remained as to whether the patient should be considered for pulmonary homograft replacement on the basis of his exercise-induced VT. Before answering, it was felt necessary to undertake an electrophysiologic study to investigate whether VT could be easily induced and sustained. A firm decision could then be made regarding whether to offer reoperation or continue with medical follow-up.*

## FINAL DIAGNOSIS

Moderate pulmonary homograft stenosis

Exercise-induced VT with some hemodynamic compromise

## PLAN OF ACTION

Electrophysiologic study

## INTERVENTION

The patient underwent electrophysiologic testing, which showed no inducible VT; neither was there inducible supraventricular tachycardia.

## OUTCOME

Following a multidisciplinary meeting and a lengthy discussion with the patient it was decided to continue with medical therapy with close monitoring of the situation. The patient was scheduled for a repeat transthoracic echocardiogram, cardiopulmonary exercise test, and a cardiac MRI in 12 months. However, the patient presented 9 months later with streptococcus viridans endocarditis on his pulmonary homograft. He responded well to a 4 week-course of intravenous antibiotics. Secondary to his endocarditis, there was further deterioration of his pulmonary homograft function, with a peak Doppler gradient of 70 mm Hg and moderate pulmonary regurgitation. He thus had elective pulmonary homograft replacement 6 months later, which was uneventful.

Two years after his redo surgery, the patient remains asymptomatic, with maintained biventricular systolic function, a well-functioning pulmonary homograft prosthesis, and no sustained arrhythmia on atenolol therapy.

### Selected References

1. Chambers JC, Somerville J, Stone S, Ross DN: Pulmonary autograft procedure for aortic valve disease: Long-term results of the pioneer series. Circulation 96:2206–2214, 1997.
2. Gatzoulis MA, Clark AL, Cullen S, et al: Right ventricular diastolic function 15–35 years after repair of tetralogy of Fallot: Restrictive physiology predicts superior exercise performance. Circulation 91:1775–1781, 1995.
3. Currie PJ, Hagler DJ, Seward JB, et al: Instantaneous pressure gradient: A simultaneous Doppler and dual catheter correlative study. J Am Coll Cardiol 7:800–806, 1986.
4. Carr-White GS, Kilner PJ, Hon JK, et al: Incidence, location, pathology, and significance of pulmonary homograft stenosis after the Ross operation. Circulation 104(12 Suppl 1):I16–I20, 2001.
5. Phillips JR, Daniels CJ, Orsinelli DA, et al: Valvular hemodynamics and arrhythmias with exercise following the Ross procedure. Am J Cardiol 87:577–583, 2001.

# Part III
# Coarctation of the Aorta

# Acute Presentation with Cerebral Hemorrhage

**Panagiotis D. Arvanitis**

**Age: 26**
**Gender: Male**
**Occupation: Engineer**
**Working diagnosis: Subarachnoid hemorrhage, suspected aortic coarctation**

## HISTORY

The patient was well throughout childhood and adolescence, without physical limitation or any health problems.

Three weeks ago he suddenly developed a severe headache associated with transient loss of consciousness. He had neck stiffness and was slightly confused. He complained of severely impaired vision bilaterally as well as impairment of his visual fields. Examination at the time showed bilateral subretinal hemorrhages. A CT scan of the brain showed diffuse subarachnoid hemorrhage.

A cerebral angiogram via the right femoral route was attempted but failed because the catheter could not be advanced past the thoracic descending aorta. Instead, the study was performed via the right brachial approach. The angiogram revealed an anterior communicating artery aneurysm.

The patient underwent right frontal craniotomy and successful clipping of the aneurysm. Postoperatively he had a left hemiparesis, which resolved over the following days.

He had smoked for 10 years and occasionally drank alcohol.

**Comments:** Twelve percent of patients presenting with sudden-onset headache with a normal neurological examination, and up to 25% of those with an abnormal examination, have a subarachnoid hemorrhage.[1] The mortality rate for a subarachnoid hemorrhage is 50%.

Risk factors for intracranial aneurysm include advanced age (>50 years), female gender, cigarette smoking, cocaine use, hypertension, head trauma, and inherited factors such as autosomal dominant polycystic kidney disease, Ehlers-Danlos syndrome, hereditary hemorrhagic telangiectasia, pseudoxanthoma elasticum, alpha$_1$-antitrypsin deficiency, aortic coarctation, Klinefelter's syndrome, Noonan syndrome, and alpha-glucosidase deficiency.[2,3]

The first-line investigation for a suspected subarachnoid hemorrhage is high-resolution CT scan of the brain. Sensitivity is 98% if done within the first 12 hours, and lower if the study is done later. Digital subtraction angiography is the gold standard for identifying the source of hemorrhage.

Treatment of a ruptured intracranial aneurysm with open craniotomy and clipping has a 2.6% mortality and 10.9% morbidity. Endovascular treatment for such aneurysms is still evolving.

The history of an intracranial aneurysm and the failure of cerebral angiogram via the right femoral route should raise strong suspicions for coarctation of the aorta (CoA). Ten percent of the patients presenting to the emergency department with ruptured intracranial aneurysm have undiagnosed coarctation.[3,4]

## CURRENT SYMPTOMS

Prior to his cerebral hemorrhage the patient denied any symptomatology.

The patient was recovering from his operation and regaining function on his left side. Vision was still incomplete.

His blood pressure was low in the immediate postoperative period but gradually became severely elevated and controlled with atenolol and amlodipine.

NYHA class: I (prior to these events)

**Comments:** Most patients with suspected CoA are asymptomatic. However, in some cases, a careful history may reveal exercise limitations compared to peers, particularly involving lower body strength and stamina.

The diagnosis of coarctation is made in most cases because of the discovery of high blood pressure.

If symptoms are present, they can be attributed either to upper body hypertension, such as headache, nose bleeding, dizziness, and tinnitus, or to lower body hypoperfusion, including abdominal angina and exertional leg fatigue. True leg claudication may suggest the presence of abdominal coarctation.

Very occasionally patients come to medical attention with symptoms of LV failure, aortic dissection, or intracranial hemorrhage, as with our patient.

## CURRENT MEDICATIONS

Atenolol 100 mg once daily

Amlodipine 10 mg once daily

## PHYSICAL EXAMINATION

BP 134/76 mm Hg (right arm), 97/46 (right leg); HR 60 bpm, oxygen saturation 99% on room air

Height 177 cm, weight 73 kg, BSA 1.89 m²

Surgical scars: Right frontal craniotomy

Neck veins: JVP is not elevated.

Lungs/chest: Chest was clear.

Heart: The rhythm was regular. The apex was not displaced. The right and left radial pulses were strong, but his femoral pulses were relatively weak and there was an appreciable radiofemoral delay. The apex was not displaced. He had a normal first and split second sound with an early systolic click and a grade 2–3/6 ejection systolic heart murmur best heard at the back.

Abdomen: Soft, nontender, nonpalpable spleen and liver, normal bowel sounds

Extremities: No clubbing of the fingers or toes, and no edema

Neurological examination: The left hemiparesis had now completely resolved.

Ophthalmologic assessment: Complete right hemianopsia. Normal visual acuity and cranial nerve function.

**Comments:** Most adults with CoA are asymptomatic, and the diagnosis is made when systemic arterial hypertension is observed in the arm(s) with diminished femoral pulses during routine physical examination.

On physical examination the cardinal sign of CoA is differential blood pressure and pulses between upper and lower extremities. The femoral pulse is weak and delayed. A systolic thrill may be palpable in the suprasternal notch, and LV enlargement may be noted. A systolic ejection murmur can be identified along the left sternal border and in the back, particularly over the coarctation. A continuous murmur caused by flow through the collateral vessels may be heard in the back. A systolic ejection click, due to bicuspid aortic valve, is very common in patients with aortic coarctation.

## LABORATORY DATA

| | |
|---|---|
| Hemoglobin | 14.7 g/dL (13.0–17.0) |
| Hematocrit/PCV | 43% (41–51) |
| MCV | 91 fL (83–99) |
| Platelet count | 194 × 10⁹/L (150–400) |
| Sodium | 138 mmol/L (134–145) |
| Potassium | 4.3 mmol/L (3.5–5.2) |
| Creatinine | 0.7 mg/dL (0.6–1.2) |
| Blood urea nitrogen | 5.1 mmol/L (2.5–6.5) |

**Comments:** No abnormal values present.

## ELECTROCARDIOGRAM

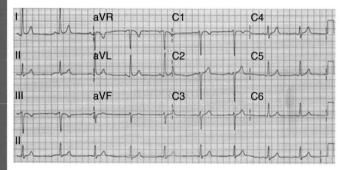

Figure 24-1 Electrocardiogram.

## FINDINGS

Heart rate: 53 bpm

PR interval: 172 msec

QRS axis: −15°

QRS duration: 105 msec

Sinus rhythm, bradycardia

The QRS duration is mildly prolonged.

The QRS axis is slightly shifted to the left.

R1 + S3 greater than 25 mm and RaVL greater than 11 mm suggest LV hypertrophy.

No LA overload

**Comments:** The sinus bradycardia reflects atenolol therapy.

## CHEST X-RAY

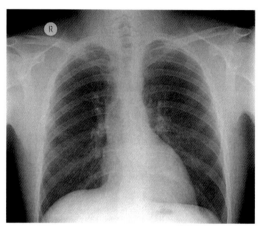

Figure 24-2 Posteroanterior projection.

## FINDINGS

Cardiothoracic ratio: 51%

The CXR shows a normal heart size. Rib notching is present in the left fifth and seventh ribs. The fullness to the right of the midline may indicate an ascending aortopathy.

**Comments:** The characteristic "figure 3 sign" delineating the dilatation of the proximal descending aorta and postcoarctation dilatation of the descending aorta creating a double contour in the region of the coarctation is also present.

In most adults with aortic coarctation rib notching is absent or unappreciated. If present, it is often most visible at the posteroinferior border of the third to eighth ribs and is caused by the impression of enlarged and tortuous intercostal collateral arteries.

## EXERCISE TESTING

Not performed

# ECHOCARDIOGRAM

## OVERALL FINDINGS

The patient had a bicuspid aortic valve with normal function. There was normal LV size and systolic function, normal function of all other valves, and no chamber enlargement.

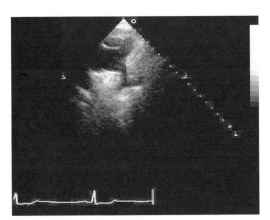

Figure 24-3 Suprasternal view, 2D image.

## FINDINGS

The suprasternal view shows localized segmental narrowing in aortic luminal diameter in the region of the ligamentum arteriosum, just distal to the left subclavian artery.

**Comments:** The site of the stenosis can only be seen properly in the suprasternal view. However, adult images are not always optimal because of artifact caused by the proximity of the left bronchus.

Even though the coarctation is near the left subclavian, there was still normal blood pressure in the left arm, as may be seen in coarctation, in contrast to the blood pressure in the legs.

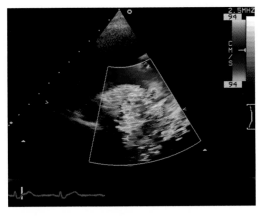

Figure 24-4 Color Doppler imaging, suprasternal view.

## FINDINGS

Turbulent flow through an area of coarctation was visible.

**Comments:** In this suprasternal view, slightly different from the prior 2D plane, there is turbulent flow into the distal aorta, although the narrowest portion of the coarctation is not as well appreciated. Color flow in the lower right could reflect artifact or turbulent flow in collateral arteries, though the former is more likely in this image.

In significant coarctation, continuous-wave Doppler will also reveal increased velocity through the descending aorta, with a diastolic "tail" (high velocities maintained during diastole). Minimal diastolic flow is seen in cine imaging here.

# MAGNETIC RESONANCE IMAGING

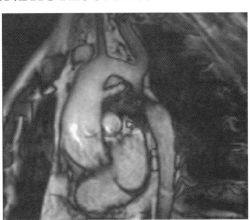

Figure 24-5 Oblique sagittal view stady-state free precession cine.

## FINDINGS

There is an abrupt, severe CoA present 18 mm distal to the origin of the left subclavian artery. There was LV hypertrophy with preserved LV function. The diameters were as follows: aortic root 40 mm, ascending aorta 39 mm, aortic arch proximal to the left subclavian artery 15 mm, coarctation 2 mm, 2 cm distal to coarctation 20 mm, aorta at the level of the diaphragm 15 mm.

**Comments:** The coarctation can easily be appreciated by MRI. MRI is also advantageous as it allows for measurement of aortic diameter throughout the thorax, quantification of flow both above and below the coarctation, assessment of col-lateralization, as well as quality imaging of the heart itself including bicuspid valve function and LV mass. Here the LV hypertrophy reflects the long-standing hypertension.

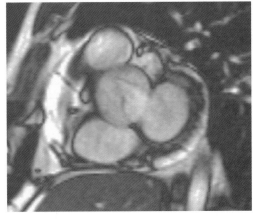

Figure 24-6 Oblique sagittal view along the short axis of the left ventricle.

### Ventricular Volume Quantification

|  | LV | (Normal range) | RV | (Normal range) |
|---|---|---|---|---|
| EDV (mL) | 116 | (77–195) | 94 | (88–227) |
| ESV (mL) | 51 | (19–72) | 33 | (23–103) |
| SV (mL) | 65 | (51–133) | 61 | (52–138) |
| EF (%) | 57 | (57–74) | 65 | (48–74) |
| EDVi (mL/m$^2$) | 68 | (68–103) | **50** | (68–114) |
| ESVi (mL/m$^2$) | 27 | (19–41) | **17** | (21–50) |
| SVi (mL/m$^2$) | **34** | (44–68) | **32** | (40–72) |
| Mass index (g/m$^2$) | **105** | (59–93) | 36 | (23–50) |

## FINDINGS

The aortic valve was bicuspid without stenosis or regurgitation. The aortic root measured 40 mm.

*Comments:* This short-axis view shows the bicuspid aortic valve leaflets closing at the end of systole. Aortic root dilatation is a common feature in patients with bicuspid aortic valves even in the absence of coarctation or valve dysfunction. It may reflect histologic/biochemical defects of the aortic wall itself.[5] Bicuspid aortic valve is present in up to 85% of patients with aortic coarctation.[6]

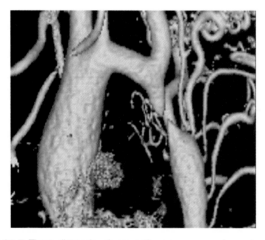

Figure 24-7 Three-dimensional magnetic resonance angiography.

## FINDINGS

The abrupt severe aortic coarctation distal to the origin of the left subclavian artery was seen. The descending aorta distal to the coarctation was filled via extensive collaterals. The internal mammary arteries and the left intercostal arteries were prominent and enlarged. The left subclavian artery had a diameter of 13 mm.

*Comments:* Angiography allows easy visualization of collateral vessels.

Flow distal to the coarctation is derived mainly from the extensive collateral circulation. Even though the angiogram suggests complete interruption of the arch, there is likely a small lumen through which a catheter could be placed.

## CEREBRAL ANGIOGRAM

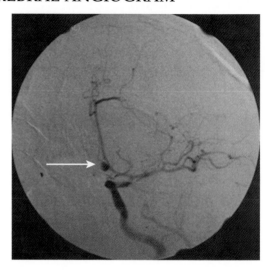

Figure 24-8 Cerebral angiogram. (From Varghese A, Gatzoulis M, Mohiaddin R: Magnetic resonance angiography of an interrupted aortic arch. Circulation 106:e9, 2002.)

## FINDINGS

A berry aneurysm (*arrow*) was seen in the left anterior cerebral artery, the likely source of the subarachnoid hemorrhage.

*Comments:* An association between berry aneurysms and coarctation is known, and estimated at as high as 10%,[6] although referral bias may make this prevalence figure artificially high. It is not certain what the association is, that is, whether it is due to shared intrinsic histopathologic vascular features or is secondary to poorly controlled hypertension.

## CATHETERIZATION

### HEMODYNAMICS

Heart rate   57 bpm

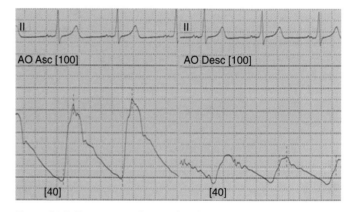

Figure 24-9 Pressure gradient registration proximal and distal to the coarctation.

|  | Pressure |
|---|---|
| LV | 79/1 |
| AO root | 77/46 mean 59 |
| AO asc | 84/50 mean 63 |
| AO desc | 59/53 mean 55 |
| Right femoral a | 68/60 mean 61 |

The catheterization was performed to establish precisely the pressures proximal and distal to the stenosis and, if possible, for therapeutic intervention. Because of the possibility of intervention, the study was done under general anesthesia.

## FINDINGS

A right femoral artery sheath was placed and a J-wire used to cross the aortic coarctation without difficulty. There was no significant pressure gradient across the aortic valve. Pressure tracings proximal and distal to the coarctation were obtained, demonstrating the significant gradient across the coarctation.

***Comments:*** Under general anesthesia all pressures were diminished. However, the pressures proximal to the coarctation here were significantly higher than those distally. The pressure difference across the coarctation is graphically represented.

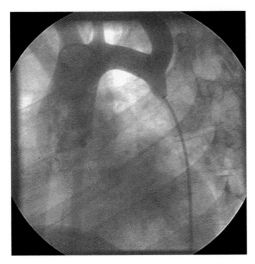

Figure 24-10 Left anterior oblique view aortic angiogram.

## FINDINGS

Near interruption of the aortic arch was seen. There was minimal collateral flow angiographically to the descending aorta. The arrangement of the head/arm vessels was normal.

***Comments:*** The severity of the aortic coarctation was confirmed with aortic angiography.

The narrowing at the site of the coarctation is so severe that the angiographic catheter completely blocks it, giving the impression of a complete interruption.

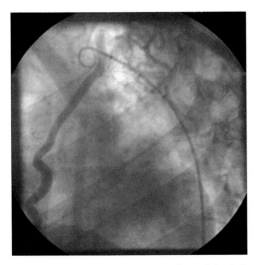

Figure 24-11 Left anterior oblique view, extensive collateral circulation.

## FINDINGS

After injection, several extensive collateral arteries were seen arising from the intercostal arteries, as well as a dilated internal mammary artery.

***Comments:*** Collateralization is common in severe coarctation, as shown also by the MR angiogram.

### FOCUSED CLINICAL QUESTIONS AND DISCUSSION POINTS

1. **If the diagnosis of aortic coarctation had been made earlier in this patient, could the cerebral event have been prevented?**

   *While berry aneurysms are a well-recognized association with CoA, routine head CT or MRI is not standard established practice. A recent paper from the Mayo Clinic showed a 10% incidence among 100 adult patients with CoA, which is at least five times higher than in the general population.[5] However, no risk factors were identified and only one patient with a large aneurysm from this series underwent elective aneurysm surgery. The diagnosis and treatment of native CoA and optimal blood pressure control are likely to improve prognosis even in patients with cerebral aneurysms.*

2. **What is the right time for repair of the aortic coarctation?**

   *Repair of aortic coarctation should not be delayed once the diagnosis has been made. The rationale for this is to relieve upper body hypertension and prevent LV dysfunction, early coronary artery disease, subarachnoid hemorrhage, and aortic dissection. This patient has already suffered a cerebral event, and correction of the coarctation should reduce the risk of further catastrophe.*

3. **Is surgical repair or transcatheter repair preferred?**

   *The choice of the procedure depends on the type of coarctation, coexisting morbidity, age of patient, and available expertise.*

   *Surgical options include end-to-end anastomosis, prosthetic interposition tube graft, subclavian flap aortoplasty (under age 1), prosthetic flap repair, and bypass tube graft.*

   *Surgery has previously been the mainstay in the treatment of a native coarctation and recoarctation. In recent years angioplasty with or without stenting has been introduced in the treatment of aortic coarctation, and the availability of stents has led to improved outcomes.[7] Very young age (in childhood), marked arch hypoplasia, and previous patch repair (for recoarctation) are relative contraindications for transcatheter repair of CoA.*

4. **What should the patient be told about future hypertension?**

   *Normalization of the blood pressure without medication generally occurs in 74% of the patients treated with angioplasty for aortic coarctation with subsequent long-term regression of LV hypertrophy. Increasing age at the time of surgical or catheter repair is an important risk factor for persisting hypertension.[8–10]*

5. **What is the significance of the bicuspid aortic valve?**

   *Up to 85% of patients with aortic coarctation have a bicuspid aortic valve. Ascending aortopathy and aortic root dilatation are features of bicuspid aortic valve and not of CoA per se. Bicuspid aortic valve function may deteriorate with time leading to aortic stenosis, aortic regurgitation, or both and merits lifelong follow-up (as does CoA).*

## FINAL DIAGNOSIS

Aortic coarctation

Bicuspid aortic valve

Intracranial berry aneurysm

# PLAN OF ACTION

Transcatheter balloon angioplasty and stenting

# INTERVENTION

The patient underwent percutaneous balloon angioplasty with stenting, done at the time of his initial catheterization.

Balloon angioplasty is a percutaneous intervention technique. Access to the vascular system is achieved by puncture of the femoral artery.

Angiography of the ascending and descending aorta will be performed as well as recording of the pressures proximal and distal to the coarctation.

# OUTCOME

The result of the intervention was excellent without any complications. There was no pressure gradient on pullback from the ascending to the descending aorta at the end of the procedure. Currently, he is only on atenolol 50 mg once daily. The patient was alerted of the risk of accelerated atherosclerosis associated with CoA and was advised to minimize his risk factors.

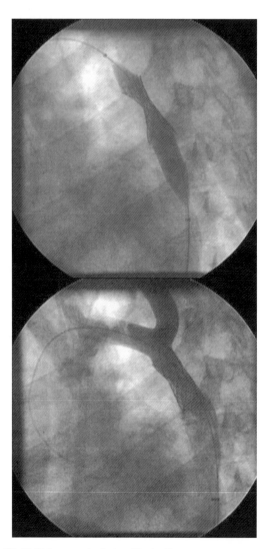

Figure 24-12 Balloon angioplasty with stenting.

# FINDINGS

Angiography during balloon inflation and immediately following shows no signs of aortic tear or rupture.

***Comments:*** The main risk of balloon angioplasty is of aortic rupture and dissection. This occurs rarely but especially in native coarctation repairs in relatively elderly patients.

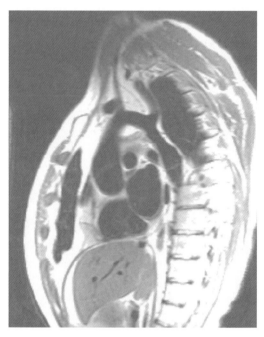

Figure 24-13 Magnetic resonance image of an oblique sagittal plane using turbo-spin imaging.

# FINDINGS

The patient had a follow-up CMR scan 1 year after initial deployment of the stent. The site of coarctation is now widely patent.

***Comments:*** Signal loss from the stent will obscure a true-FISP cine image as shown previously. Using this slightly different sequence reveals the true lumen diameter, which shows successful relief of coarctation 1 year after the initial procedure. Note persisting aortic root dilatation relating to the bicuspid aortic valve.

## Selected References

1. Edlow JA, Caplan LR: Avoiding pitfalls in the diagnosis of subarachnoid hemorrhage. N Engl J Med 342:29–36, 2000.
2. Vega C, Kwoon JV, Lavine SD: Intracranial aneurysm: Current evidence and clinical practice. Am Fam Physician 66:601–608, 2002.
3. Bederson JB, Awad IA, Wiebers DO, et al: Recommendations for the management of patients with unruptured intracranial aneurysms: A statement for healthcare professionals from the Stroke Council of the American Heart Association. Circulation 102: 2300–2308, 2000.
4. Aris A, Bonnin JO, Sole JO, et al: Surgical management of aortic coarctation associated with ruptured cerebral aneurysm. Tex Heart Inst J 13:313–319, 1986.
5. Fedak PW, de Sa MP, Verma S, et al: Vascular matrix remodeling in patients with bicuspid aortic valve malformations: Implications for aortic dilatation. J Thorac Cardiovasc Surg 126:797–806, 2003.
6. Connolly HM, Huston J, Brown RD, et al: Intracranial aneurysms in patients with coarctation of the aorta: A prospective magnetic

resonance angiographic study of 100 patients. Mayo Clin Proc 78: 1491–1499, 2003.

7. Richard A, Krasuski RA, Bashore TM: The emerging role of percutaneous intervention in adults with congenital heart disease. Rev Cardiovasc Med 6:11–22, 2005.

8. Fawzy ME, Sivanandam V, Pieters F, et al: Long-term effects of balloon angioplasty on systemic hypertension in adolescent and adult patients with coarctation of the aorta. Eur Heart J 20:827–832, 1999.

9. Swan L, Wilson N, Houston AB, et al: The long-term management of the patient with an aortic coarctation repair. Eur Heart J 19: 382–386, 1998.

10. Kaemmerer H: Aortic coarctation and interrupted aortic arch. In Gatzoulis MA, Webb GD, Daubeney PEF (eds): Diagnosis and Management of Adult Congenital Heart Disease. Philadelphia, Churchill Livingstone, 2003, pp 253–264.

# Recoarctation: Criteria for Intervention

**Richard M. Donner, Jonathan Rome, Vaikom S. Mahadevan, and Andrew Crean**

**Age: 45 years**
**Gender: Male**
**Occupation: Auto industry worker**
**Working diagnosis: Recurrent coarctation of the aorta**

## HISTORY

The patient was well at birth but presented in heart failure at 10 days of age. A diagnosis of severe coarctation of the aorta (CoA) was made by physical examination. He was stabilized with medication and underwent a primary repair at 3 years of age. The method of repair was unknown.

He remained well and was followed infrequently until 9 months ago (44 years old), when he was referred to a cardiologist with high right upper-extremity blood pressure obtained on a routine exam. Echocardiography and MRI suggested a significant recoarctation, and he was begun on antihypertensive therapy with quinapril. One week ago, he presented with an initial episode of atrial fibrillation and was successfully cardioverted. Metoprolol was added, and he was referred for further therapy.

He has no other ongoing medical problems. He is married with children. Until 7 years ago he was a regular smoker.

*Comments:* Newborn CoA with heart failure is now normally addressed with immediate surgery, eliminating some of the morbidity seen in adults with long-standing hypertension. Ductus arteriosus patency would be a temporary measure, if the distal systemic vascular bed perfusion depends on ductal flow. Although speculative, this patient's coarctation could not have been critical for him to survive to the age of 3. Probably he also developed collateral flow.

The atrial fibrillation may have been related to elevated LA and LV filling pressure due to hypertension or associated aortic valve disease.

## CURRENT SYMPTOMS

The patient is otherwise asymptomatic. He completes 45 hours of work each week without difficulty, can walk up two flights of steps without dyspnea, and enjoys hiking and camping.

NYHA class: I

*Comments:* Most patients with native or recurrent coarctation are asymptomatic. In isolated coarctation with or without mild aortic valve disease, heart failure is rare.

## CURRENT MEDICATIONS

Quinapril 20 mg once daily

Metoprolol XR 25 mg once daily

## PHYSICAL EXAMINATION

HR 44 bpm, RR 16, oxygen saturation on room air 98%

Height 178 cm, weight 92 kg, BSA 2.13 m$^2$

Pulses and blood pressures: The right radial and both femoral pulses were of equal volume with a small pulse delay between the brachial and femorals. The left radial pulse had a diminished volume in comparison with all other pulses. None were bounding. The blood pressures were obtained with appropriate-sized manual cuffs and the patient in the supine position. BP 156/70 (right forearm), 115/60 (left forearm), systolic pressure 118 mm Hg (right thigh).

Surgical scar: Left thoracotomy scar

Neck veins: Normal waveform, not elevated

Lungs/chest: Normal breath sounds

Heart: The precordium was quiet, and there was no thrill. The first heart sound was normal with no early systolic ejection click or third or fourth heart sound. The second heart sound was narrowly split. A grade 3 short, harsh systolic ejection murmur was present at the base and could be heard with less intensity in the neck (right carotid area). A long, early diastolic murmur was audible along the left sternal border. A short, harsh systolic murmur was easily appreciated over the thoracic spine, and a very faint, low-pitched continuous murmur was present in the same area.

Abdomen: No enlargement of the liver or spleen

Extremities: All were warm and well perfused with no temperature changes, mottling, or peripheral edema.

*Comments:* The low HR may be partially related to metoprolol therapy even though the dose is modest.

A recurrent coarctation is suggested by the systolic gradient of 38 mm Hg recorded from the right arm to the right thigh. The presence of equal pulse volumes with a small delay in transmission of the pulse wave may be compatible with a variety of anatomic distortions of the aortic arch but is commonly seen in the presence of arterial collateral formation. The femoral pulses may also be enhanced by the presence of aortic valve regurgitation.

Radiofemoral delay requires the presence of a collateral source of blood flow to the lower body. This is more specific for aortic coarctation than is simply a lower perfusion pressure in a leg, which could be due to local arterial disease.

The absence of an early systolic ejection click is unusual since a bicuspid aortic valve is present in this patient and should be present in at least 50% of coarctation patients. The harsh murmur at the base may reflect turbulence across the coarctation or aortic valve stenosis. The early diastolic murmur is aortic valve regurgitation that cannot be severe since the pulses are not bounding and the diastolic pressure in the right arm is low normal. However, the coarctation may minimize both of these findings, masking more significant aortic regurgitation. The coarctation can also be appreciated as the harsh murmur in the back, and the continuous murmur suggests the presence of some arterial collaterals.

It is unusual to observe alteration of the extremities in all but the most severe coarctations unless there is coexistent peripheral arterial disease.

## LABORATORY DATA

| | |
|---|---|
| Hemoglobin | 13.2 g/dL (13.0–17.0) |
| Hematocrit/PCV | 41% (41–51) |
| MCV | 87.5 fL (83–99) |
| Platelet count | $280 \times 10^9$/L (150–400) |
| Sodium | 138 mmol/L (134–145) |
| Potassium | 4.2 mmol/L (3.5–5.2) |
| Creatinine | 0.8 mg/dL (0.6–1.2) |

## ELECTROCARDIOGRAM

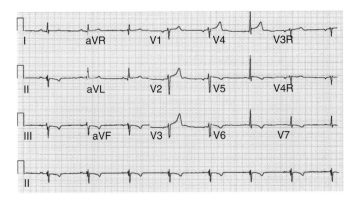

Figure 25-1 Electrocardiogram.

### FINDINGS

Heart rate: 46 bpm

PR interval: 215 msec

QRS axis: –60°

QRS duration: 95 msec

Marked sinus bradycardia with first-degree AV block. Left anterior fascicular block. Inverted T-waves inferiorly and leftward. ST segment elevation in V1–4.

***Comments:*** First-degree AV block may be related to the metoprolol, but in this patient, it predated the atrial fibrillation.

The significance of the left anterior fascicular block is unknown.

Abnormal repolarization may be part of a "left ventricular strain pattern," although there is no additional evidence here for LV hypertrophy. Even without LV hypertrophy, it suggests some abnormal state of the LV muscle. Of course, the changes may reflect coronary artery disease as well.

## CHEST X-RAY

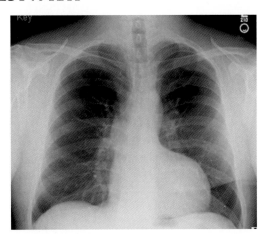

Figure 25-2 Posteroanterior projection.

### FINDINGS

Cardiothoracic ratio: 52%

While the cardiac silhouette was normal in size, there was a left ventricular configuration to the heart. The aortic arch was normal in size and on the left. The main pulmonary artery segment was small compared with the aortic arch. Pulmonary vascular markings were normal. Irregularity to the posterior fourth and fifth ribs was likely postsurgical (postthoracotomy) given the patient's history of coarctation repair.

***Comments:*** The prominent LV apex suggests some ventricular overload (hypertrophy), usually right when the apex is elevated. Distortion of the aortic arch, commonly present following coarctation repair, is not seen in this image. There is evidence of dilatation of the ascending aorta.

Rib notching is seldom seen before age 5 in patients with aortic coarctation. In looking for rib notching, one looks for sclerosis of the undersurface of the rib rather than an irregularity of the inferior margin.

# ECHOCARDIOGRAM

## Overall Findings

The LV was normal in size and function. The RV was also normal. There was no mitral or tricuspid regurgitation. The atria were of normal size. The coarctation was not seen.

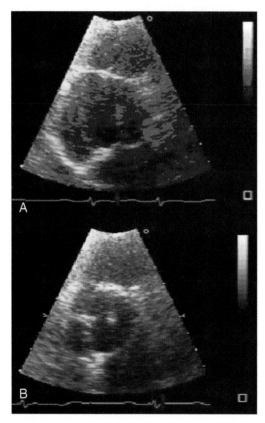

Figure 25-3 Parasternal short-axis view.

## Findings

A bicuspid aortic valve was present. Aortic regurgitation was mild. There was partial fusion of the right and noncoronary cusps (*B*) resulting in a functionally bicuspid aortic valve. The three leaflets are approximately equal in size. Aortic regurgitation was mostly central but also occurred along each of the cusps.

**Comments:** Unlike aortic arch imaging in newborns and children, coarctation in the adult may be suspected from suprasternal imaging, but the anatomy and typical flow patterns are often poorly defined.

All patients with bicuspid aortic valves should be considered at risk for coarctation, and vice versa.

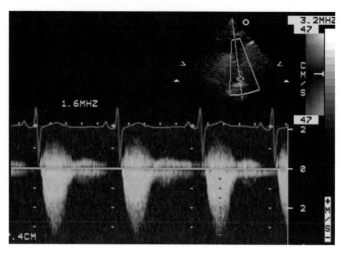

Figure 25-4 Continuous-wave Doppler through the high descending thoracic aorta, obtained from the suprasternal notch.

## Findings

The aortic arch was difficult to visualize, but continuous-wave Doppler from the suprasternal view showed a peak gradient of 47 mm Hg in the descending aorta with a detectable velocity even in diastole (diastolic spillover or diastolic tail).

**Comments:** A high gradient in the descending aorta and evidence of diastolic flow in the abdominal aorta are echocardiographic signs of significant coarctation or recoarctation.

# MAGNETIC RESONANCE ANGIOGRAPHY

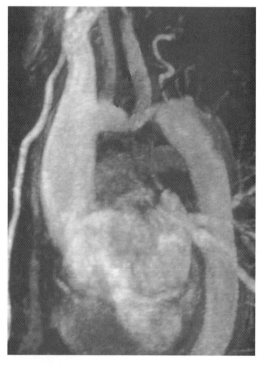

Figure 25-5 Maximal intensity projection image of the thoracic aorta and reconstructed arch from a sagittal oblique magnetic resonance angiogram.

## Findings

There was mild dilatation of the ascending aorta. There were three abnormal segments of the transverse arch:

1. The aortic arch tapered to a discrete, severe coarctation just distal to the origin of the left carotid artery.

2. Just beyond the coarctation, there was a diffusely narrowed segment from which the left subclavian artery arises.

3. There was probably another discrete narrowing at the junction of the isthmus and descending thoracic aorta.

Collateral formation was present but not extensive.

***Comments:*** The true anatomy of the coarctation is best appreciated by observing 2D (or 3D) reconstructed images viewed in a rotated sequence. The initial posteroanterior image in the sequence often fails to show any abnormality.

In this series of images there are three areas of the arch that are of concern. All must be remedied to achieve a satisfactory result. A potential source of concern is the origin of the left subclavian artery from the diffusely narrowed segment. An interventional catheterization procedure would need to address the two discrete stenoses that are separated by a considerable length of hypoplastic vessel while providing flow into the left subclavian artery. Such a procedure would also require the presence of some native aortic tissue in all of the segments. The method by which the original coarctation repair was accomplished is unknown (subclavian flap angioplasty is excluded by the presence of the left subclavian artery). However, these images do not suggest the use of a circumferential interposition graft.

## CATHETERIZATION

### HEMODYNAMICS
Heart rate    45 bpm

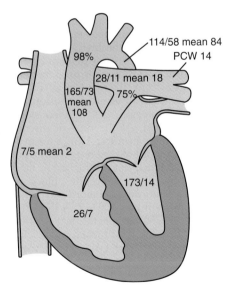

Figure 25-6 Summary of hemodynamic data obtained at cardiac catheterization prior to intervention.

Cardiac index 2.7 L/min/m$^2$

PVR 0.7 Wood units

### FINDINGS
Cardiac catheterization was performed to measure the LV filling pressure, assess the magnitude of aortic stenosis and regurgitation, assess the coronary arteries, verify the severity of the coarctation, and perform angioplasty/stenting if safe and appropriate.

The peak-to-peak aortic valve gradient was only 8 mm Hg and the coarctation gradient, 51 mm Hg. The LV filling pressure was mildly increased at 14 mm Hg. Angiography confirmed the anatomy demonstrated by MRA and showed moderate aortic regurgitation. Coronary angiography was normal. Cardiac index and pulmonary vascular resistance were normal.

***Comments:*** In the presence of a normal cardiac index and moderate aortic valve regurgitation, the aortic valve gradient is close to zero. The pulmonary capillary wedge pressure and LV end-diastolic pressure are equal, eliminating the possibility of mitral stenosis. The moderate to severe coarctation gradient accurately assesses the severity of arch obstruction since collateral formation is present but not extensive.

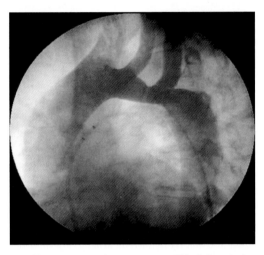

Figure 25-7 Transverse arch aortogram, 70° left anterior oblique projection.

### FINDINGS
CoA was present between the left carotid and left subclavian arteries. The narrowest segment in this projection measured approximately 8 mm. There was mild to moderate dilatation of the ascending aorta. The descending aorta distal to the left subclavian artery was also dilated.

***Comments:*** The coarctation is easily seen in this projection, and the anatomy is nearly identical to that seen on MRA.

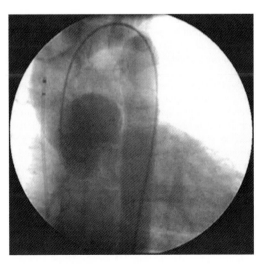

Figure 25-8 Ascending aortogram, posteroanterior projection.

# FINDINGS

There was moderate aortic regurgitation.

**Comments:** The aortic regurgitation is related to the presence of a bicuspid aortic valve. The contrast takes nearly 5 beats to clear from the LV cavity. This suggests that the degree of regurgitation is severe. However, the LV is not qualitatively enlarged (partially related to the aortic obstruction and wall hypertrophy) and the filling pressure is only mildly elevated, even in the presence of the coarctation. These observations are more consistent with moderate regurgitation. Coronary angiography was unremarkable.

As with any form of valve disease, there can often be discrepancies between different imaging modalities in the assessment of the degree of regurgitation. Variation can be due to hemodynamic differences on the study day as well as technical limitations of the various modalities. It should be remembered that recoarctation (or residual coarctation) is assessed not by a single entity but by several modalities and clinical features.

## FOCUSED CLINICAL QUESTIONS AND DISCUSSION POINTS

1. What are the severity, significance, and spectrum of disease present in this patient with residual and/or recurrent CoA?

*The presence of systolic hypertension in the right arm and a 51 mm Hg gradient across the coarctation at catheterization are consistent with moderate obstruction that is likely responsible for the clinical hypertension. Without knowledge of the patient's history or recognition of blood pressure measurements in the other extremities and the radiofemoral pulse delay, the systolic pressure of 156 mm Hg in the right arm by cuff could be mistaken for essential hypertension and treated improperly.*

*Clinical assessment of a coarctation gradient usually rests on blood pressure determinations and comparison of upper and lower limb pulses. In some patients, however, even these may be misleading, for example, in the presence of aortic insufficiency as in this case. Without further noninvasive assessment,[1] such factors may also lead to misdiagnosis.*

*The spectrum of disease in this patient includes a bicuspid aortic valve that may be part of a generalized arteriopathy affecting the aorta and its branches.[2] Consequences of this might include a higher prevalence of intracranial aneurysms,[3] aortic aneurysms,[4] and important risks and complications of catheter and surgical interventions.[5,6]*

2. What therapy or therapies are indicated?

*Relief of recoarctation to reduce the afterload on the LV and ascending aorta and to optimize systemic blood pressure control is clearly desirable. A decision to address only the coarctation depends on the severity of the aortic valve disease and the potential beneficial effects of coarctation intervention on the aortic physiology. In this patient, there was little or no aortic stenosis and aortic regurgitation was estimated to be no more than moderate.*

*A decision was made at catheterization to proceed with primary stenting based on the hope that aortic regurgitation would be improved or stabilized if the aortic obstruction were relieved.*

*A nonsurgical approach was previously discussed and ultimately was offered to the patient based on the following:*
1. *Avoidance of surgical morbidity and longer hospitalization*
2. *Similar risks (low) of aneurysm formation from catheter versus surgical relief of coarctation or recoarctation*
3. *Medium- to long-term results in native coarctation, which showed freedom from hypertension and regression of hypertrophy[7]*

*The option of primary stenting for recoarctation was also chosen based on the operator's experience and the tubular nature of the*

obstruction.[8] *Possible compromise of the left subclavian artery was considered a risk.*

# FINAL DIAGNOSIS

Moderate residual/recurrent CoA

Bicuspid aortic valve with moderate aortic regurgitation

# PLAN OF ACTION

Catheterization with primary stenting as the most likely option pending confirmation of the anatomy and assessment of the magnitude of obstruction

# INTERVENTION

Heart catheterization was undertaken, and the hemodynamic and angiographic findings described previously were obtained. It was decided that stenting of the narrowed aortic segment from a point distal to the left carotid artery to the dilated descending aortic segment would probably result in obliteration of most or all of the gradient. Bridging of the left subclavian artery would be a necessary consequence of the procedure with flow passing through the stent wall into the left arm. This was accomplished with a Palmaz 4010 stent dilated with an 18-mm high-pressure balloon. Subsequently, there was no pressure gradient recorded from the ascending to the descending aorta, and the narrowest portion of the coarctation was estimated at 16 to 17 mm, twice its original diameter. There was no obvious intimal tear, but there was some stenosis at the origin of the left subclavian artery that was bridged by the stent.

# OUTCOME

The postcatheterization course was marked by significant rebound systolic hypertension that required continued hospitalization for 3 days. During the first 24 hours, systolic blood pressure the right arm ranged from 165 mm Hg to 205 mm Hg and diastolic pressure from 65 mm Hg to 85 mm Hg. Mean arterial pressure ranged from 100 mm Hg to 140 mm Hg. This was initially controlled with esmolol infusion at rates up to 350 µg/kg/min. The infusion was weaned slowly and oral medication was restarted. At the time of discharge, systolic blood pressure in the right arm was 132/78 mean 94. Discharge medications were quinapril (30 mg once a day), metoprolol XR (25 mg once a day), and aspirin (81 mg once a day).

Three weeks following the procedure, blood pressure was taken 2 hours after the morning quinapril and metoprolol doses. Pressure in the right arm was 108/65, in the left arm 113/70, and in the right leg 132/80. Despite the near equality of the right and left arm pressure, the left brachial pulse felt slightly less prominent than the right brachial. None of the pulses were bounding. Blood pressure was subsequently followed by the family physician. Occasional dizziness appeared a few weeks later with progressive reduction of right arm blood pressure to values ranging from 88/62 mm Hg to 122/72 mm Hg. The quinapril was eventually reduced to 10 mg once a day in the morning and metoprolol 12.5 mg once a day in the evening.

**Comments:** Rebound hypertension following surgical repair of coarctation is a well-known phenomenon,[9] likely representing an abnormal autonomic system response to the augmented lowered systemic vascular bed perfusion following repair, and it is a transient phenomenon. It is rarely seen in adults, and rarely after interventional therapy.

The choice of quinapril to control rebound hypertension and reduce aortic regurgitation after discharge is arbitrary and was made to conform to his preprocedure medications. Metoprolol was continued in the hopes of preventing recurrent atrial fibrillation.

Despite what appeared to be partial compromise of flow into the left subclavian artery, blood pressure in both arms remained essentially equal. There was no measurable gradient from either arm to the legs, as evidenced by the higher leg pressure. The absence of bounding pulses and normal pulse pressure in all extremities reinforced the notion that aortic regurgitation was not severe. However, the effect of the procedure on the aortic regurgitation will need to be followed with echocardiography over time.

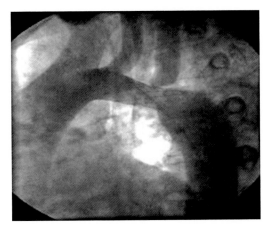

Figure 25-9 Transverse arch aortogram, 70° left anterior oblique projection.

## FINDINGS

The stent was positioned just distal to the left common carotid artery, bridging the left subclavian artery. The narrowest portion of the aorta measured 16 mm. No dissection was seen. The left subclavian artery was narrow at its origin.

***Comments:*** The three areas of concern identified on MRA imaging prior to catheterization have been expanded by the stent. This is consistent with the absence of a blood pressure gradient between the arms and legs.

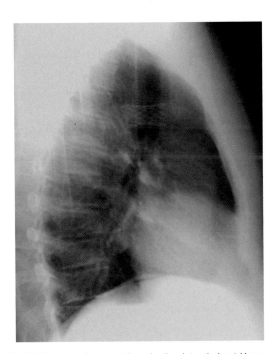

Figure 25-10 Two-month postcatheterization lateral chest X-ray.

## FINDINGS

The stent is seen in the aortic arch. Comparison with immediate postcatheterization films shows that its position has not changed. There does not appear to be any fracture or recurrent narrowing.

***Comments:*** The CXR is a useful tool to confirm that there has been no migration or fracture of the stent that might result in further recurrence of the coarctation. It is usually performed immediately after the procedure, 1 to 2 weeks later, and again at 2 to 3 months. A follow-up CXR at 1 year is also advisable.

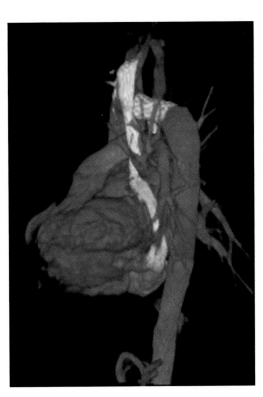

Figure 25-11 Three-month postcatheterization 3D computed tomography reconstruction.

## FINDINGS

Three-dimensional CT reconstruction showed the stent in its original position in the aortic arch. It extended from a point just distal to the left subclavian artery, beyond the origin of the left subclavian artery, and across the aortic isthmus. There was no obvious fracture or recurrent narrowing within the stent or at its margins. The origin of the left subclavian artery was mildly narrowed, but the caliber of the vessel was normal.

***Comments:*** MRI may be the most suitable method to follow patients for complications of catheter intervention.[10] However, the considerable artifact introduced by ferrous metal stents makes 3D CT a viable alternative.

## Selected References

1. Araoz PA, Reddy GP, Tarnoff H, et al: MR findings of collateral circulation are more accurate measures of hemodynamic significance than arm-leg blood pressure gradient after repair of coarctation of the aorta. J Magn Reson Imaging 17:177–183, 2003.
2. Warnes CA: Bicuspid aortic valve and coarctation: Two villains part of a diffuse problem. Heart 89:965–966, 2003.
3. Connolly HM, Huston J, III, Brown RD, Jr, et al: Intracranial aneurysms in patients with coarctation of the aorta: A prospective

magnetic resonance angiographic study of 100 patients. Mayo Clin Proc 78:1491–1499, 2003.

4. Oliver JM, Gallego P, Gonzalez A, et al: Risk factors for aortic complications in adults with coarctation of the aorta. J Am Coll Cardiol 44:1641–1647, 2004.

5. Mahadevan V, Mullen MJ: Endovascular management of aortic coarctation. Int J Cardiol 97(Suppl 1):75–78, 2004.

6. Hijazi ZM: Catheter intervention for adult aortic coarctation: Be very careful! Cathet Cardiovasc Intervent 59:536–537, 2003.

7. Fawzy ME, Sivanandam V, Pieters F, et al: Long-term effects of balloon angioplasty on systemic hypertension in adolescent and adult patients with coarctation of the aorta. Eur Heart J 20:827–832, 1999.

8. Zabal C, Attie F, Rosas M, et al: The adult patient with native coarctation of the aorta: Balloon angioplasty or primary stenting? Heart 89:77–83, 2003.

9. Sealy WC: Paradoxical hypertension after repair of coarctation of the aorta: A review of its causes. Ann Thorac Surg 50:323–329, 1990.

10. Therrien J, Thorne SA, Wright A, et al: Repaired coarctation: A "cost-effective" approach to identify complications in adults. J Am Coll Cardiol 35:997–1002, 2000.

# Pregnancy-Related Complications in Coarctation

**Anselm Uebing**

**Age: 27 years**
**Gender: Female**
**Occupation: Business manager**
**Working diagnosis: Aortic coarctation**

## HISTORY

The patient was diagnosed with aortic coarctation within the first week of life and was operated on at the age of 2 months. A left subclavian flap angioplasty was performed.

Thereafter, the patient remained asymptomatic and developed normally throughout childhood. She never experienced any chest pain and did not develop systemic hypertension. However, she did not receive regular follow-up.

As an adult the patient expressed an interest in starting a family, and sought advice at our adult congenital heart disease clinic about the safety of pregnancy. A general workup followed, and the patient was told that no interventions were required.

The patient later presented to a high-risk obstetrics service 11 weeks pregnant.

*Comments:* Generally, the earlier a patient undergoes repair for coarctation, the lower the chance of future complications from hypertension (see also Case 25). In contrast, the risk of recoarctation is higher in patients requiring angioplasty repair in infancy compared to those who undergo surgical repair of coarctation later on in childhood or during adult life.

The left subclavian flap angioplasty was first introduced in 1966 by Waldhausen and Nahrwold and involves dividing of the left subclavian artery and ligating it distally. The proximal part of the artery is then split longitudinally, turned down, and used as a flap to enlarge the stenosed portion of the descending aorta.[1] It is used primarily in patients less than 1 year of age.

Prepregnancy counseling should be offered to all women with congenital heart disease to prevent avoidable risks and crisis management.[2] Estimation of the individual pregnancy risk for these women should be based on a recent evaluation of their cardiac status and anatomy.

A patient with previous coarctation repair should be investigated before pregnancy to exclude residual coarctation, aortic aneurysm formation, and systemic hypertension.

## CURRENT SYMPTOMS

The patient presented without any symptoms and was feeling entirely well. She denied nausea, vomiting, palpitations, or shortness of breath.

NYHA class: I

*Comments:* Significant cardiovascular changes occur during pregnancy. There is a steady increase in blood volume and cardiac output until the end of the second trimester, at which time cardiac output reaches a plateau at 30% to 50% above prepregnancy levels. But at the 11th week of gestation, such changes are not yet substantial.

## CURRENT MEDICATIONS

None

## PHYSICAL EXAMINATION

BP 135/70 mm Hg (right arm), BP 110/65 mm Hg (right leg); HR 74 bpm, oxygen saturation 99%

Height 171 cm, weight 56.7 kg, BSA 1.64 m$^2$

Surgical scars: Left lateral thoracotomy

Neck veins: JVP was not elevated.

Lungs/chest: Chest was clear.

Heart: There was a normal first and a physiologically split second heart sound. There was a soft 2/6 systolic ejection murmur, but there was no diastolic murmur or murmurs over the back.

Abdomen: Normal

Extremities: There was no peripheral edema, and there were normal peripheral pulses palpable at the right arm and both legs without radiofemoral pulse delay. The left radial pulse was not palpable. The left arm was slightly smaller than the right arm.

*Comments:* An abnormal difference in upper and lower limb arterial pulses and blood pressures is the clinical hallmark of coarctation. Manual cuff blood pressure is normally about 10 to 20 mm Hg higher in the leg than arm. Reversal of this pressure pattern may be suggestive of aortic arch obstruction, a sign that is commonly used for the clinical evaluation of coarctation or recoarctation. In significant cases, pulses distal to the obstruction are diminished and/or delayed. In this patient the pressure gradient between the right arm and the right leg and the soft murmur without an obvious radiofemoral pulse difference or delay were in keeping with a diagnosis of mild residual coarctation.

Diastolic murmurs in the back would be evidence of more severe coarctation, since they indicate the development of collateral circulation to bypass significant aortic obstruction.

The left arm arterial pulse was not palpable. After surgery for aortic coarctation with a subclavian flap, blood flow to the arm is often compromised, as the subclavian artery has been sacrificed (via Waldhausen subclavian flap angioplasty). The right arm is usually the best side to measure the blood pressure proximal to the site of surgery (with the exception of patients with an aberrant right subclavian originating distal to the aortic arch and coarctation).

The loss of the subclavian artery as part of a subclavian flap angioplasty of aortic coarctation in infancy does not usually impact the growth of the left arm, as collateral arterial flow develops, and certainly symptoms of brachial ischemia are exceedingly rare.

## LABORATORY DATA

| | |
|---|---|
| Hemoglobin | 11.7 g/dL (11.5–15.0) |
| Hematocrit/PCV | 40% (36–46) |
| MCV | 90 fL (83–99) |
| Platelet count | $205 \times 10^9$/L (150–400) |
| Sodium | 139 mmol/L (134–145) |
| Potassium | 4.2 mmol/L (3.5–5.2) |
| Creatinine | 0.7 mg/dL (0.6–1.2) |
| Blood urea nitrogen | 3.1 mmol/L (2.5–6.5) |

## ELECTROCARDIOGRAM

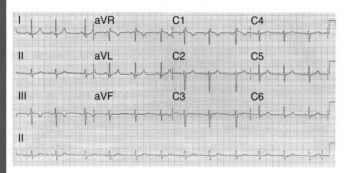

Figure 26-1 Electrocardiogram.

### FINDINGS
Heart rate: 74 bpm

PR interval: 141 msec

QRS axis: −23°

QRS duration: 82 msec

Atrial rhythm with leftward axis and incomplete RBBB

**Comments:** The QRS axis was leftward but there were no other signs of LV hypertrophy.

## CHEST X-RAY

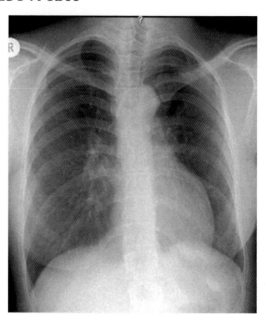

Figure 26-2 Posteroanterior projection.

### FINDINGS
Cardiothoracic ratio: 44%

The CXR was done 2 years before pregnancy.

There was situs solitus and levocardia (apex pointing to the left). There was a left aortic arch and no cardiomegaly. The aortic knuckle was abnormally prominent. Additionally, there were deformities in the left-sided ribs (ribs 2 to 4). The pulmonary vascular markings were normal.

**Comments:** This CXR showed some typical findings for a patient late after repair of coarctation. The left-sided deformities of the ribs are a typical result of left lateral thoracotomy in infancy. The prominent aortic knuckle is suspicious for aneurysm formation at the site of previous surgery. There is no obvious dilatation of the ascending aorta, making coexistence of a bicuspid aortic valve less likely.

## BLOOD PRESSURE MONITORING

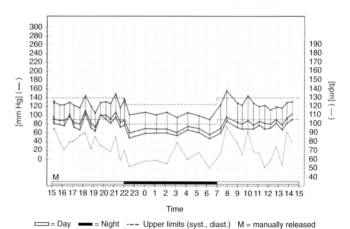

Figure 26-3 Twenty-four-hour noninvasive blood pressure monitoring.

## FINDINGS

The average blood pressure recorded in the right arm was 122/74 mm Hg. During the day, the average blood pressure was 127/79 mm Hg and at night 105/59 mm Hg.

**Comments:** This documented normal systemic blood pressure profile is reassuring and excludes systemic hypertension in this patient.

Systemic hypertension is common in patients with aortic coarctation even after successful repair of this anomaly and without residual mechanical obstruction.[3]

Systemic hypertension can develop or worsen during pregnancy and increases the risk for aortic dissection or rupture of preexisting aneurysms.[4] Furthermore, patients with coarctation of the aorta are at increased risk of preeclampsia. Meticulous blood pressure control is therefore crucial in these patients.

## EXERCISE TESTING

| Exercise protocol: | Modified Bruce |
| Duration (min:sec): | 12:12 |
| Reason for stopping: | Dyspnea and dizziness |
| ECG changes: | None |

| | Rest | Peak |
| --- | --- | --- |
| Heart rate (bpm): | 74 | 160 |
| Percent of age-predicted max HR: | | 83 |
| $O_2$ saturation (%): | 99 | 98 |
| Blood pressure (mm Hg): | 124/70 | 170/70 |
| Peak $V_{O_2}$ (mL/kg/min): | | 25.1 |
| Percent predicted (%): | | 78 |
| $V_e/V_{CO_2}$: | | 28 |
| Metabolic equivalents: | | 7.9 |

**Comments:** This exercise test had been performed before pregnancy to exclude systemic hypertension during exercise. There is evidence that after coarctation repair systemic hypertension can occur during exercise even if the blood pressure at rest is normal, although the clinical importance of this observation is not clear.[5] The peak exercise systolic blood pressure in this patient was well within normal limits (<200 mm Hg).

Documentation of this patient's blood pressure response during exercise was felt to be helpful in estimating her risk of developing systemic hypertension during pregnancy, although this is speculative. Pregnancy, nevertheless, with its increase in blood volume and cardiac output can be regarded as a state of mild to moderate exercise over its duration.

## ECHOCARDIOGRAM

### OVERALL FINDINGS

There was normal LV size with maintained systolic function and without LV hypertrophy. The RV was also normal. There was no significant valvular abnormality, and the aortic valve was tricuspid.

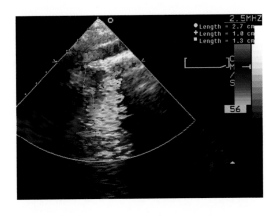

Figure 26-4 Two-dimensional suprasternal notch view (color flow image).

## FINDINGS

There was moderate hypoplasia of the distal aortic arch. The narrowest diameter measured was 10 mm. Turbulent blood flow started at this site of the aorta. There was aneurysmal dilatation of the descending aorta distal to the narrow segment.

**Comments:** In any patient with coarctation of the aorta, an echocardiogram should search extensively for other congenital abnormalities. The most common, of course, is bicuspid aortic valve, but mitral valve abnormalities and shunts can also occur.

Echocardiography is not the best modality to delineate the aortic arch anatomy. For this purpose MRI would be the technique of choice, with CT angiography as a second choice (less optimal given radiation and contrast agent exposure).

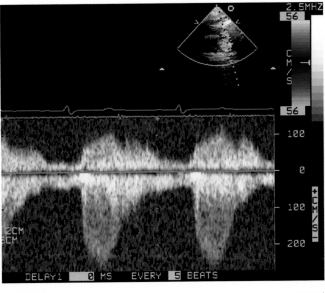

Figure 26-5 Continuous-wave Doppler recording from the suprasternal notch view.

## FINDINGS

There was a peak systolic velocity of 2.7 m/sec across the coarctation, suggesting a pressure gradient of 30 mm Hg. A borderline diastolic tail of the Doppler flow curve was present, indicating an increased forward flow velocity even during early diastole (*arrow*).

**Comments:** The peak systolic gradient across the coarctation repair site can normally be up to 20 mm Hg, but diastolic persistence is abnormal.

The velocity can underestimate the severity of obstruction if significant collateral vessels are present, and so assessment of coarctation requires the integration of several data points, including the narrowest diameter, the presence of a diastolic "tail," LV hypertrophy, as well as peak velocities.

In keeping with the clinical findings there was evidence for mild residual coarctation on echocardiography.

# MAGNETIC RESONANCE IMAGING

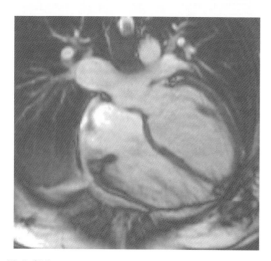

Figure 26-6 Oblique transverse four-chamber view.

## FINDINGS

This view showed pulmonary veins draining normally to the LA, and both atria were of normal size. Both AV valves were competent. The LA and RV were of normal size and function. Importantly, there was no LV hypertrophy.

**Comments:** There are no known risks of MRI in pregnancy, though the use of gadolinium is contraindicated. In this setting, MRI provides quality assessment of the entire aorta and is useful in following for changes during gestation.

Regardless of the underlying diagnosis of congenital heart disease, impaired ventricular function is a risk factor for pregnancy-related maternal death.[6,7] The absence of LV hypertrophy indicates that there was no long-standing systemic hypertension in this patient.

## Ventricular Volume Quantification

|  | LV | (Normal range) | RV | (Normal range) |
|---|---|---|---|---|
| EDV (mL) | 131 | (52–141) | 118 | (58–154) |
| ESV (mL) | 56 | (13–51) | 42 | (12–68) |
| SV (mL) | 75 | (33–97) | 76 | (35–98) |
| EF (%) | 57 | (56–75) | 64 | (49–73) |
| EDVi (mL/m²) | 80 | (65–99) | 72 | (65–102) |
| ESVi (mL/m²) | 34 | (19–37) | 26 | (20–45) |
| SVi (mL/m²) | 46 | (42–66) | 46 | (39–63) |
| Mass index (g/m²) | 76 | (47–77) | 37 | (22–42) |

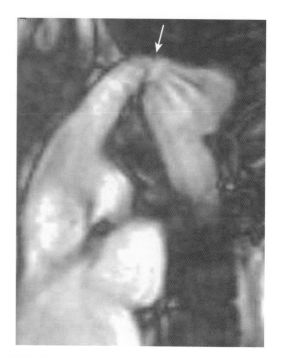

Figure 26-7 Oblique sagittal view of the aorta taken at the end of systole.

## FINDINGS

The ascending aorta was not enlarged. The aortic arch was mildly hypoplastic, and there was mild residual stenosis with a minimum diameter of $7 \times 12$ mm (*arrow*). The peak blood flow velocity at this site was 2.4 m/sec, suggesting mild residual aortic coarctation.

An aneurysm immediately distal to the site of residual coarctation was also seen, with a maximum diameter of 33 mm. Turbulent blood flow is directed into the aneurysm.

**Comments:** Repair site aortic aneurysms occur in about 5% to 9% of patients with surgically repaired coarctation.[8,9] The highest incidence is associated with the use of a patch graft technique at repair.[8]

In this patient, the site of coarctation forms a sharp angle, where the proximal portion and distal portions are nearly perpendicular to each other, making potential deployment of a stent more difficult.

### FOCUSED CLINICAL QUESTIONS AND DISCUSSION POINTS

1. Should this patient have undergone repair of the coarctation and aneurysm prior to considering pregnancy?

   *The presence of residual coarctation and of the aortic aneurysm would undoubtedly increase the risk of this pregnancy and future pregnancies for this patient. There are no well-established guidelines for when an intervention is necessary. Rupture can occur, particularly for aneurysms resulting from a Dacron graft repair.[10] Therefore, decisions regarding reintervention are based on the size of the aneurysm, the degree of recoarctation, the rate of progression, anticipated pregnancy, and considerations of the interventional options (catheter vs. surgery).*

   *When considering all the available information in this particular patient, the degree of residual coarctation was mild and would not warrant intervention in itself. The paracoarctation* aneurysm was worrisome, but it was not large enough to demand repair.

The options for correcting both her residual coarctation and distal aneurysm would be either surgery or catheter-based stent placement. Because of the 90-degree bend in the aorta at the coarctation site, catheter deployment of a stent would be challenging and would not necessarily relieve the obstruction fully. Surgically, the risks of the procedure seemed higher than even the risks of a subsequent pregnancy (provided there were no signs of aneurysmal growth).

All of these points were raised at a multidisciplinary conference following the patient's thorough assessment, and it was felt that no intervention should be offered at this time (particularly in light of the patient's clinical condition and the absence of systemic hypertension), and that pregnancy should be allowed to continue under close surveillance.

2. What are the pregnancy-related risks for the patient?

Data on the outcome of pregnancy in patients after repair of aortic coarctation are limited. The available data suggest that the overall risk for this group of patients to experience a significant cardiovascular complication such as stroke or death is low.[4] A bicuspid aortic valve—not present in this patient—has been linked with dilatation and dissection of the ascending aorta.[11]

Women who have had repair of aortic coarctation are more likely to develop systemic hypertension during pregnancy compared to healthy women, especially if some degree of residual stenosis is present.[4] Hypertension increases the risk of cardiovascular events.

In this particular patient, there is a significant aneurysmal dilatation of the aorta in the area of the surgical repair. In any woman with previous coarctation repair there is a risk of aortic dissection or rupture during pregnancy.[12] This risk certainly increases if an aneurysm at the site of repair or systemic arterial hypertension is present; however, there are few data on how significant the added risk truly is.

Finally, one should counsel the patient on the risk of recurrence of congenital heart disease in her offspring, which in this case is between 5% and 7% against a background risk of 0.8%.[13]

3. What is the optimal care for the patient during pregnancy?

Optimal care for women with unrepaired native and repaired coarctation requires a multidisciplinary team approach involving cardiologists, obstetricians, and anesthetists.

Meticulous systemic blood pressure control, using beta-blockers if required, may become crucial for this patient. The size and anatomy of the aortic aneurysm should be measured during pregnancy, ideally using serial MRIs. Regular monitoring of fetal growth is important in patients with unrepaired or residual coarctation, as systemic blood pressure in the lower part of the body is reduced if significant coarctation is present, to the potential detriment of the fetus.

4. What is the optimal mode for delivery?

Labor and delivery must be planned carefully and well in advance. Decisions about timing and the mode of delivery should be made following a multidisciplinary case discussion of the individual patient.

In general, vaginal delivery carries a lower risk of complications for both the mother and the fetus, as it causes smaller volume shifts, less hemorrhage, fewer clotting complications, as well as a lower risk of infection compared to cesarean section. However, prolonged labor, pain, and maternal pushing (Valsalva maneuver) during delivery should be avoided in a woman with an aortic aneurysm, as blood pressure may increase rapidly.

Vaginal delivery with low-dose epidural analgesia and elective instrumental delivery without maternal pushing in the second stage is usually recommended for any patient with complex congenital heart disease. If cesarean section is required, epidural analgesia can be extended in an attempt to minimize cardiovascular instability.

Elective cesarean section may be desirable in a patient with coarctation and poorly controlled systemic hypertension, severe residual or native coarctation, and marked or progressive aortic dilatation. Regardless of the mode of delivery, antibiotic cover may be prescribed in the peripartum period to prevent endarteritis.

## FINAL DIAGNOSIS

Mild residual aortic coarctation with paracoarctation aneurysm and pregnancy

## PLAN OF ACTION

Careful medical management of pregnancy and delivery

## OUTCOME

The patient's case was reviewed and discussed in a joint high-risk pregnancy and cardiology clinic, and a management plan was established and documented. Weekly blood pressure checks were recommended. Beta-blockers would be started if the proximal systolic blood pressure exceeded 140 mm Hg. The patient was advised to remain physically active for the remainder of her pregnancy but to avoid extreme exercise.

A follow-up MRI scan and an echocardiogram were scheduled to be done at the end of the second trimester, that is, after full expansion of blood volume and increase in cardiac output, to reevaluate the gradient across the coarctation and to exclude any change in the diameter and anatomy of the paracoarctation aneurysm (which remained stable). A fetal cardiac scan was planned at 14 and 20 weeks of pregnancy.[14] All these tests were performed as planned, and the results were reassuring. The patient had an uneventful course through the remainder of pregnancy and did not develop systemic hypertension.

To ensure optimal delivery avoiding any delay in her obstetric care and to secure close blood pressure monitoring at the end of pregnancy, it was decided to electively admit the patient to the obstetric inpatient ward at 38 weeks of pregnancy.

A vaginal delivery under epidural analgesia with a short second stage of labor was planned unless dramatic changes in her cardiovascular findings such as uncontrollable systemic hypertension and further distension of the aneurysm occurred, or obstetric complications arose.

Antibiotic cover during delivery was recommended.

In the 39th week of gestation she went into spontaneous labor while in the hospital. A healthy baby was delivered vaginally with low-dose epidural analgesia. Blood pressure was monitored continuously during labor and delivery. The highest blood pressure measured was 175/110 mm Hg. The patient recovered fully from delivery and was discharged home after 3 days.

One year later, baby and mother are both doing well.

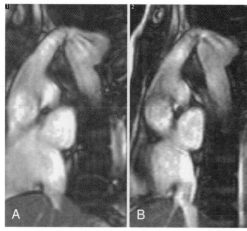

11th week of gestation     27th week of gestation

Figure 26-8 Oblique sagittal magnetic resonance images of the aorta taken at the end of systole.

## FINDINGS

An MRI done in the 27th week of pregnancy (*B*) shows the anatomy of the aorta and the paracoarctation aneurysm were unchanged. There was no increase in flow velocity at the site of the residual stenosis. The identical picture taken in early pregnancy (11th week; *A*) is shown for comparison.

**Comments:** By the end of the second trimester of pregnancy, cardiac output and blood volume have increased by 50%.

Thus, even after full-volume expansion, the paracoarctation aneurysm was stable, with no change in peak velocities across the coarctation repair site. These were clearly reassuring signs supporting the original plan for medical therapy and vaginal delivery under epidural, unless additional obstetric indications determined otherwise.

## Selected References

1. Waldhausen JA, Nahrwold DL: Repair of coarctation of the aorta with a subclavian flap. J Thorac Cardiovasc Surg 51:532–533, 1966.
2. Thorne, SA: Pregnancy in heart disease. Heart 90:450–456, 2004.
3. Leandro J, Smallhorn JF, Benson L, et al: Ambulatory blood pressure monitoring and left ventricular mass and function after successful surgical repair of coarctation of the aorta. J Am Coll Cardiol 20:197–204, 1992.
4. Beauchesne LM, Connolly HM, Ammash NM, et al: Coarctation of the aorta: Outcome of pregnancy. J Am Coll Cardiol 38:1728–1733, 2001.
5. Kaemmerer H, Oelert F, Bahlmann J, et al: Arterial hypertension in adults after surgical treatment of aortic coarctation. Thorac Cardiovasc Surg 46:121–125, 1998.
6. Siu SC, Sermer M, Harrison DA, et al: Risk and predictors for pregnancy-related complications in women with heart disease. Circulation 96:2789–2794, 1997.
7. Siu SC, Sermer M, Colman JM, et al: Prospective multicenter study of pregnancy outcomes in women with heart disease. Circulation 104:515–521, 2001.
8. Von Kodolitsch Y, Aydin MA, Koschyk DH, et al: Predictors of aneurysmal formation after surgical correction of aortic coarctation. J Am Coll Cardiol 39:617–624, 2002.
9. Oliver JM, Gallego P, Gonzalez A, et al: Risk factors for aortic complications in adults with coarctation of the aorta. J Am Coll Cardiol 44:1641–1647, 2004.
10. Parks WJ, Ngo TD, Plauth WH Jr: Incidence of aneurysm formation after Dacron patch aortoplasty repair for coarctation of the aorta: Long-term results and assessment utilizing magnetic resonance angiography with three-dimensional surface rendering. J Am Coll Cardiol 26:266–271, 1995.
11. Niwa K, Perloff JK, Bhuta SM, et al: Structural abnormalities of great arterial walls in congenital heart disease: Light and electron microscopic analyses. Circulation 103:393–400, 2001.
12. Plunkett MD, Bond LM, Geiss DM: Staged repair of acute type I aortic dissection and coarctation in pregnancy. Ann Thorac Surg 69:1945–1947, 2000.
13. Nora JJ: From generational studies to a multilevel genetic-environmental interaction. J Am Coll Cardiol 23:1468–1471, 1994.
14. Allan LD: Cardiac anatomy screening: What is the best time for screening in pregnancy? Curr Opin Obstet Gynecol 15:143–146, 2003.

# Extraanatomic Bypass Graft Repair of Coarctation

**Omer Goktekin, Darryl F. Shore, and Michael A. Gatzoulis**

**Age: 31**
**Gender: Female**
**Occupation: Nurse**
**Working diagnosis: Aortic recoarctation**

## HISTORY

When the patient was 5 years old, the diagnosis of coarctation of the aorta was made after a murmur was heard. One year later she underwent three successive operations for repair. At age 13 a bypass tube graft was implanted between the left subclavian artery and descending thoracic aorta. Through adolescence and early adulthood she felt well but had persistent systemic hypertension despite triple drug therapy.

The patient had had two spontaneous abortions. Knowing the history of her coarctation and extensive repair, her obstetrician referred her to a tertiary care center regarding the potential relationship between her coarctation and miscarriages.

**Comments:** Aortic coarctation accounts for 5% to 8% of all congenital heart defects, and it is more common in males than females by approximately 2 to 1.[1]

There are several operative techniques (Fig. 27-1) for the surgical management of aortic coarctation. These include subclavian flap aortoplasty, end-to-end anastomosis, extended anastomosis, prosthetic patch aortoplasty, interposition graft, and bypass tube graft. As is common, the surgical details of this patient's prior repairs were lost, which challenges her care as an adult. From the patient's own recollection, it seemed that most likely she had at least one interposition graft and one bypass tube graft.

Persistent systolic hypertension despite medical therapy in this young patient should suggest recoarctation or residual coarctation. The incidence of recurrent coarctation ranges between 3% and 41% in a survey of 11 major studies, and may occur with all known surgical techniques.[2] No single technique appears to be superior to the others. The risk of recoarctation is associated with smaller patient size or younger age at operation, and the presence of associated transverse arch hypoplasia. Children operated on in infancy or early childhood are at particular risk.

Many patients with recoarctation are asymptomatic[3] and can be identified with MRI screening.[4,5]

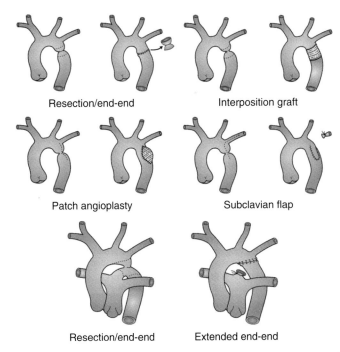

Resection/end-end

Interposition graft

Patch angioplasty

Subclavian flap

Resection/end-end

Extended end-end

Figure 27-1 Major surgical aortic coarctation repair techniques. (Modified from Rocchini AP: Coarctation of the aorta and interrupted aortic arch. In Moller JH, Hoffman JIE [eds]: Pediatric Cardiovascular Medicine. New York, Churchill Livingstone, 2000, pp 567–593.)

## CURRENT SYMPTOMS

The patient was asymptomatic. She was able to climb three flights of stairs without dyspnea or chest pain. She had not had palpitations, dizziness, or epistaxis.

NYHA class: I

# CURRENT MEDICATIONS

Atenolol 25 mg daily

Enalapril 10 mg twice daily

Hydralazine 25 mg twice daily

# PHYSICAL EXAMINATION

BP 182/79 mm Hg (right arm), 155/83 mm Hg (left arm), 145/75 mm Hg (right leg), 147/78 mm Hg (left leg); HR 50 bpm; oxygen saturation in right hand 98%

Height 165 cm, weight 48.8 kg, BSA 1.5 m²

Surgical scars: Midline sternotomy scar and a left lateral thoracotomy scar

Neck veins: JVP was not elevated, and the waveform was normal.

Lungs/chest: The chest was clear to auscultation, with normal breath sounds.

Heart: The heart rhythm was regular. There was a normal apical impulse. Auscultation revealed a normal first heart sound, a normally split second with a very soft ejection systolic murmur in the upper left sternal edge with no continuous murmur. There were no murmurs over the posterior thorax. The right and left radial pulses were equal and forceful whereas both femoral pulses were weak and delayed.

Abdomen: There was no organomegaly.

Extremities: No clubbing of the fingers and toes seen, and there was no edema.

***Comments:*** The major clinical manifestation in adults with coarctation of the aorta is a difference in resting systolic blood pressure between the upper and lower extremities (in most cases, the diastolic blood pressures are similar).[6]

The classic findings are hypertension in the upper extremities, diminished or delayed femoral pulses (relative to the radial), and lower or unobtainable arterial blood pressure in the lower extremities (normally the systolic blood pressure is higher in the leg than the arm). The mechanical obstruction to flow is thought to be largely responsible for the elevation of blood pressure in the upper extremities. In addition, renal ischemia may lead to enhanced renin secretion and "secondary" systolic hypertension.

Auscultatory findings vary and depend on the nature of any associated cardiac lesions and hemodynamic adaptations. Approximately 70% of patients have a bicuspid aortic valve, so an ejection click might be expected at this age, but was not present here.

# LABORATORY DATA

| | | |
|---|---|---|
| Hemoglobin | 12.4 g/dL | (11.5–15.0) |
| Hematocrit/PCV | 37% | (36–46) |
| MCV | 89 fL | (83–99) |
| Platelet count | 190 × 10⁹/L | (150–400) |
| Sodium | 138 mmol/L | (134–145) |
| Potassium | 3.9 mmol/L | (3.5–5.2) |
| Creatinine | 1.1 mg/dL | (0.6–1.2) |
| Blood urea nitrogen | **8.9 mmol/L** | (2.5–6.5) |

# ELECTROCARDIOGRAM

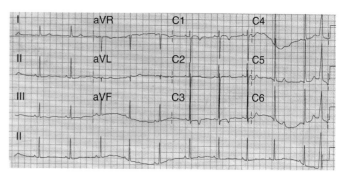

Figure 27-2 Electrocardiogram.

## FINDINGS

Heart rate: 63 bpm

QRS axis: +58°

QRS duration: 85 msec

Normal sinus rhythm with a normal axis. Voltage criteria for LV hypertrophy are present (RV4–6 > 25 mm, SV2 > 25 mm, SV1 + RV5 > 35 mm). Nonspecific T-wave inversion in V3. One ventricular premature beat is seen.

***Comments:*** The most common finding in coarctation is evidence of LV hypertrophy.

# CHEST X-RAY

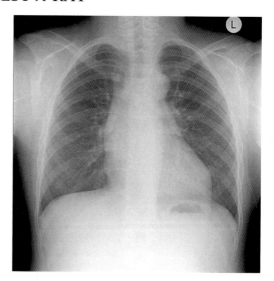

Figure 27-3 Posteroanterior projection.

## FINDINGS

Cardiothoracic ratio: 49%

Cardiac size is at the upper limit of normal, with mild dilatation of the ascending aorta. There is no obvious rib notching. The lung parenchyma is normal.

***Comments:*** Rib notching can be present from severe coarctation with extensive collateralization. It is not seen in the anterior ribs because the anterior intercostal arteries are not located in costal grooves.[1]

# EXERCISE TESTING

| | | | |
|---|---|---|---|
| Exercise protocol: | Modified Bruce | | |
| Duration (min:sec): | 11:00 | | |
| Reason for stopping: | Dyspnea | | |
| ECG changes: | Frequent bigeminy, no ST change | | |

| | Rest | Reak |
|---|---|---|
| Heart rate (bpm): | 50 | 137 |
| Percent of age-predicted max HR: | | 72 |
| $O_2$ saturation (%): | 98 | 99 |
| Left arm blood pressure (mm Hg): | 155/85 | 190/90 |
| Right arm blood pressure (mm Hg): | 180/80 | 200/90 |
| Peak $Vo_2$ (mL/kg/min): | | 17.3 |
| Percent predicted (%): | | 50 |
| $Ve/Vco_2$: | | 36 |
| Metabolic equivalents: | | 5.7 |

***Comments:*** The purpose of the test is twofold. One is to assess the patient's objective exercise tolerance, given that she feels asymptomatic. The other is to determine the blood pressure response to exercise, which may be an important consideration for some patients with repaired coarctation.

Her heart rate response was 72% of the maximal age-predicted heart rate (presumably attenuated by her beta-blocker). Her functional capacity was decreased compared to what was expected for her age and gender despite her self-reported absence of exercise limitation.

The blood pressure response to exercise here was not of concern.

# ECHOCARDIOGRAM

## OVERALL FINDINGS

The LV was of normal size and function but there was moderate LV hypertrophy. The RV was normal in size and function. There was no significant valvular abnormality, including a normal trileaflet aortic valve.

The posterior and septal walls of the LV were thickened, consistent with LV hypertrophy.

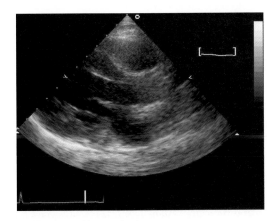

Figure 27-4 Parasternal long-axis view.

***Comments:*** Hypertrophy found here is indicative of long-standing proximal hypertension despite the use of antihypertensive therapy. Echocardiography also helps to exclude associated congenital abnormalities, with a bicuspid aortic valve being the most common.

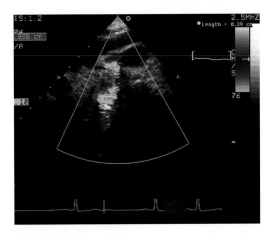

Figure 27-5 Suprasternal long-axis view.

## FINDINGS

Dilated ascending aorta, narrowing of the distal aorta immediately after the origin of the left subclavian artery. The diameter is 4 mm. The peak velocity was 4.5 m/sec.

***Comments:*** Although the aortic arch, including branching arteries, can be seen easily in infants and early childhood, visualization can be difficult in adult patients, and other modalities are required to clarify the aortic anatomy.

In this patient localized, severe narrowing was seen just beyond the left subclavian artery. This finding should be interpreted with caution given her history of multiple repairs. This narrowing may have been bypassed by a graft, which cannot be seen on the echocardiogram, and hence may not be the main flow pathway. However, the peak velocity through this narrowing does suggest a significant pressure gradient between these two portions of the aorta, and hence an obstruction must be present.

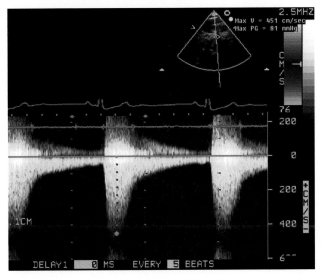

Figure 27-6 Continuous-wave Doppler.

## FINDINGS

Peak velocity through the identified narrowing is 4.5 m/sec, meaning there is a pressure gradient of 81 mm Hg. There is also a significant velocity throughout diastole, the so-called diastolic tail.[7]

***Comments:*** The presence of a detectable antegrade diastolic velocity through the narrowing is further evidence of significant obstruction. It implies the presence of a persistent gradient throughout diastole, meaning that there is not adequate runoff either through collaterals or through an extra-aortic conduit.

# MAGNETIC RESONANCE IMAGING

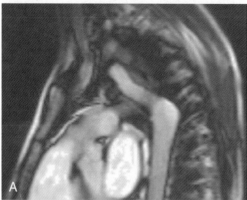

Graft 1 (patent)

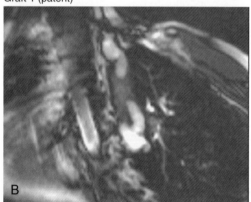

Graft 2 (occluded)

Figure 27-7 Oblique sagittal view (**A**), and oblique coronal view (**B**).

## FINDINGS

There were two aortic interposition grafts. Graft 1 was placed end to end between the isthmus and the descending aorta. It was patent but significantly stenosed at its proximal suture line. The peak flow velocity at the proximal suture line was 3.5 m/sec.

Graft 2 (presumably placed later) was a bypass conduit placed from the proximal left subclavian artery to the descending aorta just distal to the insertion of graft 1. However, graft 2 was completely obstructed by dense thrombus in its central region. The distal anastomoses of both grafts were unobstructed.

## Ventricular Volume Quantification

|  | LV | (Normal range) | RV | (Normal range) |
|---|---|---|---|---|
| EDV (mL) | 140 | (52–141) | 132 | (58–154) |
| ESV (mL) | 50 | (13–51) | 41 | (12–68) |
| SV (mL) | 90 | (33–97) | 91 | (35–98) |
| EF (%) | 64 | (57–75) | 69 | (51–75) |
| EDVi (mL/m²) | 94 | (62–96) | 88 | (61–98) |
| ESVi (mL/m²) | 33 | (17–36) | 27 | (17–43) |
| SVi (mL/m²) | 60 | (40–65) | **61** | (20–40) |
| Mass index (g/m²) | **101** | (47–77) | 39 | (20–40) |

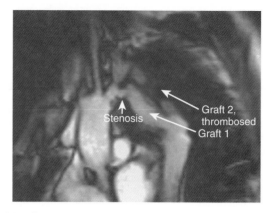

Figure 27-8 Oblique sagittal view.

## FINDINGS

There was a severe coarctation immediately distal to the origin of the left subclavian artery, which itself was stenosed at its origin.

## ADDITIONAL FINDINGS

The aortic valve was tricuspid and functioned normally. The LV was hypertrophied and markedly trabeculated, but had good systolic function.

The ascending and descending aorta were of normal size. The ascending aorta and dilated right brachiocephalic artery were unusually pulsatile, expanding to 29 mm at end systole. By comparison, the descending aorta was 13 mm in diameter at the diaphragm.

***Comments:*** MRI plays an important role in noninvasively demonstrating structure and flow in the arch region after coarctation repair. It can show the site, extent, and degree of the aortic narrowing including possible arch hypoplasia, the prestenotic and poststenotic aorta, and collateral vessels, if present. The course and patency of prosthetic bypass grafts can be depicted. In the present patient, significant residual coarctation, peak velocity 3.5 m/sec, was due to stenosis at the proximal suture line of interposition graft 1. Suture-related stenosis is a common reason for recoarctation. A second interposition graft from the left subclavian to the descending aorta was completely obstructed by thrombus.

Based on these findings, the narrowed area seen by echo is the only communication between ascending and descending aorta, and the peak velocity measured here (either by echocardiography or MRI) reflects the true pressure gradient.

### FOCUSED CLINICAL QUESTIONS AND DISCUSSION POINTS

1. How should this patient's recoarctation be addressed?

   *Although this patient is asymptomatic, she has significant hypertension and LV hypertrophy, which are risk factors for cardiovascular events over the long term.*

   *A resting pressure gradient of greater than 20 mm Hg in the setting of a coarctation should be considered a good indication for intervention.[8] Both echo and MRI confirmed significant recoarctation and LV hypertrophy, making treatment warranted.*

2. What are the risks of complications from a future pregnancy in this patient?

   *There are known potential complications of coarctation and pregnancy, including maternal death and fetal loss. In a review of 50 women undergoing 118 pregnancies, there was one maternal death reported, 11% fetal loss, and 4% prematurity. There did* not seem to be a difference in patients who had prior repair of coarctation versus those without.[9] Although in this study the fetal loss rate was similar to that for the general population, impaired lower body perfusion is a known risk factor for miscarriage, which has been a problem for this patient. Complete control of proximal hypertension may be counterproductive during pregnancy as it would lead to lower body hypotension, thus compromising placental flow.

Even after her residual coarctation has been addressed, the patient should know that, based on these limited data, there is a risk of maternal death due to aortic dissection or rupture of a cerebral aneurysm. With appropriate preconception evaluation and treatment, close attention throughout gestation, and a well-planned labor and delivery with properly trained obstetrics and anesthesia services, pregnancy should be tolerated without major problems, though there is still much to learn about this unique problem during pregnancy.

The patient should also be counseled that the overall risk of recurrence of congenital heart disease ranges between 3% and 5%, and the risk is higher (5%–10%) for left-sided obstructive lesions, including coarctation.[10]

The degree of stenosis in this patient's case is severe and may have been responsible at least in part for the history of miscarriages. There was hope but no guarantee that with improved lower-body hemodynamics the patient would have a better chance of a successful pregnancy.

3. What is the best way to repair the recoarctation?

Balloon angioplasty with primary stenting may have an important and successful role in the management of the adult with native coarctation or recoarctation.[11] In this patient, fourth-time redo surgery with a thrombosed graft in place is not an attractive option. However, in this particular case, several factors made surgical redo more attractive.

First, the angioplasty target will have to be the interposition graft (graft 1) and its suture-related stenosis. Unfortunately, the diameter of graft 1 is not large enough to allow the placement of an adequate-sized stent. Second, the risk of rupture during angioplasty is probably significant in this patient because there is stenosis at a prior suture line. Third, the recoarctation is at the origin of the left subclavian artery, which in itself has severe ostial stenosis, and there would be a high risk of losing flow to the left subclavian artery (minor point) with stent placement.

Therefore, after multidisciplinary discussion, surgical placement of a large extra-anatomic bypass graft from ascending to descending aorta, leaving the current grafts as they are, was chosen as the treatment of choice.[12]

## FINAL DIAGNOSIS

Recoarctation of proximal aortic interposition graft

Thrombosis of left subclavian to aorta bypass graft

Severe proximal stenosis of the left subclavian artery

## PLAN OF ACTION

Surgical placement of an extra-anatomic bypass graft from ascending to descending aorta

## OUTCOME

The patient had uneventful surgery via a median sternotomy approach with cardiopulmonary bypass. She was extubated on the first postoperative day, mobilized fully, and left the hospital within a week. She had complete relief of her coarctation with normalization of her blood pressure on minimal medical therapy and normal lower body perfusion. Repeat MRI showed effective relief of the proximal hypertension with a long conduit from her ascending to descending thoracic aorta functioning well with no residual pressure gradients.

The patient went on to have a successful pregnancy a year later and gave birth to a healthy male infant (weight 3 kg) by vaginal delivery under epidural anesthesia. Postnatal echocardiography on the infant showed a bicuspid aortic valve without stenosis or regurgitation. The patient herself was normotensive and off all antihypertensive medication.

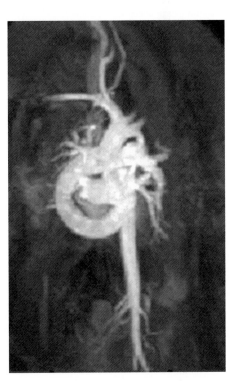

Figure 27-9 Magnetic resonance angiography of the aorta.

## FINDINGS

The new bypass graft (to the left in the image) passing from ascending to the descending aorta, is widely patent and measures 23 mm in diameter. The pressure gradient between ascending and descending aorta has been completely abolished as was the systemic hypertension.

**Comments:** Ascending to descending aortic bypass surgery for relief of complex aortic coarctation (or recoarctation) can be effective in relieving proximal hypertension. Patients, however, clearly warrant lifelong follow-up, as concerns may be raised regarding the lifelong impact of such an invasive approach for what could be, otherwise, an inoperable condition.[12]

## Selected References

1. Brickner ME, Hillis LD, Lange RA: Congenital heart disease in adults: First of two parts. N Engl J Med 342:256, 2000.
2. Cohen M, Fuster V, Steele PM, et al: Coarctation of the aorta: Long-term follow-up and prediction of outcome after surgical correction. Circulation 80:840–845, 1989.
3. Attenhofer Jost CH, Schaff HV, Connolly HM, et al: Spectrum of reoperations after repair of aortic coarctation: Importance of an individualized approach because of coexistent cardiovascular disease. Mayo Clin Proc 77:46–53, 2002.
4. Therrien J, Thorne SA, Wright A, et al: Repaired coarctation: A "cost-effective" approach to identify complications in adults. J Am Coll Cardiol 35:1003–1006, 2000.

5. Marx GR: "Repaired" aortic coarctation in adults: Not a "simple" congenital heart defect. J Am Coll Cardiol 35:997–1002, 2000.
6. Swan L, Goyal S, Hsia C, et al: Exercise systolic blood pressures are of questionable value in the assessment of the adult with a previous coarctation repair. Heart 89:89–92, 2003.
7. Carvalho JS, Redington AN, Shinebourne EA, et al: Continuous wave Doppler echocardiography and coarctation of the aorta: Gradients and flow patterns in the assessment of severity. Br Heart J 64:33–37, 1990.
8. Aboulhosn J, Child JS: Left ventricular outflow obstruction: Subaortic stenosis, bicuspid aortic valve, supravalvar aortic stenosis, and coarctation of the aorta. Circulation 114:2412–2422, 2006.
9. Beauchesne LM, Connolly HM, Ammash NM, Warnes CA: Coarctation of the aorta: Outcome of pregnancy. J Am Coll Cardiol 38:728–733, 2001.
10. Uebing A, Steer PJ, Yentis SM, Gatzoulis MA: Pregnancy and congenital heart disease. BMJ 332:401–406, 2006.
11. Harrison DA, McLaughlin PR, Lazzam C, et al: Endovascular stents in the management of coarctation of the aorta in the adolescent and adult: One year follow up. Heart 85:561–566, 2001.
12. McKellar SH, Schaff HV, Dearani JA, et al: Intermediate-term results of ascending-descending posterior pericardial bypass of complex aortic coarctation. J Thorac Cardiovasc Surg 133:1504–1509, 2007.

# Interrupted Aortic Arch in a Patient with DiGeorge Syndrome

**Sabrina D. Phillips**

**Age: 18**
**Gender: Female**
**Occupation: Student**
**Working diagnosis: Left ventricular outflow tract obstruction and DiGeorge syndrome**

## HISTORY

The patient was the product of a normal pregnancy delivered at term. She initially had symptoms of heart failure on day 10 of life. She was found to have nearly complete aortic arch interruption, a VSD, and an ASD. Before a planned operative repair, she was noted to have hypocalcemia, which was corrected. Otherwise, she underwent repair of the aortic arch, VSD closure, and ASD closure and had no operative complications. Thereafter, she grew normally.

At 10 years of age the patient again developed heart failure symptoms. She was diagnosed with severe aortic valve stenosis, and a balloon valvotomy was attempted. During that hospitalization, however, she developed a severe systemic infection with severe splenomegaly and hepatomegaly. This was eventually diagnosed as a cytomegalovirus infection. Her aortic stenosis was not relieved after the balloon valvotomy, so she was considered for operative replacement of her aortic valve. She developed a transfusion reaction during a platelet transfusion that was being administered prophylactically for thrombocytopenia prior to a diagnostic angiogram. The patient eventually had replacement of her aortic valve with a 21-mm St. Jude prosthesis. Notably, several large mediastinal lymph nodes were removed during this surgery.

The patient did well initially after her aortic valve replacement, and cardiology follow-up visits were unremarkable. She was eventually diagnosed with selective IgA deficiency and treatment was initiated with monthly IVIG infusion. In late adolescence, however, she began to feel increasingly tired. She presented at 18 years of age with increasing fatigue and reduced exercise tolerance over the prior 6 months.

**Comments:** Cardiac anomalies commonly associated with DiGeorge syndrome include tetralogy of Fallot, pulmonary atresia/VSD, truncus arteriosus, and interrupted aortic arch.[1]

Hypocalcemia in DiGeorge syndrome occurs secondary to absent parathyroid function. The term *partial DiGeorge syndrome* is applied when infants have impaired rather than absent parathyroid or thymus function,[2] as in this case.

Patients with DiGeorge syndrome manifest a deficiency in cell-mediated immunity related to thymic hypoplasia. Susceptibility to infection is variable.[2] Disorders of humoral immunity can also occur.[3]

Some patients with DiGeorge syndrome produce autoantibodies to red cells, white cells, and platelets.[2]

Fatigue is a very nonspecific symptom at any age, and late adolescence can cause psychosocial problems that can be diffi-cult to decipher against the background of complex congenital heart disease. Further, DiGeorge patients are at risk for depression and schizophrenia.[4] Still, a hemodynamic cause of deterioration must be sought.

## CURRENT SYMPTOMS

The patient had exertional fatigue. She denied dyspnea, orthopnea, and paroxysmal nocturnal dyspnea. She did not have intolerance to heat or cold, or constipation. Her menstrual cycles were regular but generally heavy. She noted that it had been very difficult to keep her INR in the therapeutic range. She also admitted that she was ambivalent about anticoagulation, as she was prohibited from some activities because of fear of injury and bleeding.

NYHA class: I–II

**Comments:** There were no typical symptoms of thyroid disease to explain her fatigue, but thyroid disease should be properly excluded by laboratory testing. Heavy menses may be associated with iron deficiency anemia, which may cause fatigue or exacerbate cardiac causes of fatigue. Selective IgA deficiency is associated with malabsorption and is another potential cause of iron deficiency anemia.[5] Malabsorption likely contributes to difficulty in controlling oral anticoagulation and results in a need for higher warfarin doses. Noncompliance certainly needs to be considered, especially in teenagers and young adults with chronic disease who may rebel against the constraints placed on them. Compliance could be increased with home INR monitoring and education.

## CURRENT MEDICATIONS

Trimethoprim/sulfamethoxazole, regular strength, orally twice daily

IVIG Polygam, every 5 weeks

Hydrocortisone prior to IVIG administration

Coumadin 9.5 mg daily (target INR 2.5–3.5)

Subacute bacterial endocarditis prophylaxis

**Comments:** Trimethoprim/sulfamethoxazole is administered prophylactically in this patient secondary to her reduced CD4 cell count. IVIG and steroids are useful in the treatment of autoantibodies to red cells, white cells, and platelets. This also provides treatment for deficiency of immunoglobulin, which this patient has demonstrated.

# PHYSICAL EXAMINATION

BP 100/70 mm Hg (arm), 100/70 mm Hg (leg); HR 80 bpm; oxygen saturation 100%

Height 151 cm, weight 39 kg, BSA 1.28 m$^2$

Head and neck: Long, narrow face with a pointed chin, narrow palpebral fissures, and small ears with overfolding of the superior helix

Surgical scars: Sternotomy

Neck veins: Normal

Lungs/chest: Decreased air entry in the right lung base

Heart: There was a regular rhythm, a 2+ LV impulse, a crescendo-decrescendo murmur heard best at the right upper sternal margin, a crisp, metallic A2, and a suprasternal thrill. The carotid upstroke was delayed.

Abdomen: Marked hepatosplenomegaly was present.

Extremities: There was no radiofemoral delay; no cyanosis, clubbing, or edema.

## PERTINENT NEGATIVES

She was not pale.

***Comments:*** The patient's height and weight are less than the third percentile when plotted on standard growth curves. Patients with DiGeorge syndrome commonly have short stature. This may be related to growth hormone deficiency or hypothyroidism, both of which have been associated with the syndrome.[3] Poor growth is also seen in children with immunoglobulin deficiency.[6]

Several "typical" facial features have been described in patients with DiGeorge or velocardiofacial syndrome. These include a small mandible, long face, large nose, narrow palpebral fissures, abnormal ear folding, and a flat malar region. However, the features described are subtle, and two separate studies have demonstrated an inability to predict whether a patient has the syndrome based on facial features.[1,7]

The cardiac exam is consistent with severe aortic valve stenosis. There was no radiofemoral delay to suggest significant coarctation. She did not appear anemic.

# LABORATORY DATA

| | |
|---|---|
| Hemoglobin | **11.3 g/dL** (11.5–15.0) |
| Hematocrit/PCV | **33.8%** (36–46) |
| MCV | **73 fL** (83–99) |
| Platelet count | **106 × 10$^9$/L** (150–400) |
| Leukocyte count | **2.0 × 10$^9$/L** (3.5–10.5) |
| Sodium | 139 mmol/L (134–145) |
| Potassium | 3.8 mmol/L (3.5–5.2) |
| Creatinine | 0.7 mg/dL (0.6–1.2) |

***Comments:*** A mild pancytopenia is present, which may be secondary to autoantibodies to red cells, white cells, and platelets. Iron deficiency is possible given the microcytic picture. The degree of anemia is unlikely to be the cause of her fatigue.

## OTHER RELEVANT LAB RESULTS

| | |
|---|---|
| TSH | 4.0 mIU/L (0.3–5) |
| Bio-Intact PTH (1-84) | **<4.0 pg/mL** (10–55) |
| Calcium | **7.7 mg/dL** (9.1–10.3) |
| Albumin | 4.6 g/dL (3.5–5.0) |
| INR | **1.9** |
| IgA | **2 mg/dL** (55–377) |
| IgM | **19 mg/dL** (56–242) |
| IgG | 1310 mg/dL (724–1611) |

***Comments:*** The low parathyroid hormone (PTH) and calcium are consistent with reduced parathyroid function.

Her INR is low. One may need to ask her about and emphasize compliance. She may need to reduce her dietary vitamin K intake. The dose of warfarin needed to maintain an adequate INR may be higher secondary to the malabsorption associated with IgA deficiency.

The levels of IgA and IgM are severely reduced, consistent with a defect in antibody-mediated immunity.

# ELECTROCARDIOGRAM

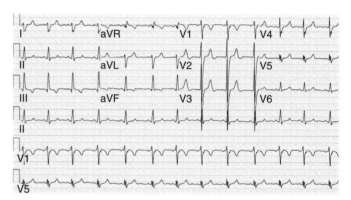

Figure 28-1 Electrocardiogram.

## FINDINGS

Heart rate: 74 bpm

QRS axis: +109°

QRS duration: 138 msec

Normal sinus rhythm with a nonspecific intraventricular conduction delay and right-axis deviation.

***Comments:*** The patient does not have clear evidence of LV hypertrophy, which should be looked for in any patient with aortic valve and/or arch stenosis.

# CHEST X-RAY

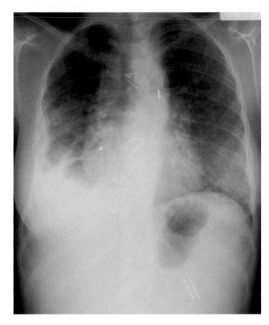

Figure 28-2 Posteroanterior projection.

## FINDINGS

Cardiothoracic ratio: 45%

Moderately dense infiltrates and pleural thickening around the right lung base were seen, as well as increased pulmonary vascularity. Epicardial leads and an aortic prosthesis were noted.

*Comments:* Often, epicardial leads were placed by surgeons at the time of other surgery for potential future use. Although the patient does not have a pacemaker, consideration of these wires is relevant when considering the utility of a MRI scan (see Fig. 28-6).

# ECHOCARDIOGRAM

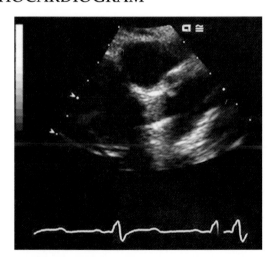

Figure 28-3 Parasternal long-axis view.

## FINDINGS

The LV was normal in size with normal systolic function, ejection fraction 62%. There was no LV hypertrophy. No evidence of residual VSD or ASD was seen.

In addition, mild RV enlargement with normal systolic function was noted. The estimated RV systolic pressure was 32 mm Hg.

*Comments:* LV hypertrophy would be expected in a patient with significant prosthetic valve stenosis.

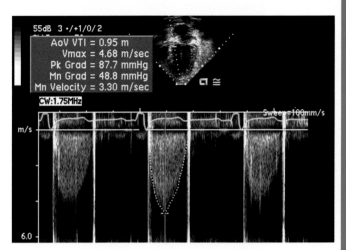

Figure 28-4 Continuous-wave Doppler of the aortic valve.

## FINDINGS

Severe aortic valve prosthetic stenosis was present. The peak velocity was 4.7 m/sec, giving a systolic gradient of 88 mm Hg. The mean systolic Doppler gradient was 49 mm Hg. There was mild prosthetic regurgitation.

*Comments:* Mechanical prosthetic aortic valve stenosis is most commonly related to pannus formation or thrombosis.[8-11] The incidence of pannus formation resulting in valve obstruction is estimated to be about 1% to 6%.[12] Thrombosis must be considered in this patient given the history of variable control of her anticoagulation.

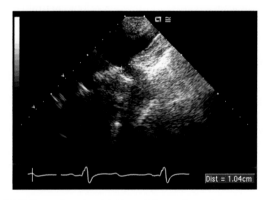

Figure 28-5 Suprasternal notch view of the aortic arch.

## FINDINGS

There was mild residual obstruction of the aortic arch just distal to the origin of the left common carotid artery, with a maximal instantaneous gradient of 21 mm Hg and a mean systolic gradient of 13 mm Hg.

*Comments:* The patient was born with an interrupted aortic arch, one of many congenital defects associated with DiGeorge syndrome. The residual narrowing here is a known long-term complication of the early repair.

# MAGNETIC RESONANCE ANGIOGRAPHY

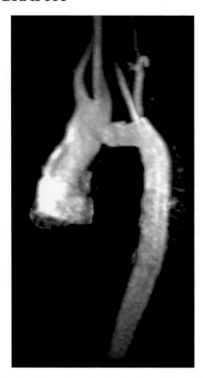

Figure 28-6 Maximal intensity projection image of the aortic arch.

## FINDINGS

There was mild residual narrowing of the aortic arch. An aberrant right subclavian artery was seen originating distal to the origin of the left subclavian artery. The course of the right subclavian artery was posterior to the esophagus.

**Comments:** Patients with type B aortic interruption and patients with DiGeorge syndrome often have an aberrant right subclavian artery related to the embryologic neural crest contribution to the vascular anatomy.[12]

It should be noted that on the CXR the patient had epicardial pacing leads, which were often left in place after cardiac surgery and commonly found in adult congenital heart disease patients even when no pacemaker is present. Such leads are considered a possible contraindication to MRI because of the potential for heating. However, more and more laboratories are challenging this contraindication. Even if no appreciable heating occurs, the wires can still cause significant artifacts. Thankfully, this angiogram was not affected by such artifact.

## FOCUSED CLINICAL QUESTIONS AND DISCUSSION POINTS

1. What is the etiology of the DiGeorge phenotype?

    *DiGeorge syndrome is the result of a microdeletion of chromosome 22q11.2. It is part of a spectrum of phenotypic expression of this deletion, which also includes velocardiofacial syndrome and conotruncal anomaly face syndrome. These syndromes have been referred to as CATCH-22 disorders (Cardiac defects, Abnormal facies, Thymic hypoplasia, Cleft palate, and Hypocalcemia) and result from developmental abnormalities of the embryonic third and fourth branchial arches and neural crest cells.[3] The 22q11.2 microdeletion is the most common deletion disorder in humans, with an incidence of approximately 1 out of 4000 births.[13]*

2. Do patients with 22q11.2 microdeletion and conotruncal abnormalities have an unfavorable surgical outcome?

    *Patients with 22q11.2 microdeletion tend to have more complex pulmonary anatomy and abnormalities of great artery anatomy when compared to patients with the same cardiac diagnosis who do not have the microdeletion. This potentially affects surgical outcome in an unfavorable manner.[1] The multisystem consequences of the microdeletion require a team approach to the surgical patient, including anesthesia, hematology, and infectious disease experts. Blood products should be irradiated in patients with the DiGeorge phenotype to reduce transfusion-related complications.[2] Laryngotracheal abnormalities are common and need to be anticipated by the anesthesiologist.*

3. When should the 22q11.2 microdeletion be suspected?

    *Patients with conotruncal abnormalities (tetralogy of Fallot, pulmonary atresia/VSD, truncus arteriosus, and interrupted aortic arch) should be suspect, especially when there is an associated right-sided aortic arch, discontinuous or hypoplastic pulmonary arteries, multiple aortopulmonary collateral arteries, a dysplastic or absent semilunar valve, or interrupted aortic arch type B.[3] Aortic arch interruptions are defined as type A, B, or C depending on the site of discontinuity of the aorta. Type A interruptions occur distal to the left subclavian artery. Type B interruptions are located between the left carotid artery and the left subclavian artery. Type C interruptions are defined as aortic interruptions between the right innominate artery and the left carotid artery. The aorta and its branches distal to the interruption are supplied by a patent ductus arteriosus.*

    *Genetic testing can be performed via several methods to detect the microdeletion. This testing is performed on peripheral blood samples from the patient, from which lymphocytes are isolated. DNA obtained from these lymphocytes is used in the testing. Fluorescence in situ hybridization with commercial probes is widely used. A multiplex ligation dependent probe amplification single tube assay can also be used. This assay is rapid and economical. Short tandem repeat segregation tests can also be used.[13] Patients with the deletion should be counseled regarding pregnancy, as each offspring will have a 50% chance of having the deletion themselves. Although genetic screening of parents of index cases is recommended, most new presentations of DiGeorge syndrome are sporadic.*

4. Why did the St. Jude prosthetic valve become obstructed?

    *The pathogenesis of obstruction of a St. Jude medical aortic valve prosthesis has been evaluated by several authors.[8–11,14] While thrombosis is often considered the culprit, pannus formation, with or without thrombosis, has been documented at operation more frequently.[8,10] Thrombosis of a mechanical prosthesis tends to occur earlier after implantation and at random, whereas pannus formation requires a larger time interval after implantation and has a delayed exponential increase in risk.[8] Thrombosis of the prosthesis is more likely to present with acute symptoms in contrast to pannus formation, which presents with increasing valve gradient over time.[8,10] The clinical distinction between pannus and thrombosis, however, is quite difficult. This patient presents with significant obstruction and a history of inadequate anticoagulation, which makes thrombosis a concern. Operation is indicated for relief of the obstruction, at which time the pathogenesis can be determined. Thrombolytic therapy is not indicated in this circumstance, as the patient is hemodynamically stable and the true cause of obstruction is unknown.*

## FINAL DIAGNOSIS

DiGeorge syndrome

Severe prosthetic aortic valve stenosis

Mild aortic arch stenosis (following repair of aortic interruption in infancy)

## PLAN OF ACTION

Aortic valve re-replacement with multidisciplinary involvement from hematology, anesthesiology, infectious disease, and endocrinology

## INTERVENTION

The patient underwent aortic valve re-replacement. The surgeon described circumferential subvalvular obstruction of the prosthesis by fibrous tissue, which was confirmed by pathology to be pannus formation without thrombosis. Dacron patch enlargement of the aortic valve annulus and implantation of a 19-mm St. Jude aortic valve prosthesis was performed.

Pannus formation is likely caused by persistent neointimal development related to a chronic inflammatory response that results in proliferation of myofibroblasts and extracellular matrix without fresh thrombus formation.[9] Pannus is often found to be circumferential and is almost exclusively found on the LV aspect of the valve.[9,10,14] The fibrous tissue most commonly restricts movement of the leaflets directly, but has been demonstrated at a distance from the valve, resulting in LVOT narrowing.[14] The cause of leaflet motion restriction in the St. Jude medical prosthesis may relate to its low-profile structure and the placement of the pivot guards. The straight edges of the leaflets are very close to the edge of the pivot guards in the fully open position. One of the pivot guards comes into contact with the ventricular wall (in either placement orientation). If pannus formation occurs, growth into the pivot guards restricts the opening of the leaflet without restricting closing of the leaflet.[10]

A 19-mm prosthesis was chosen as this was the largest prosthesis that could be implanted after Dacron patch enlargement of the aortic annulus. While this is a small prosthesis it was felt to be adequate for this small patient, as she has completed growth and has a BSA of only 1.28 m[2].

## OUTCOME

The patient's postoperative course was complicated by AV dissociation and heart failure. Hypocalcemia was noted, but correction of the hypocalcemia did not resolve the conduction system abnormalities. Permanent pacemaker implantation was performed.

Seven months after surgery, the patient presented with bacteremia and concerns for endocarditis. Serial transesophageal echocardiography revealed a normal aortic valve prosthesis. The patient had no further positive blood cultures after treatment with a 4-week course of intravenous antibiotics.

Conduction abnormalities requiring permanent pacemaker implantation after aortic valve replacement have an incidence of 5.7% but are not related to adverse long-term outcome when compared to patients with aortic valve replacement who did not need permanent pacing.[15]

## Selected References

1. Beauchesne LM, Warnes CA, Connolly HM, et al: Prevalence and clinical manifestations of 22q11.2 microdeletion in adults with selected conotruncal anomalies. J Am Coll Cardiol 45:595–598, 2005.
2. Hayward AR: Immunodeficiency. In Hay WW, Hayward AR, Levin M, Sondheimer JM (eds): Current Pediatric Diagnosis and Treatment, 16th ed. New York, McGraw-Hill Professional, 2003, pp 921–936.
3. Cuneo BF: 22q11.2 deletion syndrome: DiGeorge, velocardiofacial, and conotruncal anomaly face syndromes. Curr Opin Pediatr 13:465–472, 2001.
4. Bassett AS, Chow EWC, Husted J, et al: Clinical features of 78 adults with 22q11 deletion syndrome. Am J Med Genet 138: 307–313, 2005.
5. Spickett GP, Misbah SA, Chapel HM: Primary antibody deficiency in adults. Lancet 337:281–284, 1991.
6. Bjorkander J, Bake B, Hanson LA: Primary hypogammaglobulinaemia, impaired lung function, and body growth with delayed treatment and inadequate treatment. Eur J Respir Dis 65:529–536, 1984.
7. Becker DB, Pilgram T, Marty-Grames L, et al: Accuracy in identification of patients with 22q11.2 deletion by likely care providers using facial photographs. Plast Reconstr Surg 114:1367–1372, 2004.
8. Rizzoli G, Guglielmi C, Toscano G, et al: Reoperations for acute prosthetic thrombosis and pannus: An assessment of rates, relationship and risk. Eur J Cardio-Thor Surg 16:74–80, 1999.
9. Teshima H, Hayashida N, Yano H, et al: Obstruction of St. Jude medical valves in the aortic position: Histology and immunohistochemistry of pannus. J Thorac Cardiovasc Surg 126:401–407, 2003.
10. Aoyagi S, Nishimi M, Tayama E, et al: Obstruction of St. Jude medical valves in the aortic position: A consideration for pathogenic mechanism of prosthetic valve obstruction. Cardiovasc Surg 10:339–344, 2002.
11. Katircioglu SF, Ulus AT, Yamak B, et al: Acute mechanical valve thrombosis of the St. Jude medical prosthesis. J Card Surg 14: 164–168, 1999.
12. Bergwerff M, Verberne ME, DeRuiter MC, et al. Neural crest cell contribution to the developing circulatory system: Implications for vascular morphology? Circ Res 82:221–231, 1998.
13. Fernandez L, Lapunzina P, Arjona D, et al: Comparative study of three diagnostic approaches (FISH, STRs and MLPA) in 30 patients with 22q11.2 deletion syndrome. Clin Genet 69:373–378, 2005.
14. Kuniyoshi Y, Koja K, Miyagi K, et al: Pannus formation in aortic valve prostheses in the late postoperative period. J Artificial Organs 6:179–182, 2003.
15. Boughaleb D, Mansourati J, Genet L, et al: Permanent cardiac stimulation after aortic valve replacement: Incidence, predictive factors and long-term prognosis. Arch Mal Coeur Vaiss 87: 925–930, 1994.

Case 29

# Ebstein Anomaly and Wolff-Parkinson-White Syndrome

**Masahiro Koh, Toshikatsu Yagihara, and Hideki Uemura**

**Age: 19 years old**
**Gender: Male**
**Occupation: College student**
**Working diagnosis: Ebstein malformation and tachyarrhythmia**

## HISTORY

Soon after birth, the patient developed paroxysmal supraventricular tachycardia, which was controlled reasonably well with digoxin. The diagnosis of Wolff-Parkinson-White (WPW) syndrome was made by the presence of ventricular pre-excitation noted on his ECG.

At the age of 8 months, echocardiography confirmed the coexistence of Ebstein anomaly of the tricuspid valve and an ASD of the secundum type. He never had clinical cyanosis.

When he was 6 years old, digoxin was discontinued, and he had no further episodes of tachycardia.

Recent routine echocardiography at a local hospital demonstrated an enlarged RV, worsening tricuspid regurgitation, and a left-to-right shunt between the atria. Therefore, he was referred for further evaluation.

***Comments:*** Digoxin and its relatives were chosen in the past to control supraventricular tachycardia even in infants. Its positive inotropic effects were believed to work synergistically with its blockade of AV conduction. The actual mechanism of action was not clearly understood, however, and the narrow therapeutic window made appropriate dosing troublesome. Serum digoxin levels above the therapeutic range could be arrhythmogenic. More recently, other drugs have replaced digoxin in this role.

Ventricular pre-excitation via one or more accessory AV conduction pathway(s) is the hallmark of WPW syndrome. Such pathways, often manifest by a delta wave on the resting ECG, may conduct antegrade or retrograde, enabling AV reentrant tachycardia under certain circumstances. According to the location of the accessory pathways, several types of clinical arrhythmias may be seen. In some patients, the pre-excitation pattern is not seen on the ECG, which is called a concealed type of WPW syndrome.

Ebstein anomaly is a malformation of the tricuspid valve and RV involving incomplete separation (delamination) of portions of the valve leaflet and the endocardium. An ASD or stretched patent foramen ovale is the most common associated lesion.

The common association between Ebstein anomaly and WPW syndrome (in approximately 25% of cases) is well known. Not surprisingly, incomplete formation of the annular attachment of the tricuspid valve results in less than perfect AV orientation. Some muscle fibers bridging the atrium and the ventricle may persist and allow accessory conduction; hence multiple pathways are often found between the right atrium and the RV in Ebstein patients.

## CURRENT SYMPTOMS

The patient is entirely asymptomatic. He has no limitation in daily life, and does not experience palpitations or dizziness.

NYHA class: I

## CURRENT MEDICATIONS

None

## PHYSICAL EXAMINATION

BP 90/60 mm Hg, HR 82 bpm regular rhythm, oxygen saturation 97%

Height 171 cm, weight 66 kg, BSA 1.77 m$^2$

Surgical scars: None

Neck veins: The venous waveform was normal.

Lungs/chest: Lung sounds were clear with no rales.

Heart: The rhythm was regular. There was no RV lift. The second heart sound had a normal pulmonary component, and there was persistent splitting. A blowing 3/6 systolic murmur was heard at the fourth left intercostal space.

Abdomen: The abdomen was soft and flat, with no organomegaly.

Extremities: No edema was present, there was no clubbing.

***Comments:*** The JVP is often normal in Ebstein patients. Typically, a secundum ASD will cause fixed splitting of the second heart sound if there is a significant left-to-right shunt. Severe tricuspid regurgitation will cause closure of the pulmonary valve to occur earlier. Hence splitting may be variable.

## LABORATORY DATA

| | |
|---|---|
| Hemoglobin | 15.6 g/dL (13.5–17.0) |
| Hematocrit/PCV | 47.4% (41–51) |
| Platelet count | $229 \times 10^9$/L (150–350) |
| Sodium | 141 mmol/L (138–145) |
| Potassium | 4.4 mmol/L (3.4–4.9) |
| Creatinine | 0.8 mg/dL (0.7–1.3) |
| Blood urea nitrogen | 13 mg/dL (6–24) |

***Comments:*** No specific abnormalities were present.

## ELECTROCARDIOGRAM

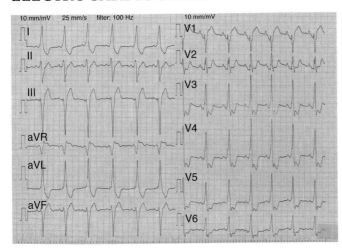

Figure 29-1 Electrocardiogram.

### FINDINGS
Heart rate: 79 bpm

QRS axis: Left axis deviation to −50°

QRS duration: 160 msec

Normal sinus rhythm with a shortened PR interval and widened QRS complex with evidence of pre-excitation. Nonspecific ST- and T-wave inversions. Voltage evidence of possible LV hypertrophy is not reliable in the context of WPW. RA overload is likely in V1–2.

24-hour Holter ECG

Repeated 24-hour ECGs showed no tachyarrhythmia.

***Comments:*** The short PR interval, slurred upstroke of the QRS complex (delta wave), and wide QRS complex make up a typical ECG pattern of WPW syndrome.

Abnormalities of repolarization (ST-T waves) are often present with abnormal depolarization and are not indicative of specific pathology.

The 24-hour ECG is helpful to exclude asymptomatic tachyarrhythmias.

## CHEST X-RAY

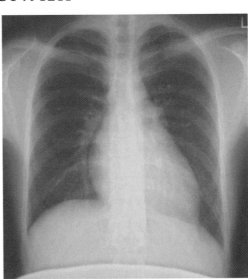

Figure 29-2 Posteroanterior projection.

### FINDINGS
Cardiothoracic ratio: 55%

Enlarged cardiac silhouette, RA enlargement, and normal pulmonary vascular markings.

***Comments:*** Patients with Ebstein anomaly have variable but sometimes severe enlargement of the cardiac silhouette on CXR because of severe enlargement of the right heart chambers. Here, the degree of cardiomegaly is modest. The aortic knuckle is small, in keeping with chronic/lifelong low systemic cardiac output.

## EXERCISE TESTING

| | |
|---|---|
| Exercise protocol: | Modified Bruce |
| Duration (min:sec): | 10:00 |
| Reason for stopping: | Leg fatigue |
| ECG changes: | Persistent ST abnormality |

| | Rest | Peak |
|---|---|---|
| Heart rate (bpm): | 82 | 184 |
| Percent of age-predicted max HR: | | 92 |
| $O_2$ saturation (%): | 97 | 94 |
| Blood pressure (mm Hg): | 90/60 | 176/80 |
| Peak $Vo_2$ (mL/kg/min): | | 36.4 |
| Percent predicted (%): | | 68 |
| Metabolic equivalents: | | 10.0 |

***Comments:*** The patient's exercise tolerance was mildly reduced. The oxygen saturation dropped slightly with exercise, possibly due to tricuspid regurgitation raising right atrial pressure and facilitating a mild right-to-left shunt. However, this small saturation decline is most likely clinically irrelevant.

# ECHOCARDIOGRAM

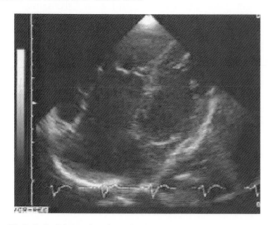

Figure 29-3 Apical four-chamber view.

## FINDINGS

The LV was normal in size and had normal function. There was a relatively small RV. The annular attachment of the septal and posterior leaflets of the tricuspid valve was displaced downward toward the apex by 4.2 cm, with severe tricuspid regurgitation.

There was a 2 × 3 cm secundum ASD, with a left-to-right shunt. The IVC was mildly dilated and did not collapse with normal inspiration.

**Comments:** The septal attachment of the tricuspid valve should not be more than approximately 1 to 2 cm toward the apex relative to the mitral valve, whereas this was over 4 cm. Most commonly, Ebstein anomaly involves the septal leaflet or posterior leaflet, and the leaflets may be adherent to the internal surface of the ventricle. The ventricular muscle of the affected part—the atrialized part of the RV—is thin walled.

The dilated IVC and lack of inspiratory collapse indicate elevated RA pressure.

## CATHETERIZATION

### HEMODYNAMICS

| | Pressure | Saturation (%) |
|---|---|---|
| SVC | mean 10 mm Hg | 72 |
| IVC | | 77 |
| RA | mean 10 | 78 |
| RV | 30/15 | |
| PA | 23/10 mean 16 | 86 |
| LA | mean 11 | 97 |
| LV | 120/16 | |
| Aorta | 118/81 mean 97 | 97 |

**Calculations**

| | |
|---|---|
| Qp (L/min) | 9.41 |
| Qs (L/min) | 4.75 |
| Cardiac index (L/min/m$^2$) | 2.68 |
| Qp/Qs | 1.98 |
| PVR (Wood units) | 0.53 |
| SVR (Wood units) | 18.30 |

**Comments:** Although utility of cardiac catheterization has been reduced nowadays, still some institutions employ catheterization whenever surgical treatments are considered in children or adolescents with complicated cardiac malformations.

Catheterization showed an important left-to-right shunt at the atrial level with Qp/Qs ratio quantified as 2:1. Pulmonary arterial pressure was not raised. Estimated RV volumes from ventriculography were small, because of the displacement of the tricuspid leaflets, and the tricuspid regurgitation was severe.

## FOCUSED CLINICAL QUESTIONS AND DISCUSSION POINTS

1. **When and how should WPW be treated in this case?**

   *Asymptomatic WPW does not necessarily justify intervention. Despite the history of tachyarrhythmia in infancy and childhood, this patient was arrhythmia free without medication throughout adolescence. Prophylactic catheter ablation for asymptomatic WPW syndrome remains controversial, and observation without invasive catheter ablation has been justified in this setting.[1,2]*

   *However, when surgical intervention for other reasons is contemplated, the effect of surgery and cardiopulmonary bypass and/or the use of inotropic drugs can all induce arrhythmia and complicate the postoperative course. In turn, some antiarrhythmic drugs can depress ventricular function. Therefore, for both short- and long-term benefit, accessory pathway ablation prior to or at the time of surgery may be considered.*

   *In WPW associated with Ebstein anomaly, there are often several accessory pathways. Electrophysiological study with mapping is mandatory to locate as many as possible. Catheter ablation is not always successful in a dilated atrialized ventricle but can greatly improve the surgical procedure using a less invasive strategy and is worth pursuing. Surgical division of additional pathways may be considered as a backup if catheter ablation is not definitive.[3-6]*

2. **Should the other anatomical defects be addressed?**

   *Normally, closure of an isolated ASD such as this, with a left-to-right shunt of 2:1 and normal pulmonary vascular resistance, would be straightforward and indicated.[7]*

   *In contrast, surgical treatment of Ebstein anomaly is much less straightforward. Tricuspid valve replacement is problematic because of the abnormal annular position. At the same time, an echocardiogram suggested that repair would not be an option in this patient because there was excessive displacement of the septal leaflet insertion and because the anterior leaflet was not large enough to be employed for reconstructing the tricuspid valve.*

   *In general, tricuspid valve surgery is indicated for congestive heart failure, deteriorating exercise capacity, or cyanosis (arterial saturation of less than 90% at rest or with exercise).[8,9] In this patient, none of these indications apply. If the interatrial communication were smaller (Qp/Qs < 1.5:1), many providers would opt for no intervention at this stage.*

   *However, the lesions must be considered together, and treated concurrently. One strategy is to perform combined transcutaneous interventional procedures; that is, catheter ablation of the accessory pathways for WPW syndrome concomitantly with ASD closure using a catheter closure device. Offloading the right heart by closing the ASD, even without treatment of tricuspid insufficiency, may be favorable and has the obvious advantage of being minimally invasive. If the initial catheter interventions do not improve the measured exercise capacity, surgical intervention on the Ebstein anomaly of the tricuspid valve can be considered later. For this patient, catheter-based ASD closure was not yet available.*

# FINAL DIAGNOSIS

Ebstein malformation with severe tricuspid regurgitation

ASD (secundum type)

WPW syndrome

# PLAN OF ACTION

Electrophysiologic study and catheter ablation, followed by surgical closure of the ASD and repair or replacement of the tricuspid valve

# INTERVENTION

An electrophysiologic study was performed, and three accessory AV pathways were detected. One was located at the right posterior part of the septum, and two others at the posterior and the lateral aspects of the RV free wall. Radio-frequency ablation was applied to all three, and the procedure was thought to have been successful. The preprocedural delta wave (Fig. 29-4A) was no longer present, and the QRS axis had been altered (Fig. 29-4B).

PREPROCEDURAL ECG

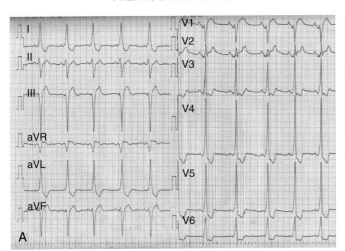

POSTCATHETER ABLATION

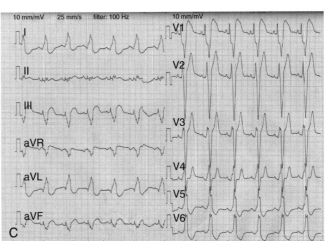

POSTCATHETER ABLATION

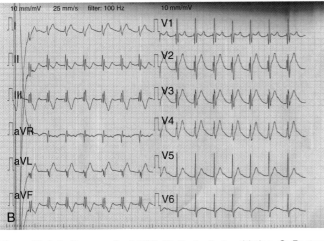

ATRIAL FLUTTER 3 YEARS AFTER SURGERY

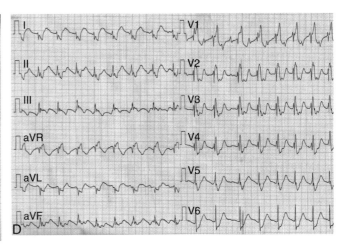

Figure 29-4 **A,** Preprocedural ECG. **B,** Postcatheter ablation. **C,** Postcatheter ablation. **D,** Atrial flutter 3 years after surgery.

# OUTCOME

Two days after the radiofrequency catheter ablation, the delta wave reappeared together with abnormal ventricular depolarization (Fig. 29-4C). The patient had a recurrence of supraventricular tachycardia. Therefore, we arranged surgical division of residual accessory pathways concomitantly with intracardiac reparative surgery. This entailed tricuspid valvuloplasty with plication of the atrialized RV (Carpentier's sliding procedure), ASD closure, and a Sealy procedure (epicardial division of the accessory pathway with endocardial cryoablation).

At surgery, through a median sternotomy and on cardiopulmonary bypass, division of accessory pathways at the free wall was achieved by the epicardial approach. To secure electrical inactivity of these pathways as well as to ablate the other pathway on the septal side, endocardial cryoablation was employed.[3–6] Subsequently, tricuspid valvuloplasty was performed using the Carpentier technique.[10] The ASD was closed using an autologous pericardial patch.

The postoperative course was uneventful. A mild degree of residual tricuspid regurgitation was noted on echo. The electrocardiogram showed regular sinus rhythm without preexcitation but with the appearance of RBBB.

Three years after surgery, the patient had an episode of atrial flutter (Fig. 29-4D) requiring direct current cardioversion. A 24-hour ECG subsequently showed first-degree AV block but no evidence of arrhythmia. Echocardiography showed moderate to severe tricuspid regurgitation and RA dilatation.

The patient's exercise capacity and hemodynamics were reassessed at 1 and 3 years postoperatively (see table below). As a whole, the patient's functional status did not improve. He continuously complained of general fatigue and exercise intolerance. His quality of life did not improve, and he eventually gave up his educational pursuits.

The deterioration could not be accounted for by his resting hemodynamics. There was no change in RA or LA pressure. His cardiac output was stable, his right ventricular ejection fraction improved.

Theoretically, his functional capacity should have improved from ASD closure, even in the presence of residual tricuspid insufficiency. Disappointingly, however, surgical intervention did not provide an improved functional outcome.

There may be several reasons for this; the most likely is worsening tricuspid regurgitation despite repair. His RV end-diastolic volumes had increased, which may account for his "improved" RVEF.

Further, close follow-up is clearly needed, and the patient may well come to require tricuspid valve replacement in the future.

In retrospect, the option of medical management without surgical intervention at that point in time may have been a better choice.

| | Preop | 1 yr | 3 yr |
|---|---|---|---|
| **Exercise Testing** | | | |
| Duration (min) | 10:00 | 9:00 | 9:00 |
| Peak HR (bpm) | 184 | 184 | 189 |
| Peak Vo$_2$ (mL/kg/min) | 36.4 | 30.1 | 21.7 |
| AT (mL/kg/min) | 17.9 | 18.9 | 13.9 |
| **Catheterization** | | | |
| Mean RA (mm Hg) | 10 | 8 | 8 |
| PA (mm Hg) | 23/10 mean 16 | 17/5 mean 11 | 19/7 mean 11 |
| Mean LA (mm Hg) | 11 | 7 (PCWP) | 7 (PCWP) |
| LV (mm Hg) | 120/16 | 110/11 | 110/8 |
| Ao (mm Hg) | 118/81 mean 97 | 108/70 mean 88 | 106/68 mean 85 |
| CO (L/min) | 4.4 | 4.6 | 4.2 |
| CI (L/min/m$^2$) | 2.6 | 2.7 | 2.5 |
| **Ventriculography** | | | |
| RVEDV (mL) | 67 | 78 | 105 |
| RVEF (%) | 24 | 46 | 50 |
| LVEDV (mL) | 152 | 115 | 147 |
| LVEF (%) | 45 | 72 | 52 |

## Selected References

1. Pappone C, Manguso F, Santinelli R, et al: Radiofrequency ablation in children with asymptomatic Wolff-Parkinson-White syndrome. N Engl J Med 351:197–205, 2004.
2. Campbell RM, Strieper MJ, Frias PA, et al: Survey of current practice of pediatric electrophysiologists for asymptomatic Wolff-Parkinson-White syndrome. Pediatrics 111:245–247, 2003.
3. Misaki T, Watanabe G, Iwa T, et al: Surgical treatment of patients with Wolff-Parkinson-White syndrome and associated Ebstein's anomaly. J Thorac Cardiovasc Surg 110:702–707, 1995.
4. Huang CJ, Chiu IS, Lin FY, et al: Role of electrophysiological studies and arrhythmia intervention in repairing Ebstein's anomaly. Thorac Cardiovasc Surg 48:47–50, 2000.
5. Lazorishinets VV, Glagola MD, Stychinsky AS, et al: Surgical treatment of Wolf-Parkinson-White syndrome during plastic operations in patients with Ebstein's anomaly. Eur J Cardiothorac Surg 18:87–90, 2000.
6. Sealy WC, Hattler BG, Jr, Blumenschein SD, Cobb FR: Surgical treatment of Wolff-Parkinson-White syndrome. Ann Thorac Surg 8:1–11, 1969.
7. Gatzoulis MA, Redington AN, Somerville J, Shore DF: Should atrial septal defects in adults be closed? Ann Thorac Surg 61:57–59, 1996.
8. Celermajer DS, Bull C, Till JA, et al: Ebstein's anomaly: Presentation and outcome from fetus to adult. J Am Coll Cardiol 23:70–76, 1994.
9. ACC/AHA guidelines for the management of patients with valvular heart disease: A report of the American College of Cardiology/American Heart Association. Task Force on Practice Guidelines (Committee on Management of Patients with Valvular Heart Disease). J Am Coll Cardiol 32:1486–1588, 1998.
10. Carpentier A, Chauvaud S, Mace L, et al: A new reconstructive operation for Ebstein's anomaly of the tricuspid valve. J Thorac Cardiovasc Surg 96:92–101, 1988.

# Ebstein Anomaly and Sudden Cardiac Death

**Konstantinos Dimopoulos**

**Age: 33 years**
**Gender: Male**
**Occupation: Accountant**
**Working diagnosis: Ebstein malformation, previous artial septal defect repair**

## HISTORY

The patient was found to have a murmur at age 6, which led to the diagnosis of an ASD with Ebstein malformation of the tricuspid valve. At age 7 he underwent surgical closure of the ASD. He had a normal recovery, but after age 15 had no further cardiologic follow-up. He reports feeling well during those years.

At the age of 32, he experienced palpitations. He was hospitalized at an outside institution with fast atrial fibrillation. He was started on amiodarone and his rate was controlled. He was also found to have abnormal liver function tests at that time. An echocardiogram showed severe Ebstein anomaly of the tricuspid valve with severe tricuspid regurgitation. He underwent a liver biopsy to clarify the etiology of the liver enzyme abnormalities. He was referred for possible heart transplantation.

***Comments:*** About half of all patients with Ebstein anomaly have an ASD or a stretched patent foramen ovale. These are the Ebstein patients who are cyanotic at rest or perhaps become cyanotic only with exertion. As a rule, the cyanotic patient with Ebstein anomaly should not have the ASD closed. A minority of these patients, such as this patient, benefit from ASD closure either to eliminate a large left-to-right shunt or to prevent exertional desaturation causing exercise intolerance.

Atrial flutter, less commonly atrial fibrillation, is common in Ebstein anomaly when the RA is very large. Such arrhythmias may be poorly tolerated and should be carefully treated. If recurrent, an ablative procedure or even cardiac surgery may be required.

## CURRENT SYMPTOMS

The patient is short of breath with moderate exertion, such as walking uphill. However, he still does low-intensity aerobic workouts, such as cycling, on a regular basis.

He denies any lightheadedness, dizziness, or syncope.

He is a nonsmoker and drinks alcohol on rare social occasions.

NYHA class: II

## CURRENT MEDICATIONS

Amiodarone 200 mg daily

Warfarin (target INR of 2–3)

## PHYSICAL EXAMINATION

BP 112/76 mm Hg, HR 70 bpm, oxygen saturation 98%

Height 178 cm, weight 61 kg, BSA 1.74 m$^2$

Surgical scars: Median sternotomy scar

Neck veins: Visible neck veins 8 cm above the sternal angle, with a dominant V-wave and Y descent

Lungs/chest: Clear

Heart: Irregular rhythm. Right ventricular lift. Split S1 with a loud tricuspid component. Normal S2. Grade 2/6 systolic murmur at the lower left parasternal edge, which did not increase with inspiration. No diastolic murmurs. Normal peripheral pulses.

Abdomen: Moderate hepatomegaly with soft, nontender, pulsatile liver

Extremities: No edema

***Comments:*** Even though the systolic murmur seems to be due to tricuspid regurgitation, it did not increase on inspiration. This may be due to RV impairment, such that the RV cannot increase its stroke volume despite increased RV preload.

A V-wave is typically not visible at the level of the neck veins due to low-pressure tricuspid regurgitation and a large, compliant RA. This patient is an exception to this rule.

The split first heart sound with loud tricuspid component is called the "sail sign." It occurs because the large, sail-like anterior tricuspid leaflet takes more time to reach the closed position.

## LABORATORY DATA

| | |
|---|---|
| Hemoglobin | 14.9 g/dL (13.0–17.0) |
| PCV | 46% (41–51) |
| MCV | 94 fL (83–99) |
| Platelet count | **91 × 10⁹/L** (150–400) |
| WBC | 6 × 10⁹/L (3.6–9.2) |
| Sodium | 140 mmol/L (134–145) |
| Potassium | 4.2 mmol/L (3.5–5.2) |
| Creatinine | 0.92 mg/dL (0.6–1.2) |
| Blood urea nitrogen | 5.2 mmol/L (2.5–6.5) |
| Total bilirubin | **29 µmol/L** (3–24) |
| ALP | 82 U/L (38–126) |
| ALT | 19 U/L (8–40) |
| Total protein | 70 g/L (62–82) |
| Albumin | 41 g/L (37–53) |

### OTHER RELEVANT LAB RESULTS

Liver biopsy: Some hepatocyte replacement with fibrosis, indicative of early cirrhosis.

**Comments:** Total bilirubin was mildly elevated, but the remaining liver function parameters were within normal limits. The abnormal liver enzymes reported at the other facility may have been due to raised right-sided pressure at the time of rapid atrial fibrillation.

# ELECTROCARDIOGRAM

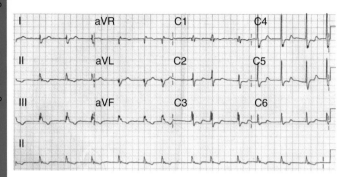

Figure 30-1 Electrocardiogram.

## FINDINGS
Heart rate: 70 bpm

QRS axis: Right-axis deviation of initial forces

QRS duration: 136 msec

Atrial fibrillation. Right-axis deviation of initial forces with terminal, complete RBBB.

**Comments:** Arrhythmias are a common reason for adults with Ebstein anomaly to come to medical attention. Atrial flutter, atrial fibrillation, and reentrant tachycardias related to accessory pathways may be encountered.

A Q-wave in the V1 lead is characteristic of Ebstein anomaly. This is due to the large RA and leftward rotation of the heart causing V1 to record RV intracavitary potentials. For the same reason V1 may resemble the aVR lead.

# CHEST X-RAY

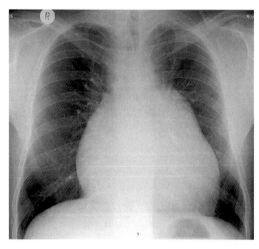

Figure 30-2 Posteroanterior projection.

## FINDINGS
Cardiothoracic ratio: 63%

Situs solitus, levocardia, left aortic arch. Very large cardiac silhouette. The RVOT and/or main pulmonary artery were prominent. Pulmonary blood flow seemed normal or diminished.

**Comments:** The cardiothoracic ratio may range from normal to grossly enlarged in patients with Ebstein anomaly. If increased, as is usual, the dilation is due to enlarged right heart chambers. Pulmonary blood flow is normal or decreased unless there is a sizable left-to-right shunt through an ASD, which may cause increased pulmonary vascular markings. The aortic arch or knuckle is typically small due to a chronically low cardiac output.

# EXERCISE TESTING

| Exercise protocol: | Modified Bruce |
|---|---|
| Duration (min:sec): | 10:38 |
| Reason for stopping: | Dyspnea |
| ECG changes: | Atrial fibrillation throughout |

|  | Rest | Peak |
|---|---|---|
| Heart rate (bpm): | 70 | 151 |
| Percent of age-predicted max HR: |  | 81 |
| $O_2$ saturation (%): | 98 | 98 |
| Blood pressure (mm Hg): | 112/76 | 145/80 |
| Peak $Vo_2$ (mL/kg/min): |  | 23 |
| Percent predicted (%): |  | 67 |
| VE/$Vco_2$: |  | 26 |
| Metabolic equivalents: |  | 6.5 |

**Comments:** The patient's exercise tolerance was surprisingly good (67% of predicted) and well above the recommended level for consideration of heart transplantation in patients with LV dysfunction (14 mL/kg/min). The test results are consistent with the patient's self-reported exercise tolerance and his regular exercise routine. He has a good chronotropic response despite atrial fibrillation.

The Ve/$Vco_2$ slope is a measure of ventilatory efficiency. Ventilation–perfusion mismatch and enhanced ventilatory reflex sensitivity are thought to be the major determinants of the Ve/$Vco_2$ slope. Recently, a Ve/$Vco_2$ slope of 38 or above was identified as a marker of adverse outcome in noncyanotic adults with congenital heart disease.[1]

# ECHOCARDIOGRAM

## OVERALL FINDINGS
LV size and function were normal. The mitral valve functioned normally, and the LA was not enlarged.

The RV cavity was enlarged, and the septal leaflet of the tricuspid valve inserted closer to the apical septum.

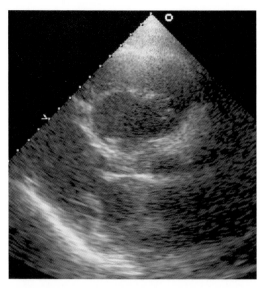

Figure 30-3 Parasternal long-axis view.

## FINDINGS

Normal LV size and function with RV enlargement.

**Comments:** The anomalies of the tricuspid valve are best seen in other views. Much of the RV cavity seen here is probably the atrialized portion.

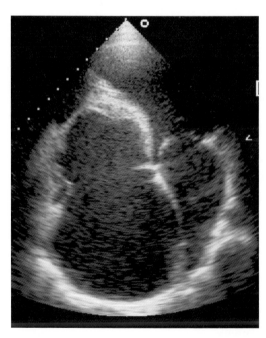

Figure 30-4 Apical four-chamber view.

## FINDINGS

The attachment of the septal leaflet of the tricuspid valve was displaced nearly 6 cm toward the apex from the level of the mitral valve. The tricuspid valve was severely regurgitant. There was a large atrialized portion of the RV. The RA was severely dilated, measuring almost 10 cm in diameter.

**Comments:** These findings show an extreme example of Ebstein anomaly. The tricuspid leaflets do not coapt properly, resulting in severe regurgitation.

In reality, the displacement of the tricuspid valve leaflet attachment is apparent only because the leaflets are tethered to the underlying ventricular wall. Tethering is most common for the posterior and septal leaflets, the latter being the typical and most commonly identified echocardiographic feature of Ebstein anomaly.[2] In this case, a typical large, sail-like anterior leaflet tethered to the RV free wall was also present.

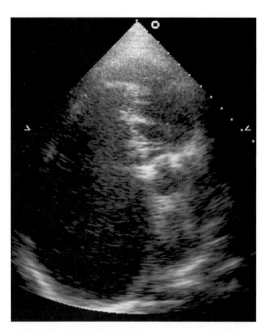

Figure 30-5 Parasternal short-axis view.

## FINDINGS

Again, the severely dilated RA was prominently seen. The aortic valve in short axis is in the center of the image. In the RVOT at the top of the image the insertion of the septal leaflet was seen.

**Comments:** The severity of the Ebstein malformation in this case can be appreciated here. The valve leaflets are actually in the outflow tract, meaning that the true right ventricular cavity is extremely small.

## MAGNETIC RESONANCE IMAGING

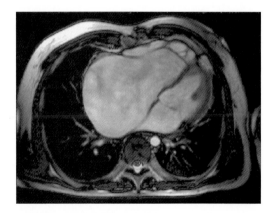

Figure 30-6 Oblique transaxial section, four-chamber view.

## FINDINGS

There is extreme apical displacement of the septal leaflet of the tricuspid valve, and the very small RV cavity is not wholly appreciated in this view. The RA was severely dilated. The regurgitant fraction was 31%.

The LV and LA were normal in size.

### Ventricular Volume Quantification

|  | LV | (Normal range) | RV | (Normal range) |
|---|---|---|---|---|
| EDV (mL) | 159 | (77–195) | 210 | (88–227) |
| ESV (mL) | 72 | (19–72) | 83 | (23–103) |
| SV (mL) | 87 | (51–133) | 127 | (52–138) |
| EF (%) | **55** | (57–75) | 60 | (50–76) |
| EDVi (mL/m²) | 92 | (66–101) | **121** | (65–111) |
| ESVi (mL/m²) | 41 | (18–39) | **48** | (18–47) |
| SVi (mL/m²) | 50 | (43–67) | 73 | (39–71) |

***Comments:*** These findings confirm the echocardiographic data. Volume measurement of the actual RV cavity in severe Ebstein malformation can be difficult using the traditional short-axis stack and Simpson's rule. Instead, transaxial cuts more similar to the section shown here (Fig. 30-6) more clearly delineate the RV cavity from the atrialized RV portion. In this case, the end-diastolic volume calculated for the RV was at the upper limits of normal despite a large portion of the RV being atrialized. This was due to inclusion in the calculations of the expanded RVOT.

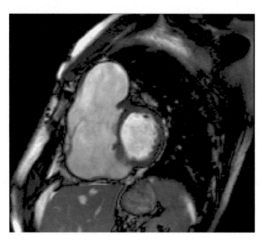

Figure 30-7 Outflow tract view.

***Comments:*** The tricuspid valve is displaced within the RVOT, leaving a very small true ventricular cavity, which is limited to the outflow portion of the anatomic RV.

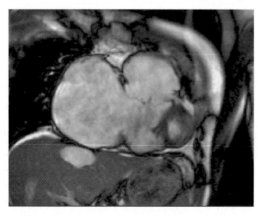

Figure 30-8 Coronal plane trueFISP cine image.

## FINDINGS

The RA was severely dilated. The tricuspid valve was seen in the RVOT.

***Comments:*** This view coincides with a CXR projection, and the large RA can be appreciated. Again, the tricuspid valve is displaced within the RVOT, and the remaining RV is small.

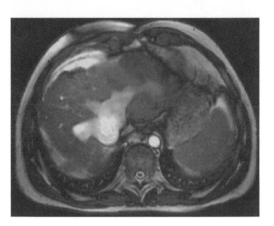

Figure 30-9 Transaxial plane.

## FINDINGS

The IVC and hepatic vein were severely dilated. Ascites was present. The liver appeared slightly nodular.

***Comments:*** The effects on the liver of severe tricuspid regurgitation and elevated RA pressure are evident here, and it is not surprising that abnormalities were seen by liver biopsy in response to the elevated hepatic venous pressure. Similar changes can occur in patients with Fontan physiology (see Cases 62 and 65).

## CATHETERIZATION

### HEMODYNAMICS

Heart rate    70 bpm

|  | **Pressure** | **Saturation** (%) |
|---|---|---|
| SVC | mean 15 | 70 |
| IVC | mean 16 | 65 |
| RA | mean 15, v wave 22 | 68 |
| RVOT | 26/16 | 71 |
| PA | 27/18 mean 20 | 72 |
| PCWP | mean 14 | |
| LV | 122/14 | 97 |
| Aorta | 125/76 mean 91 | 96 |

**Calculations**

| | |
|---|---|
| Qp (L/min) | 4.41 |
| Qs (L/min) | 4.05 |
| Cardiac index (L/min/m²) | 2.33 |
| Qp/Qs | 1.09 |
| PVR (Wood units) | 1.36 |
| SVR (Wood units) | 18.78 |

***Comments:*** Cardiac catheterization was performed as part of the preoperative assessment. Assessment of pulmonary artery pressures is especially important when a bidirectional Glenn anastomosis is considered (one and a half ventricle repair, see Fig. 30-10). In this instance, a mean pulmonary artery pressure of 20 mm Hg would preclude the use of a bidirectional

Glenn shunt as part of Ebstein repair surgery. LV filling and indirect LA pressures are mildly elevated for reasons likely due to ventricular-ventricular interaction. The cardiac output and index are mildly reduced.

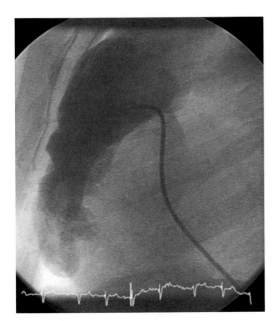

Figure 30-10 Lateral right ventricular outflow tract angiogram.

## FINDINGS

In this view the apical displacement of the tricuspid valve is evident. The true RV is limited to the RVOT. Contrast also delineates the large atrialized portion of the RV due to the severe tricuspid regurgitation.

### FOCUSED CLINICAL QUESTIONS AND DISCUSSION POINTS

1. **Is there a need for heart surgery, and, if so, what are the surgical options for this patient?**

*Current indications for intervention in Ebstein anomaly include poor exercise capacity (NYHA class > II), right heart failure, large heart size (cardiothoracic ratio > 64%), important cyanosis (resting oxygen saturation < 90%), severe symptomatic tricuspid regurgitation, transient ischemic attack, or stroke due to a paradoxic embolus, sustained atrial flutter, or fibrillation and atrial arrhythmias secondary to an accessory pathway.[3] The in-hospital perioperative mortality rate is reported at 6% with a 10-year mortality rate of 8% and a 15-year reoperation rate of 20%.[4] Therefore, this patient meets criteria for intervention, and a suitable procedure should be offered.*

*However, given the severity of his condition, the options are not straightforward. The choice to replace rather than repair the valve depends on the anatomy of the tricuspid valve as well as the experience and skill of the surgeon. Creation of a monocusp valve from the larger anterior leaflet has been reported and can be performed with low mortality and low reoperation rates, with substantial long-term improvement of functional performance and clinical status (see Case 31). However, the surgeon felt that repair was not likely to be possible here.*

*The most likely surgical scenario would be to replace the tricuspid valve with a bioprosthetic valve at the level of the normal tricuspid valve annulus. One has to accept that a large portion*

*of the resulting RV will be dysfunctional (i.e., the previously atrialized portion).*

*This patient certainly did not fulfill indications for cardiac transplantation.*

2. **What is the risk of life-threatening arrhythmia, and is there a role for any further arrhythmia investigation or intervention?**

*Tachyarrhythmias occur in approximately 30% of patients with Ebstein anomaly. These can be atrial flutter (less often fibrillation), supraventricular tachycardia due to bypass tracts, or even ventricular tachycardia. Ablation in the electrophysiology laboratory may be helpful in some patients. In some patients, surgical ablation may be offered in addition to tricuspid valve repair or replacement. Sudden cardiac death has been described in numerous series of Ebstein patients, both operated and unoperated. There are no data on the use of ICD devices or other therapies to prevent sudden death in these patients. Predictors of death due to all causes are functional class, increased cardiothoracic ratio (>64%), age, and severity of tricuspid regurgitation.[5,6] In one study, all Ebstein patients who developed atrial fibrillation died within 5 years.[6]*

*At the time of reparative surgery, a concomitant biatrial maze procedure should be considered in patients with chronic atrial fibrillation. This was planned in this case.*

3. **What is the cause of this patient's hepatomegaly?**

*This patient has hepatomegaly by clinical examination, as well as mild hyperbilirubinemia, and previous transient elevation of liver enzymes. Further, a liver biopsy showed changes consistent with early cirrhosis, with fibrosis replacing hepatocytes. The implications are that chronically elevated right heart failure is causing portal hypertension and liver dysfunction. Whether correction of the right atrial pressure will alter the course is uncertain. Hepatitis serology should also be checked in such a patient, especially if the previous heart surgical procedure had been done prior to 1995.*

## FINAL DIAGNOSIS

Severe Ebstein anomaly of the tricuspid valve

Chronic atrial fibrillation

Prior ASD closure

## PLAN OF ACTION

Tricuspid valve replacement with a bioprosthetic valve at the normal AV junction, combined with biatrial surgical maze procedure

## OUTCOME

Elective surgery was planned following the multidisciplinary discussion. Unfortunately, 1 month later, the patient reported feeling slightly unwell to his relatives. The following day he was found unresponsive on his bathroom floor after taking a shower. Attempts at resuscitation failed and he was pronounced dead at the scene. A postmortem examination was not performed.

The likely cause of sudden cardiac death was arrhythmia. The patient was certainly at risk of further arrhythmia, including ventricular tachycardia, and had been treated with amiodarone. It may be that this unfortunate outcome could have been avoided if surgery had been offered earlier. Patient selection and timing of surgery for patients with Ebstein anomaly or other forms of congenital heart disease who are "stable" remain challenging, especially in some countries with relatively long surgical waiting lists. Furthermore, this case reiterates the difficulties of risk stratification and risk modification for sudden cardiac death.

## Selected References

1. Dimopoulos K, Okonko DO, Diller GP, et al: Abnormal ventilatory response to exercise in adults with congenital heart disease relates to cyanosis and predicts survival. Circulation 113:796–802, 2006.
2. Patel V, Nanda NC, Rajdev S, et al: Live/real time three-dimensional transthoracic echocardiographic assessment of Ebstein's anomaly. Echocardiography 22:47–54, 2005.
3. Therrien J, Dore A, Gersony W, et al: Canadian Cardiovascular Society: CCS Consensus Conference 2001 update: Recommendations for the management of adults with congenital heart disease—Part II. Can J Cardiol 17:940–959, 2001.
4. Sondergaard L, Cullen S: Ebstein anomaly. In Gatzoulis MA, Webb GD, Daubeney PE (eds): Diagnosis and Management of Adult Congenital Heart Disease. Philadelphia, Churchill Livingstone, 2003, pp 283–288.
5. Attie F, Rosas M, Rijlaarsdam M, et al: The adult patient with Ebstein anomaly: Outcome in 72 unoperated patients. Medicine (Baltimore) 79:27–36, 2000.
6. Gentles TL, Calder AL, Clarkson PM, Neutze JM: Predictors of long-term survival with Ebstein anomaly of the tricuspid valve. Am J Cardiol 69:77–81, 1992.

## Bibliography

Augustin N, Schmidt-Habelmann P, Wottke M, et al: Results after surgical repair of Ebstein anomaly. Ann Thorac Surg 63:650–656, 1997.
Augustin N, Schreiber C, Wottke M, Meisner H: Ebstein anomaly: When should a patient have operative treatment? Herz 23:87–92, 1998.
Celermajer DS, Bull C, Till JA, et al: Ebstein anomaly: Presentation and outcome from fetus to adult. J Am Coll Cardiol 23:70–76, 1994.
Chauvaud S: Ebstein malformation: Surgical treatment and results. Thorac Cardiovasc Surg 48:20–23, 2000.
Giuliani ER, Fuster V, Brandenburg RO, Mair DD: Ebstein anomaly: The clinical features and natural history of Ebstein anomaly of the tricuspid valve. Mayo Clin Proc 54:63–73, 1979.
Perloff JK: Ebstein anomaly of the tricuspid valve. In Perloff JK (ed): The Clinical Recognition of Congenital Heart Disease, 5th ed. Philadelphia, Saunders, 2003, pp 194–215.

# Successful Tricuspid Valve Repair of Ebstein Anomaly

**George Krasopoulos, Pedro A. Catarino, and Hideki Uemura**

Age: 22 years
Gender: Female
Occupation: Mother
Working diagnosis: Ebstein anomaly of the tricuspid valve

## HISTORY

The patient was diagnosed early in infancy with Ebstein anomaly of the tricuspid valve, ASD, and RVOT obstruction. At 1 year of age she underwent a successful balloon dilatation of the obstructed RVOT.

She remained well and asymptomatic until 2 years ago (20 years old) when she had a successful pregnancy but suffered a stroke after delivery, from which she fully recovered. Following this she underwent a successful device closure of the ASD, which was thought to have been the cause of a paradoxical embolus.

Her exercise tolerance remained normal up until 6 months prior to presentation. During this time her major complaint was shortness of breath on mild to moderate exertion. She was referred for further evaluation.

*Comments:* Ebstein anomaly has a prevalence of 5 per 100,000 live births (0.5% of congenital heart disease). Most cases are sporadic, although familial cases have been reported. A predisposing factor may be maternal use of lithium carbonate during pregnancy.

Ebstein anomaly is defined as apical displacement of the septal and often mural leaflets of the tricuspid valve. Associated abnormalities include the presence of an ASD or stretched PFO, conduction system abnormalities, RVOT obstruction, and other cardiac defects.

Pregnancy in women with Ebstein anomaly can be well tolerated in the absence of significant cyanosis, arrhythmia, and/or heart failure.

As patients become older, tachyarrhythmia becomes a frequent and often disabling complication. Arrhythmia is usually supraventricular but can also be ventricular in origin and may lead to sudden cardiac death.

## CURRENT SYMPTOMS

Shortness of breath on exertion is the patient's primary complaint. For example, she was unable to run after her 2-year-old son. The patient also described sporadic episodes of dizzy spells associated with palpitations. She denied chest pain or syncope.

NYHA class: II–III

*Comments:* Despite the risk of arrhythmia, heart failure, and cyanosis, many patients with Ebstein anomaly surviving to adulthood maintain a good NYHA class I–II for many years.

## CURRENT MEDICATIONS

Aspirin 75 mg, once daily (for thromboprophylaxis)

## PHYSICAL EXAMINATION

Looking healthy, pink, and well perfused

BP 110/70 mm Hg, HR 78 bpm, oxygen saturation 98% on room air

Height 165 cm, weight 67 kg, BSA 1.75 $m^2$

Neck veins: 3–4 cm above the sternal angle

Lungs/chest: Clear lung sounds

Heart: The rhythm was regular. A mild RV lift was present. Normal first and second heart sounds were heard, with a 3/6 pan-systolic murmur at the lower left sternal edge. A soft ejection systolic murmur was also heard.

Abdomen: Normal

Extremities: Normal palpable peripheral pulses, with no radiofemoral delay detected. There was no edema.

### PERTINENT NEGATIVES
None

*Comments:* The JVP can remain low or normal despite severe tricuspid regurgitation due to severe enlargement of the very compliant RA.

Typical auscultatory findings in Ebstein anomaly include wide splitting of the first (the second portion sometimes referred to as a sail-like sound) and second sounds (due to RBBB), a gallop rhythm, and a holosystolic murmur.

The systolic ejection murmur was probably due to mild residual RVOT obstruction.

## LABORATORY DATA

| | |
|---|---|
| Hemoglobin | 13.9 g/dL (11.5–15.0) |
| Hematocrit/PCV | 39% (36–46) |
| MCV | 89 fL (83–99) |
| MCHC | 34 g/dL (31–35) |
| Platelet count | $210 \times 10^9$/L (150–400) |
| Sodium | 141 mmol/L (134–145) |
| Potassium | 3.6 mmol/L (3.5–5.2) |
| Creatinine | 0.91 mg/dL (0.6–1.2) |
| Blood urea nitrogen | 4.7 mmol/L (2.5–6.5) |
| ALP | 53 U/L (38–126) |
| ALT | 9 IU/L (8–40) |

## ELECTROCARDIOGRAM

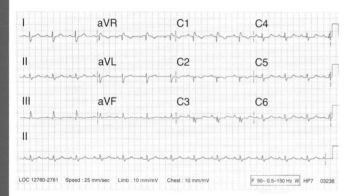

Figure 31-1 Electrocardiogram.

### FINDINGS

Heart rate: 80 bpm

QRS axis: +131°

QRS duration: 113 msec

Sinus rhythm with borderline first-degree heart block

Right bundle branch block. Poor R progression. Unusual Q-waves V2–3. No frank RA overload. Generally low-voltage ECG.

24-hour Holter ECG: Sinus rhythm with sinus arrhythmia, and occasional supraventricular and ventricular ectopics.

**Comments:** The ECG in Ebstein anomaly is highly variable. The most common findings are first-degree block, RBBB, low voltage, and RA overload.

The apical displacement of the septal tricuspid valve leaflet is associated with discontinuity of the central fibrous body, creating a potential substrate for multiple accessory AV pathways invariably located in the atrialized portion of the RV. If an accessory pathway is present, it is usually mapped and obliterated either surgically or preoperatively using percutaneous radiofrequency ablation techniques. On this occasion there was no evidence of pre-excitation.

## CHEST X-RAY

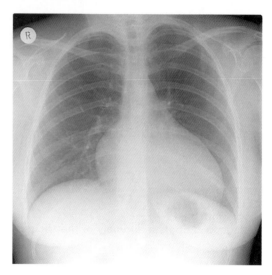

Figure 31-2 Posteroanterior projection.

### FINDINGS

Cardiothoracic ratio: 60%

Cardiomegaly with RA enlargement. There is no evidence of pulmonary hypertension. The lung fields are normal.

**Comments:** The prominent bulging of the right cardiac border indicates right atrial enlargement, as is often seen in Ebstein patients.

The findings largely depend on the severity of the disease. The cardiac silhouette may vary but is generally of a globular shape due to RA enlargement and dilatation of the RV infundibulum. The aortic knuckle is often small, reflecting the chronically low cardiac output in many of these patients.

## EXERCISE TESTING

### Treadmill Stress Test

| | |
|---|---|
| Exercise protocol: | Modified Bruce |
| Duration (min:sec): | 9:12 |
| Reason for stopping: | Dyspnea |
| ECG changes: | None |

| | Rest | Peak |
|---|---|---|
| Heart rate (bpm): | 78 | 165 |
| Percent of age-predicted max HR: | | 83 |
| O₂ saturation (%): | 98 | 81 |
| Blood pressure (mm Hg): | 110/40 | 145/70 |
| Peak Vo₂ (mL/kg/min): | | 14 |
| Percent predicted (%): | | 43 |
| Ve/Vco₂: | | 31 |
| Metabolic equivalents: | | 4.7 |

**Comments:** In a patient with potential intracardiac shunting, exercise testing should include saturation measurement to screen for hypoxemia that may not be present at rest.

It is somewhat surprising that this patient desaturates at peak exercise, despite device ASD closure. Desaturation may reflect a residual ASD and/or intrapulmonary "shunting."

# ECHOCARDIOGRAM

## OVERALL FINDINGS

There was severe Ebstein anomaly of the tricuspid valve, with severe tricuspid regurgitation and RA enlargement. There was normal RV free wall contraction. There was mild to moderate pulmonary regurgitation. Good left ventricular function was seen, with a normal mitral and aortic valve. The ASD closure device was well positioned.

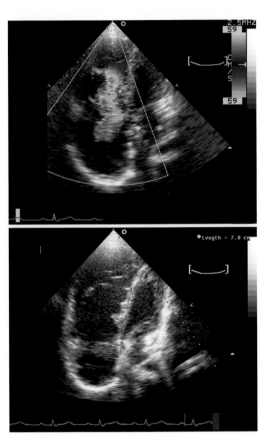

Figure 31-3 Apical four-chamber 2D Doppler.

## FINDINGS

Severe Ebstein-type anomaly of the tricuspid valve, with 70-mm apical displacement of the septal leaflet and a sail-like mural (anterior) leaflet. There was severely impaired coaptation of the tricuspid valve leaflets with a large central gap during systole leading to severe tricuspid regurgitation. The peak velocity through this valve was 2.5 m/sec, suggesting an estimated RV pressure of approximately 25 mm Hg. The RVOT was dilated.

**Comments:** Echocardiography is the investigation of choice for the assessment of the severity of the tricuspid displacement and interatrial shunting. It can also be useful for assessing for associated congenital defects and RV function, although quantification of RV function is difficult.

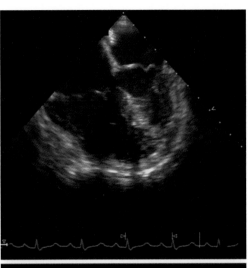

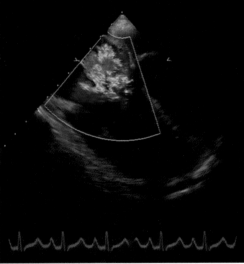

Figure 31-4 Mid-esophageal four-chamber view.

## FINDINGS

The RV was dilated but with good systolic function. The tricuspid valve septal leaflet was displaced apically, with severe lack of coaptation resulting in severe tricuspid regurgitation.

**Comments:** Transesophageal echocardiography is both an invaluable tool for preoperative assessment of valvular lesions and a necessary resource perioperatively, as it can provide information on the quality of surgical repair and its hemodynamic impact.

Transesophageal echocardiography was done to obtain a better view of the extent of leaflet displacement to make a decision about the possibility of repair. It is particularly important to pay attention to the septal leaflet and its insertion relative to the RVOT. One notes here that the septal leaflet insertion is not as apical as seen from the transthoracic images. As a result, the likelihood of successful repair is higher.

# MAGNETIC RESONANCE IMAGING

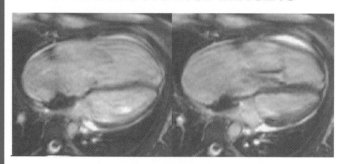

Figure 31-5 Steady state free precession cine, axial (diastole and systole).

## FINDINGS

Again, there was severe apical displacement of the tricuspid valve with severe tricuspid regurgitation. The tricuspid regurgitant fraction was 58%. Flow through the pulmonary valve by velocity map was 68 mL/beat, which is consistent with the left ventricle stroke volume.

### Ventricular Volume Quantification

|  | LV | (Normal range) | RV | (Normal range) |
|---|---|---|---|---|
| EDV (mL) | 96 | (52–141) | 283 | (58–154) |
| ESV (mL) | 32 | (13–51) | 124 | (12–68) |
| SV (mL) | 64 | (33–97) | 159 | (35–98) |
| EF (%) | 67 | (56–75) | 56 | (49–73) |
| EDVi (mL/m²) | 55 | (65–99) | 161 | (65–102) |
| ESVi (mL/m²) | 18 | (19–37) | 71 | (20–45) |
| SVi (mL/m²) | 37 | (42–66) | 91 | (39–63) |
| Mass index (g/m²) | 45 | (47–77) |  | (22–42) |

***Comments:*** MRI is sometimes helpful for quantifying RV size and function in Ebstein, but it is not necessary for making a decision about tricuspid valve repair/replacement.

Systolic signal loss on cine MRI deep within the right ventricular cavity correctly indicated the presence of an abnormally positioned and incompetent tricuspid valve. All characteristic abnormalities can be seen and analyzed well. Signal loss from the ASD closure device is easily seen.

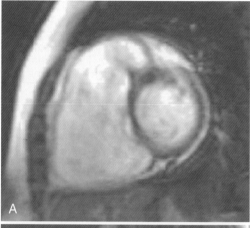

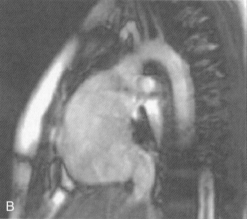

Figure 31-6 Steady state free precession cine, short axis (**A**) and oblique sagittal (right ventricular outflow tract view) (**B**).

## FINDINGS

There was atrialization of the inlet part of the RV, with a rather dilated RVOT. Overall, there was normal RV systolic function.

***Comments:*** The challenge of quantifying RV volume persists even with MRI. Given the difficulty of seeing the rather complex valve plane properly in short axis, volume measurements made from axial slices often give the most reliable results (see Case 30). This allows one to differentiate the atrialized portion more clearly from the functional RV.

### FOCUSED CLINICAL QUESTIONS AND DISCUSSION POINTS

1. When should a patient with Ebstein anomaly be offered surgical intervention on the tricuspid valve?

*Observation alone is advised for asymptomatic patients or for patients with no right-to-left shunting and mild cardiomegaly only. Surgery should be considered if there is moderate cardiomegaly[1] on chest radiography, substantial exercise intolerance due to tricuspid regurgitation, cyanosis, or a history of sustained atrial flutter or fibrillation.*

*Once symptoms progress to NYHA class III or IV, medical management has little to offer, and surgical risks increase sharply although surgery is commonly discussed. Biventricular reconstruction may be possible, but if ventricular dysfunction is more than mild, especially involving the LV, cardiac transplantation may be a better option.*

*This patient has a young child to care for, and a serious operation can be disruptive at best. However, in light of her cardiomegaly and exercise limitation it is appropriate to consider her for elective surgery and discuss the relative risks-to-benefits ratio.*

*Device closure of the atrial communication should be undertaken in Ebstein patients only after careful review and discussion. If this were done in many Ebstein patients, acute and/or chronic right heart failure could be precipitated.*

2. **What is the preferred surgical approach to Ebstein anomaly and why?**

*In 1988 Carpentier et al[2] proposed tricuspid valve repair involving mobilization of the anterior tricuspid valve leaflet. For certain subtypes, however, temporary detachment of the anterior leaflet and the adjacent part of the posterior leaflet was complemented by longitudinal plication of the atrialized ventricle and the adjacent RA, repositioning of the anterior and posterior leaflets to cover the orifice area at a normal level, and remodeling and reinforcement of the tricuspid annulus with a prosthetic ring.*

*Kiziltan et al[3] from the Mayo Clinic reviewed 293 Ebstein patients and found no statistically significant difference between tricuspid valve repair and replacement with regard to freedom from reoperation 12 years after index surgery. Similarly, there was no difference between bioprosthetic and mechanical valve prostheses with regard to freedom from reoperation in this series. Our bias has been for valve repair, when feasible, over valve replacement because repair has the potential to be more durable over a lifetime. Some of our early patients are doing well and are free from reoperation for more than 20 years after surgery.*

*We prefer bioprostheses over mechanical prostheses, and reserve the latter for a small number of selected adults who are already on warfarin for other indications.[4] Bioprostheses are preferred for two reasons, especially in pediatric patients: (1) They avoid the inconvenience and risks of long-term warfarin anticoagulation, and (2) there is no evidence at present that mechanical valves have greater freedom from reoperation than have bioprostheses in the tricuspid position in Ebstein patients.*

3. **Should we remove the ASD occluding device and proceed into closing the ASD surgically?**

*This may be considered only if there is a residual ASD. It is important not to extend the surgical time beyond that absolutely necessary, making an already technically demanding operation more difficult. At the same time, it is important to identify and address all significant anatomical and hemodynamic abnormalities while in theater. Modification of atrial arrhythmia risk prompts additional work within the atria in the form of a modified and extended maze procedure.*

## FINAL DIAGNOSIS

Severe Ebstein anomaly of the tricuspid valve

Prior ASD device closure

## PLAN OF ACTION

Surgical repair of Ebstein anomaly of the tricuspid valve and plication of the RV (atrialized portion)

## INTERVENTION

The heart was exposed via a full-sized median sternotomy with a standard skin incision. Cardiopulmonary bypass was established with cannulation of the ascending aorta, SVC, and IVC via the RA, followed by ascending aortic cross-clamp. Cold blood antegrade cardioplegia was infused via the aortic root cannula. Access was obtained via the RA. The anterior tricuspid valve leaflet was large and in continuity with the inferior (posterior) tricuspid valve leaflet. The inferior leaflet had short cords leading to short and underdeveloped papillary muscles (incomplete plastering). The inferior part of the RV wall, although not atrialized, was markedly thinned. The inferior leaflet of the tricuspid valve was detached from its annular attachment. The thin ventricular wall, including the atrialized portion, was plicated from inside and outside the heart. The tricuspid valvar orifice was reduced to a diameter of 30 to 32 mm. The anterior and the inferior leaflets were reattached to the true tricuspid valve annulus. The tricuspid valve was water tested, and there was no obvious regurgitation. Routine de-airing was performed. The patient came off bypass in sinus rhythm with no inotropic support. Routine hemostasis and closure were performed.

## OUTCOME

The patient had an uneventful recovery and was discharged home on the sixth postoperative day, having been put on warfarin for 3 months.

At her 3-year postop follow-up at the joint adult congenital heart clinic at her local hospital, she had a reduced cardiothoracic ratio on her CXR, reported sustained improvement in her functional capacity, and said she was freely able to care for her young son.

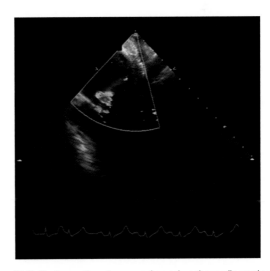

Figure 31-7 Postoperative transesophageal echocardiography. Midesophageal four-chamber view with reduced depth, concentrating at the tricuspid valve.

## FINDINGS

Normal systolic function of the RV and LV. Good tricuspid valve coaptation, with trivial tricuspid regurgitation. There was no RVOT obstruction.

***Comments:*** The transesophageal echocardiogram shows favorable results following surgery.

## Selected References

1. Theodoro DA, Danielson GK, Porter CJ, Warnes CA: Right-sided Maze procedure for right atrial arrhythmias in congenital heart disease. Ann Thorac Surg 65:149–154, 1998.
2. Carpentier A, Chauvaud S, Mace L, et al: A new reconstructive operation for Ebstein anomaly of the tricuspid valve. J Thorac Cardiovasc Surg 96:92–101, 1988.
3. Dearani JA, Danielson GK: Ebstein anomaly of the tricuspid valve. In Mavroudis C, Backer C (eds): Pediatric Cardiac Surgery, 3rd ed. Philadelphia, Mosby, 2003, pp 524–536.
4. Kiziltan HT, Theodoro DA, Warnes CA, et al: Late results of bioprosthetic tricuspid valve replacement in Ebstein anomaly. Ann Thorac Surg 66:1539–1545, 1998.

## Bibliography

Attenhofer Jost CH, Connolly HM, Edwards WD, et al: Ebstein anomaly—review of a multifaceted congenital cardiac condition. Swiss Med Wkly 135:269–281, 2005.

Chauvaud S: Ebstein malformation surgical treatment and results. Thorac Cardiovasc Surg 48:220–223, 2000.

Chen JM, Mosca RS, Altmann K, et al: Early and medium-term results for repair of Ebstein anomaly. J Thorac Cardiovasc Surg 127:990–998; discussion 998–999, 2004.

Danielson GK, Maloney JD, Devloo RAE: Surgical repair of Ebstein anomaly. Mayo Clin Proc 54:185–192, 1979.

Ebstein W: Ueber einen sehr seltenen Fall von Insufficienz der Valvula tricuspidalis, bedingt durch eine angeborene hochgradige Missbildung derselben. Arch F Anat Physiol Wissensch Med Leipz, 238–255, 1866.

Hetzer R, Nagdyman N, Ewert P, et al: A modified repair technique for tricuspid incompetence in Ebstein anomaly. J Thorac Cardiovasc Surg 115:857–868, 1998.

Quaegebeur JM, Sreeram N, Fraser AG, et al: Surgery for Ebstein anomaly: The clinical and echocardiographic evaluation of a new technique. J Am Coll Cardiol 17:722–728, 1991.

Takagaki M, Ishino K, Kawada M, et al: Total right ventricular exclusion improves left ventricular function in patients with end-stage congestive right ventricular failure. Circulation 108(Suppl 1):II226–229, 2003.

Tanaka M, Ohata T, Fukuda S, et al: Tricuspid valve supra-annular implantation in adult patients with Ebstein anomaly. Ann Thorac Surg 71:582–586, 2001.

Wu Q, Huang Z: A new procedure for Ebstein anomaly. Ann Thorac Surg 77:470–476; discussion 476, 2004.

# Ebstein Anomaly and Prepregnancy Counseling

**Lorna Swan**

**Age: 37 years**
**Gender: Female**
**Working diagnosis: Childhood cyanosis**

## HISTORY

The patient had been investigated as a child for episodes of possible cyanosis. She had been referred to a teaching hospital and followed until her teenage years. The patient remained well throughout this time and believed her previous cyanotic episodes settled. Neither she nor her family could recall the details of the problem or any investigations, though she was certain she never had surgery.

Over the next 20 years the patient remained asymptomatic and did regular aerobic exercise without limitation. After initiating discussions regarding pregnancy with her family doctor and relating this uncertain history of cyanosis, she was referred to an ACHD clinic. Despite several attempts, it was not possible to retrieve any clinical notes from either her original family doctor or the tertiary referral center.

*Comments:* In the past it was often routine policy for many units to destroy old case records after an interval of non-attendance. In patients with ACHD this often meant the unfortunate loss of old operation notes and results of previous investigations. Detailed discussions, including written documentation, with patients and their families will hopefully prevent similar shortcomings in the future.

Very few cardiac lesions cause intermittent cyanosis and then improve or are apparently cured. This history would tend to suggest a small right-to-left shunt rather than a progressive disorder with pulmonary vascular disease or impaired pulmonary blood flow.

Although being asymptomatic with a congenital cardiac disorder is reassuring, the absence of reported symptoms does not exclude important cardiac conditions that may impact on long-term outcome or the ability, for example, to carry a pregnancy safely.

## CURRENT SYMPTOMS

The patient was entirely asymptomatic. She was able to exercise on a treadmill for 30 minutes with no difficulty. The patient had never experienced significant palpitations.

NYHA class: I

## CURRENT MEDICATIONS

None

## PHYSICAL EXAMINATION

BP 104/68 mm Hg, HR 72 bpm, oxygen saturation on room air 100%

Height 162 cm, weight 65 kg, BSA 1.71 m$^2$

Surgical scars: None

Neck veins: A normal, nonelevated waveform was seen.

Lungs/chest: Clear to auscultation

Heart: Rhythm was regular. There was a widely split first heart sound. No murmurs were heard. Normal peripheral pulses were present.

Extremities: Nonedematous. There was no visible cyanosis. The nail beds were not clubbed in the hands or feet.

*Comments:* This patient was fully saturated at rest, but it is possible that desaturation/cyanosis might occur only during exercise. Right-to-left shunting at the atrial level may occur either through a PFO or an ASD, and occurs when RA pressure rises above LA pressure in the presence of a septal defect.

The normal neck veins are reassuring, but neck veins may be normal even when significant pathology is present, such as tricuspid regurgitation into a large RA with increased compliance.

The first heart sound is persistently split because of delayed closure of the tricuspid valve. This can be due to the presence of congenital abnormalities of the tricuspid valve itself or conduction abnormalities such as LBBB, or an ASD.

All professionals caring for congenital heart patients would be advised to check specifically for clubbing in the feet (see Case 17).

## LABORATORY DATA

| | |
|---|---|
| Hemoglobin | 14.6 g/dL (11.5–15.0) |
| Hematocrit/PCV | 42% (36–46) |
| MCV | 88 fL (83–99) |
| Platelet count | 237 × 10$^9$/L (150–400) |
| Sodium | 142 mmol/L (134–145) |
| Potassium | 4.2 mmol/L (3.5–5.2) |
| Creatinine | 0.8 mg/dL (0.6–1.2) |
| Blood urea nitrogen | 3.9 mmol/L (2.5–6.5) |

***Comments:*** The laboratory results showed no evidence of erythrocytosis, which indicates that even transient cyanosis is not likely.

## ELECTROCARDIOGRAM

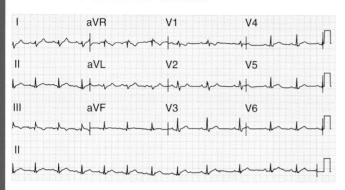

Figure 32-1 Electrocardiogram.

### FINDINGS

Heart rate: 73 bpm

PR interval: 195 msec

QRS axis: +127°

QRS duration: 135 msec

Sinus arrhythmia. Borderline first-degree AV block. Right-axis deviation. Atypical, complete RBBB. Generally low voltage.

***Comments:*** The findings here suggest abnormalities of the RV and perhaps the RA. This could be consistent with volume overload conditions such as an ASD or Ebstein anomaly of the tricuspid valve. P-waves that are tall and peaked may be due to RA enlargement. AV block is common in many conditions, as are accessory pathways (25% of Ebstein anomaly patients). Low-voltage QRS complexes can be due to large body habitus, fluid retention states, and pulmonary disease and are commonly seen in Ebstein anomaly.

## CHEST X-RAY

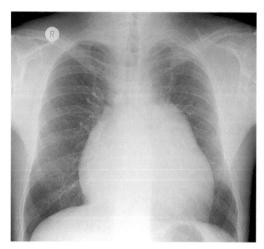

Figure 32-2 Posteroanterior projection.

### FINDINGS

Cardiothoracic ratio: 63%

Cardiomegaly with enlargement of the RA. Prominent main pulmonary artery. Normal lung parenchyma and mediastinum.

***Comments:*** The CXR in this setting confirms gross right atrial enlargement, more so than might be expected from an ASD alone. Furthermore, and in contrast to ASDs, the pedicle of the heart is small, in keeping with the reduced pulmonary and systemic forward flow and cardiac output. This combination is much more suggestive of Ebstein anomaly. The CXR may vary greatly depending on the lesion severity. The heart may adopt a globular appearance due to the dilated RA. The cardiothoracic ratio is a good indicator of severity and may be useful as a serial measurement to assess disease progression.

## EXERCISE TESTING

Exercise protocol:        Modified Bruce
Duration (min:sec):       13:38
Reason for stopping:      Stopped by technician
ECG changes:              None

|                              | Rest   | Peak    |
| ---------------------------- | ------ | ------- |
| Heart rate (bpm):            | 72     | 168     |
| Percent of age-predicted max HR: |    | 92      |
| O$_2$ saturation (%):        | 100    | 96      |
| Blood pressure (mm Hg):      | 104/68 | 153/108 |

***Comments:*** Formal effort tolerance testing provided valuable information regarding performance, exercise saturations, and arrhythmias. Again, this is a useful serial measurement to access symptoms and progress in a variety of conditions.

This patient had an excellent effort capacity and did not significantly desaturate at peak exercise.

## ECHOCARDIOGRAM

### OVERALL FINDINGS

The insertion of the septal leaflet of the tricuspid valve was displaced approximately 5 cm toward the apex. The RA was markedly dilated and the residual RV was small but had maintained function. The ventricular septum was bowed over toward the small, "squashed" LV. Despite the marked abnormality of the tricuspid valve there was only very mild tricuspid regurgitation. No septal defects were seen, and there were no other abnormalities.

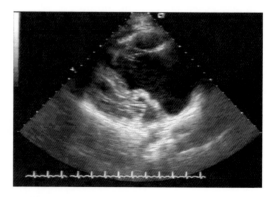

Figure 32-3 Modified long-axis view.

### FINDINGS

Parasternal view of the RV and RA clearly demonstrated the tricuspid valve abnormality and confirmed the diagnosis of Ebstein anomaly. This was best seen on the modified long-axis view with the transducer pointing down toward the right heart.

***Comments:*** Ebstein anomaly often may be seen in association with other defects including VSD, PDA, and CCTGA.

The diagnosis of Ebstein is made if there is more than 8 mm per m² of BSA apical displacement of the tricuspid valve.

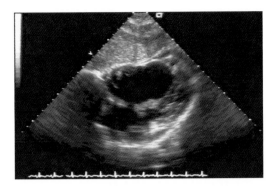

Figure 32-4  Subcostal four-chamber view.

## FINDINGS

The subcostal view again demonstrated the dominance of the right heart and the tricuspid valve displacement.

***Comments:*** From this image it is not difficult to see the importance of ventricular-ventricular interactions in determining cardiac output.

## MAGNETIC RESONANCE IMAGING

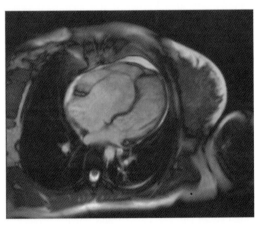

Figure 32-5  Oblique axial plane steady-state free precession cine (four-chamber view).

### Ventricular Volume Quantification

|  | LV | (Normal range) | RV | (Normal range) |
|---|---|---|---|---|
| EDV (mL) | 111 | (52–141) | 98 | (58–154) |
| ESV (mL) | 46 | (13–51) | 41 | (12–68) |
| SV (mL) | 65 | (33–97) | 57 | (35–98) |
| EF (%) | 59 | (57–75) | 58 | (51–75) |
| EDVi (mL/m²) | 65 | (62–96) | 57 | (61–98) |
| ESVi (mL/m²) | 27 | (17–36) | 24 | (17–43) |
| SVi (mL/m²) | 38 | (40–65) | 33 | (38–62) |
| Mass index (g/m²) | 47 | (47–77) | 38 | (20–40) |

## FINDINGS

The four-chamber view confirmed the degree of apical displacement with images similar to echocardiography. Ventricular size

and function were quantified. There was a large RA with an atrialized portion of the RV. Importantly, no ASD was present.

The LV was deformed and compressed by the large atrialized portion of the RV, giving it a sigmoid or "banana" shape.

***Comments:*** Cardiac MRI aspires to be the gold standard for determining ventricular volumes. Even so, it can be extremely challenging to do so in Ebstein anomaly, because the valve plane may be difficult to see in short axis. Often, axial views are obtained for proper RV volume calculations. The RV here is small because the volume excludes the atrialized portion. The stroke volume difference is small, reflecting only mild tricuspid valve regurgitation.

Despite the extreme displacement of the septal leaflet, the degree of tricuspid regurgitation is surprisingly low. This underscores the wide variation seen with Ebstein anomaly. Likely the absence of severe regurgitation is a large factor in the patient's lack of symptoms.

Note: The opening of the tricuspid valve is not visible in this view but is located more superiorly toward the RVOT.

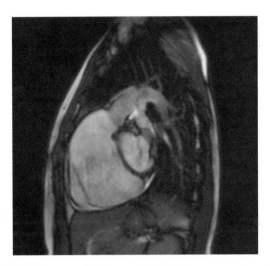

Figure 32-6  Oblique sagittal plane steady-state free precession cine.

## FINDINGS

The LV was dwarfed by the dominant right heart. The small residual RV was seen beyond the abnormal tricuspid valve in this sagittal plane. Note the aneurysmal, dilated RVOT.

Additional MRI findings included pulmonary arteries of a reasonable size, normal outflow valves, and an IVC that was not dilated.

***Comments:*** LV function is often abnormal in this patient group. There are several reasons for this, including chronic low cardiac output from the right heart, ventricular-ventricular interactions, and the presence of cyanosis.

MRI is particularly useful for demonstrating the outflow portion of the RV and offering a 3D look at the complex deformed valve.

### FOCUSED CLINICAL QUESTIONS AND DISCUSSION POINTS

1. Is this patient's presentation unusual for Ebstein anomaly?

The history of intermittent cyanosis in childhood and the absence of any other symptoms for over 20 years is unusual. Nevertheless, many infants with this condition may be cyanotic soon after birth, although this usually improves with time when pulmonary vascular resistance falls and, thus, right-to-left shunting through the patent foramen ovale diminishes.

There is a wide spectrum of clinical presentation of Ebstein. The anomaly may present in utero or in early life with severe cardiomegaly leading to lung hypoplasia.[1] Alternatively, the anomaly may be an incidental finding in the elderly. ASDs are very common and in the presence of moderate to severe Ebstein lead to cyanosis, which, however, would persist beyond childhood (not the case with our patient). Poor cardiac output can also be a cause of peripheral cyanosis.

It is somewhat surprising to find only a mild degree of tricuspid regurgitation despite gross structural deformation of the valve. The degree of regurgitation can be difficult to assess with any modality, though both the echo and MRI were in agreement that only mild regurgitation was present. Although valve competency does not necessarily correlate with the degree of apical displacement of the septal leaflet, this case seems more the exception rather than the rule.

2. What are the maternal and fetal risks of pregnancy in uncorrected Ebstein anomaly?

The two largest clinical series of pregnancy and Ebstein anomaly (n = 42 pregnancies and n = 111 pregnancies) suggest that in the absence of cyanosis or palpitations, maternal outcome is excellent. Possible complications to watch for might include symptoms of right heart failure or atrial arrhythmia. There is, however, an increased risk of miscarriage and prematurity. The recurrence risk for congenital cardiac defects in offspring is 4% to 6%.[2] Thus, one would not necessarily need to offer the patient much more than proper education in anticipation of pregnancy.

3. Should this patient have cardiac surgery to correct her abnormality irrespective of potential pregnancy?

The current indications for cardiac surgery in Ebstein anomaly usually include substantial exercise intolerance and/or cyanosis. This may or may not correlate with the severity of regurgitation. Right-sided heart failure, paradoxical embolism, a cardiothoracic ratio > 64%, and troublesome arrhythmias are other indications.

Tricuspid valve repair is preferable to replacement, but it is often technically difficult in these patients with grossly abnormal valves (see Case 31), and may not lead to satisfactory results. The addition of a bidirectional Glenn (SVC anastomosis to the pulmonary artery) may be needed when the small right heart is incapable of coping with full venous return. Atrial maze procedures, interventional ablative procedures, and surgical/electrophysiology treatment of accessory pathways, if present, should be anticipated before any contemplated surgery and performed when necessary.

Despite the anatomical severity of her tricuspid valve septal displacement, this patient represents the milder end of the wide spectrum encountered with Ebstein anomaly. She does not, at present, have a hard indication for surgery, even considering a potential future pregnancy, but careful follow-up with further serial data on cardiac size will be required over the coming years.

## FINAL DIAGNOSIS

Ebstein anomaly with no additional defects

## PLAN OF ACTION

Continued outpatient follow-up

Supportive care for any future pregnancy

## INTERVENTION

None

## DISCUSSION/OUTCOME

The patient was seen in follow-up at a joint obstetric/cardiac clinic. Issues regarding potential arrhythmia, cyanosis, right ventricular failure, and recurrence risk of congenital heart disease were discussed at length with the patient, but no intervention was felt necessary.

The patient felt somewhat surprised to discover that her congenital problem had not resolved as she had believed. Although many of the findings were reassuring and she was asymptomatic, the patient and partner wanted to reconsider their plans for conception.

After several further regular follow-up visits she remains asymptomatic. She also knows that specialized care will be available if and when she decides to start a family.

## Selected References

1. Celermajer DS, Bull C, Till JA, et al: Ebstein's anomaly: Presentation and outcome from fetus to adult. J Am Coll Cardiol 23:170–176, 1994.
2. Nora JJ, Nora AH: Familial risk of congenital heart defect. Am J Med Genet 29:231, 233, 1988.

## Bibliography

The Canadian Cardiovascular Society's Consensus Document. Recommendations for the Management of Adult Patients with Congenital Heart Disease. Part I. Can J Cardiol 17:940–959, 2001.

The Canadian Cardiovascular Society's Consensus Document. Recommendations for the Management of Adult Patients with Congenital Heart Disease. Part II. Can J Cardiol 17:1029–1050, 2001.

The Canadian Cardiovascular Society's Consensus Document. Recommendations for the Management of Adult Patients with Congenital Heart Disease. Part III. Can J Cardiol 17:1135–1158, 2001.

Connolly HM, Warnes CA: Ebstein's anomaly: Outcome of pregnancy. J Am Coll Cardiol 23:1194–1198, 1994.

Donnelly JE, Brown JM, Radford DJ: Pregnancy outcome and Ebstein's anomaly. Br Heart J 66:368–371, 1991.

# Pregnancy and Fetal Death in a Patient with Ebstein Anomaly

**Beatriz Bouzas**

**Age: 32 years**
**Gender: Female**
**Occupation: Part-time secretary**
**Working diagnosis: Ebstein anomaly of the tricuspid valve, 32 weeks pregnant**

## HISTORY

The patient was diagnosed with Ebstein anomaly of the tricuspid valve at the age of 2 years. She has remained well throughout her life, with a good exercise capacity and only occasional palpitations. She was told she may have Wolff-Parkinson-White (WPW) syndrome and had been started on digoxin and a beta-blocker.

Recently she became pregnant. She had been followed regularly by her local obstetrician and local cardiologist. The pregnancy had been uncomplicated, but the patient was more recently found to have high blood pressure and proteinuria. She was referred again for tertiary cardiology and obstetric advice at 32 weeks of pregnancy.

**Comments:** Ebstein anomaly of the tricuspid valve is characterized by apical displacement of the septal leaflet of the tricuspid valve. The subvalvar apparatus is often affected as well, with abnormal tethering of the chordae to the ventricular wall. The tricuspid valve is usually regurgitant, and less frequently stenotic.

Patients with mild to moderate Ebstein anomaly may remain asymptomatic for decades. However, symptoms occur earlier in life when the lesion is more severe. The diagnosis may be established in infancy because of a heart murmur. Alternatively, children or young adults may present with arrhythmia. When the anomaly is severe it may manifest itself with cyanosis at birth, or even with fetal hydrops or intrauterine death ("wall-to-wall heart").[1]

Preeclampsia is defined as new-onset hypertension and proteinuria (>300 mg over 24 or ++ in two urine samples). High blood pressure during pregnancy is one of the leading causes of both maternal and perinatal morbidity and mortality.[2]

## CURRENT SYMPTOMS

The patient had no specific complaints. Her exercise tolerance was good and without obvious limitation. She described occasional palpitations, lasting a few seconds only and never associated with other symptoms such as shortness of breath or fainting.

NYHA class: I

**Comments:** Pregnancy is generally well tolerated in patients with Ebstein anomaly. In a report of 44 mothers under-going 111 pregnancies, there were no maternal deaths or major cardiovascular complications.[3] However, if an ASD is present and the patient is cyanotic, cardiovascular complications are more likely.[4]

Palpitations may be due to ectopic beats, atrial fibrillation, or flutter or reentrant tachycardia. Accessory pathways (WPW syndrome) are a common association with Ebstein anomaly (~25%) and may lead to supraventricular tachycardia.

## CURRENT MEDICATIONS

Atenolol 50 mg daily

Digoxin 250 µg daily

**Comments:** Beta-blockers have a relatively good safety profile during pregnancy, although there is a perceived risk of growth retardation for the fetus. This may also relate to the underlying condition for which the beta-blockers are prescribed, as many patients with native or operated congenital heart disease have a low systemic cardiac output. Digoxin is safe to use during pregnancy. However, it is not certain whether these drugs are either needed or effective in this particular patient.

## PHYSICAL EXAMINATION

BP 142/72 mm Hg, HR 70 bpm, oxygen saturation on room air 96%

Height 158 cm, weight 63 kg, BSA 1.66 m$^2$

Surgical scars: None

Neck veins: The JVP was elevated to 6 cm above the sternal angle with a large V-wave visible.

Lungs/chest: Lungs were clear.

Heart: The heart rhythm was regular. There was an RV lift. There was a normal first sound and a normally split second sound. A 2–3/6 holosystolic murmur was audible at the lower left sternal border.

Abdomen: Gravid uterus, appropriate for dates

Extremities: There was trace pedal edema.

**Comments:** There is mild systolic hypertension.

The elevated JVP with presence of V-waves in the neck pulse is indicative of substantial tricuspid regurgitation. It should be noted that the jugular veins of most patients with Ebstein anomaly are normal in both height and waveform, the tricuspid regurgitation not being transmitted to the jugular veins by the very compliant and large RA (and liver).

The right ventricular lift reflects RV dilatation, and the holo-systolic murmur is indicative of tricuspid regurgitation.

## LABORATORY DATA

| | |
|---|---|
| Hemoglobin | **15.8 g/dL** (11.5–15.0) |
| Hematocrit/PCV | 46% (36–46) |
| MCV | 91 fL (83–99) |
| Platelet count | $269 \times 10^9$/L (150–400) |
| Sodium | 136 mmol/L (134–145) |
| Potassium | 4.4 mmol/L (3.5–5.2) |
| Creatinine | 0.64 mg/dL (0.6–1.2) |
| Blood urea nitrogen | 3.2 mmol/L (2.5–6.5) |

### OTHER RELEVANT LAB RESULTS

| | |
|---|---|
| Protein | 2.2 µmol/dL (0.3–2.4) |
| Albumin | 4.2 g/dL (3.7–5.3) |
| Urinalysis | 2+ protein |

***Comments:*** Usually hemoglobin/hematocrit will fall during pregnancy as blood volume expands. The slightly elevated hemoglobin here is unusual; it may reflect mild secondary erythrocytosis, due to a small right-to-left shunt during exercise through an interatrial communication or a PFO.

Serum protein levels remained normal despite preeclampsia.

## ELECTROCARDIOGRAM

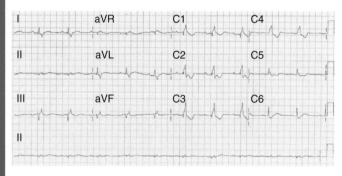

Figure 33-1 Electrocardiogram.

### FINDINGS
Heart rate: 64 bpm

PR interval: 218 msec

QRS duration: 167 msec

Sinus rhythm with first-degree heart block

Left-axis deviation of initial forces and RBBB. Nonspecific repolarization changes related to RBBB. Reduced overall ECG voltages.

***Comments:*** First-degree heart block is found in up to 50% of patients with Ebstein anomaly and may relate to right atrial dilatation and stretch. The RBBB and low ECG voltages are typical in this condition.

Up to 25% of patients with Ebstein anomaly have an accessory AV pathway (WPW) due to discontinuity of the central fibrous body. The accessory pathway might be the substrate for supraventricular tachycardia.

There was no pre-excitation (delta wave) to suggest WPW in this patient. A 24-hour ECG showed no evidence of sustained arrhythmia.

## CHEST X-RAY

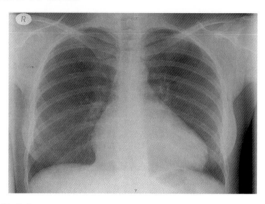

Figure 33-2 Posteroanterior projection.

### FINDINGS
Cardiothoracic ratio: 62%

Cardiomegaly is present with RA enlargement. A small pulmonary trunk and a small aortic knuckle are noted.

***Comments:*** This CXR had been taken prior to conception. The cardiomegaly is due to dilatation of the RA and atrialized portion of the RV, and is anticipated in patients with Ebstein anomaly; it can be dramatic in extreme cases (wall-to-wall hearts).

A small aortic knuckle is also a common finding in Ebstein anomaly, because of the chronically low cardiac output in many patients.

## EXERCISE TESTING

| | |
|---|---|
| Exercise protocol: | Modified Bruce |
| Duration (min:sec): | 7:28 |
| Reason for stopping: | Fatigue |
| ECG changes: | None |

| | Rest | Peak |
|---|---|---|
| Heart rate (bpm): | 70 | 155 |
| Percent of age-predicted max HR: | | 82 |
| O₂ saturation (%): | 96 | **85** |
| Blood pressure (mm Hg): | 114/72 | 126/80 |
| Peak Vo₂ (mL/kg/min): | | 17.1 |
| Percent predicted (%): | | 56 |
| Ve/Vco₂: | | **61** |
| Metabolic equivalents: | | 6.1 |

***Comments:*** Exercise testing was performed prior to pregnancy as a way of assessing the patient's risks for cardiovascular complications during pregnancy.

Oxygen saturation decreased during exercise from 96% to 85%. This was due to a raised RA pressure during exercise with right-to-left shunting through a presumed PFO or ASD.

It was a good prognostic sign for this patient that no sustained atrial or ventricular arrhythmia occurred during exercise.

Although the patient denied physical limitations, there was an objective reduction of her functional capacity (56% of predicted) compared to matched healthy controls. Ideally, a woman ought to have a higher peak oxygen consumption to feel confident in an ability to carry a pregnancy safely. The patient was told she was at increased risk of complications related to pregnancy, but that there was no need for surgical or other intervention beforehand.

## ECHOCARDIOGRAM

### Overall Findings
Ebstein anomaly of the tricuspid valve with displacement of the septal leaflet toward the apex by 47 mm. The RV and RA were enlarged when compared with the left-sided chambers.

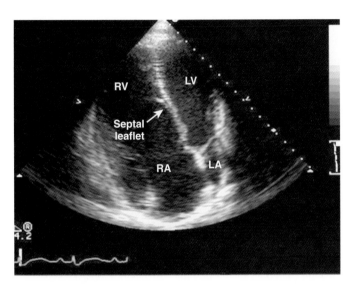

Figure 33-3 Four-chamber view.

***Comments:*** The tricuspid annulus normally should insert within about 15 mm of the mitral septal insertion (8 mm per m² of BSA).

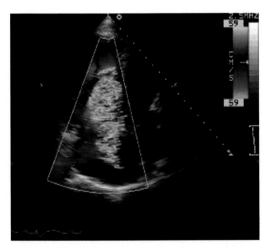

Figure 33-4 Four-chamber view, 2D color Doppler.

### Findings
Severe tricuspid regurgitation was present.

***Comments:*** Note the origin of the regurgitant jet that is well within the RV, close to the apex, because of the apical displacement of the leaflets.

## MAGNETIC RESONANCE IMAGING

### Overall Findings
Ebstein anomaly of the tricuspid valve was confirmed with severe tricuspid regurgitation. The RV (nonatrialized portion) was enlarged (end-diastolic volume 325 mL, indexed end-diastolic volume 213 mL/m², end-systolic volume 161 mL, indexed end-systolic volume 106 mL/m²), as was the RA. RV function was preserved (ejection fraction 50%), with a high stroke volume of 164 mL (indexed 108 mL/m²) due to severe TR. By comparison, the stroke volume of the LV was 51 mL (indexed 33 mL/m²). LVEF was normal (69%).

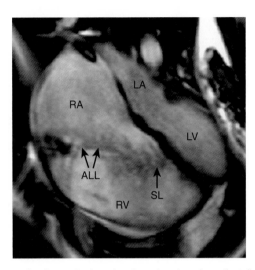

Figure 33-5 Gradient echo imaging, four-chamber view, diastolic frame.

### Findings
The septal leaflet of the tricuspid valve was displaced apically about 50 mm. The anterolateral leaflet (*arrows*) was inserted normally at the AV junction but there was abnormal tethering of this leaflet to the ventricular wall. The severely enlarged RA can easily be seen, including the atrialized portion of the RV. In this view the RV is reduced to the apical portion. The left ventricle is relatively small and the asynchronous paradoxical motion of the nonapical part of the interventricular septum can be seen.

***Comments:*** MRI is safe during pregnancy. It allows one to carefully assess the extent of the deformity, determine the volume of the RV, and estimate the regurgitant fraction. The ejection fraction of the RV should be high (artificially so, since ejection is substantially into a low impedance chamber, i.e., the RA) in the setting of severe tricuspid regurgitation, as in this case.

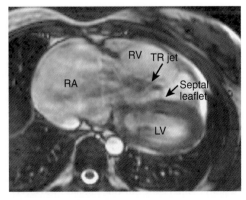

Figure 33-6 Gradient echo imaging, transverse view, systolic frame.

## FINDINGS

There was a turbulent jet of severe tricuspid regurgitation reaching the top of the RA.

Despite atrialization of the inlet portion of the RV, true RV volumes were increased mainly due to RVOT dilatation.

***Comments:*** Associated anomalies such as ASD or LVOT obstruction (uncommon) can also be documented, if present.

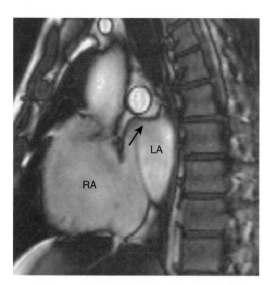

Figure 33-7 Gradient echo steady-state free precession imaging, sagittal view.

## FINDINGS

The RA was enlarged. A small PFO (*arrow*) was present with right-to-left shunting.

***Comments:*** A shunt at the atrial level (ASD or PFO) is found in 50% of patients with Ebstein anomaly of the tricuspid valve. The shunt may be primarily left to right at rest, and right to left with exercise. In functionally small RVs with significant tricuspid regurgitation and elevated RA pressures there is often a predominant right-to-left shunt through the defect. This shunt leads to oxygen desaturation (as was seen during exercise in this patient) but helps to maintain the systemic cardiac output, albeit at the expense of cyanosis. Also, there is an increased risk of paradoxical embolism, particularly if atrial flutter or fibrillation occurs.

### FOCUSED CLINICAL QUESTIONS AND DISCUSSION POINTS

1. What is the risk of pregnancy-related complications in this patient?

*Pregnancy in women with Ebstein anomaly is usually well tolerated provided there is no maternal cyanosis, arrhythmia, or right-sided heart failure. The largest series involving 44 mothers and 111 pregnancies reported no maternal mortality.[3] As in any other cyanotic condition, this risk is much higher when resting oxygen saturations are below 85%.[4] However, one must also consider the risk to the fetus, including prematurity, lower birth weight, and fetal loss, which can be as high as 19% of nonaborted pregnancies[3] particularly in cyanotic mothers (the miscarriage rate among healthy women is roughly 10%).*

*When addressing this particular patient, the risk of maternal complications during pregnancy was considered to be mild to*

moderate. *There was no cyanosis at rest but oxygen saturation dropped to 85% during exercise. Biventricular function was good, though function of the RV was difficult to assess given the abnormal morphology and the TR. Importantly, there were no signs of right-sided heart failure. Arrhythmias are another source of morbidity, but this patient had neither documented arrhythmias nor evidence for an accessory conduction pathway.*

2. Is preeclampsia related to her cardiovascular problem?

*Coexistent congenital heart disease does not increase the risk of preeclampsia. However, the presence of preeclampsia will significantly increase the overall risk of maternal complications during pregnancy and may compromise further the fetal prospects.*

3. Are there interventions that should be made to make pregnancy and delivery safer?

*Given this patient's desaturation with exertion, excessive exercise might best be avoided. Beta-blockers and digoxin do not necessarily need to be discontinued. At this point in time, the patient's management should focus on treating preeclampsia.*

*Although Ebstein anomaly is not associated with any known genetic defects, fetal echocardiography is a useful screening tool; there is probably a risk of recurrence of congenital heart disease in offspring of 5%.*

*Despite a common assumption to the contrary, vaginal delivery with epidural anesthesia—and assisted delivery with forceps or ventouse extraction when necessary (to shorten the duration of the second stage of labor)—is safer and preferable for patients with stable heart disease. Elective cesarean section has the advantage of avoiding the physical stress of labor and of being able to plan the procedure, but there may be hemodynamic instability related to anesthesia and assisted ventilation and, as well, there is an increased risk of bleeding, venous thromboembolism, and infection associated with it.*

*Therefore, close cardiac follow-up for the remainder of pregnancy was recommended, particularly close monitoring for signs of heart failure, worsening hypoxemia, or maternal sustained arrhythmia—with optimal management of her preeclampsia by a high-risk obstetric team.*

4. Should this patient have a repair of the tricuspid valve after delivery?

*As a rule, the asymptomatic patient with Ebstein anomaly should be left alone. Interventions on the tricuspid valve are difficult and give mixed results (see Cases 30 and 31). The surgical options are tricuspid valve repair when feasible or valve replacement (often with RA plication).[5] When the functional RV is small and the pulmonary arterial pressures not elevated (mean < 16 mm Hg), a bidirectional cavopulmonary connection may be considered. When right heart function is grossly impaired and there is also advanced LV dysfunction, heart transplantation may be a better option. In most cases the PFO should not be closed in isolation (without repair of the tricuspid valve); it functions as a safety valve to maintain cardiac output, and if closed the patient may become pink temporarily but suffers from right heart failure and low cardiac output (see Case 34).*

*There is no clear indication for surgery on the tricuspid valve in this patient at this point in time.[6,7] She is asymptomatic with a reasonable exercise capacity and maintained right and left systolic ventricular function. The patient should undergo regular follow-up with special attention to the onset of functional deterioration, sustained arrhythmias, worsening hypoxemia, or heart failure, all of which should prompt consideration of surgery.*

*If reentrant tachycardia occurs, the accessory pathway should be mapped and ablated. However, there may be multiple accessory pathways, and the rate of success of ablation is lower than for patients with WPW without Ebstein anomaly.[8] Onset of sus-*

*tained arrhythmia, which may be difficult to control by other means, may also lead to surgery on the tricuspid valve (combined with a modified maze procedure).*[9]

# FINAL DIAGNOSIS

Ebstein anomaly of the tricuspid valve

Severe tricuspid regurgitation

PFO, preeclampsia

35 weeks pregnant

# PLAN OF ACTION

Management of preeclampsia and delivery as per obstetric need

Close cardiologic support and follow-up after delivery

Thrombophylaxis for the peripartum period

# OUTCOME

At 35 weeks a fetal scan showed retarded intrauterine growth. The patient was admitted for closer observation. Two days after hospital admission, there was marked deceleration of fetal heart rate during fetal heart monitoring, which prompted a cesarean section under epidural anesthesia. The patient tolerated the operation well, but the baby was a stillborn. No cardiac anomalies were found on postmortem examination.

In retrospect, it is difficult to know what might have been done to avoid the tragic outcome for this pregnancy. There may have been a delay in delivering the baby; unfortunately, fetal loss is high in preeclampsia, which seems to have been an important risk factor in this case on top of the low cardiac output and variable hypoxemia associated with Ebstein anomaly of the tricuspid valve.

The patient attended a joint cardiology/obstetric clinic at a different center for further counseling regarding future pregnancy. The recommendation was, again, that no surgical intervention is necessary at this point in time given her current clinical state, even if she were to attempt another pregnancy. She should, however, be managed very closely, possibly with third trimester hospital admission, close monitoring of fetal growth and heart rate, minimal exertion, and perhaps a low threshold for early delivery if in doubt.

## Selected References

1. Celermajer DS, Bull C, Till JA, et al: Ebstein's anomaly: Presentation and outcome from fetus to adult. J Am Coll Cardiol 23:170–176, 1994.
2. Task Force on the Management of Cardiovascular Diseases during Pregnancy of the European Society of Cardiology. Expert consensus document on management of cardiovascular diseases during pregnancy. Eur Heart J 24:761–781, 2003.
3. Connolly HM, Warnes CA: Ebstein's anomaly: Outcome of pregnancy. J Am Coll Cardiol 23:1194–1198, 1994.
4. Presbitero P, Somerville J, Stone S, et al: Pregnancy in cyanotic congenital heart disease: Outcome of mother and fetus. Circulation 89:2673–2676, 1994.
5. Carpentier A, Chauvaud S, Mace L, et al: A new reconstructive operation for Ebstein's anomaly of the tricuspid valve. J Thorac Cardiovasc Surg 96:92–101, 1988.
6. Danielson GK, Driscoll DJ, Mair DD, et al: Operative treatment of Ebstein's anomaly. J Thorac Cardiovasc Surg 104:1195–1202, 1992.
7. Gentles TL, Calder AL, Clarkson PM, Neutze JM: Predictors of long-term survival with Ebstein's anomaly of the tricuspid valve. Am J Cardiol 69:377–381, 1992.
8. Smith WM, Gallagher JJ, Kerr CR, et al: The electrophysiologic basis and management of symptomatic recurrent tachycardia in patients with Ebstein's anomaly of the tricuspid valve. Am J Cardiol 49:1223–1234, 1982.
9. Attenhofer Jost CH, Connolly HM, Dearani JA, et al: Ebstein's anomaly. Circulation 115:277–285, 2007.

# Cyanosis in Ebstein Anomaly and Catheter Closure of Atrial Septal Defect

**Martin St. John Sutton, Howard C. Herrmann, and Richard M. Donner**

**Age: 47 years**
**Gender: Female**
**Occupation: Secretary**
**Working diagnosis: Ebstein anomaly**

## HISTORY

The patient presented with presyncope 14 months earlier, having been asymptomatic and well all her life. She was found to be in complete heart block and a dual chamber DDD pacemaker was placed. Echocardiography, performed to rule out structural heart disease, demonstrated a previously unknown diagnosis of Ebstein anomaly of the tricuspid valve with a small secundum ASD or PFO. Except for some diaphragmatic pacing she was extremely well. However, over the ensuing 5 months she complained of slowly progressive shortness of breath on exertion (one flight of stairs), mild orthopnea, and increasing fatigue. Further investigation was recommended to assess the possibility and severity of right-to-left shunting at rest and the possible role of percutaneous closure of the defect in the inter-atrial septum.

There was no known maternal exposure to lithium during her gestation. She was followed with uterine fibroids, a mild anxiety syndrome, and a smoking history of 20 pack-years. She had no known allergies.

**Comments:** Only a small percentage of patients with Ebstein anomaly require pacing.[1]

Maternal lithium use is a risk factor for Ebstein anomaly in the fetus.

## CURRENT SYMPTOMS

The patient complains of shortness of breath climbing one flight of stairs and with other modest activities. She has no other symptoms.

NYHA class: II

## CURRENT MEDICATIONS

None

## PHYSICAL EXAMINATION

Well-developed white female in no apparent distress

BP 110/70 mm Hg, HR 86 bpm and regular, oxygen saturation (upright and recumbent) 93%

Height 162 cm, weight 59.2 kg BSA 1.63 m$^2$

Surgical scars: None

Neck veins: JVP was elevated to 10 cm with a prominent V-wave.

Lungs/chest: Respiratory excursion was symmetric, and breath sounds were normal.

Heart: The pulse was regular. The apical impulse was normal; there was a left parasternal RV lift. The heart sounds were normal, and there was a soft holosystolic murmur at the lower left sternal border that became louder with inspiration.

Abdomen: The liver was enlarged and mildly pulsatile.

Extremities: There was no lower extremity edema. Peripheral arterial pulses were normal and equal bilaterally.

**Comments:** RV volume overload caused by tricuspid valve regurgitation is responsible for the RV lift. It is unusual for the JVP to be frankly elevated in patients with Ebstein anomaly.

## LABORATORY DATA

| | |
|---|---|
| Hemoglobin | **16.3 g/dL** (11.5–15.0) |
| Hematocrit/PCV | 45% (36–46) |
| MCV | 97 fL (83–99) |
| MCHC | 34 g/dL (31–35) |
| Platelet count | $157 \times 10^9$/L (150–400) |
| Sodium | 139 mmol/L (134–145) |
| Potassium | 4.1 mmol/L (3.5–5.2) |
| Creatinine | 0.9 mg/dL (0.6–1.2) |
| Blood urea nitrogen | 10 mg/dL (6–24) |

**Comments:** The elevated hemoglobin concentration presumably represents secondary erythrocytosis, and suggests that despite the mildly reduced resting oxygen saturation, the patient presumably desaturates further with exercise.

# ELECTROCARDIOGRAM

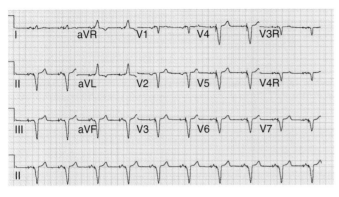

Figure 34-1 Electrocardiogram.

## FINDINGS

Dual chamber pacing (A paced–V paced) with 160 msec AV interval at low rate of 60 bpm.

*Comments:* In this paced rhythm, there is no AV conduction across a right-sided bypass tract that is present in some patients with Ebstein anomaly.

Pacing is from the RV, with a LBBB conduction pattern.

# CHEST X-RAY

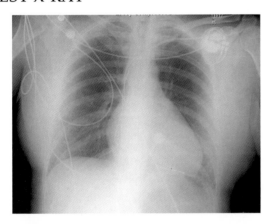

Figure 34-2 Posteroanterior projection.

## FINDINGS

Cardiothoracic ratio: 52%

There is mild cardiomegaly. The mediastinum is unremarkable.

The lungs are clear. A left subclavian transvenous pacemaker is present with tips overlying the RA and RV. The RA is prominent. The left heart border is straight, likely from RV and RVOT dilation.

*Comments:* The cardiomegaly is mainly due to RA enlargement. The normal appearance of the pulmonary arteries argues against a significant left-to-right shunt, but does not exclude a right-to-left shunt as a cause of her low oxygen saturation.

# EXERCISE TESTING

### Stress/Echo Study

| | |
|---|---|
| Exercise protocol: | Modified Bruce |
| Duration (min:sec): | 8:45 |
| Reason for stopping: | Dyspnea |
| ECG changes: | Not diagnostic |

| | Rest | Peak |
|---|---|---|
| Heart rate (bpm): | 86 | 150 |
| Percent of age-predicted max HR: | | 87 |
| O$_2$ saturation (%): | 93 | 87 |
| Blood pressure (mm Hg): | 110/70 | 166/82 |
| Peak Vo$_2$ (mL/kg/min): | | 13.3 |
| Metabolic equivalents: | | 4.6 |

Resting PA systolic pressure: 30 mm Hg

Peak PA systolic pressure: 60 mm Hg

*Comments:* This exercise study was done as part of a stress echocardiogram. The major finding of the study was low-normal arterial saturation at rest with mild additional arterial desaturation at peak exercise. The dyspnea that terminated exercise was probably related to the low saturation and to reaching the upper ventricular response rate of the pacemaker.

It is postulated that the normal increase of RV peak pressure during exercise (estimated at 60 mm Hg) results in increased tricuspid valve regurgitation and RA pressure, promoting right-to-left shunting across the atrial septum.

# ECHOCARDIOGRAM

## OVERALL FINDINGS

Ebstein anomaly of the tricuspid valve. There was no RVOT obstruction. The RA and RV were mildly enlarged with abnormal interventricular septal motion. Peak pulmonary systolic pressure estimated by Doppler was 29 mm Hg above the RA V-wave. Tricuspid regurgitation was moderate. The LV was small by comparison but had normal function.

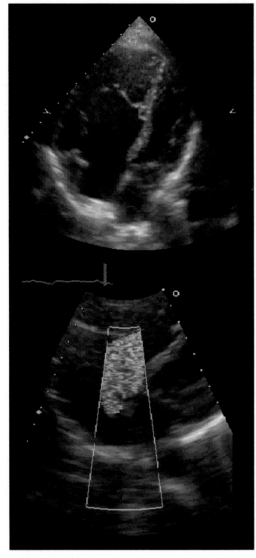

Figure 34-3 Apical four-chamber view (2D and Doppler).

## FINDINGS

Ebstein malformation of the tricuspid valve is present with downward displacement of the septal leaflet from the annulus and a very large sail-like anterior leaflet. There was moderate tricuspid regurgitation.

**Comments:** The four-chamber views typically image the displaced septal leaflet and the nondisplaced, sail-like anterior leaflet. The true tricuspid valve annulus may be seen with no valve tissue in it. A portion of the RV between the true annulus and the commissure is often referred to as the "atrialized RV."

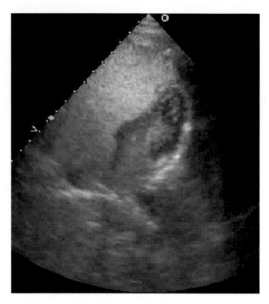

Figure 34-4 Two-chamber contrast echocardiogram.

## FINDINGS

Following the injection of contrast, there is opacification of the LA and LV, consistent with a right-to-left shunt across the atrial septum.

**Comments:** The presence of an atrial shunt is an important observation to make in a patient with Ebstein anomaly. The relatively higher RA pressures can lead to right-to-left shunt and desaturation. Decisions to close such a defect must be carefully considered in this clinical situation (see "Focused Clinical Questions and Discussion Points").

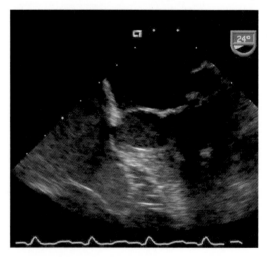

Figure 34-5 Transesophageal echocardiogram (24°).

## FINDINGS

Ebstein malformation of the tricuspid valve. Note how the septal leaflet of the tricuspid valve is "plastered down" the RV aspect of the ventricular septum (*left lower panel*) compared with the mitral valve (*right mid panel*).

**Comments:** The transesophageal four-chamber view demonstrates tethering of the septal leaflet that displaces the valve's commissure into the body of the RV.

## CATHETERIZATION

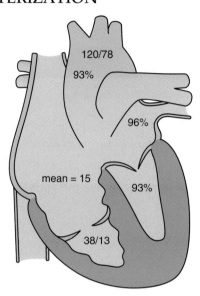

Figure 34-6 Schema showing right and left heart hemodynamics and oxygen saturations.

## FINDINGS

RA and RV filling pressures are elevated. There is right-to-left shunting across the atrial septum.

### FOCUSED CLINICAL QUESTIONS AND DISCUSSION POINTS

1. What is the complete anatomic cardiac diagnosis?

   *The complete diagnosis is Ebstein anomaly of the tricuspid valve, moderate tricuspid regurgitation, and PFO with bidirectional shunting.*

   *Ebstein anomaly of the tricuspid valve is a relatively uncommon lesion accounting for less than 1% of congenital heart disease. It is generally considered to be a complex abnormality with extremely variable presentations and treatment options.[2] In about 50% of all cases of Ebstein anomaly there is an intracardiac shunt at the atrial level, either a PFO or a secundum ASD. This patient had a PFO and an associated interatrial septal aneurysm that, during ventricular systole, deviated to the left, stretching the PFO widely open and facilitating brisk right-to-left shunting that was unequivocally demonstrated by all modes of echocardiography.*

   *The diagnostic imaging modality of choice in Ebstein anomaly is transthoracic and transesophageal Doppler echocardiography. The diagnostic features are demonstrated in the apical four-chamber view and relate to the anatomic disposition of the three leaflets of the tricuspid valve. The cardinal diagnostic feature in Ebstein anomaly is apical displacement of the insertion of the septal and posterior leaflets by more than 8 mm/m$^2$ and a large redundant anterior leaflet.[3] The leaflets may be dysplastic and tethered by chordal attachments to the right ventricular free wall and septum preventing leaflet coaptation such that the origin of the tricuspid jet appears to originate within the body of the RV. The apical displacement of the tricuspid valve divides the RV into a thin-walled atrialized portion and the small apical true RV. The degree of tricuspid regurgitation determines the degree of RA and RV enlargement and influences the direction and magnitude of atrial shunting. RVOT obstruction may be caused by displacement of the tricuspid valve leaflets into the RVOT. Although uncommon, this should be excluded by Doppler echocardiography, as it may increase tricuspid valve regurgitation.*

2. Is high-degree AV block a frequent finding in Ebstein anomaly of the tricuspid valve?

   *Complete heart block is seldom a feature of Ebstein anomaly, although it can occur.[1] The QRS morphology may be within normal limits, although the most frequent findings include first-degree AV block, RBBB, and RA enlargement.*

   *At the other extreme, approximately 20% of patients have evidence of pre-excitation due to accessory right-sided bypass tract(s). Arrhythmic events including reciprocating tachycardia (when bypass tracts are present), atrial flutter, and atrial fibrillation (reflecting tricuspid regurgitation) occur commonly in the natural history of Ebstein anomaly.[4,5]*

3. What is the cause/mechanism of the hypoxia, and does this explain progressive dyspnea and justify percutaneous device closure?

   *The mechanism for the hypoxia was elevation of RA pressure due to tricuspid regurgitation in ventricular systole. This forced the atrial septal aneurysm to the extreme left (>20 mm beyond the midline), stretching the PFO and maintaining its patency throughout ventricular systole. The pressure differential across the PFO during ventricular systole was the driving force that determined the direction of shunt flow from right to left, producing systemic desaturation. In ventricular diastole, the pressure relationship changes and shunting may be left to right. Stress testing showed that when the patient's pulmonary artery systolic pressure increased to 60 mm Hg, systemic oxygen saturation fell further with associated dyspnea and fatigue, terminating her exercise test. This hypoxemia is considered a contributor to exercise intolerance in the setting of only moderate tricuspid valve regurgitation[6] and was the rationale for considering percutaneous closure of the PFO. Right-sided heart failure was also absent in this patient. Primary surgical valve repair or replacement is reserved for more severe anatomy and symptomatology and may be recommended if there is little or no clinical improvement following PFO closure.[7] A variety of surgical options are available.[8-11]*

4. Why did the patient develop exercise intolerance at this point in her life?

   *Right-to-left shunting through a PFO or ASD in Ebstein patients can be seen as a benefit or a curse. Some patients with Ebstein anomaly need the right-to-left shunt to maintain right heart compensation. If an ASD were to be closed in such a patient, acute right heart decompensation can result. Accordingly, closure of an atrial communication in Ebstein anomaly should be undertaken only after careful consideration and discussion, usually in a patient with a high resting oxygen saturation.*

   *A variety of factors may be responsible for the appearance of significant right-to-left shunting with exercise, the major cause of exercise intolerance in this patient. These include progression of tricuspid regurgitation and the natural increase in pulmonary vascular resistance with aging.*

## FINAL DIAGNOSIS

Ebstein anomaly of the tricuspid valve with right-to-left atrial shunting across a PFO

# PLAN OF ACTION

Percutaneous closure of the PFO

# INTERVENTION

The first attempted closure procedure was performed using intracardiac echocardiography (ICE) guidance. A 33-mm diameter CardioSeal VSD occluder device (off-label utilization) was deployed. When the RA clamshell was opened, it entrapped the atrial pacemaker lead as it coursed toward the RA appendage. It could not be disengaged and the entire device was removed from the septum. During removal from the right femoral vein, the device detached from the deployment/delivery catheter necessitating surgical removal by a local cut-down on the femoral vein by a vascular surgeon. This was achieved without incident.

***Comments:*** Prior to the procedure, the risks and benefits were discussed thoroughly with the patient. These included dislodgement with need for removal of the CardioSeal device, embolization, bleeding, infection, and the possibility that the defect would not be satisfactorily closed, requiring the need for surgical closure at which time strong consideration would be given to repairing or replacing the tricuspid valve. It was also important to discuss the possibility that complete occlusion of the PFO would not result in any improvement of her symptoms.

# OUTCOME

The following day, she awoke with a neurologic event characterized as sudden left-sided facial weakness, slurred speech, and possible left hemiagnosia/neglect. The neurology stroke service suggested that the neurologic stigmata most likely represented a paradoxical embolism (presumably from the site of her femoral vein vascular surgery the day before) through the PFO. The prognosis was good, and thrombolysis was not recommended.

After the stroke, permission was obtained from the institutional review board for compassionate use of an Amplatzer PFO occluder device that was believed less likely to become entrapped in the RA pacemaker lead. Three days after removal of the CardioSeal device, a 35-mm Amplatzer PFO occluder was successfully deployed from the left femoral vein under ICE guidance without entrapment or dislodgement of the atrial pacing electrode. Postprocedure ICE showed that the device was fully deployed but a small residual bidirectional shunt remained at the superior aspect of the device. The patient was discharged on aspirin 81 mg/day for 3 months, and her previous medications.

Follow-up at 1 month demonstrated complete recovery from her stroke. Her symptoms of dyspnea had improved, and she had an oxygen saturation of 99% on room air at rest. A transthoracic echocardiogram showed moderate tricuspid valve regurgitation with minimal right-to-left shunting. Two years following the procedure, there were no complaints of dyspnea on exertion, and oxygen saturation at the time of outpatient visits was always 95% or greater. Repeat stress testing was not performed. Echocardiography demonstrated increasing tricuspid regurgitation.

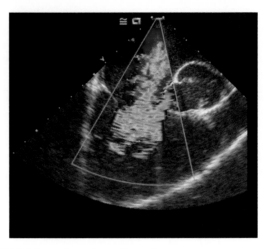

Figure 34-7 Intracardiac echocardiography.

## FINDINGS

There was moderate tricuspid regurgitation.

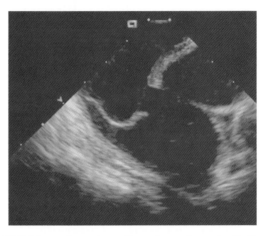

Figure 34-8 Intracardiac echocardiography performed with the transducer in the right atrium during the initial attempted closure of the atrial communication with a CardioSeal occlusion device.

## FINDINGS

The atrial septum was greatly mobile, and there was a variably sized interatrial communication located adjacent to the SVC. The largest defect during the cardiac cycle measured approximately 12 mm.

***Comments:*** In this ICE, the RA is in the upper left and the LA is in the lower right. The interatrial communication features a mobile, "aneurysmal" septum secundum that loses its continuity with the segment of septum primum located adjacent to the SVC. The defect is transiently closed with no permanent deficiency of tissue. Therefore, this is likely to represent a PFO. An occluder delivery device enters the LA through the defect but does not appear to stent the defect open. In some frames, a pacing wire is seen entering the RA from the SVC.

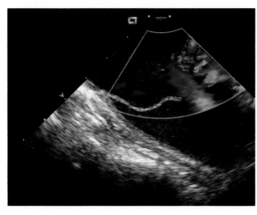

Figure 34-9 Intracardiac echocardiography color Doppler of the right heart chambers.

## FINDINGS

With the transducer in the RA, shunting across the PFO is bidirectional.

*Comments:* Shunting across the PFO from right to left is shown in dark blue. It is low velocity since the mobile atrial septum is pushed far into the LA during ventricular systole when tricuspid valve regurgitation occurs. This creates a large, unobstructed passage.

Shunting across the PFO from left to right is shown in red and yellow. It is high velocity since the PFO is nearly closed in ventricular diastole.

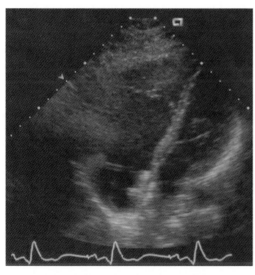

Figure 34-10 Transthoracic echocardiography performed 7 months after deployment of the Amplatzer device. Apical four-chamber view.

## FINDINGS

The Amplatzer device is deployed on the atrial septum and is in good position. There appears to be a small right-to-left shunt by contrast echocardiography. However, no contrast is noted in the LA.

*Comments:* The presence of contrast in the LV is consistent with right-to-left shunting across the Amplatzer device. The magnitude of right-to-left shunting is less, consistent with the patient's improvement.

## Selected References

1. Allen MR, Hayes DL, Warnes CA, et al: Permanent pacing in Ebstein's anomaly. Pacing Clin Electrophysiol 20:1243–1246, 1997.
2. Spitaels SE: Ebstein's anomaly of the tricuspid valve complexities and strategies. Cardiol Clin 20:431–439, vii, 2002.
3. Frescura C, Angelini A, Daliento L, et al: Morphological aspects of Ebstein's anomaly in adults. Thorac Cardiovasc Surg 48:203–208, 2000.
4. Jaiswal PK, Balakrishnan KG, Saha A, et al: Clinical profile and natural history of Ebstein's anomaly of tricuspid valve. Int J Cardiol 46:113–119, 1994.
5. Attie F, Rosas M, Rijlaarsdam M, et al: The adult patient with Ebstein anomaly: Outcome in 72 unoperated patients. Medicine (Baltimore) 79:27–36, 2000.
6. MacLellan-Tobert SG, Driscoll DJ, Mottram CD, et al: Exercise tolerance in patients with Ebstein's anomaly. J Am Coll Cardiol 29:1615–1622, 1997.
7. Chauvaud S, Berrebi A, d'Attellis N, et al: Ebstein's anomaly: Repair based on functional analysis. Eur J Cardiothorac Surg 23:525–531, 2003.
8. Danielson GK, Driscoll DJ, Mair DD, et al: Operative treatment of Ebstein's anomaly. J Thorac Cardiovasc Surg 104:1195–1202, 1992.
9. Kiziltan HT, Theodoro DA, Warnes CA, et al: Late results of bioprosthetic tricuspid valve replacement in Ebstein's anomaly. Ann Thorac Surg 66:1539–1554, 1998.
10. Wu Q, Huang Z: A new procedure for Ebstein's anomaly. Ann Thorac Surg 77:470–476, 2004.
11. Attenhofer Jost CH, Connolly HM, Dearani JA, et al: Ebstein's anomaly. Circulation 115:277–285, 2007.

# Right Ventricular Outflow

# Congenital Pulmonary Stenosis Turned to Pulmonary Regurgitation

**Beatriz Bouzas and Craig S. Broberg**

**Age: 41 years**
**Gender: Male**
**Lifestyle information: Aggressive sportsman**
**Working diagnosis: Pulmonary regurgitation**

## HISTORY

The patient underwent a successful surgical valvotomy for pulmonary valve stenosis at the age of seven.

He had a splenectomy following a motor-cross motorbike accident in his early 20s. He receives an annual pneumococcal vaccine and a small dose of penicillin prophylaxis daily.

He was well leading a full life until about 2 years ago, when he had his first episode of what was probably atrial fibrillation triggered by an upper respiratory tract infection. He was started on sotalol and converted spontaneously to sinus rhythm. Given the absence of arrhythmias on subsequent 24-hour ECG tape recordings, the medication was stopped.

He remained asymptomatic until 2 months ago, when he presented with chest pain and palpitations. He had a supraventricular tachycardia, and sotalol 80 mg twice daily was reintroduced.

Since then the patient has experienced palpitations clearly related to exercise and always resolving with rest. The symptoms did not improve after increasing the dose of sotalol. Eventually this was stopped and replaced with amiodarone 200 mg daily.

**Comments:** The patient was born with pulmonary valve stenosis. Surgical valvotomy was widely employed in the 1960s and 1970s. More recently, balloon valvuloplasty has become the treatment of choice for pulmonary valve stenosis. Surgical valvotomy is nowadays reserved for extremely dysplastic valves and patients with sub- or supravalvular stenosis.

Some degree of pulmonary regurgitation is found after surgical or balloon valvuloplasty of a stenotic pulmonary valve in up to 70% of cases,[1,2] and is reported to be moderate or severe in 25% of them.

In these patients, as in patients with repaired tetralogy of Fallot, chronic severe pulmonary regurgitation may cause right ventricular dilatation and dysfunction, reduced exercise capacity, atrial and ventricular arrhythmias, and sudden cardiac death.

## CURRENT SYMPTOMS

The patient complained of palpitations, most of which were clearly related to exertion and resolved with rest. Sometimes he would wake from sleep with a fast, irregular heart rate.

He also noted worsening of his exercise capacity. Although previously very fit, he was now becoming breathless after climbing one flight of stairs.

NYHA class: II

**Comments:** Pulmonary regurgitation is usually well tolerated, and patients remain symptom-free for many years. When patients become symptomatic, right ventricular systolic dysfunction is likely and may be irreversible.

## CURRENT MEDICATIONS

Amiodarone 200 mg daily

**Comments:** The efficacy of amiodarone for maintaining sinus rhythm in patients with nonischemic heart disease appears to be better than that of sotalol[3]; amiodarone does, however, have more side effects, especially long term. Class I antiarrhythmic agents (such as flecainide and propafenone) may also be useful in preventing atrial fibrillation, but experience with this treatment is limited and some advocate against their use for patients with structural heart disease.

## PHYSICAL EXAMINATION

BP 128/78 mm Hg, HR 85 bpm, oxygen saturation 99% on room air

Height 183 cm, weight 87 kg, BSA 2.1 m$^2$

Surgical scars: Sternotomy, laparotomy

Neck veins: Normal waveform, 2 cm above the sternal angle

Lungs/Chest: Clear

Heart: There was an RV lift. The heart rhythm was regular. There was a normal first heart sound and single second sound with no audible pulmonary component. A 2/6 systolic ejection murmur and a low-pitched early ending diastolic murmur were audible at the left sternal edge.

Abdomen: Normal

Extremities: Normal

***Comments:*** An RV heave reflects RV dilatation. The absence of the pulmonary component of the second sound may reflect an absent, defective, or stenotic pulmonary valve. The systolic murmur reflects some degree of residual turbulence through the RVOT. The diastolic murmur of pulmonary regurgitation is best heard with the bell at the second or third left intercostal space. It is a low frequency murmur with a delayed onset after the second sound; its duration seems to be inversely related to the severity of pulmonary regurgitation. A short diastolic murmur, therefore, with an RV heave suggests severe pulmonary regurgitation and a dilated RV.

There were no signs of congestion in this patient. Elevated jugular pressure, hepatic enlargement, and peripheral edema can be present when there is established right ventricular dysfunction with decompensated heart failure.

## LABORATORY DATA

| | |
|---|---|
| Hemoglobin | 14.9 g/dL (13.0–17.0) |
| Hematocrit/PCV | 43% (41–51) |
| MCV | 93 fL (83–99) |
| Platelet count | $285 \times 10^9$/L (150–400) |
| Sodium | 140 mmol/L (134–145) |
| Potassium | 4.3 mmol/L (3.5–5.2) |
| Creatinine | 0.9 mg/dL (0.6–1.2) |
| Blood urea nitrogen | 6.1 mmol/L (2.5–6.5) |

***Comments:*** No abnormalities were detected.

## ELECTROCARDIOGRAM

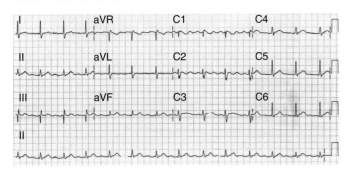

Figure 35-1 Electrocardiogram.

### FINDINGS
Heart rate: 84 bpm

QRS axis: +15°

QRS duration: 105 msec

Atrial flutter at a rate of 255 bpm and with 3:1 conduction. A degree of RBBB is present.

***Comments:*** The patient was in atrial flutter with a normal ventricular rate at rest. Macroreentrant atrial tachycardias can often be atypical and subtle in ACHD, and the provider should be careful to inspect the ECG carefully.

It is speculative, but his AV conduction probably increases during exercise, accounting for his exertional palpitations. The atrial rate is slower than the usual atrial flutter rate of 300 bpm because the patient is on amiodarone.

## CHEST X-RAY

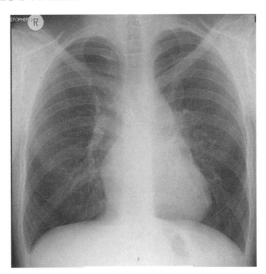

Figure 35-2 Posteroanterior projection.

### FINDINGS
Cardiothoracic ratio: 48%

Mild cardiomegaly, with normal pulmonary vascular markings. Straightening of the left heart border due to dilation of the RVOT and the main pulmonary artery. RA enlargement. Prior sternotomy.

***Comments:*** RV enlargement and dilatation of the pulmonary trunk are the hallmarks of pulmonary regurgitation, though better appreciated on lateral projections (not available for this patient).

## EXERCISE TESTING

| | |
|---|---|
| Exercise protocol: | Modified Bruce |
| Duration (min:sec): | 8:26 |
| Reason for stopping: | Tachycardia |
| ECG changes: | Tachycardia |

| | Rest | Peak |
|---|---|---|
| Heart rate (bpm): | 85 | 170 |
| Percent of age-predicted max HR: | | 95 |
| $O_2$ saturation (%): | 99 | 100 |
| Blood pressure (mm Hg): | 128/78 | 140/80 |
| Peak $\dot{V}o_2$ (mL/kg/min): | | 15 |
| Percent predicted (%) | | 42 |
| Ve/$\dot{V}co_2$ | | 49 |
| Metabolic equivalents: | | 4.9 |

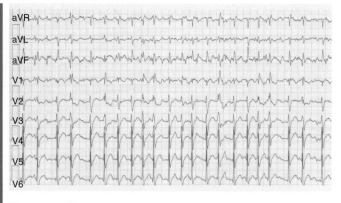

Figure 35-3 Electrocardiogram.

**Comments:** Even though many patients with RV dysfunction may be asymptomatic, some degree of objective exercise intolerance can usually be found on exercise testing.[4]

The test showed a much reduced functional capacity, only 42% of predicted for his age and gender. The elevated $Ve/Vco_2$ slope shows an inefficient ventilatory response.

The patient did the exercise test while on sotalol. He accelerated his ventricular response during the test, with the same symptoms he had previously reported during exercise.

## ECHOCARDIOGRAM

### OVERALL FINDINGS

There was normal LV systolic function and a dilated RV with mildly reduced systolic function.

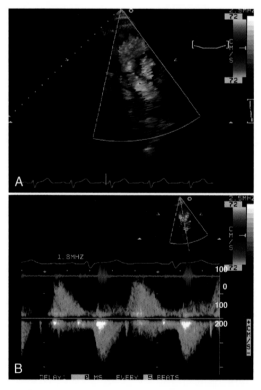

Figure 35-4 Color (**A**) and continuous-wave (**B**) Doppler performed in the parasternal short axis at the level of the pulmonary valve.

### FINDINGS

There was retrograde flow of pulmonary regurgitation with a wide jet (17 mm) indicative of severe pulmonary regurgitation (*A*) and diastolic regurgitant flow with a fast decay lasting about two thirds of diastolic time (*B*). There was a mild increase in systolic peak velocity explained by an increase in stroke volume across the pulmonary valve.

**Comments:** Good agreement between duration of pulmonary regurgitant flow (expressed as a percentage of the total diastolic time on continuous-wave Doppler) and CMR-derived pulmonary regurgitant fraction has been reported.[5,6] Diastolic flow lasting less than 60% of the diastolic time and pulmonary pressure with a half-time less than 100 msec are indicative of severe pulmonary regurgitation.

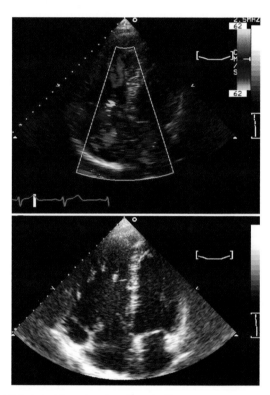

Figure 35-5 Apical four-chamber 2D color Doppler.

### FINDINGS

There was mild tricuspid regurgitation.

**Comments:** The function of the tricuspid valve often becomes compromised following dilatation of the RV. Tricuspid regurgitation, in turn, causes RA enlargement and thus possible atrial flutter variants. It is somewhat surprising that the degree of regurgitation seen in this patient is only mild, but RV adaptation to volume overload and remodeling vary from patient to patient.

# MAGNETIC RESONANCE IMAGING

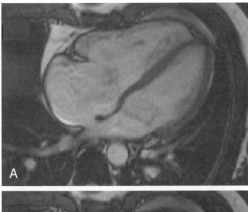

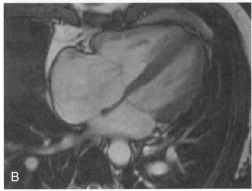

Figure 35-6 Gradient echo cine imaging, four-chamber view in diastole (**A**) and systole (**B**).

## FINDINGS

### Ventricular Volume Quantification

|  | LV | (Normal range) | RV | (Normal range) |
|---|---|---|---|---|
| EDV (mL) | 157 | (77–195) | 498 | (88–227) |
| ESV (mL) | 63 | (19–72) | 280 | (23–103) |
| SV (mL) | 94 | (51–133) | 218 | (52–138) |
| EF (%) | 60 | (58–75) | 44 | (52–77) |
| EDVi (mL/m$^2$) | 75 | (64–99) | 237 | (62–108) |
| ESVi (mL/m$^2$) | 30 | (17–38) | 104 | (16–45) |
| SVi (mL/m$^2$) | 45 | (42–66) | 133 | (39–71) |
| Mass index (g/m$^2$) |  |  |  | (21–48) |

There was mild tricuspid regurgitation. The RA was moderately dilated. LV volumes and ejection fraction were within the normal range.

***Comments:*** The RV was severely dilated; furthermore, end-systolic volumes were well above the normal range suggesting RV systolic dysfunction beyond what the ejection fraction would suggest.

The RA is enlarged, presumably due to tricuspid regurgitation. The stretching of the RA wall has contributed to atrial flutter. Again, only mild tricuspid regurgitation was present, and there was no ASD.

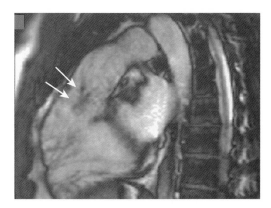

Figure 35-7 Oblique sagittal steady-state free precession cine (right ventricular outflow tract view [diastole]).

## FINDINGS

There was free pulmonary regurgitation (*arrows*). The RVOT and pulmonary trunk were dilated (40 mm and 38 mm, respectively). The pulmonary arteries were of normal size with no significant stenoses.

***Comments:*** Due to the small pressure difference between the pulmonary artery and RV in diastole, the jet of pulmonary regurgitation might not appear as evident by MRI as, for example, a jet of aortic regurgitation.

The pulmonary arteries were of normal size, which is important given that branch pulmonary artery stenosis may worsen pulmonary regurgitation.[7]

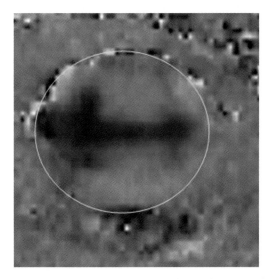

Figure 35-8 Non–breath-hold through-plane phase velocity mapping transecting the right ventricular outflow tract immediately below the pulmonary valve (*circle*).

## FINDINGS

The dark pixels show the regurgitant stream in diastole. The arrow-shaped dark area represents the regurgitant orifice. The pulmonary regurgitant fraction was 54%.

There was no significant pulmonary valve stenosis.

***Comments:*** A regurgitant fraction of about 40% is typical of free or nearly free pulmonary regurgitation. There is only partial valve action with a large regurgitant orifice, in this patient more marked at the level of the right-sided commissure.[5,6]

## Focused Clinical Questions and Discussion Points

### 1. When is the optimal time to replace the pulmonary valve in a patient with severe pulmonary regurgitation?

*There is considerable controversy about this question. We believe the following comments are generally well accepted. Pulmonary valve replacement (PVR) surgery should be performed in the context of severe pulmonary regurgitation to alleviate attributable exercise intolerance, after the occurrence of sustained ventricular tachycardia or atrial flutter, and when severe right ventricular dilation is present. Young adults undergoing PVR are likely to require further surgery as bioprosthetic valves have a limited lifespan. The therapeutic goals of PVR are reduction of ventricular volumes and preservation of RV function,[8] improved functional capacity and quality of life, risk modification for arrhythmia and sudden cardiac death, and overall improved prognosis.[9,10]*

### 2. What are the surgical options?

*Bioprosthetic valves (homograft or porcine) have a lower complication rate compared with mechanical prosthesis in the pulmonary position and thus are the valves of choice.[11] The 10-year freedom from repeat PVR increases with increasing age of the patient at time of pulmonary valve implantation. These valves should last much longer than 10 years in most adult patients.*

*There is a lot of excitement about percutaneous implantation of a bovine valve mounted in a stent in the pulmonary position.[12] This approach, although experimental, was considered for this patient but was not suitable because of the marked dilatation of the RVOT (when more than 22 mm, percutaneous valve implantation is not feasible at present; see Case 42).*

### 3. Will PVR prevent further arrhythmia?

*The combination of cryoablation and other antiarrhythmic surgery with PVR at the time of the surgery has been shown to reduce the incidence of atrial and ventricular arrhythmia in patients with repaired tetralogy of Fallot and severe pulmonary regurgitation. These data may be relevant to nontetralogy patients with pulmonary regurgitation,[13] but there are no specific data on patients such as this one. Of course, therapy for both atrial and ventricular arrhythmias can also be delivered in the interventional electrophysiology laboratory. The most important principle is that both the arrhythmia and its underlying hemodynamic substrate should be treated as definitively as possible.*

*Alternatively, the patient could have a modified RA maze cryoablative procedure with removal of the RA appendage, as marked RA dilatation was thought to be the likely arrhythmogenic substrate here.*

## FINAL DIAGNOSIS

Congenital pulmonary valvar stenosis

Surgical pulmonary valvotomy

Residual severe pulmonary regurgitation

Sustained atrial flutter

## PLAN OF ACTION

PVR with a bioprosthetic valve plus arrhythmia mapping and ablation

## OUTCOME

The patient underwent catheter electrophysiologic study with successful ablation of his atrial flutter. One month later he underwent PVR with a 25-mm homograft prosthesis. His postoperative course was uneventful, and he left the hospital on the fourth postoperative day in sinus rhythm. He was encouraged to physically recondition himself.

A follow-up cardiac MRI (1 year from surgery) showed normal function of the pulmonary homograft with no evidence of valvar stenosis and only trivial regurgitation. There was mild supravalvar stenosis located about 15 mm above the pulmonary valve leaflets, probably at a suture line, with peak recorded velocity at 2.9 m/sec. The RV was still mildly dilated at end systole, but overall RV size normalized and systolic function improved—EDV 202 mL (RVEDVi 96 mL/m$^2$), ESV 106 mL, stroke volume 96 mL, ejection fraction 48%.

Two years after surgery the patient presented with sustained atrial flutter requiring direct current cardioversion. Currently he is maintained in sinus rhythm with flecainide (intolerant of beta-blockers) and warfarin.

Otherwise, the patient feels better now than before his operation, having more energy and being less easily breathless.

## Selected References

1. Chen CR, Cheng TO, Huang T, et al: Percutaneous balloon valvuloplasty for pulmonic stenosis in adolescents and adults. N Engl J Med 335:21–25, 1996.
2. Hayes CJ, Gersony WM, Driscoll DJ, et al: Second natural history study of congenital heart defects: Results of treatment of patients with pulmonary valvar stenosis. Circulation 87(2 Suppl):I28–37, 1993.
3. Singh BN, Singh SN, Reda DJ, et al: Sotalol Amiodarone Atrial Fibrillation Efficacy Trial (SAFE-T) Investigators: Amiodarone versus sotalol for atrial fibrillation. N Engl J Med 352:1861–1872, 2005.
4. Fredriksen PM, Therrien J, Veldtman G, et al: Aerobic capacity in adults with tetralogy of Fallot. Cardiol Young 12:554–559, 2002.
5. Li W, Davlouros PA, Kilner PJ, et al: Doppler-echocardiographic assessment of pulmonary regurgitation in adults with repaired tetralogy of Fallot: Comparison with cardiovascular magnetic resonance imaging. Am Heart J 147:165–172, 2004.
6. Silversides CK, Veldtman GR, Crossin J, et al: Pressure half-time predicts hemodynamically significant pulmonary regurgitation in adult patients with repaired tetralogy of Fallot. J Am Soc Echocardiogr 16:1057–1062, 2003.
7. Ilbawi MN, Idriss FS, DeLeon SY, et al: Factors that exaggerate the deleterious effects of pulmonary insufficiency on the right ventricle after tetralogy repair: Surgical implications. J Thorac Cardiovasc Surg 93:36–44, 1987.
8. Vliegen HW, van Straten A, de Roos A, et al: Magnetic resonance imaging to assess the hemodynamic effects of pulmonary valve replacement in adults late after repair of tetralogy of Fallot. Circulation 106:1703–1707, 2002.
9. Caldarone CA, McCrindle BW, Van Arsdell GS, et al: Independent factors associated with longevity of prosthetic pulmonary valves and valved conduits. J Thorac Cardiovasc Surg 120:1022–1030, 2000.
10. Bouzas B, Kilner PJ, Gatzoulis MA: Pulmonary regurgitation: Not a benign lesion. Eur Heart J 26:433–439, 2005.
11. Kawachi Y, Masuda M, Tominaga R, Tokunaga K: Comparative study between St. Jude Medical and bioprosthetic valves in the right side of the heart. Jpn Circ J 55:553–562, 1991.
12. Khambadkone S, Coats L, Taylor A, et al: Percutaneous pulmonary valve implantation in humans: Results in 59 consecutive patients. Circulation 112:1189–1197, 2005.
13. Therrien J, Siu SC, Harris L, et al: Impact of pulmonary valve replacement on arrhythmia propensity late after repair of tetralogy of Fallot. Circulation 103:2489–2494, 2001.

# Syncope in a Patient with Noonan Syndrome

**William Alazawi**

**Age: 32 years**
**Gender: Female**
**Occupation: Retail manager**
**Working diagnosis: Noonan syndrome**

## HISTORY

The patient was diagnosed with pulmonary stenosis and Noonan syndrome at birth in 1972 and underwent open pulmonary valvotomy at the age of 11 months. Her childhood and adolescent development were relatively normal, with the expected manifestations of Noonan syndrome. Her level of physical activity was not limited by shortness of breath, and she performed well academically at school. Her social development and interactions were normal.

In her early 20s, she noticed increasing shortness of breath with less exertion. Workup showed progressive pulmonary stenosis, and she underwent balloon valvuloplasty with a good result.

Since then she had no further dyspnea. She underwent a sterilization procedure at the time of her marriage, 4 years ago, without complication. Her career progressed and she held a number of posts in middle-level retail management.

Apart from hypothyroidism she has had no other medical problems. She is a nonsmoker and drinks alcohol only occasionally.

Two months ago the patient began to experience nonexertional dizziness and lightheadedness on occasion. She had two brief syncopal episodes with minimal exertion, which she recovered from spontaneously. At the same time, she noted some limitation in pursuing activities of daily living and was short of breath on minimal exertion. She presented for further workup.

**Comments:** Noonan syndrome is a common autosomal dominant condition characterized by dysmorphic facies, short stature, and congenital heart disease. Most commonly, the patients have pulmonary stenosis. The incidence is estimated at between 1 in 1000 and 1 in 2000 live births.[1]

Up to three quarters of male infants with Noonan syndrome may have undescended testes.[2] Cryptorchidism, in turn, may adversely affect fertility. In the presence of normally descended testes, men with Noonan syndrome are likely to be fertile. Pubertal development is delayed is both sexes, and fertility does not appear to be affected in females.

## CURRENT SYMPTOMS

The patient complained of episodic light-headedness and dizziness without palpitations. She was no longer able to climb the stairs in her house.

NYHA class: III

## CURRENT MEDICATIONS

Thyroxine 200 µg daily by mouth

## PHYSICAL EXAMINATION

Pink, comfortable at rest, characteristic facies of Noonan syndrome

BP 115/75 mm Hg, HR 75 bpm, oxygen saturation 96%

Height 135 cm, weight 50 kg, BSA 1.37 m$^2$

General: The patient had a webbed neck, low-set ears, and low hairline.

Surgical scars: Midline sternotomy scar

Neck veins: JVP was not elevated and was normal in character.

Lungs/chest: Chest was clear.

Heart: A grade 3 ejection systolic murmur was audible in the aortic area, radiating to the carotids, and a grade 3 ejection systolic murmur was also heard in the pulmonary area radiating to the back.

Abdomen: Soft with no palpable organs

Extremities: Warm and well perfused. The patient was not clubbed.

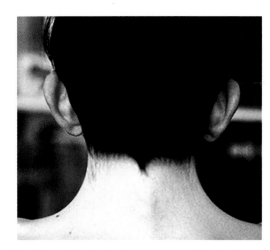

Figure 36-1 The webbed neck, low-set ears, and low hairline are typical features of Noonan syndrome. (From Digilio MC, Marino B: Clinical manifestations of Noonan syndrome. Images Paediatr Cardiol 7:19–30, 2001.)

***Comments:*** The normal jugular venous contour is notable in any patient with suspected right heart abnormalities.

It can be difficult to distinguish a murmur of aortic stenosis from pulmonary stenosis, particularly if both are loud. Position of the murmur differs, as well as duration of the murmur relative to the second heart sound. While right-sided heart murmurs and sounds typically may be augmented by inspiration, this may be difficult to appreciate when the murmur is loud. Murmurs due to pulmonary stenosis radiate more to the back than murmurs due to aortic stenosis, because of the more anteroposterior direction of the main pulmonary artery, compared to the ascending aorta.

## LABORATORY DATA

| | |
|---|---|
| Hemoglobin | 13.7 g/dL (11.5–15.0) |
| Hematocrit/PCV | 40% (36–46) |
| MCV | 88 fL (83–99) |
| Platelet count | $251 \times 10^9$/L (150–400) |
| Sodium | 139 mmol/L (134–145) |
| Potassium | 3.8 mmol/L (3.5–5.2) |
| Creatinine | 0.6 mg/dL (0.6–1.2) |
| Blood urea nitrogen | 4.0 mmol/L (2.5–6.5) |

***Comments:*** The patient was not anemic or erythrocytotic.

## ELECTROCARDIOGRAM

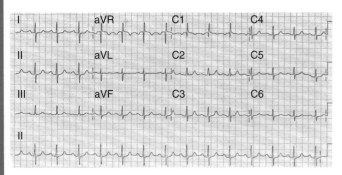

Figure 36-2 Electrocadiogram.

### FINDINGS
Heart rate: 77 bpm

QRS axis: –95°

QRS duration: 80 msec

Normal sinus rhythm, indeterminate axis, tall R-wave in V1

***Comments:*** The dominant R-wave in V1 and deep S-wave in V6 are consistent with RV hypertrophy due to pressure overload. There are no signs of LV hypertrophy. The superior axis is characteristic of patients with Noonan syndrome.

## CHEST X-RAY

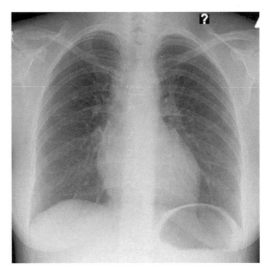

Figure 36-3 Posteroanterior projection.

### FINDINGS
Cardiothoracic ratio: 49%

Sternal wiring indicated a previous median sternotomy. There is no significant cardiomegaly, and the pulmonary vascular markings were normal.

***Comments:*** Findings on CXR in a patient with Noonan syndrome depend on associated lesions. Significant pulmonary stenosis with severe RV hypertrophy, AVSDs, and hypertrophic cardiomyopathy can all give cardiomegaly, while coarctation of the aorta will produce characteristic findings of the aortic knuckle (see Case 24).

## EXERCISE TESTING

Not performed

## ECHOCARDIOGRAM

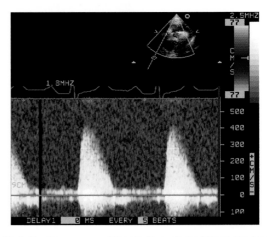

Figure 36-4 Continuous-wave Doppler through the left ventricular outflow tract (suprasternal notch view).

## FINDINGS

Suboptimal acoustic windows limited visualization of the cardiac chambers. There was normal LV size and systolic function, with no dynamic LVOT obstruction (Noonan patients may have hypertrophic obstructive cardiomyopathy). However, peak aortic valve velocity obtained by continuous wave Doppler in the apical four-chamber view was 3 m/sec (peak gradient of 36 mm Hg).

***Comments:*** Echocardiography is at times imperfect as a 2D imaging tool, as in this case. Doppler can be more sensitive, and a careful sonographer can identify key Doppler patterns in expected regions even when the 2D data are incomplete.

The flow acceleration found here is noteworthy. LVOT obstruction (most often secondary to asymmetric septal hypertrophy) is well described in patients with Noonan syndrome, though less common than RVOT obstruction. However, the Doppler pattern is not suggestive of dynamic LVOT obstruction (i.e., it does not have the relatively slow rise or late peak of velocity as is sometimes seen with hypertrophic obstructive cardiomyopathy). The 2D imaging was of insufficient quality to assess the cause of the obstruction.

# MAGNETIC RESONANCE IMAGING

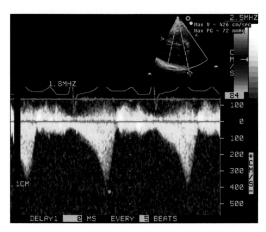

Figure 36-5  Continuous-wave Doppler.

## FINDINGS

The pulmonary valve was not well visualized in this patient's 2D images.

Continuous wave Doppler assessment across the pulmonary valve showed a maximal velocity of more than 4 m/sec, corresponding to a peak systolic gradient of over 70 mm Hg. There was mild pulmonary regurgitation.

***Comments:*** Both the RVOT and LVOT deserve careful scrutiny in any patient with Noonan syndrome and syncope.

Visualization of the pulmonary valve is more difficult in an adult than in children, but its anatomy may usually be appreciated from the parasternal short-axis view or sometimes the parasternal long-axis RV outflow view. A thickened and dysplastic appearance of the pulmonary valve is typical of Noonan syndrome.

For isolated pulmonary valve stenosis, Doppler-derived peak systolic gradient shows a good correlation with catheter peak-to-peak gradient. However, the modified Bernoulli equation is less reliable in the presence of multiple stenoses at various levels, as can sometimes be the case in this and other forms of congenital heart disease.

Still, the gradient suggested by these Doppler measurements is considerable. The late peaking jet suggests a dynamic component to the obstruction.

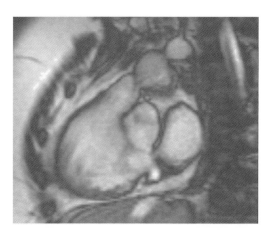

Figure 36-6  Magnetic resonance image.

## FINDINGS

There was RV hypertrophy with vigorous systolic function. The RVOT was narrowed at several levels. There was mild dynamic infundibular stenosis with a peak velocity of 1.7 m/sec. The pulmonary valve was stenosed with a maximal velocity of 2.5 m/sec. The sinotubular junction also appeared relatively narrow. There was mild pulmonary regurgitation. In mid systole, signal loss (black) was appreciated proximal to the valve leaflets within the infundibular area.

***Comments:*** This view of the RVOT demonstrates a discrete narrowing in the main pulmonary artery just above the pulmonary valve, as well as within the valve itself. Obstruction in Noonan syndrome may occur at any level of the RVOT. The pattern of turbulence seen here represents infundibular stenosis in addition to stenosis at other levels of the RVOT.

### Ventricular Volume Quantification

|  | LV | (Normal range) | RV | (Normal range) |
|---|---|---|---|---|
| EDV (mL) | 131 | (52–141) | 95 | (58–154) |
| ESV (mL) | 48 | (13–51) | 17 | (12–68) |
| SV (mL) | 83 | (33–97) | 78 | (35–98) |
| EF (%) | 63 | (57–75) | **82** | (51–75) |
| EDVi (mL/m²) | 96 | (62–96) | 69 | (61–98) |
| ESVi (mL/m²) | 35 | (17–36) | **12** | (17–43) |
| SVi (mL/m²) | 61 | (40–65) | 57 | (38–62) |
| Mass index (g/m²) | 76 | (47–77) | **65** | (20–40) |

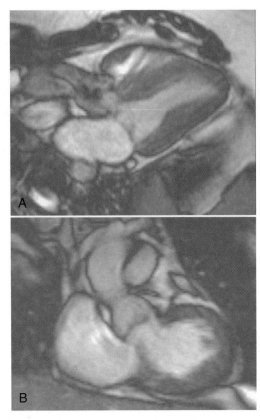

Figure 36-7 Oblique transaxial view, midsystole (**A**) and oblique coronal view (**B**).

## FINDINGS

During systole, the aortic valve leaflets were restricted and there was signal loss at the valve level. Above the aortic valve was a narrowing at the sinotubular junction, the site of supravalvular stenosis, with turbulence visible. In addition, there was evidence of narrowing at the sinotubular junction and of LV hypertrophy.

***Comments:*** These orthogonal views of the LVOT again indicate obstruction at three levels. The serial LVOT obstruction serves as a reminder that coexisting defects are often seen in congenital heart disease. Although less common, Noonan syndrome can also involve obstruction of the LVOT, usually with dynamic septal motion. Whether any of these, or their combination, could explain the patient's syncope is difficult to determine.

Although MRI allows quantification of velocity at a given plane, there is motion of that plane throughout the cardiac cycle, making accurate assessment of the velocity at each par-

ticular level challenging. Furthermore, Bernoulli's assumptions about velocity and pressure are less accurate when multiple stenoses are present.

## CATHETERIZATION

### HEMODYNAMICS

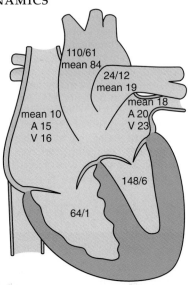

Figure 36-8 Hemodynamic data.

**Calculations**

| | |
|---|---|
| Qp (L/min) | 3.29 |
| Qs (L/min) | 3.13 |
| Cardiac index (L/min/m$^2$) | 2.28 |
| Qp/Qs | 1.05 |
| PVR (Wood units) | 0.30 |
| SVR (Wood units) | 23.67 |

### FINDINGS

Cardiac catheterization was done to formally measure hemodynamics and clarify the exact pressure gradients at the various levels of obstruction and obtain information on end-diastolic ventricular pressures.

The pressure gradient on slow withdrawal of the catheter across the RVOT was 50 to 60 mm Hg. The gradient across the LVOT was 30 mm Hg. The coronary arteries were normal.

***Comments:*** The findings confirmed the echo and MRI findings of gradients across both the RVOT and LVOT.

There was also a gradient between the mean wedge pressure (18 mm Hg) and the measured LV end-diastolic pressure (6 mm Hg).

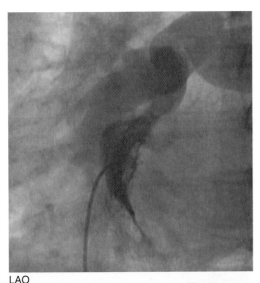

LAO

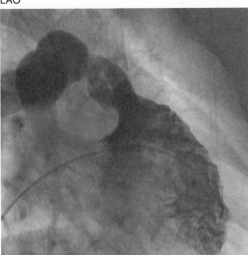

RAO

Figure 36-9 Right ventriculogram.

## FINDINGS

There was significant subvalvular and supravalvular RVOT stenosis.

**Comments:** The findings confirm the MRI and echo data. Ventriculography was not necessary here, but instructive nonetheless.

### FOCUSED CLINICAL QUESTIONS AND DISCUSSION POINTS

1. **What are the typical features of Noonan syndrome?**

*Noonan and Ehmke described the condition in the 1960s as an association between pulmonary stenosis and characteristic facial anomalies, short stature, webbed neck, chest deformity, and undescended testes. Facial features characteristic of Noonan syndrome are hypertelorism, epicanthic folds, slanted palpebral fissures, ptosis, flat nasal bridge, micrognathia, and low-set rotated ears with a thick helix. Pulmonary stenosis is the most common cardiac abnormality (40%); however, other associations include AVSDs (13.8%), coarctation of the aorta (12.5%), and hypertrophic cardiomyopathy (8.8%).[3] Obstruction of LV outflow is much less common and usually takes the form of asymmetric*

septal hypertrophy rather than valvular or supravalvular obstruction.[4]

*Easy bruising and abnormal bleeding are frequently reported and are due, at least in part, to partial deficiency of factor XI and anomalies of factors VIII and XII. The majority of children with Noonan syndrome have normal mental capacity and perform normally at school.*

*Fifty percent of cases are caused by missense mutations in the PTPN11 gene on chromosome 12, resulting in a gain of function of the protein SHP-2.[5] SHP-2 is involved in epidermal growth factor receptor-mediated signaling during semilunar valvulogenesis[6]; however, it has numerous other functions acting as both a positive and negative regulator of Jak-STAT and NF-kB signaling, hence the multisystem nature of the syndrome.*

2. **What is the cause of this patient's syncope?**

*It is very difficult to be certain which of the serial stenoses is responsible for the patient's symptoms. Aortic valve stenosis is a more likely cause of syncope than RV outflow obstruction. However, given that the LV-Ao gradient in this case was only 40 mm Hg, it seems hard to ascribe her syncopal events to this degree of obstruction alone. It may be that the combination of the serial right and LV outflow obstruction was significant enough to reduce cardiac output and result in syncope, and certainly larger gradients are created with exertion. Furthermore, patients with pulmonary stenosis in the setting of tetralogy have been shown to have an abnormal autonomic nervous system,[7] and this may also have contributed to syncope in this patient.*

*The other consideration is whether a transient arrhythmia could be responsible for her attacks, but there was no other evidence to suggest this, and a 24-hour ECG failed to show any arrhythmia.*

3. **Should the patient undergo a mechanical intervention?**

*This patient had already undergone both an open and a closed pulmonary valvotomy in the past, and now had significant restenosis across the RVOT. Isolated pulmonary valvuloplasty at this time would not be ideal, particularly given the serial stenoses at other levels in the RVOT and would be unlikely to significantly alter the hemodynamics. Surgical relief with implantation of a bioprosthetic valve in the pulmonary position was felt to be the way forward.*

*As repair of the RVOT may increase transpulmonary blood flow and accentuate the LVOT obstruction, it was again felt that the LVOT obstruction should be addressed concurrently.*

*The ultimate decision as to whether either valve could be repaired rather than replaced would eventually rest with the surgeon after directly inspecting each valve during surgery.*

## FINAL DIAGNOSIS

Noonan syndrome

Multilevel RVOT obstruction (infundibular, valvular, and supravalvular)

Multilevel LVOT obstruction (valvular and supravalvular)

## PLAN OF ACTION

Surgical relief of both RVOT and LVOT obstruction

## INTERVENTION

Intraoperatively, the findings overall were consistent with the preoperative assessment. The pulmonary valve was rigid and fibrosed. An RVOT repair was performed using a Gore-Tex valved prosthesis. Myotomy of the hypertrophied RV infundibulum was also performed.

The LVOT was very unusual. The aortic valve comprised four leaflets, unequal in size, aligned at different levels in a sort of spiral configuration, explaining the multiple levels of obstruction seen. One leaflet in particular appeared responsible for the majority of the obstruction, and was thus resected. The aortic root was reconstructed in such a way as to allow for repair of a competent aortic valve without obstruction. By TEE there was no further RVOT or LVOT obstruction at the conclusion of the procedure.

## OUTCOME

The postoperative recovery was complicated by recurrent episodes of laryngeal spasm that caused significant difficulty in extubation and in weaning from ventilatory support. However, her cardiovascular hemodynamics were excellent. After a prolonged stay in the intensive care unit, the patient recovered well and returned home. Her convalescence was otherwise unremarkable.

The patient returned back to her full-time work 3 months after her surgery. At 1-year follow-up she was in sinus rhythm with good biventricular function, no significant LVOT or RVOT stenosis, and a competent aortic valve. After 2 years the patient has had no further syncope and her exercise function has completely returned to normal.

The patient knows that she will require and benefit from lifelong cardiac follow-up.

## Selected References

1. Allanson JE: Noonan syndrome. J Med Genet 24:9–13, 1987.
2. Theintz G, Savage MO: Growth and pubertal development in five boys with Noonan's syndrome. Arch Dis Child 57:13–17, 1982.
3. Digilio MC, Marino B: Clinical manifestations of Noonan syndrome. Images Paediatr Cardiol 7:19–30, 2001.
4. Burch M, Sharland M, Shinebourne E, et al: Cardiologic abnormalities in Noonan syndrome: Phenotypic diagnosis and echocardiographic assessment in 119 patients. J Am Coll Cardiol 22: 1189–1192, 1993.
5. Tartaglia M, Mehler EL, Goldberg R, et al: Mutations in PTPN11, encoding the protein tyrosine phosphatase SHP-2, cause Noonan syndrome. Nat Genet 29:465–468, 2001.
6. Chen B, Bronson RT, Klaman LD, et al: Mice mutant for Egfr and Shp2 have defective cardiac semilunar valvulogenesis. Nat Genet 24:296–299, 2000.
7. Davos CH, Davlouros PA, Wensel R, et al: Global impairment of cardiac autonomic nervous activity late after repair of tetralogy of Fallot. Circulation 106(12 Suppl 1):I69–75, 2002.

# Dyspnea in a Patient with a Loud Murmur

Periklis A. Davlouros, Ageliki A. Karatza, and Dimitrios Alexopoulos

**Age: 39 years**
**Gender: Male**
**Occupation: Manufacturer**
**Working diagnosis: Heart murmur**

## HISTORY

The patient had been found to have a murmur at the age of 14. The character of the murmur was felt most compatible with a small, restrictive PDA. The patient felt well and was followed clinically for 25 years. The only advice he was given was endocarditis prophylaxis. He was asymptomatic and not limited with exertion.

Over the last 6 months, however, he began experiencing progressive exercise intolerance manifested as easy fatigability and exertional dyspnea. An echocardiogram failed to demonstrate the PDA, and the patient was referred for further evaluation.

He is a smoker, with mild hyperlipidemia and no other risk factors for coronary heart disease. There was no family history of congenital heart disease.

**Comments:** The typical murmur of a PDA is continuous and "machinery-like." It is usually quite characteristic. Many patients with small PDAs will not need intervention. If the shunt is very large in a baby, pulmonary hypertension may develop, eventually leading to reversed shunt and differential cyanosis (bluer toes than fingers).

The lack of a demonstrable PDA by echo is somewhat surprising, since the lesion, especially if small and restrictive as presumed here, is usually seen on color Doppler. However, one must also consider that the childhood diagnosis was incorrect, and that other explanations for both a murmur and worsening dyspnea must be entertained.

There are only a few hemodynamically significant congenital heart lesions that may first be diagnosed during adult life, either incidentally or due to the appearance of symptoms. More common among these is an ASD or, less commonly, Ebstein anomaly or significant pulmonary stenosis.[1–3]

## CURRENT SYMPTOMS

Although the patient continues to work full time, he becomes tired easily and needs to take rests more frequently than in the past. He notes feeling breathless more easily with mild exertion such as climbing two flights of stairs. He denies chest pain, palpitations, or syncope. He has never noticed cyanosis or ankle swelling.

NYHA class: II

## CURRENT MEDICATIONS

None

## PHYSICAL EXAMINATION

BP 130/80 mm Hg, HR 90 bpm, oxygen saturation 97% on room air (right hand)

Weight 90 kg, height 180 cm, BSA 2.12 m$^2$

Surgical scars: None

Neck veins: There was a prominent jugular A-wave. The central venous pressure was mildly elevated.

Lungs/chest: Chest was clear.

Heart: There was an RV lift and a palpable systolic thrill at the second left intercostal space. The first heart sound was normal, the second heart sound was widely split at the second left intercostal space, and a right-sided (augmented by inspiration) fourth heart sound was audible. There was a loud and harsh ejection murmur peaking late in systole, heard all over the precordium with maximum intensity (4/6) at the second left intercostal space and radiating to the back. There was no ejection click.

Abdomen: There was no ascites or hepatomegaly.

Extremities: There was no lower extremity edema. The skin was warm and dry.

**Comments:** There is no cyanosis at rest. Isolated pulmonary stenosis is not a cyanotic lesion, per se. However, arterial desaturation and cyanosis are not uncommon in patients with severe pulmonary stenosis due to right-to-left shunting through a patent foramen ovale or a coexisting ASD at rest and or during exercise.[3] Such patients may have a degree of secondary erythrocytosis, which in itself may suggest the presence of a right-to-left shunt.

A prominent A-wave is due to forceful right atrial contraction essential to fill a hypertrophied noncompliant RV due to increased RV afterload. A V-wave may be indicative of significant tricuspid regurgitation, which may appear late in the course of the disease, when a pressure overloaded RV decompensates and RV failure ensues. The murmur here is conspicuously not that of a PDA, and there were no signs of pulmonary hypertension. Instead, the systolic thrill at the second left intercostal space indicates turbulence in the RVOT. It is present in all but the mildest forms of pulmonary stenosis.[3] In this case, the characteristics and site of maximal intensity of the murmur indicate valvular stenosis, whereas infundibular stenosis is typically heard best at the third or fourth intercostal space.

Several characteristics indicate severe pulmonary stenosis: (1) A right-sided fourth heart sound, indicative of a hypertrophied and noncompliant RV; (2) a splitting of the second heart sound, which becomes wider in severe pulmonary stenosis due to delayed contraction of the infundibulum resulting in high pressure that delays valve closure (the pulmonary component is often not audible, however); (3) the lack of a systolic ejection click (the systolic ejection click may diminish in severe pulmonary stenosis); and (4) the long and late-peaking systolic ejection murmur. In cases of mild or moderate pulmonary stenosis, a loud ejection click is heard as the valve opens to its domed position. It has been suggested that in severe pulmonary stenosis with a hypertrophied, noncompliant RV, atrial systole may open the pulmonary vein to its "domed" position, and hence the ejection click will no longer be present. Inspiration with its increased systemic venous return may have a similar effect.[3]

## ELECTROCARDIOGRAM

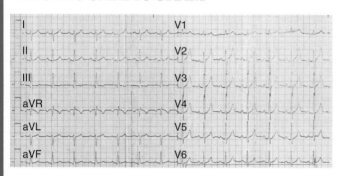

Figure 37-1 Electrocardiogram.

### FINDINGS

Heart rate: 84 bpm

PR interval: 160 msec

QRS axis: +110°

QRS duration: 85 msec

Normal sinus rhythm. Right-axis deviation to +110°. First-degree AV block. Dominant R-wave in lead V1 compatible with RV hypertrophy. No RA overload.

***Comments:*** A QRS axis of 110 degrees or more, an R/S ratio greater than 1 in lead V1 or V3R, an S-wave less than 2 mm in lead V1, and onset of intrisicoid deflection in V1 35 to 55 msec—all features of the current ECG—are considered to be indicative of RV hypertrophy.[4] The Sokolow-Lyon criteria of RV hypertrophy (R in V1 + S in V5 or V6 > 10.5 mm) are less specific. The first two criteria mentioned on the current ECG (the QRS axis and R/S in V1) have an accuracy of 78% for RV hypertrophy.[4]

There is a correlation between the ECG findings and the degree of pressure overload of the RV in patients with pulmonary stenosis.[3,4] More specifically, with peak Doppler gradients less than 60 mm Hg, the ECG may be entirely normal in 50% of cases. With more severe pulmonary stenosis, most ECGs show signs of RV hypertrophy. Patients with R-waves in lead V1 greater than 20 mm almost always demonstrate gradients greater than 100 mm Hg and vice versa. However, the ECG is only indicative of the degree of pressure overload of the RV. This correlation is even less satisfactory in other types of congenital lesions.[4] P-waves may be tall in inferior leads denoting RA hypertrophy.

## CHEST X-RAY

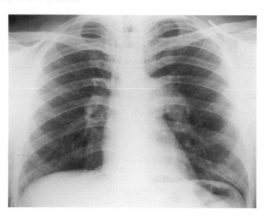

Figure 37-2 Posteroanterior projection.

### FINDINGS

Situs solitus, levocardia, left aortic arch, marked enlargement of the main and left pulmonary arteries, normal cardiothoracic ratio, normal peripheral pulmonary vascular markings.

***Comments:*** The rather prominent main pulmonary artery (PA) and the dilated left PA (perhaps due to preferential turbulent flow toward the latter through the stenotic pulmonary valve orifice) are the main features of the frontal chest radiograph in patients with pulmonary stenosis. The normal heart size is consistent with the absence of RV failure. However, RV enlargement may be evident in the lateral film.[1] Pulmonary vascularity is also normal, which precludes pulmonary oligemia as happens in patients with a right-to-left shunt through an ASD, or in patients with severely reduced RV cardiac output or RV failure.[3]

## LABORATORY FINDINGS

| | |
|---|---|
| Hemoglobin | 15 g/dL (13.0–17.0) |
| Hematocrit/PCV | 48% (41–51) |
| MCV | 90 fL (83–99) |
| Platelet count | $300 \times 10^9$/L (150–400) |
| Sodium | 139 mmol/L (134–145) |
| Potassium | 3.7 mmol/L (3.5–5.2) |
| Creatinine | 0.9 mg/dL (0.6–1.2) |
| Blood urea nitrogen | 5.0 mmol/L (2.5–6.5) |

***Comments:*** Most patients have normal blood chemistry. Secondary erythrocytosis may be present in patients with a right-to-left shunt through an ASD.[3]

## EXERCISE TESTING

| | |
|---|---|
| Exercise protocol: | Modified Bruce |
| Duration (min:sec): | 8:00 |
| Reason for stopping: | Dyspnea and chest pain |
| ECG changes: | None |

| | Rest | Peak |
|---|---|---|
| Heart rate (bpm): | 90 | 160 |
| Percent of age-predicted max HR: | | 88 |
| O$_2$ saturation (%): | 97 | 99 |
| Blood pressure (mm Hg): | 130/80 | 175/85 |

***Comments:*** Exercise capacity may be reduced in patients with significant RVOT obstruction, due to a fixed RV stroke volume and inadequate cardiac output (stroke volume × heart rate) during exercise.[5,6] Relief of the obstruction can be expected to lead to a significant improvement in cardiopulmonary performance.

# ECHOCARDIOGRAM

## OVERALL FINDINGS

There was severe RV hypertrophy but maintained RV systolic function. The LV was normal. Mild tricuspid regurgitation was present with an estimated RV systolic pressure of 65 mm Hg. There was significant flow acceleration across the RVOT (Vmax = 4.7 m/sec). The RA was mildly dilated. The LA was normal. The aortic and mitral valves were normal. There were no signs of a PDA. An ostium secundum ASD was suspected (faint jet of left-to-right shunting on subcostal interrogation of the interatrial septum with color Doppler) but not clearly demonstrated.

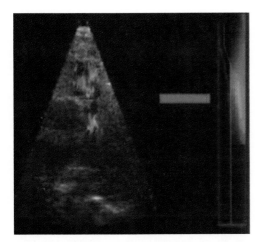

Figure 37-3 Parasternal short-axis view at the level of the great vessels (aortic valve seen in short axis).

## FINDINGS

The RVOT is superior with the main pulmonary trunk to the right of the image and the Doppler jet seen from top to bottom.

There is turbulent flow (color aliasing) across the RVOT, mainly at the level of the pulmonary vein. The valve itself, however, was difficult to visualize.

***Comments:*** Transthoracic echocardiography suggests the presence of a significant obstruction at the level of the RVOT. However, the poor echocardiographic window here did not allow for a clear assessment of the nature of the obstruction and the anatomy of the pulmonary vein and pulmonary arteries.

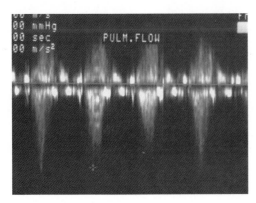

Figure 37-4 Continuous-wave Doppler tracing derived from the parasternal short-axis view at the level of the great vessels.

## FINDINGS

Peak velocity through the RVOT is 4.7 m/sec (under the curve, as the direction of flow is from top to bottom), suggesting an estimated peak pressure gradient between the RV and the main PA of approximately 88 mm Hg.

***Comments:*** Pulmonary stenosis is confirmed. Subvalvar stenosis is seen in approximately 40% of cases of valvar pulmonary stenosis due to infundibular hypertrophy. Ventricular "crosstalk" via altered RV geometry or bowing of the ventricular septum may also be evident, with resultant LV dysfunction or LV outflow obstruction, although uncommon.[3,7]

# MAGNETIC RESONANCE IMAGING

## OVERALL FINDINGS

Normal RV function and LV function. Dilated RA with a signal void toward it during ventricular systole (indicative of an ASD with left-to-right shunting), normal aorta and aortic arch, and an estimated pulmonary/systemic flow ratio (Qp/Qs) of 1.2:1.

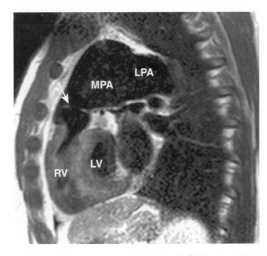

Figure 37-5 Spin echo sequences (black blood). Oblique sagittal plane.

### Ventricular Volume Quantification

|  | LV | (Normal range) | RV | (Normal range) |
|---|---|---|---|---|
| EDV (mL) | 138 | (77–195) | 184 | (88–227) |
| ESV (mL) | 46 | (19–72) | 74 | (23–103) |
| SV (mL) | 92 | (51–133) | 110 | (52–138) |
| EF (%) | 67 | (57–75) | 60 | (50–76) |
| EDVi (mL/m²) | 65 | (66–101) | 87 | (65–111) |
| ESVi (mL/m²) | 22 | (18–39) | 35 | (18–47) |
| SVi (mL/m²) | 43 | (43–67) | 52 | (39–71) |

## FINDINGS

The RV is hypertrophied and the pulmonary vein is thickened and doming during systole (*arrow*). There is severe dilatation of the main pulmonary trunk (55 mm, normally less than 27 mm) and of the left PA (40 mm, normally less than 25 mm).

***Comments:*** Due to the difficulties viewing the pulmonary vein clearly and the RVOT with echocardiography, a CMR scan was scheduled to clarify this patient's anatomy, particularly whether stenosis was valvular or subvalvular.

Valve thickening and doming during systole are the hallmarks of congenital pulmonary valve stenosis (PVS). Poststenotic dilatation of the main and left PA is present in most cases of valvar pulmonary stenosis regardless of the severity of stenosis.[1,8] This lack of correlation of PA dilatation with the severity of pulmonary stenosis is not well understood, but there may be some resemblance to the aortopathy seen with a bicuspid aortic valve. Intrinsic abnormalities of the medial wall of the great arteries have been shown in a wide spectrum of ACHD patients (including pulmonary stenosis), suggesting a possible genetic predisposition toward dilatation.[9]

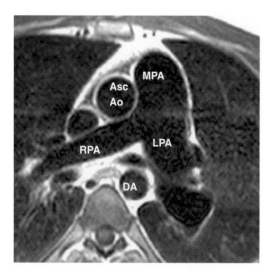

Figure 37-6 Transverse (transaxial) plane at the level of the pulmonary artery. Asc Ao, ascending aorta.

***Comments:*** Dilatation of the left PA is presumably due to preferential flow of blood toward the PA through the stenotic valve and the turbulence beyond it.[1,8] There are reports of spontaneous rupture of severely dilated pulmonary arteries (aneurysms) in the context of pulmonary stenosis, although this must be exceedingly rare in the absence of pulmonary hypertension.[10]

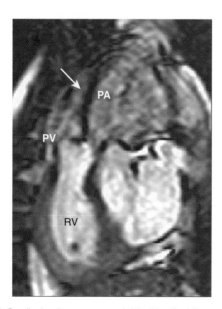

Figure 37-7 Gradient echo sequences (white blood), oblique sagittal view, mid systole.

## Findings

A long signal void (*arrow*) is shown, extending from the stenotic pulmonary vein to the "roof" of the main pulmonary trunk and toward the left PA.

***Comments:*** Pulmonary stenosis may be associated with other lesions. In our patient, an ASD (secundum type) was present. Signal void (loss of white color) in gradient echo sequences is similar to turbulent flow due to aliasing in color flow Doppler echocardiography. However, the size or intensity of CMR signal void does not reflect the magnitude of flow acceleration and thus the severity of the lesion (a large signal void does not reflect necessarily a great pressure difference between the two chambers). The long signal void can be "followed" from the pulmonary vein up to the main and left PA, where it "hits" against the arterial walls, perhaps explaining the preferential dilatation of these vessels.

The Qp/Qs of only 1.2:1 suggests either a small-sized ASD, or equalization of atrial pressures, or both.

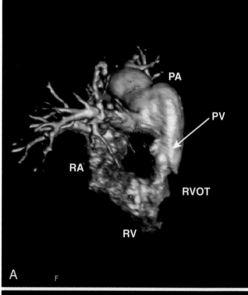

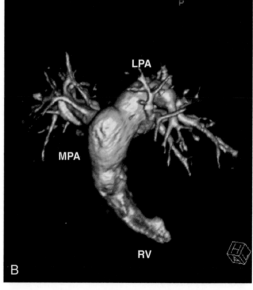

Figure 37-8 Three-dimensional reconstruction of cardiac magnetic resonance angiography (after gadolinium injection through a peripheral vein). **A,** The image corresponds to right anterior oblique projection of right ventricular angiocardiography. **B,** Modified left anterior oblique projection. PA, pulmonary artery.

## FINDINGS

Doming of the thickened pulmonary valve (*arrow*) and severely dilated main and left pulmonary arteries are seen in *A*. Dilatation of the main pulmonary trunk and left pulmonary artery is evident in *B*.

***Comments:*** MRA with gadolinium injection through a peripheral vein is a useful tool for the study of great vessel anatomy, for example, coarctation of the aorta, aortic and pulmonary arterial aneurysms, and so on.[11] Advances in postprocessing software allow the 3D reconstruction of images, which can be rotated by the workstation user in various directions. This aids in better understanding of the anatomy and detailed planning of the interventions needed.

## CATHETERIZATION

### HEMODYNAMICS

Heart rate: 80 bpm

| | Pressure | Saturation (%) |
|---|---|---|
| SVC | | 81 |
| IVC | | 77 |
| RA | mean 15 | |
| RV | 88/15 | |
| PA | 23/15 mean 19 | 81 |
| PCWP | mean 5 | |
| Aorta | 125/80 mean 92 | 98 |

**Calculations**

| | |
|---|---|
| Qp (L/min) | 7.95 |
| Qs (L/min) | 7.95 |
| Cardiac index (L/min/m²) | 3.75 |
| Qp/Qs | 1.00 |
| PVR (Wood units) | 1.76 |
| SVR (Wood units) | 9.68 |

## FINDINGS

Due to the patient's age and risk factors for coronary artery disease, coronary angiography was performed to assess coronary artery anatomy before cardiac surgery. Right heart catheterization (optional) was also performed to assess intracardiac and pulmonary arterial pressures and Qp/Qs.

The coronary arteries were normal. Mean right atrial pressure was normal. The RV systolic pressure was elevated (88 mm Hg). RV end-diastolic pressure was only mildly elevated (15 mm Hg) underlining the absence of severe RV failure. The pullback gradient through the RVOT was 65 mm Hg. Pulmonary arterial pressure and vascular resistance were normal. There was no shunt.

***Comments:*** The degree of RV hypertension reflects the severity of pulmonary stenosis. A RV systolic pressure of 60 to 100 mm Hg reflects at least moderate pulmonary stenosis.[3] The pullback gradient represents the peak-to-peak gradient between the two chambers and is somewhat less than the continuous-wave Doppler determined peak instantaneous gradient.

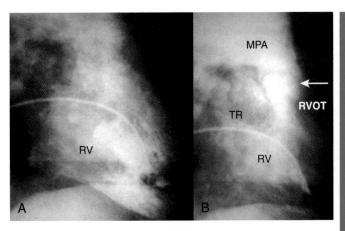

Figure 37-9 Right ventriculogram, right anterior oblique view, end diastole (**A**) and end systole (**B**).

## FINDINGS

RV systolic function is normal. There is mild tricuspid regurgitation. Secondary infundibular narrowing (RVOT) is present. The translucent area between the RVOT and main PA (*arrow*) represents the thickened and domed PV leaflets. The pulmonary annulus is of normal size. There is dilatation of the pulmonary trunk (MPA).

***Comments:*** RV angiography does not add particular anatomic or functional information in this patient, who has had thorough noninvasive imaging to assess pulmonary stenosis.

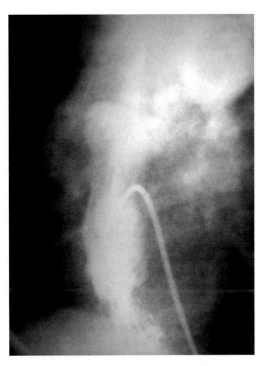

Figure 37-10 Right ventriculogram, left anterior oblique projection, end systole.

# FINDINGS

The pulmonary vein is thickened and domed, with a normal-sized pulmonary annulus. Secondary infundibular narrowing is present. Note a "small" hypertrophied RV at the end of systole.

## FOCUSED CLINICAL QUESTIONS AND DISCUSSION POINTS

1. What is the anatomical diagnosis?

*The patient has PVS, which represents 7% to 10% of CHD.[3,8] This lesion may be associated with other defects, as in our case, in which the patient had an ostium secundum ASD.[8]*

*Obstruction (stenosis) of the RVOT is usually classified as subvalvar, valvar, or supravalvar. In most cases of valvar pulmonary stenosis the pulmonary vein leaflets are fused, resulting in a dome-shaped valve. Some patients (10%–15%) demonstrate severe thickening of the leaflets, which however are not fused. Such valves are called "dysplastic" and are seen in the majority of patients with Noonan syndrome.[1,3,8] Williams and Alagille syndromes may also involve valvular pulmonary stenosis. Familial occurrence of valvar pulmonary stenosis has been described, and the probability of recurrence in siblings of affected patients is approximately 3%.[8] Acquired PVS is very rare in the context of rheumatic or carcinoid heart disease.*

*PVS usually progresses with time. However, this is a very slow process, and in some cases of mild to moderate stenosis it may even regress.[12] If the disease is mild in adulthood, it is unlikely the patient will ever need an intervention. This may not be true for neonates or infants, where disease progression can be faster.[13,14] Lifelong infrequent cardiac follow-up is, nevertheless, recommended even for the adult patient with mild pulmonary stenosis.*

2. What are the hemodynamic and clinical consequences for this patient?

*The RV remodels with hypertrophy to sustain the large pressure gradient across the valve. The RV stroke volume is thus maintained, however at the expense of an increased RV workload (RV strain). The RV stroke volume is relatively fixed due to the anatomic obstacle, so the only way to sustain an adequate cardiac output during exercise is an increase in heart rate (cardiac output = stroke volume × heart rate). The RV may sustain the increased workload for many years before dilatation and RV failure ensue. It is estimated that moderate pulmonary stenosis will progress to severe in approximately 10% of patients and usually happens at an early age, up to 12 years.[3]*

*Our patient remained asymptomatic for many years, having the erroneous diagnosis of a patent arterial duct. In asymptomatic patients pulmonary stenosis is usually discovered on routine clinical examination. If symptoms develop, they may be chest pain (RV demand ischemia), exercise-induced syncope (fixed RV stroke volume with inadequate increase in heart rate), exertional fatigue and dyspnea (inadequate RV cardiac output), or even cyanosis (right-to-left shunting through an ASD or a PFO if there is increased RA pressure). Patients with RV pressures lower than 60 mm Hg usually live normal lives.[3] Whereas patients with moderate to severe pulmonary stenosis may survive into adulthood, RV failure eventually ensues (usually after the fourth decade), and this is the most common cause of death. Survival is similar to the general population if appropriate intervention is performed in a timely fashion.[15] Atrial arrhythmias may appear later in life suggesting a change in the hemodynamic substrate (usually RV pressure overload and tricuspid regurgitation). However, sudden death is very rare.[3]*

3. Should the stenosis be relieved? What are the indications for intervention? Should the ASD be closed and the pulmonary arterial aneurysm addressed?

*The onset of symptoms (exertional dyspnea, angina, syncope, or presyncope), increasing RV hypertrophy on serial ECGs and echocardiograms, an RV systolic pressure higher than 55 to 60 mm Hg, and a peak-to-peak pulmonary transvalvular gradient higher than 50 mm Hg suggest that elective relief should be offered.[1,3,16] The last criterion is considered sufficient even for asymptomatic patients.[1] Our patient's ASD seemed hemodynamically insignificant; however, the Qp/Qs may be erroneously low due to high RA pressures during ventricular systole. After relief of PS this could potentially become a significant lesion. The aneurysmal dilatation of the PA has a theoretical risk of rupture, although this has to be exceedingly small in the absence of pulmonary hypertension.[10]*

4. Is the patient a good candidate for balloon valvuloplasty? What is the best approach to manage isolated severe pulmonary stenosis in the adult?

*Balloon valvuloplasty, first introduced in 1982,[17] is the treatment of choice for classic valvar pulmonary stenosis in both children and adults, with good short- and long-term results.[18–21] It is a safe procedure (<1% complications), less invasive and expensive than surgery, and can be repeated if needed, and resultant pulmonary regurgitation is rarely severe.[22] However, balloon valvuloplasty may be unsuccessful if the pulmonary vein is severely calcified or dysplastic (thickened leaflets without fusion). Surgical valvotomy and pulmonary vein replacement are the alternative options in such cases. Surgery is also preferred in cases of associated lesions that cannot be addressed percutaneously. Surgical pulmonary valvotomy is associated with lower residual pressure gradients and less need for reintervention compared to balloon valvuloplasty.[23]*

*In our case, the large main and left PA aneurysmal dilatation and the elective decision to perform reduction angioplasty on both influenced the decision for surgical treatment. We accept, however, that an alternative strategy could have been to balloon-dilate the stenosed pulmonary vein and choose not to intervene on the dilated pulmonary arteries.[10]*

# FINAL DIAGNOSIS

Isolated PVS

Severe "poststenotic" pulmonary arterial dilatation (aneurysm)

Ostium secundum ASD

# PLAN OF ACTION

Surgical repair and ASD closure

# INTERVENTION

The patient was operated on through a median sternotomy with systemic hypothermia (32° C) and cardioplegic circulatory arrest. An open pulmonary commissurotomy was performed. Pulmonary arterial plastic reconstruction was done to deal with the aneurysmal dilatation. A diamond-shaped part of the dilated main and left PA was excised and the vessel sutured. A longitudinal right atriotomy was done and the ostium secundum ASD was closed with a pericardial patch. The patient was rewarmed, and normal sinus rhythm returned spontaneously.

# OUTCOME

The patient had an uneventful postoperative course and was discharged home the fifth postoperative day. On the first follow-up visit in a week's time the patient was asymptomatic on regular walking and was looking well. He had a grade I–II systolic murmur of residual pulmonary stenosis, and his chest radiograph did not show a prominent main and left PA. His ECG did not differ substantially from the preoperative ECG. His echocardiogram disclosed RV hypertrophy with an RVOT pressure gradient of 29 mm Hg and no sign of pulmonary regurgitation. On the third follow-up visit in a month's time the patient had returned to regular everyday activity and reported greatly improved exercise capacity without exertional dyspnea. His exercise test was much improved (duration 14 minutes, maximum heart rate 180 bpm, peak blood pressure 170 mm Hg, no signs of ischemia, no arrhythmias, no symptoms). His ECG was almost the same apart from a QRS axis of 90°. There was mild RV hypertrophy on echocardiographic examination.

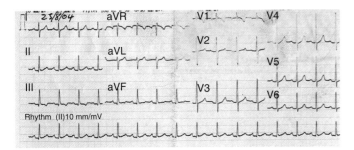

Figure 37-11 Postoperative electrocardiogram.

## FINDINGS

This ECG shows normal sinus rhythm, first-degree AV block (PR 200 msec), axis of 90° (improved), normal QRS duration (85 msec) with an RSr' morphology and negative T-waves in lead V1 and a tall R-wave in lead V2.

**Comments:** The ECG is suggestive of mild RV hypertrophy.

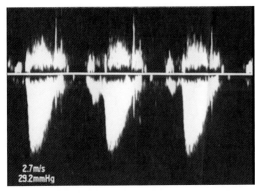

Figure 37-12 Continuous-wave Doppler at the right ventricular outflow tract level.

## FINDINGS

There is residual pulmonary stenosis (Vmax = 2.7 m/sec, PGmax = 29.2 mm Hg), but no pulmonary regurgitation.

**Comments:** This residual gradient is to be expected after either surgical or balloon valvotomy. However, in some cases a certain degree of residual gradient may be due to preexistent infudibular muscular hypertrophy. This infudibular hypertrophy regresses with time leading to a lower pressure gradient.[20,24]

## Selected References

1. Dore A: Pulmonary stenosis. In Gatzoulis M, Webb G, Daubeney P (eds): Diagnosis and Management of Adult Congenital Heart Disease. Philadelphia, Churchill Livingstone, 2003, pp 299–303.
2. Rigby ML: Atrial septal defect. In Gatzoulis M, Webb G, Daubeney P (eds): Diagnosis and Management of Adult Congenital Heart Disease. Philadelphia, Churchill Livingstone, 2003, pp 163–170.
3. Tynan M, Anderson RH: Pulmonary stenosis. In Anderson RH, Baker EJ, Macartney FJ, et al (eds): Paediatric Cardiology. London, Harcourt, 2002, I:1461–1479.
4. Chou T, Knilans T: Right ventricular hypertrophy. In Chou T, Knilans T (eds): Electrocardiography in Clinical Practice: Adult and Pediatric. Philadelphia, WB Saunders, 1996, pp 54–69.
5. Koenig PR, Mays W, Khoury P, et al: The use of exercise testing as a noninvasive measure of the severity of pulmonary stenosis. Pediatr Cardiol 18:453–454, 1997.
6. Steinberger J, Moller JH: Exercise testing in children with pulmonary valvar stenosis. Pediatr Cardiol 20(1):27–31; discussion 32, 1999.
7. Valdes-Cruz LM, Cayre RO: Anomalies of the right ventricular outflow tract and pulmonary arteries. In Valdes-Cruz LM, Cayre RO (eds): Echocardiographic Diagnosis of Congenital Heart Disease: An Embryologic and Anatomic Approach. Philadelphia, Lippincott-Raven, 1999, pp 325–348.
8. Rocchini AP, Emmanouilides GC: Anomalies of the right ventricular outflow tract and pulmonary arteries. In Emmanouilides GC, Allen HD, Riemenschneider TA, Gutgesell HP (eds): Heart Disease in Infants, Children, and Adolescents. Baltimore, Williams and Wilkins, 1995, II:930–962.
9. Niwa K, Perloff JK, Bhuta SM, et al: Structural abnormalities of great arterial walls in congenital heart disease: Light and electron microscopic analyses. Circulation 103:393–400, 2001.
10. Tami LF, McElderry MW: Pulmonary artery aneurysm due to severe congenital pulmonic stenosis. Case report and literature review. Angiology 45:383–390, 1994.
11. Geva T, Greil GF, Marshall AC, et al: Gadolinium-enhanced 3-dimensional magnetic resonance angiography of pulmonary blood supply in patients with complex pulmonary stenosis or atresia: Comparison with x-ray angiography. Circulation 106:473–478, 2002.
12. Gielen H, Daniels O, van Lier H: Natural history of congenital pulmonary valvar stenosis: An echo and Doppler cardiographic study. Cardiol Young 9:129–135, 1999.
13. Anand R, Mehta AV: Natural history of asymptomatic valvar pulmonary stenosis diagnosed in infancy. Clin Cardiol 20:377–380, 1997.
14. Rowland DG, Hammill WW, Allen HD, et al: Natural course of isolated pulmonary valve stenosis in infants and children utilizing Doppler echocardiography. Am J Cardiol 79:344–349, 1997.
15. Hayes CJ, Gersony WM, Driscoll DJ, et al: Second natural history study of congenital heart defects. Results of treatment of patients with pulmonary valvar stenosis. Circulation 87(2 Suppl): I28–I37, 1993.
16. Bonow RO, Carabello B, de Leon AC, Jr, et al: Guidelines for the management of patients with valvular heart disease: Executive summary. A report of the American College of Cardiology/American Heart Association Task Force on Practice Guidelines (Committee on Management of Patients with Valvular Heart Disease). Circulation 98:1949–1984, 1998.
17. Kan JS, White RI, Jr, Mitchell SE, et al: Percutaneous balloon valvuloplasty: A new method for treating congenital pulmonary-valve stenosis. N Engl J Med 307:540–542, 1982.
18. Chen CR, Cheng TO, Huang T, et al: Percutaneous balloon valvuloplasty for pulmonic stenosis in adolescents and adults. N Engl J Med 335:21–25, 1996.
19. Lip GY, Singh SP, de Giovanni J: Percutaneous balloon valvuloplasty for congenital pulmonary valve stenosis in adults. Clin Cardiol 22:733–737, 1999.
20. Sharieff S, Shah-e-Zaman K, Faruqui AM: Short- and intermediate-term follow-up results of percutaneous transluminal balloon valvuloplasty in adolescents and young adults with congenital pulmonary valve stenosis. J Invasive Cardiol 15:484–487, 2003.
21. Teupe CH, Burger W, Schrader R, et al: Late (five to nine years) follow-up after balloon dilation of valvular pulmonary stenosis in adults. Am J Cardiol 80:240–242, 1997.

22. Poon LK, Menahem S: Pulmonary regurgitation after percutaneous balloon valvoplasty for isolated pulmonary valvar stenosis in childhood. Cardiol Young 13:444–450, 2003.

23. Peterson C, Schilthuis JJ, Dodge-Khatami A, et al: Comparative long-term results of surgery versus balloon valvuloplasty for pulmonary valve stenosis in infants and children. Ann Thorac Surg 76:1078–1082; discussion 1082–1083, 2003.

24. Tabatabaei H, Boutin C, Nykanen DG, et al: Morphologic and hemodynamic consequences after percutaneous balloon valvotomy for neonatal pulmonary stenosis: Medium-term follow-up. J Am Coll Cardiol 27:473–478, 1996.

# Arrhythmia and Syncope in a Patient with a Childhood Murmur

**Ross J. Hunter, Arif Anis Khan, and Michael J. Mullen**

**Age: 47 years**
**Gender: Female**
**Occupation: Social worker**
**Working diagnosis: Childhood murmur**

## HISTORY

The patient had been followed for a murmur noted in childhood. After reaching adult life no further follow-up had been recommended. She felt well.

In her mid-40s, she visited her family doctor with episodes of palpitations and one syncopal episode, but no workup was ensued. Previously, she had had a hysterectomy for fibroids, but no other medical history. She did not smoke or drink. She had no other health problems, though recalled a tender swelling in her neck around a year ago that resolved spontaneously.

Over the preceding 6 months she complained of increasing frequency of syncopal episodes that seemed to be precipitated by exertion. Flecainide was prescribed empirically with little effect. She had increasing exertional breathlessness and fatigue, and was barely able to walk 100 m without stopping. She had had to quit work a month earlier and had not left the house for 2 weeks.

*Comments:* Innocent murmurs in childhood are common; echocardiography was not available in the 1960s and, thus, was not employed in our patient for evaluation of the murmur as is usually done today. As decades pass from a childhood diagnosis, patients are often understandably ill informed of an anatomical diagnosis or its pathological significance.

Unless the cause of syncope can be clearly established on clinical grounds, such as vasovagal syncope, a cardiac workup is indicated.

Empiric antiarrhythmic therapy is not recommended prior to the nature of arrhythmia or the cause of syncope being fully assessed and identified.

## CURRENT SYMPTOMS

The patient mainly complained of increasing breathlessness with exertion. She had syncopal episodes after mild exertion. She complained of swollen ankles and had gained 20 kg in weight over the last year. She had general constitutional upset, with malaise, fatigue, nausea, and vomiting.

NYHA class: III

*Comments:* In this context, a cardiac cause of syncope should be the primary concern. Syncope can occur due to supraventricular or ventricular tachycardia, or with episodes of bradycardia or heart block. Syncope on exertion may also suggest a structural cardiac cause such as aortic stenosis or hypertrophic obstructive cardiomyopathy.

## CURRENT MEDICATIONS

Flecainide 100 mg twice daily

Aspirin 75 mg daily

## PHYSICAL EXAMINATION

BP 100/60 mm Hg, HR 108, afebrile, oxygen saturation 94% on room air

Height 170 cm, weight 104 kg, BSA 2.22 m$^2$

Surgical scars: Hysterectomy scar was present, but no others.

Neck veins: Visible 3 cm above the sternal angle, with occasional cannon A-waves

Lungs/chest: Normal vesicular breath sounds throughout both lung fields

Heart: The rhythm was irregular. There was no right ventricular heave. There were no added heart sounds or murmurs. Both heart sounds were normal.

Abdomen: The patient was obese. The abdomen was not tender, and no organomegaly was noted.

Extremities: Mild bilateral pedal edema. Peripheral pulses were all palpable with normal pulse volume.

### PERTINENT NEGATIVES

There was no cyanosis or clubbing, and no splinter hemorrhages or any stigmata of endocarditis.

*Comments:* The patient has an irregular tachycardia and is mildly hypoxic.

The absence of a murmur limits the differential diagnosis, though severe regurgitant or even stenotic lesions can be inaudible.

## LABORATORY DATA

| | |
|---|---|
| Hemoglobin | 14.0 g/dL (11.5–15.0) |
| Hematocrit/PCV | 41% (36–46) |
| MCV | 92 fL (83–99) |
| Platelet count | $268 \times 10^9$/L (150–400) |
| Sodium | 135 mmol/L (134–145) |
| Potassium | 4.5 mmol/L (3.5–5.2) |
| Creatinine | 1.2 mg/dL (0.6–1.2) |
| Blood urea nitrogen | **7.3 mmol/L** (2.5–6.5) |
| Magnesium | 0.92 mmol/L (0.7–1.0) |

### OTHER RELEVANT LAB RESULTS

| | |
|---|---|
| TSH | **>100 pmol/L** (0.5–5) |
| Free T4 | **3.3 pmol/L** (7.5–21.0) |
| Thyroid peroxidase (Other autoantibodies all negative) | **1136 IU/mL** (<60) |
| Alanine transferase | **106 IU/L** (8–40) |
| Alkaline phosphatase | **148 U/L** (38–126) |
| Bilirubin | **2.4 μmol/dL** (3–24) |
| Albumin | **4.3 g/dL** (37–53) |

***Comments:*** The weight gain, fatigue, and malaise seemed likely to be a mixed picture of cardiac failure (although the normal JVP shows there is no right heart decompensation at present), rhythm disturbance, and hypothyroidism. The episode of tender neck swelling in the past suggests the patient may have subacute thyroiditis.

Hypothyroidism can occur in conjunction with Addison's disease as part of an organ-specific autoimmune disease (notably polyglandular autoimmune syndrome type II, which is hypo-adrenalism with either hypothyroidism and/or type I diabetes). Thyroxine replacement in an Addisonian state can precipitate Addisonian crisis. With the borderline low random cortisol level (which is difficult to interpret), a cortisol stimulation test was needed to rule out adrenal insufficiency, and in this case was normal. A raised alkaline phosphatase and other liver dysfunction are often present in hypothyroidism.

## ELECTROCARDIOGRAM

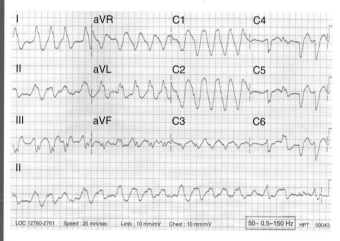

Figure 38-1 Electrocardiogram.

## FINDINGS

Heart rate: 117 bpm

QRS axis: −38°

QRS duration: 206 msec

There is an irregular, wide complex tachycardia, with widespread ST–T-wave abnormalities.

***Comments:*** The very broad QRS complex is suggestive of possible metabolic toxicity. Though the irregularity is very suspicious for atrial fibrillation, it can be difficult to distinguish whether a broad complex tachycardia is a ventricular or supraventricular tachycardia with a ventricular conduction defect.

Hypothyroidism can cause bradycardia and a prolonged QT interval and, if severe, can cause variable degree of AV block and bundle branch block.[1] Rapid atrial fibrillation is more common with hyperthyroidism.

## CHEST X-RAY

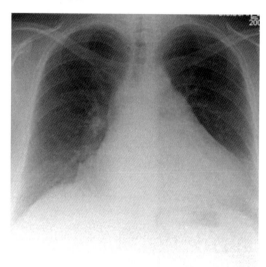

Figure 38-2 Anteroposterior projection.

## FINDINGS

Cardiomegaly with a cardiothoracic ratio of 60% and a straight left heart border.

***Comments:*** The opacity adjacent to the lower right heart border is more lucent than the adjacent cardiac tissue and likely represents a fat pad. One cannot exclude a pericardial effusion, as can be seen in hypothyroidism. Otherwise, the CXR and physical examination indicate that hypothyroidism is not the only cause of the patient's symptoms.

# ECHOCARDIOGRAM

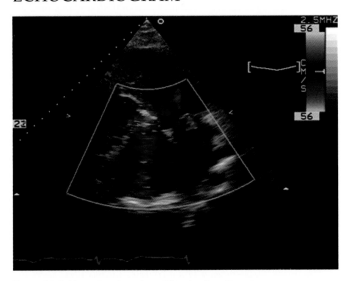

Figure 38-3 Four-chamber view, 2D color flow Doppler.

## FINDINGS

Normal LV and LA. The RV was severely hypertrophied with normal function. The RA was severely enlarged, and the atrial septum was bowed toward the left, indicating that RA pressure was greater than the left.

There was doming of the tricuspid valve during diastole, and moderate tricuspid regurgitation during systole.

**Comments:** The patient has structural tricuspid valve disease, demonstrating stenosis and regurgitation. The absence of an audible murmur is somewhat surprising, although atrial fibrillation would make this more difficult to detect. At the time of this echocardiogram, however, the patient was back in sinus rhythm.

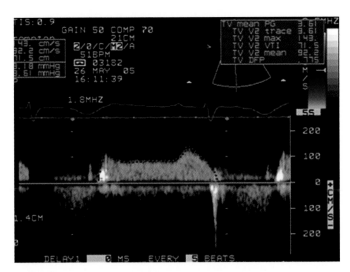

Figure 38-4 Pulsed-wave Doppler across tricuspid valve.

## FINDINGS

Sinus rhythm is present. Pulsed-wave Doppler across the tricuspid valve showed a pressure gradient throughout diastole. The mean velocity was 0.9 m/sec.

**Comments:** The Doppler data are consistent with mild tricuspid stenosis. The importance of sinus rhythm can be

appreciated here with the prominent A-wave following the P-wave on the ECG trace. There is considerable flow across the stenotic valve during atrial contraction.

Tricuspid stenosis is most commonly caused by rheumatic fever (in which case there is "always" other valve disease). Other causes include endocarditis with an obstructing vegetation, carcinoid syndrome, endomyocardial fibrosis, systemic lupus, trauma, and rarely congenital abnormalities. It occurs in less than 1% of patients in Western countries but is more common in parts of the world where rheumatic fever remains endemic. Symptoms are usually those of exertional fatigue due to reduced cardiac output, and peripheral edema and ascites due to elevated systemic venous pressure. Symptoms may rapidly worsen due to the onset of atrial fibrillation or flutter.

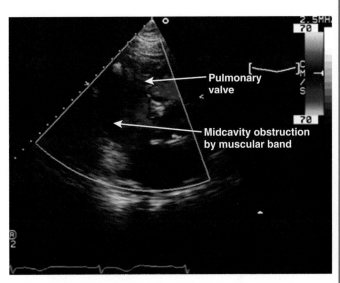

Figure 38-5 Parasternal short-axis view.

## FINDINGS

There was RV midcavity obstruction on 2D color flow Doppler. The peak velocity was 4.3 m/sec. There was no VSD.

**Comments:** The patient has another obstruction on the right side, this time a midcavity stenosis due to large trabecular bands across the infundibulum. This is consistent with a double-chamber RV.

A VSD can be difficult to detect. Because of the elevated pressure in the RV, which approaches systolic LV pressure, there is little gradient to drive flow across a VSD, which therefore may not be visible.

# MAGNETIC RESONANCE IMAGING

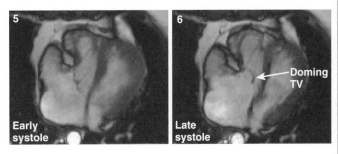

Figure 38-6 Oblique axial plane, four-chamber view.

## Ventricular Volume Quantification

| | LV | (Normal range) | RV | (Normal range) |
|---|---|---|---|---|
| EDV (mL) | 116 | (52–141) | 103 | (58–154) |
| ESV (mL) | 48 | (13–51) | 41 | (12–68) |
| SV (mL) | 68 | (33–97) | 62 | (35–98) |
| EF (%) | 59 | (58–76) | 60 | (53–77) |
| EDVi (mL/m²) | **52** | (59–93) | **46** | (57–94) |
| ESVi (mL/m²) | 22 | (16–34) | 19 | (14–40) |
| SVi (mL/m²) | **31** | (39–63) | **28** | (37–61) |
| Mass index (g/m²) | **45** | (48–77) | **40** | (19–39) |

## FINDINGS

The test was performed after sinus rhythm had been restored. RV and LV function was normal, but the RV was hypertrophied. There was doming of the tricuspid valve during early diastole.

***Comments:*** Note that the insertion point of the septal leaflet is in the normal position. Hence this is not Ebstein anomaly (see Case 31), but instead a different type of tricuspid abnormality.

The RV has an odd appearance, with much of it extending beyond the AV groove. The RV is hypertrophied. The RA is dilated, and in particular the RA appendage is quite prominent in this view.

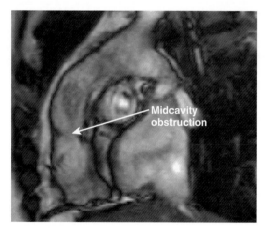

Figure 38-7 Sagittal view.

## FINDINGS

There was RV midcavity obstruction. No VSD was found.

***Comments:*** CMR can be invaluable in defining the anatomy of a complex RV, as in this case. The infundibular obstruction is easily seen, consistent with a double-chamber RV.

### FOCUSED CLINICAL QUESTIONS AND DISCUSSION POINTS

1. What is the anatomical diagnosis?

*The patient has congenital dysplasia of the tricuspid valve with tethering of the anterosuperior tricuspid valve leaflet to the septum. The RA is enlarged due to mixed tricuspid valve disease (stenosis and regurgitation).*

*In addition, there is muscular midcavity obstruction causing a double-chamber RV with a small functional RV and impaired RV outflow. The condition may cause progressive RV outflow tract obstruction and RV failure. It presents with a murmur, or with symptoms of exertional fatigue and edema.*

*In congenital tricuspid stenosis there can be varying abnormalities of the valves and chordae, sometimes with displacement of the valvular apparatus. Similarly, there are numerous subtypes of RV division, the most common of which is the double-chambered RV.[2] This is usually due to a thick muscular band that extends from the septum to the anterior RV wall below the level of the tricuspid valve. Occasionally, this may be caused by fibromuscular tissue or AV valve tissue. The defect is commonly associated with a membranous VSD (up to 90%), RVOT obstruction, or subaortic stenosis with LVOT obstruction.[3]*

*There is no clear explanation why this patient has these two abnormalities, as this combination is not a recognized entity.*

2. What is the original arrhythmia and what is its etiology?

*The initial ECG shows a broad complex tachycardia. There are no capture beats or fusion beats, no extreme axis deviation or positive concordance. The rate is irregular, and either P-waves or flutter waves can probably be seen in some leads (notably II). It is hard to see for certain whether the waves are associated with the QRS complexes or not, although it appears the waves are visible at regular points on the QRS complex. There is also an association between tricuspid valve disease (in particular Ebstein anomaly) and accessory pathways, so it is also worth considering an AV reentrant tachycardia.[4] It was thought on balance that this was likely to be atrial flutter with variable block and a wide QRS complex. An electrophysiology study could have clarified the nature of the arrhythmia, and should have been done.*

*The wide QRS must be explained. Electrolyte abnormalities such as hypomagnesemia, hyperkalemia, and hypocalcemia can sometimes be associated with abnormal depolarization, particularly QT prolongation,[5] although these were not found in this case. Hypothyroidism can alter the depolarization complex though not to this degree.*

*The patient is taking flecainide, and the QRS prolongation may be due to flecainide toxicity. Flecainide is a class Ic antiarrhythmic (Vaughan Williams classification). It is a potent blocker of fast sodium channels and is used for the suppression of supraventricular and ventricular tachycardias. It is a second-line agent to suppress supraventricular tachycardia in patients with a structurally normal heart without ischemic heart disease. Flecainide toxicity can occur with elevated or therapeutic levels, and includes nausea and vomiting, QRS prolongation and arrhythmia, hypotension, and dyspnea. Although there is no previous record of any interaction between the two, it is possible that the profound hypothyroidism may have contributed synergistically to flecainide toxicity.*

3. What are the management options?

*The first approach ought to be to clarify and treat the abnormal heart rhythm by withholding potentially harmful drugs (such as flecainide), correcting the metabolic abnormality, and restoring sinus rhythm. The patient is hemodynamically stable, so initial anticoagulation with low molecular weight heparin and other medication for rate control such as beta-blockers might be appropriate. Amiodarone might exacerbate both the thyroid problem and QRS deformity and should be avoided. Direct current cardioversion carries a risk of thromboembolism but should obviously be considered for patients with hemodynamically compromising tachyarrhythmias.*

*Thyroxine must be started slowly, as it may unmask subclinical ischemic heart disease and precipitate angina. A low dose is therefore started and slowly titrated up. Intravenous thyroxine is used only in cases of hypothyroid coma.*

*For the anatomical lesions, short-term symptomatic relief may be achieved with diuretics. Definitive treatment of tricuspid valve disease can be surgical commissurotomy or valve replacement. Less invasive methods include balloon valvuloplasty and percutaneous tricuspid valve replacement being performed experimentally in animals.[6]*

*Treatment for double-chamber RV treatment is surgical relief, although recently alcohol ablation of the tissue has been reported.[7] Indications for surgery may vary, although this is a progressive disease, and if a moderate or severe degree of stenosis is present, elective repair should be offered. In our patient, the unusual combination of serial right-sided stenoses and the development of symptoms (exertional dyspnea and fatigue, arrhythmia, and syncope) suggest that a surgical strategy may be required.*

## FINAL DIAGNOSIS

Congenital tricuspid stenosis

Double-chambered RV

Profound hypothyroidism secondary to subacute thyroiditis

Atrial flutter with variable ventricular response

Metabolic QRS repolarization abnormality due to presumed flecainide toxicity

## PLAN OF ACTION

Correction of toxic/metabolic abnormalities, rhythm control, followed by reassessment of hemodynamics

## INTERVENTION

None

## OUTCOME

The flecainide level on admission was 1530 µg/L (normal range 200–700). After 48 hours of withholding the drug, the patient's QRS complexes had returned to near normal duration and flutter waves were more clearly visible with a ventricular rate of over 100 bpm (Figs. 38-8 and 38-9). At this stage metoprolol was started at a low dose of 25 mg twice daily to control her ventricular response. Thyroid replacement was also started under endocrinologic guidance.

Despite rate control, the patient remained unwell, light-headed on exertion, and borderline hypotensive. With the degree of RA enlargement and the anatomical problems, it was thought that further rate control would not be successful. More definitive arrhythmia treatment in the form of atrial flutter ablation was pursued next.

The patient underwent an invasive electrophysiologic study and ablation of atrial flutter 6 days after admission and was converted to normal sinus rhythm (see Fig. 38-9).

While in sinus rhythm her blood pressure and lightheadedness improved. Her constitutional symptoms and lethargy also seem to vanish during the ensuing weeks. She was no longer lightheaded or presyncopal. She was able to walk around the hospital ward normally. She was discharged on metoprolol 25 mg twice daily and thyroxine 25 µg daily. The dose was titrated up to 75 µg over the next month before rechecking thyroid function.

It was agreed that repeat imaging and objective exercise capacity (including $MVo_2$) would be obtained and reviewed in 6 months' time with a view to assessing further the need

for surgery on the tricuspid valve and the double-chambered RV.

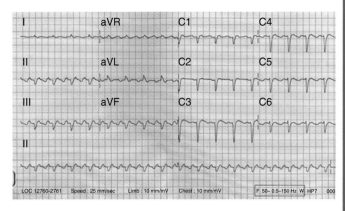

Figure 38-8 ECG 3 days after flecainide cessation.

## FINDINGS

The QRS duration is reduced to 120 msec, and flutter waves are now clearly visible. The ventricular rate remains fast at 103 bpm. There is also poor R-wave progression and T-wave inversion across anterior and lateral chest leads.

**Comments:** The flecainide toxicity has rapidly resolved and hence the normalization of the QRS complexes. There is still atrial flutter with a fairly rapid ventricular response. The thyroid abnormality would not be corrected this quickly, and thus it is less likely that thyroid disease was contributing to the problem.

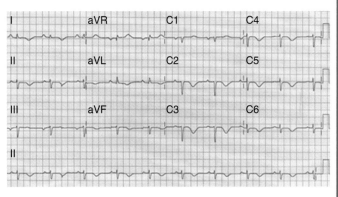

Figure 38-9 ECG after isthmus ablation 6 days after flecainide cessation.

## FINDINGS

Normal sinus rhythm at 57 bpm. There is a first-degree heart block. The QRS duration is normal at 93 msec. There is poor R-wave progression with left-axis deviation (axis −72°) and inverted T-waves anterolaterally. QT prolongation is also present.

**Comments:** The isthmus (atrial flutter) ablation has restored sinus rhythm, and the QRS duration has returned to normal 6 days after stopping flecainide. The first-degree heart block could be due to the low dose of beta-blocker, or more likely due to hypothyroidism. There is no evidence of RA hypertrophy or RV strain.

A case series of ECGs in double-chamber RV showed that ECG changes were largely dependent on the coexisting abnormalities such as VSD.[8] RV hypertrophy was common, but in nearly half the only sign was an upright T-wave in RV3. In this case the tricuspid stenosis may have protected the right heart from strain.

## Selected References

1. Slovis C, Jenkins R: ABC of clinical electrocardiography: Conditions not primarily affecting the heart. BMJ 325:259, 2002.
2. Restivo A, Cameron AH, Anderson RH, Allwork SP: Divided right ventricle: A review of its anatomical varieties. Pediatr Cardiol 5:197–204, 1984.
3. Vogel M, Smallhorn JF, Freedom RM, et al: An echocardiographic study of the association of ventricular septal defect and right ventricular muscle bundles with a fixed subaortic abnormality. Am J Cardiol 61:857–860, 1988.
4. Smith WM, Gallagher JJ, Kerr CR, et al: The electrophysiologic basis and management of symptomatic recurrent tachycardia in patients with Ebstein's anomaly of the tricuspid valve. Am J Cardiol 49:1223–1234, 1982.
5. Golzari H, Dawson NV, Speroff T, Thomas C: Prolonged QTc intervals on admission electrocardiograms: Prevalence and correspondence with admission electrolyte abnormalities. Conn Med 71:389–397, 2007.
6. Boudjemline Y, Agnoletti G, Bonnet D, et al: Steps toward the percutaneous replacement of atrioventricular valves: An experimental study. J Am Coll Cardiol 46:360–365, 2005.
7. Tsuchikane E, Kobayashi T, Kirino M, et al: Percutaneous myocardial ablation in double chamber right ventricle. Catheter Cardiovasc Interv 49:97–101, 2000.
8. Goitein KJ, Neches WH, Park SC, et al: Electrocardiogram in double chamber right ventricle. Am J Cardiol 45:604–608, 1980.

# Right Ventricular Outflow Obstruction in a Pregnant Woman

Nigel E. Drury, Christoph Kiesewetter, and Gruschen R. Veldtman

**Age: 19 years**
**Gender: Female**
**Occupation: Waitress**
**Working diagnosis: Ventricular septal defect**

## HISTORY

The patient originally presented at 2 weeks of age with heart failure and a murmur. A perimembranous VSD was diagnosed on echocardiography, and she responded well to medical treatment with diuretics and digoxin. The VSD partially closed spontaneously, and medication was ceased at 18 months of age. The patient thrived and had regular follow-up during her childhood.

Three years ago (16 years old) she reported breathlessness on exercise with an associated cough. She had had several admissions with wheezing and had a strong family history of atopy. An echocardiogram showed that the perimembranous VSD was still present with a left-to-right ventricular pressure gradient of 66 mm Hg and no evidence of volume loading of the left heart. Exercise stress testing was normal. Following this assessment, she did not attend further follow-up appointments.

She is a smoker.

*Comments:* VSD is the most common congenital heart defect (2 out of 1000 live births), representing more than 30% of cardiac malformations. However, more than 50% of patients undergoing surgery for a primary VSD have an associated lesion, either congenital or acquired.[1]

Patients with small defects may never need intervention, and, for this reason, it is tempting to discharge them from follow-up. Nevertheless, continued surveillance may be useful for the detection of acquired complications including aortic regurgitation, unexpected left ventricular volume loading, subaortic fibromuscular stenosis[2] (see Case 21), or RVOT obstruction (3%–10% of cases).[3] Of note, in adults, the RVOT is often difficult to image and the associated obstructive lesion may be missed.

## CURRENT SYMPTOMS

The patient presented again at 19 years of age, when she was 16 weeks pregnant, with increasing dyspnea on exertion, having to sit down to catch her breath after climbing two flights of stairs. She experienced exertional palpitations but denied chest pain, syncope, or ankle swelling.

NYHA class: II

*Comments:* The presence of worsening symptoms should alert the physician to the development of other problems.

Although pregnancy itself may precipitate dyspnea, symptom onset in early gestation is suspicious of underlying hemodynamic compromise. Signs suggestive of important right ventricular outflow obstruction in patients with a VSD include cyanosis as well as exertional fatigue and dyspnea.

## CURRENT MEDICATIONS

None

## PHYSICAL EXAMINATION

BP 110/70 mm Hg, HR 95 bpm, oxygen saturation 98%

Height 147 cm, weight 52 kg, BSA 1.46 m$^2$

Surgical scars: None

Neck veins: JVP was elevated to 4 cm above the sternal angle with a prominent A-wave.

Lungs/chest: Chest was clear.

Heart: There was an RV lift with a palpable thrill at the upper left sternal edge. A grade 4 ejection systolic murmur was heard at the upper left sternal edge in addition to a softer holosystolic systolic murmur lower down the sternal edge. The ejection systolic murmur relatively obscured the holosystolic murmur. Peripheral pulses were normal.

Abdomen: A gravid uterus was palpable.

### PERTINENT NEGATIVES
There was no peripheral edema, clubbing, RV third or fourth heart sounds, or hepatomegaly.

*Comments:* Oxygen saturations were normal, indicating either a left-to-right shunt or no significant shunt.

In pregnancy, the central venous pressures may be increased due to volume loading. However, in this patient the waveform was abnormal suggesting raised RV end-diastolic pressure and RV hypertrophy. The absence of a prominent CV-wave implied that any tricuspid regurgitation was insignificant or chronic.

A loud, harsh ejection systolic murmur, peaking in intensity near midsystole and loudest in the mid to upper left precordium, is characteristic of a double-chambered RV. The auscultatory characteristics of the VSD are determined by its location in relation to the RV cavity obstruction. If the VSD opens into the high-pressure proximal chamber, the "VSD" murmur may be softer or absent.

## LABORATORY DATA

| | |
|---|---|
| Hemoglobin | **11.3 g/dL** (11.5–15.0) |
| Hematocrit | **33%** (36–46) |
| MCHC | 33.5 g/dL (32–36) |
| MCV | 91 fL (83–99) |
| Platelet count | 280 × 10⁹/L (150–400) |
| Sodium | 136 mmol/L (134–145) |
| Potassium | 3.5 mmol/L (3.5–5.2) |
| Creatinine | 0.63 mg/dL (0.6–1.2) |
| Blood urea nitrogen | 2.7 mmol/L (2.5–6.5) |

***Comments:*** Red cell mass increases in a linear fashion throughout pregnancy; however, plasma volume expands more rapidly, producing a decline in hemoglobin concentration, hematocrit, and red cell count, particularly during the second trimester (see also Case 75). The mean corpuscular hemoglobin concentration remains constant. These physiological changes in oxygen carrying capacity may become more significant when cardiac reserve is limited. The relatively low hemoglobin was also consistent with the absence of a resting or exercise-induced right-to-left shunt.

## ELECTROCARDIOGRAM

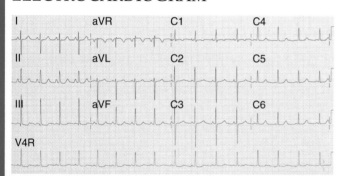

Figure 39-1 Electrocardiogram.

### FINDINGS

Heart rate: 95 bpm

PR interval: 158 msec

QRS axis: +106°

QRS duration: 62 msec

There was sinus rhythm with prominent P-waves in I and II, which were also peaked in V2 and V3 (right atrial overload). The QRS axis was deviated to the right. There were dominant, almost pure R-waves in V4R and V1.

***Comments:*** The electrocardiogram showed a right dominant picture with RA overload, right-axis deviation, and RV hypertrophy, as suggested by the dominant R-waves in V4R and V1. These abnormalities cannot be explained by a small VSD, where the ECG would be normal. The RV hypertrophy suggests important RVOT obstruction in the absence of pulmonary hypertension.

## CHEST X-RAY

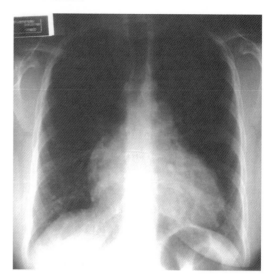

Figure 39-2 Posteroanterior projection.

### FINDINGS
Cardiothoracic ratio: 64%

The cardiac silhouette was enlarged. There was prominence of the RA. The main pulmonary artery may be enlarged. There were no features of cardiac failure, and the lungs and pleural spaces were clear.

***Comments:*** RA enlargement reflects RV hypertrophy and raised RV end-diastolic pressure and perhaps tricuspid regurgitation.

## ECHOCARDIOGRAM

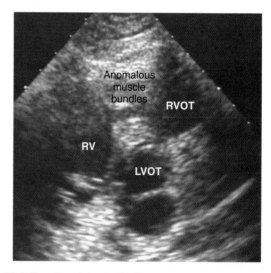

Figure 39-3 Parasternal short-axis view.

### FINDINGS
There was a discrete ridge at the infundibular os giving rise to a tight stenosis. RV systolic pressure was estimated at 145 mm Hg, from a tricuspid regurgitant jet having assumed an RA pressure of 10 mm Hg. The RV was hypertrophied with good systolic function.

A small perimembranous VSD was visible with some aortic override. There was no LA or LV volume overload. There was a small discrete subaortic membrane but no significant resting gradient. There was no aortic valve cusp prolapse.

**Comments:** The patient can be said to have a "double-chambered" RV. Essentially, there are proximal muscle bundles within the body of the RV producing an area of stenosis. Proximal to this the RV is under high pressure and hypertrophied, and distal to this the RV and the RVOT are under low pressure and may dilate. The presence of severe stenosis was confirmed with suprasystemic RV pressures in the proximal chamber.

A double-chambered RV is a condition commonly associated with a VSD, as in this case. If the VSD is proximal to the obstruction, there may be little shunt, as the RV and LV pressures may be equal.

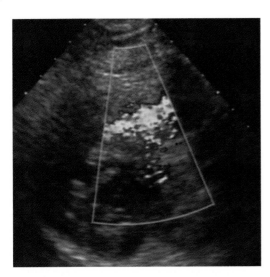

Figure 39-4 Parasternal short-axis view, 2D color Doppler.

## FINDINGS

There was turbulent flow between the proximal and distal RV chambers across the stenosis. Color flow was also seen through the VSD with a left-to-right shunt into the distal chamber.

**Comments:** The VSD communicated with the low-pressure distal RV compartment allowing continuation of the modest left-to-right shunt through the VSD.

Echocardiography is a valuable tool in the diagnosis of double-chambered RV in adults. TEE or MRI may be used as an adjunctive investigation, giving enhanced definition of the lesion and improving diagnostic accuracy.[4]

## MAGNETIC RESONANCE IMAGING

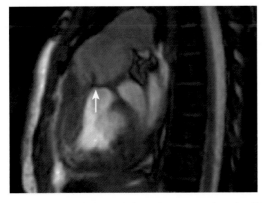

Figure 39-5 Oblique sagittal steady-state free precession cine (right ventricular outflow tract view).

## FINDINGS

The RV was severely hypertrophied but had maintained systolic function. A double-chambered RV type of stenosis with a dense band of muscles spanning the lower RVOT was seen, with a discrete jet of turbulence created by the muscle bands (above the *arrow*).

**Comments:** Again, the RV appears divided into two chambers above and below the thick muscle band, and in this entity there are always ventricular trabeculations in the distal chamber.

The VSD is not seen in this view.

### FOCUSED CLINICAL QUESTIONS AND DISCUSSION POINTS

1. **How common is a double-chambered RV in adults? What other lesions are associated with it?**

   *A double-chambered RV most commonly presents in infancy and early childhood but has a prevalence of 2% among adult congenital heart disease patients.[5] It is typically associated with a perimembranous VSD in more than 75% of cases, although the diagnosis may be missed if the murmur is not differentiated from that caused by the VSD. It is also reported in conjunction with other congenital defects including discrete subaortic stenosis, valvar pulmonary stenosis, tetralogy of Fallot, and double-outlet RV.[6]*

2. **What are the anatomical and pathophysiological features of double-chambered RV?**

   *Double-chambered RV is a form of RVOT obstruction characterized by anomalous muscle bundles that divide the RV into a high-pressure proximal chamber and a low-pressure distal chamber. These abnormal hypertrophic bundles usually arise from the septomarginal trabeculation and pass across the RV to the anterior free wall.[7] There are two basic morphological patterns with the bundles running either diagonally across the apical component of the RV or horizontally higher across the outflow tract. While the abnormal location of the prominent muscle bands is probably congenital, hemodynamic perturbations resulting from associated lesions such as a VSD lead to progressive hypertrophy and acquired obstruction.[6] As the VSD may communicate with either the proximal or distal chamber of the RV, the shunt may become right to left in some patients.*

3. **What are the hemodynamic effects of pregnancy in RVOT obstruction? How should this patient be managed?**

   *During pregnancy, cardiac output increases by approximately 40%, an absolute increase of 1.5 L/min, primarily during the first trimester. In the absence of a VSD, RV outflow obstruction can precipitate RV failure and reduce LV preload, particularly during labor when aortocaval compression and vasodilatation associated with neuraxial sympathetic block may be encountered. In our patient, left-to-right shunting through the VSD augmented pulmonary flow and LV preload, thereby reducing the relative risk of pregnancy.*

   *Antenatal management includes optimization of maternal medical status including correction of any anemia. From the cardiac point of view, early recognition and management of atrial arrhythmias will assist in completing the pregnancy. The development of RV dysfunction and failure may require early delivery. Peripartum management should be in a tertiary center, with adult congenital cardiology and anesthesia support. Delivery may be vaginal with an assisted second stage. Use of epidural anesthesia should be judicious to avoid hypotension; adequate preloading is preferential to ephedrine-based preparations, which may exacerbate the RV outflow obstruction. Arterial and central venous pressure monitoring may be useful in some patients.*

*Ideally, any outflow tract obstruction should be relieved before pregnancy is initiated. Appropriate contraceptive advice should therefore be given (see Cases 32 and 83). Following repair, patients are at low risk of pregnancy-associated complications.[6]*

4. **What are the indications for intervention in adults with double-chambered RV?**

*RVOT obstruction tends to progress fairly rapidly in adolescents and young adults, with the gradient increasing by a mean of over 6 mm Hg per year on echocardiography.[5] As the obstruction is anatomical, usually without a dynamic component, there is little place for medical therapy in most patients.[6] Surgical repair is recommended when symptoms or associated lesions are present or when there is significant asymptomatic obstruction with a peak pressure gradient equal to 40 mm Hg.[8] Resection yields excellent hemodynamic and functional short- and long-term results, with reoperation seldom being needed.[9,10]*

## FINAL DIAGNOSIS

Double-chambered RV with a perimembranous VSD and pregnancy

## PLAN OF ACTION

Observe elective delivery with assisted second stage of labor and arterial monitoring

## INTERVENTION

Delayed cardiac surgery

## OUTCOME

Management objectives were to maintain stable cardiac function, detect cardiac complications precipitated by the hemodynamic changes of pregnancy, and deliver a healthy term or near-term infant under controlled conditions before proceeding to maternal cardiac surgical repair.

The patient was admitted at 24 weeks gestation with progressive dyspnea for a period of observation and strict bed rest. She was asymptomatic at rest, and her blood pressure was steady around 90 mm Hg systolic without medication.

She remained hemodynamically stable and had an uneventful delivery at 36 weeks gestation by cesarean section for obstet-

ric reasons. A subsequent echocardiogram demonstrated well-preserved RV systolic function and no worsening of tricuspid regurgitation.

Approximately 1 year following her pregnancy, surgical correction of the double-chambered RV was performed electively. On-table TEE was used to further assess her anatomy. Surgery was uneventful with relief of the RVOT obstruction and closure of the perimembranous VSD. The patient made a good recovery, complicated only by a superficial sternal wound infection. A postoperative echocardiogram showed laminar flow in the RVOT with no residual obstruction.

The patient remains well and asymptomatic 3 years after surgery, without any evidence of recurrence of the obstruction.

## Selected References

1. Walters HL III, Delius RE. Ventricular septal defect. In Tang A, Ohri SK, StephensonLW (eds): Key Topics in Cardiac Surgery. London, Taylor & Francis, 2005, pp 254–257.
2. Vogel M, Smallhorn JF, Freedom RM, et al: An echocardiographic study of the association of ventricular septal defect and right ventricular muscle bundles with a fixed subaortic abnormality. Am J Cardiol 61: 857–860, 1988.
3. Pongliglione G, Freedom RM, Cook D, Rowe RD: Mechanisms of acquired right ventricular outflow tract obstruction in patients with ventricular septal defect: An angiocardiographic study. Am J Cardiol 50: 776–780, 1982.
4. Hoffman P, Wójcik AW, Rózanski J, et al: The role of echocardiography in diagnosing double chambered right ventricle in adults. Heart 90: 789–793, 2004.
5. Oliver JM, Garrido A, Gonzalez A, et al: Rapid progression of midventricular obstruction in adults with double-chambered right ventricle. J Thorac Cardiovasc Surg 126:711–717, 2003.
6. McElhinney DB, Goldmuntz E: Double-chambered right ventricle. In Gatzoulis MA, Webb GD, Daubeney PEF (eds): Diagnosis and Management of Adult Congenital Heart Disease. Edinburgh, Churchill Livingstone, 2003, pp 305–311.
7. Alva C, Ho SY, Lincoln CR, et al: The nature of obstructive muscular bundles in double-chambered right ventricle. J Thorac Cardiovasc Surg 117: 1180–1189, 1999.
8. McElhinney DB, Chatterjee KM, Reddy VM: Double-chambered right ventricle presenting in adulthood. Ann Thorac Surg 70: 124–127, 2000.
9. Galal O, Al-Halees Z, Solymar L, et al: Double-chambered right ventricle in 73 patients: Spectrum of the disease and surgical results of transatrial repair. Can J Cardiol 16: 167–174, 2000.
10. Hachiro Y, Takagi N, Koyanagi T, et al: Repair of double-chambered right ventricle: Surgical results and long-term follow-up. Ann Thorac Surg 72: 1520–1522, 2001.

# Part III
# Tetralogy of Fallot

# Late Repair of Tetralogy of Fallot

**Henryk Kafka**

**Age: 60 years**
**Gender: Female**
**Occupation: Seamstress**
**Working diagnosis: Tetralogy of Fallot**

## HISTORY

This patient was born during the closing days of World War II. She was noted to be cyanosed at birth. During childhood she had periods of breathlessness and was noted to squat. Because of severe breathlessness with exercise, she was referred for a right Blalock shunt at age 11. The right pulmonary artery could not be identified and the procedure was abandoned in the belief that she had pulmonary atresia.

Clinical examination at age 15 supported a diagnosis of TOF. Her ECG showed RV hypertrophy but no RBBB. At that time, cardiac catheterization confirmed an 18-mm VSD, subinfundibular stenosis, as well as valvular and supravalvular pulmonary stenoses. The pulmonary trunk measured 23 mm distal to the stenosis with both branches measuring 15 mm in diameter. The following year, she had a successful left-sided BT shunt procedure with a significant improvement in her exercise tolerance.

By the age of 25 she had adopted a lifestyle that avoided physical exertion. She underwent cardiac catheterization again in consideration of repair for her TOF. This revealed an infundibular gradient of 25 mm Hg and a valvular gradient of 70 mm Hg with good biventricular function. She was felt to be a good candidate for repair but she decided not to proceed with surgery.

She experienced a general decrease in her exercise tolerance over the next several years and increasingly relied on use of a wheelchair. Despite that, she was satisfied with her symptomatic status and was reluctant to consider any further surgery.

At age 45, echocardiography showed a right-sided aortic arch with a large aortic root overriding a subaortic VSD. The pulmonary valve was narrowed as was the proximal pulmonary trunk. The left Blalock shunt was reported as "apparently patent." The echocardiogram showed mild RV enlargement with mild RV dysfunction but a normal-sized LV with good systolic function. The recommendation was made to proceed to cardiac catheterization and angiography as a prelude to reparative surgery. Despite this recommendation, the patient declined further intervention.

At age 50, she was seen in routine follow-up and complained of palpitation and was noted to have paroxysms of supraventricular and ventricular tachycardia. She was started on amiodarone with significant improvement in the palpitation but with the subsequent development of hyperthyroidism. The amiodarone was stopped, and good rhythm control was maintained on sotalol. Exercise testing at that time showed her walking on the Bruce protocol for 5:52, stopping with dyspnea (metabolic equivalents = 3). Oxygen saturation was 83% at rest, falling to 68% at peak exercise and recovering to 78% postexercise.

By age 60 she had noticed marked worsening in her ability to simply walk around the house. She attended the clinic on a routine annual visit and told her physician that she had stopped her sotalol 2 months earlier because of the dyspnea and fatigue. Despite stopping her medication, she had seen no improvement in her symptoms.

**Comments:** Life expectancy for unrepaired TOF is not encouraging. More than 95% are dead by the fourth decade, whereas after successful repair in childhood, 30-year survival has exceeded 90%. Palliated patients may develop pulmonary hypertension as a result of the arterial shunt procedure. For both palliated and unrepaired patients, the residual, large VSD will result in pressure overload of the RV and often in volume overload of the LV. This may lead to biventricular dysfunction and failure, exercise intolerance, and arrhythmias. The late course may be further complicated by thrombotic events or cerebral abscess. Death may result from congestive heart failure or may be sudden due to arrhythmia.

In adults being considered for complete repair of tetralogy, workup must involve assessment of right and left ventricular size and function as well as pulmonary artery (PA) size. Imaging to visualize major aortopulmonary collaterals is necessary. If these are identified they may be closed percutaneously before the reparative surgery. Assessment of PA pressure is especially important in individuals with previous palliation procedures because of the risk that iatrogenic pulmonary hypertension may have developed. Coronary artery origin anomalies (especially origin of the left anterior descending from the right coronary) can be documented by cardiovascular MRI, but careful consideration should be given to coronary angiography to rule out significant acquired coronary disease in the older patient.

The unrepaired heart in TOF develops RV pressure overload and sometimes LV volume overload with subsequent potential dysfunction of those chambers. These changes, over time, can form the basis for ventricular arrhythmias. Likewise, secondary enlargement of the atria provides the substrate for the atrial arrhythmia. Atrial arrhythmias are not well tolerated, and every effort should be made to maintain sinus rhythm. Unfortunately, late repair in these patients may not necessarily decrease their risk of ventricular and supraventricular arrhythmias.[1]

## CURRENT SYMPTOMS

The patient complained of terrible fatigue and breathlessness with even mild exertion. She had occasional palpitations but otherwise no symptoms at rest.

NYHA class: III

## CURRENT MEDICATIONS

No medications. (She had recently stopped her sotalol.)

## PHYSICAL EXAMINATION

Thin, kyphotic woman with marked clubbing and cyanosis

BP 130/80 mm Hg (right arm), HR 40 bpm, oxygen saturation 77%

Height 170 cm, weight 43 kg, BSA 1.42 m²

Surgical scars: Bilateral infrascapular thoracotomy scars

Neck veins: JVP at 6 cm with intermittent cannon A-waves

Lungs/chest: Kyphoscoliosis. Lung fields are clear.

Heart: Rhythm regular; RV lift. S1 normal; S2 single; 3/6 long systolic murmur along the left upper sternal border with a 2/6 diastolic murmur.

Abdomen: Liver was not enlarged.

Extremities: Mild peripheral edema

### PERTINENT NEGATIVES
The thyroid was not enlarged.

**Comments:** The patient was small. Her body mass index is 14.9 kg/m², which is very low, and clearly classifies her as cachectic by any criteria. Cachexia has been linked to survival in congenital heart disease patients.[2]

Intermittent cannon A-waves show that the RA is contracting against a closed tricuspid valve, indicating loss of the usual AV association. This physical sign of AV dissociation may occur in the setting of ventricular tachycardia, complete heart block, or a paced ventricular rhythm. In this situation, that is, of a patient with bradycardia, the cannon A-waves provided clinical evidence of complete heart block. A first heart sound of variable intensity may be anticipated.

## LABORATORY DATA

| | | |
|---|---|---|
| Hemoglobin | **18.9 g/dL** | (11.5–15.0) |
| Hematocrit/PCV | **57%** | (36–46) |
| MCV | **101 fL** | (83–99) |
| Platelet count | **75 × 10⁹/L** | (150–400) |
| Sodium | 139 mmol/L | (134–145) |
| Potassium | 4.0 mmol/L | (3.5–5.2) |
| Creatinine | 0.78 mg/dL | (0.6–1.2) |

**Comments:** An elevated hemoglobin is not only common but desirable in the patient with cyanosis. A hemoglobin in the normal range is inappropriate in such patients. If such a patient were relatively anemic, and if the patient were found to have iron deficiency, iron replacement should be initiated. Thrombo-

cytopenia is frequently present in patients with cyanotic heart disease and may be associated with hemostatic abnormalities, which may occur in up to 20% of cyanotic patients. Decreased clotting factors, elevated INR and activated partial thromboplastin time, as well as thrombocytopenia have been encountered, with no clinical consequences in some patients and life-threatening hemorrhage in others.[3]

## ELECTROCARDIOGRAM

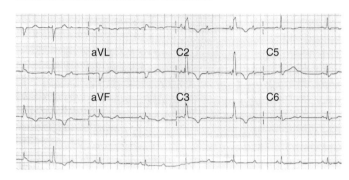

Figure 40-1 Electrocardiogram.

### FINDINGS
Heart rate: 48 bpm

QRS axis: +118°

QRS duration: 160 msec

Sinus rhythm with third-degree AV block. Right-axis deviation and RBBB with associated ST and T anomalies. RA overload in V1.

**Comments:** Data on ECG prognostic markers and long-term follow-up in unrepaired patients are not available. The development of complete heart block was presumably responsible for her declining functional capacity.

## CHEST X-RAY

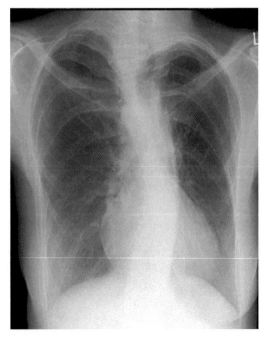

Figure 40-2 Posteroanterior projection.

## FINDINGS
Cardiothoracic ratio: 63%

Kyphoscoliosis is present with a consequent relative reduction in left lung volume. The aortic arch is right sided. There is some prominence of the right heart border in keeping with RA enlargement, but this appearance may just be related to the kyphoscoliosis.

***Comments:*** The cardiothoracic ratio is likely misleading here because of the scoliosis and thin body habitus. Scoliosis has been associated with cyanotic ACHD whether or not the patient has undergone previous thoracotomy or sternotomy. There have been a number of theories put forward including the role of cyanosis, the potential effect of abnormal pulsatile flows, or even common genetic pathways affecting both cardiac and skeletal development with cyanotic congenital heart defects and scoliosis, respectively. In some patients the skeletal abnormality may become a major source of disability, and, in that case, corrective surgery for the scoliosis should be appropriately considered.[4] Nevertheless, careful assessment of the benefits of corrective surgery and the cardiac risks of orthopedic surgery in such patients is necessary.

## ECHOCARDIOGRAM

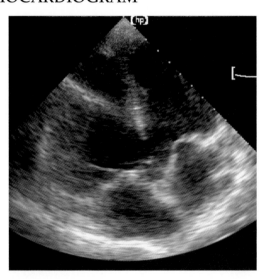

Figure 40-3 Apical four-chamber view in systole. The left ventricle and left atrium are on the right side of the figure.

## FINDINGS
The echo showed a large subaortic VSD measuring 20 mm across. The RV was moderately dilated with RV hypertrophy and with only a mild reduction in RV function. The LV was mildly enlarged with only a mild decrease in LV systolic function. The RA was dilated. The LA was of normal size. There was no ASD.

Severe valvular, subvalvular, and supravalvular pulmonary stenosis was present with a peak gradient of 104 mm Hg. RV pressure was estimated at 120 mm Hg (it would have to be the same as her systolic blood pressure). The aortic valve was slightly thickened with mild aortic regurgitation but no aortic stenosis.

***Comments:*** All of these findings are consistent with tetralogy of Fallot as originally described, namely RV hypertrophy, VSD with overriding aorta, and pulmonary stenosis. The true hallmark of this abnormality is displacement of the outlet septum anteriorly and superiorly, that is, into the normal RVOT, causing obstruction.

In a patient with unrepaired tetralogy, RV systolic pressure will equal LV systolic pressure.

### FOCUSED CLINICAL QUESTIONS AND DISCUSSION POINTS

1. **What factors may have contributed to her prolonged survival without definitive repair of the TOF?**

   *Without definitive repair, the average life expectancy in patients with tetralogy of Fallot is 12 years, with fewer than 5% surviving to their 40s. Therefore, this 60-year-old woman is exceptional.*

   *In the few cases of long survival without repair described in the literature, there have been some common features, including a hypoplastic pulmonary artery, LV hypertrophy, and extracardiac shunts, such as a patent ductus arteriosus or extensive aortopulmonary collaterals.[5]*

   *In our case, it seems that the patient had acceptable pulmonary blood flow, which was further augmented with her left BT shunt. Furthermore, she had no secondary PAH, which, in itself, would have been a risk factor.*

   *In view of the acceptable perioperative mortality in the adolescent and adult age group, careful consideration should be given to the question of repair for patients who were not repaired in childhood.*

   *There may be adults, like this patient, who are hemodynamically good candidates for repair but who refuse to consider such surgery. The physician must ensure that the patient fully understands the recommendations and the risks and benefits of an intervention, and must be aware of other factors that may affect the patient's decision. These factors may include the inability to comprehend the situation (intellectual impairment), inability to make a decision for herself (lifetime dependency on others such as parents), and depression.[6,7] Although it is important to respect a patient's decision in such matters, it is also important to ensure that the decision has been freely and rationally arrived at by an individual who is capable of making an informed choice.*

2. **What was the role of heart block in this patient's symptoms?**

   *The AV node is normally located in patients with TOF. Usually this area is of greatest concern at the time of VSD closure. In unrepaired patients, conducting system failure is a consequence of the hemodynamic derangements and the associated scarring.*

   *As ventricular function falls, cardiac output is increasingly reliant on being able to increase heart rate. Marked bradycardia and loss of AV synchrony may aggravate an already poor exercise tolerance. Permanent pacemaker insertion is certainly indicated in this situation. One important question is whether one should consider an epicardial system because of the patient's large VSD and potential paradoxical emboli.[8]*

   *It is difficult to anticipate how much symptomatic relief could be expected from restoring AV synchrony with pacing, and discussions with the patient should not be overly optimistic.*

3. **Should late repair of tetralogy of Fallot be considered in adult patients?**

   *The optimal time for repair of TOF is infancy with excellent early results—there have been no perioperative deaths in 92 patients under 12 months[9] and good long-term survival.[10] Despite this emphasis on early detection and intervention, there are still rare patients who have reached adulthood without repair of TOF.*

   *Early surgical results in adult patients were disappointing. In a group of 104 adults operated on between 1958 and 1977, the combined perioperative and first-year mortality was 32%.[11] Despite that, the long-term follow-up of these 1-year survivors showed excellent life expectancy.*

*Early surgical outcomes in adults have improved significantly with more recent series reporting perioperative mortality rates of 16%[12] to 3%.[13] Patients repaired in adulthood can now expect prolongation of life expectancy as well as improvement in symptoms and functional class.[1] Therefore, definitive repair of TOF should be considered for all adult patients with suitable anatomy and adequate ventricular function. Age alone should not be a deterrent to definitive repair[14] as long as the patient's comorbidities do not add unacceptably to the risks of the procedure.[5]*

*To illustrate this, a recent report detailed the autopsy findings in an 84-year-old woman who had undergone repair of TOF at the age of 50. She eventually died of complications from pneumonia 34 years after her cardiac surgery.[15] Nevertheless, repair does not mean cure. Patients must be informed that there are late complications after repair,[16] notably arrhythmia, heart failure, and sudden death, and that close long-term follow-up and perhaps additional therapy will be necessary.[17]*

## FINAL DIAGNOSIS

Unrepaired TOF

Complete heart block

## PLAN OF ACTION

Permanent pacemaker insertion

## INTERVENTION

The patient and her mother wanted more time to consider their options and decided to go home. Therefore, no intervention could be carried out.

## OUTCOME

Two weeks later, the patient collapsed at home. She was found in respiratory arrest. In the emergency room, she was not breathing spontaneously and was intubated. She was brady-cardic and hypotensive. A temporary pacemaker was inserted. There was a good response to these interventions initially, and she was stabilized in the intensive care unit. Unfortunately, after admission she developed septicemia and renal failure and died a few days later. An autopsy was performed.

The heart was enlarged and weighed 440 g with RV and LV hypertrophy. The cardiomegaly was particularly noteworthy given that the patient weighed only 43 kg in the year prior to her death. Temporary pacing wires were in good position in the RA and RV. There was infundibular hypertrophy with narrowing of the outflow tract. The pulmonary valve was bicuspid with thickened leaflets and large dilated sinuses. The orifice of the valve measured 10 mm in diameter. The main pulmonary artery measured 40 mm in diameter at the bifurcation but only 15 mm above the valve. The overriding aorta was enlarged but the aortic valve was structurally normal. A large perimembranous VSD (20 mm in diameter) was present with direct continuity between the aortic valve and the tricuspid valve, with some prolapse of the aortic leaflets. No vegetations were found.

There were four major aortopulmonary collaterals noted on the right and two on the left. A surprising finding was that of a surgical shunt into a left major aortopulmonary collateral artery. It appears that, 45 years earlier, the Blalock shunt had been placed into a left-sided major aortopulmonary collateral artery, rather than the left PA. The shunt was large and patent at autopsy.

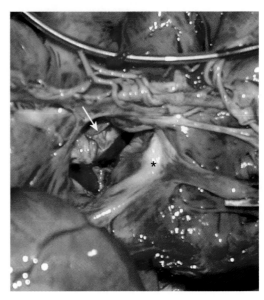

Figure 40-4 Postmortem image of the right ventricle.

### FINDINGS

View from the RV showing a large perimembranous VSD in the center of the image with an aortic cusp prolapsing through the VSD (*arrow*). The tricuspid valve (*asterisk*) has been pulled back to demonstrate the VSD.

**Comments:** Aortic regurgitation had been noted on the echocardiogram and clinically there had been a diastolic murmur on examination. At autopsy, the aortic valve was structurally normal but did prolapse into the VSD. This was probably the mechanism of her aortic regurgitation. Follow-up of unrepaired patients with VSD requires careful attention to the severity of any aortic regurgitation.

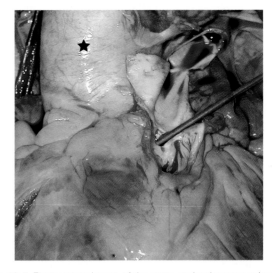

Figure 40-5 Postmortem image of the aorta and pulmonary valve.

### FINDINGS

A probe was passed through the pulmonary valve, demonstrating the very small orifice and the severe stenosis. Note is made of the dilated overriding aorta (*star*).

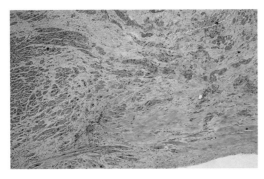

Figure 40-6 Photomicrograph of a section taken from the RV wall.

## FINDINGS

On the right-hand side of the slide, there is almost complete replacement of cardiac myocytes by fibrosis.

**Comments:** Myocardial fibrosis has been documented by late gadolinium enhancement MR scanning of systemic RVs and the RVs of patients following repair of TOF. Although fibrosis has been noted at the sites of surgical scarring, a third of the patients had evidence of fibrosis at locations unexplained by surgical intervention.[18] It has been postulated that these areas of fibrosis may be linked to later development of arrhythmias and might be a prognostic factor for late morbidity and mortality.

## ACKNOWLEDGMENT

I would like to thank Dr. Mary Sheppard for her assistance and advice with the pathology specimens.

## Selected References

1. Atik FA, Atik E, da Cunha CR, et al: Long-term results of correction of tetralogy of Fallot in adulthood. Eur J Cardio-Thoracic Surg 25:250–255, 2004.
2. Vonder Muhll IF, Dimopoulos K, Lawrance RA, et al: Cachexia as a predictor of mortality among an outpatient population of adults with congenital heart disease. J Am Coll Cardiol 49(9 Suppl A):263A, 2007.
3. Therrien J, Warnes C, Daliento L, et al: CCS Conference 2001 update: Recommendations for the management of adults with congenital heart disease Part III. Can J Cardiol 17:1137–1158, 2001.
4. Coran D, Rodgers WB, Keane JF, et al: Spinal fusion in patients with congenital heart disease: Predictors of outcome. Clin Orthop Relat Res 364:99–107, 1999.
5. Yang X, Freeman LJ, Ross C: Unoperated tetralogy of Fallot: Case report of a natural survivor who died in his 73rd year; is it ever too late to operate? Postgrad Med J 81:133–134, 2005.
6. Popelova J, Slavik Z, Skovranek J: Are cyanosed adults with congenital cardiac malformations depressed? Cardiol in the Young 11:379–384, 2001.
7. Bassett AS, Chow EWC, Husted J, et al: Clinical features of 78 adults with 22q11 deletion syndrome. Am J Med Genetics 138:307–313, 2005.
8. Khairy P, Landzberg MJ, Gatzoulis MA, et al: Transvenous pacing leads and systemic thromboemboli in patients with congenital heart disease and intracardiac shunts: A multicenter study. Circulation 113:2391–2397, 2006.
9. Van Arsdell GS, Maharaj GS, Tom J, et al: What is the optimal age for repair of tetralogy of Fallot? Circulation 102:III123–129, 2000.
10. Knott-Craig CJ, Elkins RC, Lane MM, et al: A 26-year experience with surgical management of tetralogy of Fallot: Risk analysis for mortality or late reintervention. Ann Thorac Surg 66:506–511, 1998.
11. Nollert G, Fischlein T, Bouterwek S, et al: Long-term results of total repair of tetralogy of Fallot in adulthood: 35 years follow-up in 104 patients corrected at the age of 18 or older. Thorac Cardiovasc Surgeon 45:178–181, 1997.
12. Dittrich S, Vogel M, Dahnert I, et al: Surgical repair of tetralogy of Fallot in adults today. Clin Cardiol 22:460–464, 1999.
13. Erdogan BE, Bozbuga N, Kayalar N, et al: Long-term outcome after total correction of tetralogy of Fallot in adolescent and adult age. J Card Surg 20:119–123, 2005.
14. Hu DCK, Seward JB, Puga FJ, et al: Total correction of tetralogy of Fallot at age 40 years and older: Long-term follow-up. J Am Coll Cardiol 5:40–44, 1985.
15. Gerlis LM, Ho SY, Sheppard MN: Longevity in the setting of tetralogy of Fallot: Survival to the 84th year. Cardiol Young 14:664–666, 2004.
16. Van Doorn, C: The unnatural history of tetralogy of Fallot: Surgical repair is not as definitive as previously thought. Heart 88:447–448, 2002.
17. Babu-Narayan SV, Gatzoulis MA: Management of adults with operated tetralogy of Fallot. Curr Treat Options Cardiovasc Med 5:389–398, 2003.
18. Babu-Narayan SV, Kilner PJ, Li W, et al: Ventricular fibrosis suggested by cardiovascular magnetic resonance in adults with repaired tetralogy of Fallot and its relationship to adverse markers of clinical outcome. Circulation 113:405–413, 2006.

## Bibliography

Gatzoulis MA, Balaji S, Webber SA, et al: Risk factors for arrhythmia and sudden cardiac death late after repair of tetralogy of Fallot: A multicentre study. Lancet 356:975–981, 2000.

Heit JA: Risk factors for venous thromboembolism. Clin Chest Med 24:1–12, 2003.

Khan AA, Diller GP, Sutton R, et al: Complications associated with cardiac pacing in congenital heart disease patients (Abstract). Eur Heart J 26:310, 2005.

# Timing of Pulmonary Valve Replacement

**Sonya V. Babu-Narayan and Elliot A. Shinebourne**

**Age: 31 years**
**Gender: Female**
**Occupation: Teacher**
**Working diagnosis: Tetralogy of Fallot**

## HISTORY

The patient was diagnosed at birth with TOF. At age 3 (1976) primary repair was performed, with reconstruction of the RVOT with a transannular pericardial patch.

Although she was asymptomatic, serial echocardiograms showed progressive pulmonary regurgitation, which was noted to be mild when she was 11 years old, moderate by age 27, and severe by age 30.

Otherwise, the patient noted only occasional symptoms of palpitations, which were described as "missed beats," or a few seconds of awareness of her heartbeat.

In the last 18 months she noted a more noticeable "slowing down" in her usual activities, as well as occasional episodes of fast, regular palpitations lasting 30 seconds at a time.

***Comments:*** Transannular patching (whereby the annulus of the pulmonary valve is incised and hence disrupted) is necessary when the pulmonary valve and artery are very small; in this case they were perioperatively described as being a quarter of the size of the aorta, whereas typically they are very similar in size. The surgical approach to repair of tetralogy has evolved over the years. Early cohorts underwent repair through a right ventriculotomy, whereas now repair through the RA and pulmonary artery is the norm. In this patient, the pulmonary annulus was sufficiently restrictive to necessitate the use of a transannular patch for complete relief of the RVOT obstruction, which created the potential for free pulmonary regurgitation.

In the modern era, it has become apparent that there are detrimental long-term effects of right ventriculotomy and chronic pulmonary regurgitation on RV function, the propensity to arrhythmia, and sudden cardiac death. Current surgery uses a combined transatrial/transpulmonary approach allowing both closure of the VSD and relief of the RVOT obstruction to be carried out from the right atrium and the pulmonary artery. If there is no disruption of the pulmonary valve annulus, any subvalvular patch is termed an RVOT patch.

## CURRENT SYMPTOMS

Although noting reduced exertional stamina compared to prior years, the patient was able to work full time and did not expe-rience breathlessness in her usual activities. There were no specific symptoms of chest pain, syncope, or breathlessness on exertion.

NYHA class: I

***Comments:*** It may be that in the context of pulmonary regurgitation late after repair of TOF, waiting for the patient to become clearly symptomatic may risk deferring pulmonary valve surgery too long.

## CURRENT MEDICATIONS

None

## PHYSICAL EXAMINATION

BP 110/70 mm Hg, HR 70 bpm, oxygen saturation 100%

Height 158 cm, weight 86 kg, BSA 1.94 m$^2$

Surgical scars: Midline sternotomy scar

Neck veins: Normal JVP was seen.

Lungs/chest: Clear to auscultation

Heart: The heart rate was regular. There was an RV heave. Auscultation revealed a normal first heart sound, a systolic ejection murmur at the left upper sternal border, and a short early diastolic murmur at the left sternal edge. There was a single second heart sound. Peripheral pulses were palpable and equal.

Abdomen: No abnormality detected

Extremities: No abnormality detected

***Comments:*** An RV lift or heave in such a patient is due to RV pressure or volume overload. Volume overload is much more common, and usually associated with severe pulmonary regurgitation and possibly tricuspid regurgitation. Pressure overload would be due to RV outflow or pulmonary arterial obstruction, or pulmonary hypertension.

The murmur of low-pressure pulmonary regurgitation is usually 2+ and seldom 3+ in intensity. Augmentation by inspiration is worth looking for. When pulmonary regurgitation is severe, the murmur may be minimal or even absent. The systolic ejection type murmur is due to increased flow through the valve during systole. A more harsh systolic murmur may indicate residual stenosis in the RVOT. The single second heart sound is the aortic component because in repaired TOF there is often no audible closure of the pulmonary valve.

## LABORATORY DATA

| | |
|---|---|
| Hemoglobin | 13.7 g/dL (11.5–15.0) |
| Hematocrit/PCV | 39% (36–46) |
| MCV | 86 fL (83–99) |
| Platelet count | $242 \times 10^9$/L (150–400) |
| Sodium | 139 mmol/L (134–145) |
| Potassium | 4.1 mmol/L (3.5–5.2) |
| Creatinine | **0.75 mg/dL** (0.6–1.2) |
| Blood urea nitrogen | 3.3 mmol/L (2.5–6.5) |

*Comments:* No abnormalities detected.

## ELECTROCARDIOGRAM

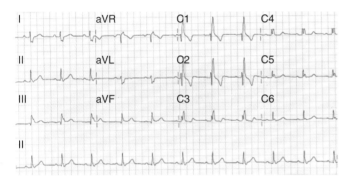

Figure 41-1 Electrocardiogram.

### FINDINGS
Heart rate: 64 bpm

QRS axis: +117°

QRS duration: 138 msec

Normal sinus rhythm with RBBB.

24-hour ECG recording: Rare supraventricular and ventricular ectopics, no arrhythmia, no ECG abnormalities were seen at the time of reported symptoms of palpitations.

*Comments:* RBBB pattern is almost universal in patients who have undergone a right ventriculotomy.

## CHEST X-RAY

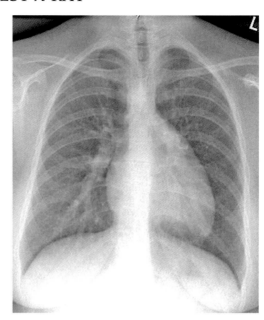

Figure 41-2 Posteroanterior projection.

### FINDINGS
Cardiothoracic ratio: 53%

Right aortic arch. The appearance of the left heart border suggests a dilated RVOT.

*Comments:* Right aortic arch, defined by the position of the arch in relation to the trachea, is commonly associated with TOF and may be seen in up to 30% of patients. When right aortic arch is associated with other anomalies of the aortic arch vessels, the probability of 22q11 microdeletion is high.

## EXERCISE TESTING

| | |
|---|---|
| Exercise protocol: | Modified Bruce |
| Duration (min:sec): | 9:30 |
| Reason for stopping: | Dyspnea |
| ECG changes: | None |

| | Rest | Peak |
|---|---|---|
| Heart rate (bpm): | 70 | 166 |
| Percent of age-predicted max HR: | | 88 |
| $O_2$ saturation (%): | 100 | 100 |
| Blood pressure (mm Hg): | 110/70 | 140/80 |

| | |
|---|---|
| Peak $Vo_2$ (mL/kg/min): | 18.8 |
| Percent predicted (%): | 48 |
| Ve/Vco$_2$: | 34.8 |
| Metabolic equivalents: | 7.8 |

*Comments:* In our institution this $Vo_2$ in absolute terms is below the mean for repaired TOF with pulmonary regurgitation. (Out of 92 prospectively studied repaired TOF patients with pulmonary regurgitation who reached a respiratory quotient [RQ] greater than 1, the mean peak $Vo_2$ obtained was $25.6 \pm 7.8$ mL/kg/min and the mean Ve/Vco$_2$ slope was $30.3 \pm 8.3$.)

# ECHOCARDIOGRAM

## OVERALL FINDINGS
The RV was severely dilated but had normal function. LV function was normal.

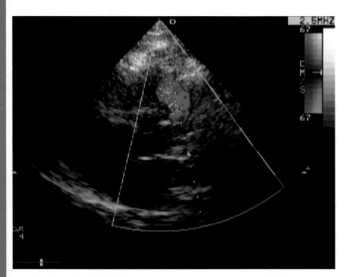

Figure 41-3 Parasternal short-axis view of the right ventricular outflow tract, with Doppler showing pulmonary regurgitant jet.

## FINDINGS
Severe pulmonary valve regurgitation was present.

**Comments:** Note the relative lack of color represented in the regurgitant jet. Instead, there is near laminar flow in diastole consistent with free pulmonary regurgitation. The murmur heard in this patient was soft, which is consistent with the Doppler finding.

It can be difficult to see the free wall of the RV by echocardiography when the RV is enlarged, and thus a true estimation of the degree of enlargement can be difficult. For this reason, MRI is really the imaging of choice for this purpose.

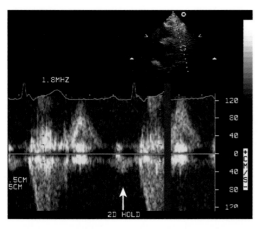

Figure 41-4 Pulsed-wave Doppler through the right ventricular outflow tract.

## FINDINGS
The peak velocity during systole was 1.8 m/sec (*not shown*). During diastole, there was regurgitant flow ending in mid dias-

tole. Following the A-wave on the ECG tracing, forward flow is seen in the RVOT (*arrow*).

**Comments:** This finding of forward diastolic flow through the RVOT is consistent with a restrictive RV. The RV fills early in diastole, and no further regurgitation occurs (consistent with the early diastolic murmur heard). With atrial contraction, the RV cannot fill further, and the atrial contribution of volume translates into forward flow into the pulmonary artery even before ventricular systole begins.

Observations suggest that the presence of restriction is favorable in this circumstance. Restriction may prevent further dilatation and hence RV dysfunction.[1]

Note also the relative delay between the QRS complex and the systolic flow. Electromechanical delays result from the widened QRS.

# MAGNETIC RESONANCE IMAGING

## OVERALL FINDINGS
The RV was moderately dilated with normal systolic function. The LV was normal in size and function. The atria were not enlarged, and there was normal function of the mitral and tricuspid valves. There was severe pulmonary valve regurgitation. By stroke volume difference, the pulmonary artery regurgitant fraction was 46%.

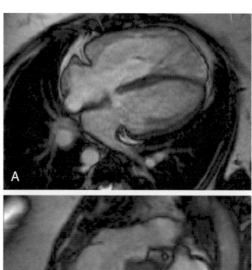

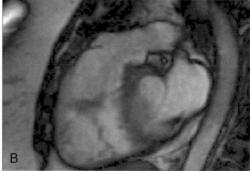

Figure 41-5 Still frames from steady-state free procession cine cardiac magnetic resonance image in an end-diastolic four-chamber view (**A**) and right ventricular outflow tract view (**B**).

## FINDINGS
The RV was enlarged but had normal function. There was absence of significant pulmonary valve leaflets with only a small rim of possible valve tissue. There was only a small, akinetic thin area of myocardium below the pulmonary valve. Such areas are commonly seen following repair of TOF.[2] The septum maintains its normal configuration (concave toward the LV) throughout the cardiac cycle in this patient, which is not always the case in TOF.

## Ventricular Volume Quantification

|  | LV | (Normal range) | RV | (Normal range) |
|---|---|---|---|---|
| EDV (mL) | 116 | (52–141) | **244** | (58–154) |
| ESV (mL) | 32 | (13–51) | **88** | (12–68) |
| SV (mL) | 84 | (33–97) | **156** | (35–98) |
| EF (%) | 72 | (57–75) | 64 | (51–75) |
| EDVi (mL/m²) | 60 | (62–96) | **126** | (61–98) |
| ESVi (mL/m²) | **16** | (17–36) | **45** | (17–43) |
| SVi (mL/m²) | 43 | (40–65) | **80** | (38–62) |
| Mass index (g/m²) | 47 | (47–77) | **49** | (20–40) |

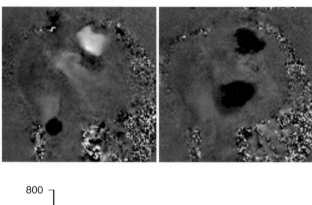

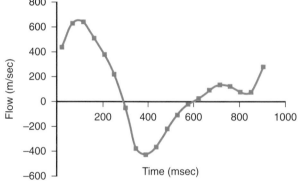

Figure 41-6 Phase-contrast velocity mapping of the main pulmonary artery above left (systole) appearing white and above right (diastole) appearing black. The resultant plotted flow curve (below) can be calculated once the region of interest, here the pulmonary trunk, has been planimetered in each phase of the cardiac cycle.

## FINDINGS

There is free pulmonary regurgitation, which lasts for a short time in diastole.

The pulmonary regurgitant fraction was 48%. At the end of diastole there is again forward flow during atrial contraction (a pulmonary A-wave).

However, these data are derived from non–real time non–breath hold velocity mapping and although this may prove a reliable method to quantify restrictive RV physiology, caution should be exercised in assuming that this finding is always exactly equivalent to the original definition based on echocardiography of an A-wave present throughout the respiratory cycle on pulsed-wave Doppler through the RVOT.

***Comments:*** Phase velocity map in systole (left top image) and diastole (right top image). Forward pulmonary artery flow in this example is white and reverse flow is black. As was seen on the echocardiographic Doppler trace, the regur-

gitation ends in mid diastole, and instead there is forward flow into the pulmonary artery before systole, consistent with a restrictive RV.

The pulmonary regurgitant fraction was calculated as follows: The region of interest (the pulmonary artery) is planimetered in each phase of the velocity map acquired. The mean velocity in the region of interest is multiplied by the area of the region of interest to derive flow in each phase of the cardiac cycle, which is plotted as a curve as shown below the phase velocity map (bottom image). By integrating the area under the flow curve in systole and diastole a pulmonary regurgitant fraction can be derived.

The total forward volume should correlate with the measured RV stroke volume, and the net forward volume should correlate with the measured LV stroke volume, in the absence of any other valve regurgitation.

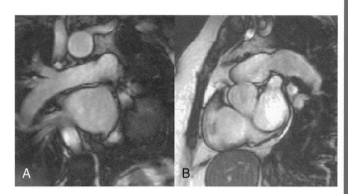

Figure 41-7 Still frames from steady state free precession cine cardiac magnetic resonance image showing right pulmonary artery (**A**) and left pulmonary artery (**B**) in systole.

## FINDINGS

Both the right and left pulmonary arteries were unobstructed and dilated.

***Comments:*** CMR can visualize the branch pulmonary arteries. In this case they were unobstructed. Pulmonary artery stenoses are fairly common in patients with repaired tetralogy; they can worsen pulmonary regurgitation and may need to be addressed surgically or in the interventional catheterization laboratory.

## CATHETERIZATION

Not performed

### FOCUSED CLINICAL QUESTIONS AND DISCUSSION POINTS

1. **What are the current indications for pulmonary valve replacement (PVR) after primary repair of TOF?**

   *Pulmonary regurgitation is very common after repair of TOF; it tends to increase with time and become clinically important some 20 to 30 years after repair. It is one of the most common problems encountered in the care of adults with congenital heart disease.*

   *In essence, the goal is to time surgery sufficiently early to avoid irreversible RV dilation and dysfunction. This has to be weighed against the absence of perfect bioprostheses. Currently available valves have a finite longevity, so PVR in younger patients may be the first of more than one reoperation.*

   *There are no universally accepted criteria for determining the optimal timing of PVR for this condition. However, there is a widespread view that in the past, operations were offered too late in some of these patients, and the trend in recent years has been to reoperate earlier. Based mainly on retrospective studies, there is a general consensus that PVR should be offered in the setting of a very large RV, attributable symptoms, or the onset of sustained atrial or ventricular arrhythmia.*

*Timing of surgery in asymptomatic patients, therefore, remains particularly challenging and more controversial in the absence of data from large prospective series reporting long-term follow-up from different approaches. In published series, there is heterogeneity in patient characteristics and hemodynamic status. Most of the presently available data come from retrospective studies summarized by Davlouros et al.[3] One of the criteria for PVR in the Leiden series[4] was important RV dilatation as defined by end-diastolic RV to LV volume ratio equal to 2:1. In addition to this important prospective series described by Vliegen and colleagues, further prospective studies have also shown a decrease in RV volumes[5,6] and improvement in other adverse prognostic markers following PVR.[6] Of note, it appears that all described series include patients that have undergone RVOT resection of aneurysmal/akinetic areas.*

2. Should this patient undergo PVR?

*This patient reported a change, though subtle, in her exercise tolerance. Defining symptoms may be difficult in this population and they may not be overt. Interpretation of this patient's symptoms caused some debate. Her exercise tolerance was well below the mean for this cohort (mixed gender) in our institution. Her pulmonary regurgitation was clearly severe on CMR and progressive on echo over the previous years, and the right heart was already dilated, measuring nearly three times that of the LV in diastole. Therefore she was offered valve replacement.*

3. What other treatment options are currently available?

*There are few data to suggest the use of pharmacotherapy for pulmonary regurgitation. The only randomized controlled trial in this setting suggests a potential limited role for ACE inhibitors.[7,8] Use of beta-blockers and other drugs would be empiric.*

*There has been novel research into newer interventional strategies[9] whereby a stented bovine jugular venous valve is inserted with a transcatheter approach. Results appear promising, particularly in patients with an existing conduit, but no long-term data are available. In older patients the reconstructed outflow tract may be too large for a valved stent (see Case 42), and the akinetic area typically below the pulmonary valve would not be addressed. If the outflow tract remains contractile it may stress the stent itself and cause dysfunction and/or embolization. However, midterm results are encouraging, and this may prove an attractive, less invasive approach for treatment of pulmonary regurgitation in selected patients.*

## FINAL DIAGNOSIS

Severe pulmonary regurgitation and RV dilatation late after repair of TOF

## PLAN OF ACTION

Surgical PVR

## INTERVENTION

The main pulmonary artery was opened and the incision extended to the previous patch. This was completely calcified. The previous patch was excised and a 23-mm pulmonary homograft was inserted.

## OUTCOME

The patient reported an immediate benefit from surgery, finding that her breathing was "easier." On her 6-week follow-up at the clinic she noted an improvement in her exercise tolerance, reporting that she was able to climb two to three flights of stairs without stopping.

One year later she continues to feel well with more energy than she had previously.

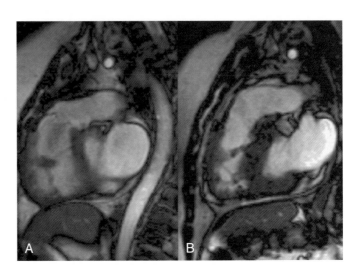

Figure 41-8 Still images taken from cine views of the right ventricular outflow tract (RVOT) in a close to sagittal orientation. Both frames are taken from the same phase of the cardiac cycle. RVOT view in early diastole (**A**) shows pulmonary regurgitation. **A**, Preop view. **B**, Postop view.

## FINDINGS

Postoperative cine imaging demonstrated a competent pulmonary valve. Velocity mapping confirmed the absence of pulmonary regurgitation. The RV volume had decreased considerably.

***Comments:*** The favorable changes of the RV are expected, as well as an indication that valve replacement was not offered too late.

## Selected References

1. Gatzoulis MA, Clark AL, Cullen S, et al: Right ventricular diastolic function 15–35 years after repair of tetralogy of Fallot: Restrictive physiology predicts superior exercise performance. Circulation 91:1775–1781, 1995.
2. Davlouros PA, Kilner PJ, Hornung TS, et al: Right ventricular function in adults with repaired tetralogy of Fallot assessed with cardiovascular magnetic resonance imaging: Detrimental role of right ventricular outflow aneurysms or akinesia and adverse right-to-left ventricular interaction. J Am Coll Cardiol 40:2044–2052, 2002.
3. Davlouros PA, Karatza AA, Gatzoulis MA, Shore DF. Timing and type of surgery for severe pulmonary regurgitation after repair of tetralogy of Fallot (Review). Int J Cardiol 97(Suppl 1):91–101, 2004.
4. Vliegen HW, van Straten A, de Roos A, et al: Magnetic resonance imaging to assess the hemodynamic effects of pulmonary valve replacement in adults late after repair of tetralogy of Fallot. Circulation 106:1703–1707, 2002.
5. Oosterhof T, van Straten A, Vliegen HW, et al: Preoperative thresholds for pulmonary valve replacement in patients with corrected tetralogy of Fallot using cardiovascular magnetic resonance. Circulation 116:545–551, 2007.
6. Frigiola A, Tsang V, Bull C, et al: Biventricular response after pulmonary valve replacement for right ventricular outflow tract dysfunction: Is age a predictor of outcome? Circulation 118(14 Suppl):S182–S190, 2008.

7. Babu-Narayan SV, Uebing A, Davlouros PA, et al: ACE inhibitors for potential prevention of the deleterious effects of pulmonary regurgitation in adults with tetralogy of Fallot repair—the appropriate study—a randomised, double-blinded, placebo-controlled trial in adults with congenital heart disease. 79th Annual Scientific Session of the American Heart Association, Chicago, IL. Circulation 114:413, 2006.

8. Babu-Narayan SV, Uebing A, Kilner PJ, et al: ACE inhibition improves systolic LV function in patients with pulmonary regurgitation and restrictive RV physiology late after repair of tetralogy of Fallot—A subgroup analysis of the appropriate study (ACE inhibitors for potential prevention of the deleterious effects of pulmonary regurgitation in adults with tetralogy of Fallot repair). 80th Annual Scientific session of the American Heart Association, Orlando, FL. Circulation 116:700, 2007.

9. Coats L, Tsang V, Khambadkone S, et al: The potential impact of percutaneous pulmonary valve stent implantation on right ventricular outflow tract re-intervention. Eur J Cardiothorac Surg 27:536–543, 2005.

## Bibliography

Bove EL, Kavey RE, Byrum CJ, et al: Improved right ventricular function following late pulmonary valve replacement for residual pulmonary insufficiency or stenosis. J Thorac Cardiovasc Surg 90:50–55, 1985.

Eyskens B, Reybrouck T, Bogaert J, et al: Homograft insertion for pulmonary regurgitation after repair of tetralogy of Fallot improves cardiorespiratory exercise performance. Am J Cardiol 85:221–225, 2000.

Gatzoulis MA, Balaji S, Webber SA, et al: Risk factors for arrhythmia and sudden cardiac death late after repair of tetralogy of Fallot: A multicentre study. Lancet 356:975–981, 2000.

Hazekamp MG, Kurvers MM, Schoof PH, et al: Pulmonary valve insertion late after repair of Fallot's tetralogy. Eur J Cardiothorac Surg 19:667–670, 2001.

Therrien J, Provost Y, Merchant N, et al: Optimal timing for pulmonary valve replacement in adults after tetralogy of Fallot repair. Am J Cardiol 95:779–782, 2005.

Therrien J, Siu SC, McLaughlin PR, et al: Pulmonary valve replacement in adults late after repair of tetralogy of Fallot: Are we operating too late? J Am Coll Cardiol 36:1670–1675, 2000.

Van Huysduynen BH, van Straten A, Swenne CA, et al: Reduction of QRS duration after pulmonary valve replacement in adult Fallot patients is related to reduction of right ventricular volume. Eur Heart J 26:928–932, 2005.

Warner KG, Anderson JE, Fulton DR, et al: Restoration of the pulmonary valve reduces right ventricular volume overload after previous repair of tetralogy of Fallot. Circulation 88(5 Pt 2):II189–197, 1993.

Yemets IM, Williams WG, Webb GD, et al: Pulmonary valve replacement late after repair of tetralogy of Fallot. Ann Thorac Surg 64:526–530, 1997.

# Catheter Implantation of Stented Pulmonary Valve

**Louise Coats, Sachin Khambadkone, and Philipp Bonhoeffer**

**Age: 22 years**
**Gender: Female**
**Occupation: Student**
**Working diagnosis: Tetralogy of Fallot with pulmonary atresia**

## HISTORY

This patient presented in early infancy when she was noticed to be cyanosed by a home health visitor. Following investigation, the diagnosis of pulmonary atresia with VSD was made. Palliative surgery, namely bilateral placement of modified BT shunts, was performed in infancy and early childhood to enhance pulmonary blood flow.

This surgery permitted the patient to develop and grow normally such that definitive surgical repair could then be performed. At the age of 6, restoration of continuity between the RV and pulmonary arteries was established with a 17-mm homograft conduit. A further 11-mm homograft conduit was used to augment and attach the left pulmonary artery to the reconstructed outflow tract. The VSD was closed. The operation was uncomplicated, but recovery was slow with a long period in intensive care. Following surgery, the patient had an uneventful childhood.

At age 18, she started her university education and became aware of increasing fatigue and breathlessness with moderate exertion. Over the ensuing years the problem became more noticeable. She returned for follow-up.

***Comments:*** Pulmonary atresia with VSD is a variant of TOF, and is sometimes called complex pulmonary atresia. The pulmonary blood supply is dependent initially on patency of the ductus arteriosus, and later on the presence of aortopulmonary collateral arteries.

The BT shunt, first performed in 1944 by Alfred Blalock and Vivian Thomas, marked the beginning of rapid development in surgery for ACHD. This progress has resulted in a marked improvement in prognosis for patients with congenital heart defects with more than 85% of patients now surviving into adult life.[1]

## CURRENT SYMPTOMS

The patient has noticed increasing tiredness and shortness of breath on moderate exertion. She did not complain of palpitations, light-headedness, or chest pains.

NYHA class: II

***Comments:*** Here the symptoms most likely represent conduit failure—either conduit stenosis or regurgitation. Pulmonary valve regurgitation, present in many patients with

TOF, has detrimental effects on RV function[2] and exercise capacity[3] and can increase the risk of arrhythmia and sudden death.[4] Most often it is found in patients with prior transannular patch repair of classic TOF. The presence of branch pulmonary artery stenosis in this situation increases the regurgitant load on the RV and is associated with accelerated clinical deterioration.[5]

## CURRENT MEDICATIONS

None

## PHYSICAL EXAMINATION

BP 110/70 mm Hg, HR 74 bpm, oxygen saturation 97%

Height 155 cm, weight 73 kg, BSA 1.77 m$^2$

Surgical scars: Median sternotomy and bilateral thoracotomy

Neck veins: Not distended

Lungs/chest: Clear to auscultation

Heart: Regular rate and rhythm were present, with the apex beat displaced to the left. There was an RV heave. A 3/6 ejection systolic murmur was heard at the left sternal edge radiating to the back and to the left axilla. Also, a 2/4 early diastolic murmur at the left sternal edge was present.

Abdomen: No abnormalities detected

Extremities: No peripheral edema or cyanosis was seen.

## LABORATORY DATA

| | |
|---|---|
| Hemoglobin | 13.3 g/dL (11.5–15.0) |
| Hematocrit | 40% (36–46) |
| White cell count | $10.2 \times 10^9$/L (4.5–13.5) |
| Platelet count | $257 \times 10^9$/L (150–400) |
| Sodium | 140 mmol/L (134–145) |
| Potassium | 3.7 mmol/L (3.5–5.2) |
| Creatinine | 0.63 mg/dL (0.6–1.2) |
| Urea | 3.5 mmol/L (2.5–6.5) |
| PT | 31 sec (26–38) |
| APTT | 10.7 sec (9.9–12.5) |

***Comments:*** Normal blood results.

# ELECTROCARDIOGRAM

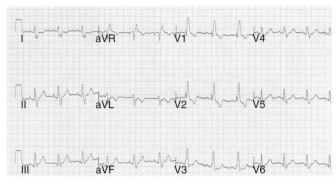

Figure 42-1   Electrocardiogram.

## FINDINGS

Heart rate: 77 bpm

Rhythm: Sinus rhythm

QRS axis: Right-axis deviation (+110°)

QRS duration: 150 msec

RBBB pattern

**Comments:** QRS duration correlates with RV volume in patients with repaired tetralogy. A QRS duration on the resting ECG of at least 180 msec is a predictor of life-threatening ventricular arrhythmia.[6]

# CHEST X-RAY

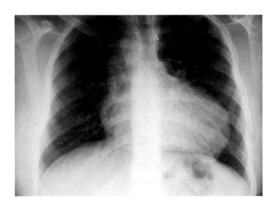

Figure 42-2  Posteroanterior projection.

## FINDINGS

Cardiothoracic ratio: 62%

Moderate cardiomegaly, cardiac shape consistent with RV hypertrophy. The inapparent pulmonary trunk fits with the diagnosis of tetralogy. Calcification of the homograft and left pulmonary artery can be seen. There is a surgical clip relating to previous shunt ligation. There is a right aortic arch (boot-shaped heart). The lung fields are clear.

**Comments:** CXR is useful for identifying the presence of circumferential homograft/conduit calcification. If transcathe-

ter intervention is considered, this finding is encouraging as it indicates the potential for device stability.

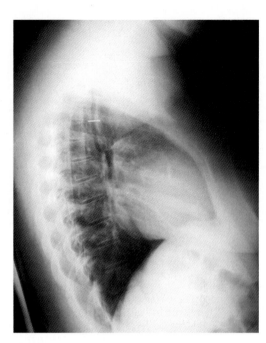

Figure 42-3  Lateral view.

## FINDINGS

Cardiomegaly with retrosternal filling consistent with RV hypertrophy and/or a retrosternal conduit. Surgical clip relating to previous shunt ligation. The lung fields are clear.

# EXERCISE TESTING

| | |
|---|---|
| Exercise protocol: | Ramp protocol |
| Peak workload: | 90 Watts |
| Reason for stopping: | Dyspnea and leg pain |
| ECG changes: | RBBB, frequent ectopic beats |

| | Rest | Peak |
|---|---|---|
| Heart rate (bpm): | 74 | 153 |
| Percent of age-predicted max HR: | | 77 |
| $O_2$ saturation (%): | 97 | 98 |
| Blood pressure (mm Hg): | 110/70 | 155/80 |
| Peak $Vo_2$ (mL/kg/min): | | 19 |
| Percent predicted (%): | | 62 |
| Ve/Vco$_2$: | | 32 |
| Metabolic equivalents: | | 6.9 |

**Comments:** Poor cardiopulmonary exercise capacity identifies ACHD patients at risk of hospitalization or death.[7] Cardiopulmonary exercise capacity can improve following restoration of pulmonary valvar competency.[8,9]

# ECHOCARDIOGRAM

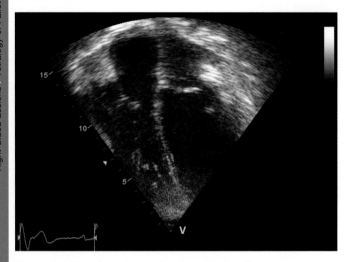

Figure 42-4 Two-dimensional apical four-chamber view.

## FINDINGS

A moderately dilated, hypertrophied RV was seen with mildly impaired function. The LV was normal except for paradoxical septal motion. There was trivial tricuspid regurgitation, with a peak regurgitant velocity of 3.8 m/sec. There was mild dilation of the RA. The IVC collapsed normally with respiration.

**Comments:** There was evidence of RV volume overload, although the central venous pressure was normal.

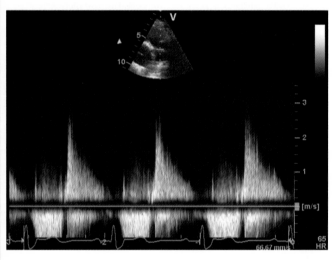

Figure 42-5 Continuous-wave Doppler across the calcified homograft demonstrating pulmonary regurgitant flow signal.

## FINDINGS

The calcified homograft was seen with degeneration of the valve leaflets. The peak gradient was 45 mm Hg, with a mean gradient of 21 mm Hg.

There was moderate pulmonary regurgitation lasting 71% of the diastolic duration. The pressure half-time was 122 msec. Diastolic flow reversal was present in the branch pulmonary arteries, and there was a proximal left pulmonary artery stenosis.

**Comments:** The pressure half-time was less than 100 msec[10] and duration of pulmonary regurgitation was less than 77% diastolic duration[11] on continuous-wave Doppler

echocardiography correlated with severe pulmonary regurgitation as quantified by MRI. However, these measurements should be interpreted with caution, as they can be influenced by RV end-diastolic dysfunction (restriction).

# MAGNETIC RESONANCE IMAGING

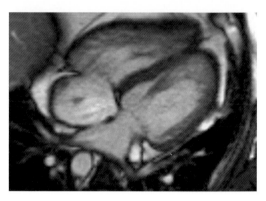

Figure 42-6 Two-dimensional single slice to b–steady-state free precession cine image, four-chamber view.

## FINDINGS

The main pulmonary artery measured 17 mm at its narrowest point. The left pulmonary artery measured 3 mm proximally and 11 mm distally. The pulmonary regurgitant fraction was 20%.

### Ventricular Volume Quantification

|  | LV | (Normal range) | RV | (Normal range) |
|---|---|---|---|---|
| EDV (mL) | 131 | (52–141) | 171 | (58–154) |
| ESV (mL) | 51 | (13–51) | 70 | (12–68) |
| SV (mL) | 80 | (33–97) | 101 | (35–98) |
| EF (%) | 61 | (56–75) | 59 | (49–73) |
| EDVi (mL/m²) | 74 | (65–99) | 96 | (65–102) |
| ESVi (mL/m²) | 29 | (19–37) | 39 | (20–45) |
| SVi (mL/m²) | 45 | (42–66) | 57 | (39–63) |

**Comments:** MR offers reliable quantitation of RV volume and function. In this case, the degree of RV dilation is mild despite the conduit dysfunction. RV function is normal.

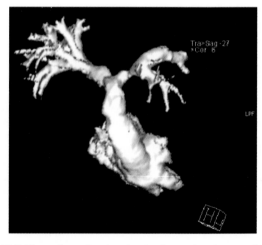

Figure 42-7 Three-dimensional contrast-enhanced angiogram of the right ventricular outflow tract and pulmonary arteries.

## FINDINGS

Mildly narrowed homograft conduit. Moderate proximal left pulmonary artery stenosis. Mild kinking of the right pulmonary artery origin.

***Comments:*** Care should be taken when measuring dimensions from 3D MR angiography, as images are not ECG-gated and are thus an average of the dimensions throughout the cardiac cycle. In addition, signal dropout can occur in regions of fast-moving blood, leading to possible overestimation of stenoses. Nevertheless, 3D reconstruction provides important additional information for planning of surgical or interventional procedures.[12]

# CATHETERIZATION

## HEMODYNAMICS

Heart rate    75 bpm

|  | Pressure | Saturation (%) |
|---|---|---|
| RA | mean 9 | 74 |
| RV | 55/4 | 72 |
| PA | 31/16 mean 21 | 66 |
| LPA | 16/6 mean 11 |  |
| PCWP | mean 10 |  |
| Aorta | 90/49 mean 63 | 98 |
| Cardiac output | 4.27 L/min |  |
| Cardiac index | 2.6 L/min/m$^2$ |  |

**Calculations**

| | |
|---|---|
| Qp (L/min) | 3.47 |
| Qs (L/min) | 4.63 |
| Cardiac index (L/min/m$^2$) | 2.61 |
| Qp/Qs | 0.75 |
| PVR (Wood units) | 3.17 |
| SVR (Wood units) | 11.66 |

## FINDINGS

Cardiac catheterization demonstrated severe homograft regurgitation in addition to moderate left pulmonary artery stenosis.

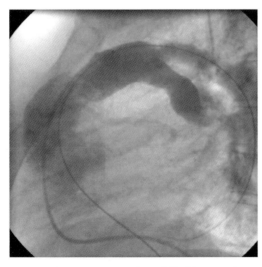

Figure 42-8 Lateral angiogram showing calcified homograft conduit with free pulmonary regurgitation.

## FINDINGS

To assess the RVOT for potential percutaneous pulmonary valve implantation, a 25-mm PTS Sizing Balloon was inflated.

This showed a dimension of 18 mm × 21 mm, with a clear stenotic segment in the center.

Significant pulmonary regurgitation was present with moderate homograft obstruction and moderate stenosis of the smaller homograft joining to the left pulmonary artery.

***Comments:*** This image is necessary for sizing the RVOT in consideration for percutaneous PVR. Percutaneous pulmonary valves can be implanted into outflow tracts up to 22 mm in diameter. Balloon sizing is commonly performed in borderline cases to document the distensibility of the potential site for implantation.

### FOCUSED CLINICAL QUESTIONS AND DISCUSSION POINTS

1. **Is there an indication for intervention in this patient?**

   *Pulmonary regurgitation is the most important residual lesion in repaired TOF, correlating with RV size, exercise intolerance, and serious ventricular arrhythmias. Pulmonary valve replacement has beneficial effects on these parameters provided it is performed before irreversible myocardial dysfunction occurs. Associated lesions, particularly branch pulmonary artery stenosis, aggravate pulmonary and tricuspid regurgitation, which further affect RV size and function.*

   *However, surgically implanted valves have limited longevity and are likely to degenerate with time, committing patients to further operations.[13] The decision to operate should, therefore, be based on the balance between progressive ventricular dilatation, exercise intolerance, symptoms, arrhythmias, and that further reoperations will be needed.*

   *Prospective follow-up of this patient group with exercise testing and assessment of RV size and function should better define the natural history of the disease and provide firm guidelines for timing especially in asymptomatic patients.[14]*

   *The recent development of transcatheter alternatives may change the balance between medical and surgical intervention. It may be that earlier, safer intervention will protect the RV from adverse remodeling. Thus the transcatheter approach may facilitate the growing inclination for earlier intervention without the risks associated with repeat sternotomy and cardiopulmonary bypass.*

   *This patient has a combination of moderate conduit stenosis and regurgitation and objective evidence of exercise intolerance with gradual onset of symptoms of shortness of breath and fatigue. These constitute criteria for elective intervention, albeit RV (and LV) systolic function seem to be maintained at rest.*

2. **What are the options for intervention?**

   *Surgical repair with a bifurcated homograft is one management approach for this patient. She is symptomatic, with objective evidence of exercise impairment and RV dilatation. However, operative intervention must be undertaken with the understanding that surgery may again be required in the future if homograft degeneration occurs. As an alternative, a valved conduit using a xenograft valve would be used in many centers in association with a left pulmonary arterioplasty.*

   *The conventional transcatheter management of this case would involve placement of a left pulmonary artery stent and a bare stent in the main pulmonary artery homograft to relieve the pressure load on the RV. While this approach can improve symptoms and reduce RV pressure,[15] it is not optimal, as the patient would continue to have free pulmonary regurgitation.*

   *The third option is transcatheter PVR and stenting of the homograft left pulmonary artery stenosis. Though a newer technique, it has obvious advantages for the properly selected patient.*

3. What are the limitations of transcatheter valve replacement?

*Percutaneous pulmonary valve replacement provides a novel transcatheter approach to this condition. The device is a bovine jugular venous valve mounted inside a platinum iridium stent that can be deployed in the same manner as a bare stent but with the additional benefit of restoring pulmonary valve competence. The procedure has been performed in more than 700 patients worldwide and has been associated with early clinical improvement, reduction in right ventricular volumes, and 98% freedom from pulmonary regurgitation at 1 year.[9]*

*Percutaneous pulmonary valve implantation is currently limited to those patients whose RVOTs are not larger than 22 mm. Furthermore, the presence of circumferential calcification or some degree of stenosis is desirable, as it is likely to aid device stability. At present, therefore, this procedure is rarely suitable for patients who have pulmonary regurgitation in association with patch augmentation of the RVOT, which was a common approach to repair in the past. Other patients may be excluded if vascular access is difficult, such as patients with azygos continuity of the IVC, although the procedure can be performed via an internal jugular approach. Documentation of coronary anatomy prior to proceeding is essential as stent implantation can cause external compression of a coronary artery if in close proximity (i.e., intramural or intra-arterial course of the left anterior descending).*

*At present, although early results are promising, the long-term fate of the valved stent remains unknown.[9] Stent fracture can occur and has been associated with clinical events such as in-stent stenosis and stent migration in a minority.[16] Nevertheless, the procedure is less invasive and has fewer complications than conventional surgery.[17]*

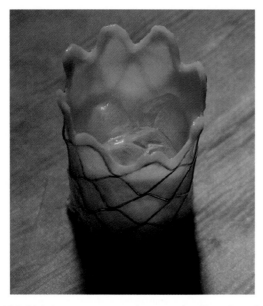

Figure 42-9 Melody percutaneous pulmonary valve. (From Coats L, Tsang V, Khambadkone S, et al: The potential impact of percutaneous pulmonary valve stent implantation on right ventricular outflow tract re-intervention. Eur J Cardiothorac Surg 27:536–543, 2005.)

## FINAL DIAGNOSIS

Late homograft degeneration associated with pulmonary regurgitation and RVOT obstruction

Proximal left pulmonary artery stenosis

## PLAN OF ACTION

Percutaneous pulmonary valve implantation and left pulmonary artery stent

## INTERVENTION

The procedure was performed from a right femoral venous approach under general anesthesia. An ultra-stiff guide wire was stabilized in the distal right pulmonary artery to facilitate delivery of the device. The percutaneous pulmonary valve was crimped onto a 22-mm Balloon in Balloon (BiB) delivery system. The device was conveyed and deployed without complication in the narrowest portion of the main homograft. Subsequently, the wire position was changed to the left pulmonary artery and a 29/10 Genesis premounted stent on a 10-mm balloon was delivered to the smaller homograft conduit. There were no immediate complications.

## OUTCOME

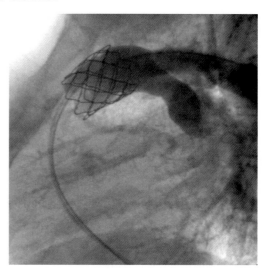

Figure 42-10 Lateral angiogram post–percutaneous pulmonary valve implantation showing relief of outflow tract obstruction and abolition of regurgitation.

### FINDINGS

Hemodynamics postprocedure were:

|  | **Pressures** |
|---|---|
| RV | 46/10 |
| PA | 36/8 mean 20 |
| LPA | 23/8 mean 5 |
| Aorta | 116/63 mean 82 |

***Comments:*** In the postintervention pulmonary angiogram no regurgitation was seen through the valved stent. Percutaneous pulmonary valve implantation has been successfully combined with other transcatheter procedures such as ASD closure and VSD closure.

The patient experienced an early improvement in clinical symptoms and was NYHA class I by 3 months. A progressive improvement in cardiopulmonary exercise capacity was noted.

|  | Pre | 1 mo post | 1 yr post |
|---|---|---|---|
| VO$_2$ max (mL/kg/min) | 19.0 | 24.3 | 27.1 |
| AT (mL/kg/min) | 10.4 | 11.8 | 14.1 |
| Workload (Watts) | 90 | 130 | 125 |
| Peak heart rate (bpm) | 153 | 180 | 176 |
| Peak blood pressure (mm Hg) | 155/80 | 170/80 | 180/70 |
| Respiratory exchange ratio | 1.06 | 1.05 | 1.16 |

Echocardiography confirmed absence of pulmonary regurgitation with a peak gradient of 31 mm Hg (mean gradient 16 mm Hg) across the percutaneous pulmonary valve and a peak velocity of 1.8 m/sec across the left pulmonary artery stent at 1 year.

MRI at 1 year showed a substantial reduction in RV volume (preprocedure values are shown in parentheses in the table below).

**Ventricular Volume Quantification**

|          | LV  | (Prior data) | RV  | (Prior data) |
|----------|-----|--------------|-----|--------------|
| EDV (mL) | 131 | (131)        | 137 | (171)        |
| ESV (mL) | 49  | (51)         | 55  | (70)         |
| SV (mL)  | 82  | (80)         | 82  | (101)        |
| EF (%)   | 63  | (61)         | 60  | (59)         |

***Comments:*** Percutaneous pulmonary valve replacement results in a reduction in RV volume and leads to an early improvement in symptoms and objective exercise capacity.[9]

# ACKNOWLEDGMENT

The MR images were contributed by Dr. Andrew Taylor, MRCP, MD, FRCR.

# Selected References

1. Moller JH, Taubert KA, Allen HD, et al: Cardiovascular health and disease in children: Current status. Circulation 89:923–930, 1994.
2. Bove EL, Byrum CJ, Thomas FD, et al: The influence of pulmonary insufficiency on ventricular function following repair of tetralogy of Fallot. Evaluation using radionuclide ventriculography. J Thorac Cardiovasc Surg 85:691–696, 1983.
3. Carvalho JS, Shinebourne EA, Busst C, et al: Exercise capacity after complete repair of tetralogy of Fallot: Deleterious effects of residual pulmonary regurgitation. Br Heart J 67:470–473, 1992.
4. Gatzoulis MA, Balaji S, Webber SA, et al: Risk factors for arrhythmia and sudden cardiac death late after repair of tetralogy of Fallot: A multicentre study. Lancet 356:975–981, 2000.
5. Chaturvedi RR, Kilner PJ, White PA, et al: Increased airway pressure and simulated branch pulmonary artery stenosis increase pulmonary regurgitation after repair of tetralogy of Fallot. Real-time analysis with a conductance catheter technique. Circulation 95:643–649, 1997.
6. Gatzoulis MA, Till JA, Somerville J, Redington AN: Mechanoelectrical interaction in tetralogy of Fallot. QRS prolongation relates to right ventricular size and predicts malignant ventricular arrhythmias and sudden death. Circulation 92:231–237, 1995.
7. Diller GP, Dimopoulos K, Okonko D, et al: Exercise intolerance in adult congenital heart disease: Comparative severity, correlates, and prognostic implication. Circulation 112:828–835, 2005.
8. Eyskens B, Reybrouck T, Bogaert J, et al: Homograft insertion for pulmonary regurgitation after repair of tetralogy of Fallot improves cardiorespiratory exercise performance. Am J Cardiol 85:221–225, 2000.
9. Khambadkone S, Coats L, Taylor AM, et al: Transcatheter pulmonary valve implantation in humans—Initial results in 59 consecutive patients. Circulation 112:1189–1197, 2005.
10. Silversides CK, Veldtman GR, Crossin J, et al: Pressure half-time predicts hemodynamically significant pulmonary regurgitation in adult patients with repaired tetralogy of Fallot. J Am Soc Echocardiog 16:1057–1061, 2003.
11. Li W, Davlouros PA, Kilner PJ, et al: Doppler-echocardiographic assessment of pulmonary regurgitation in adults with repaired tetralogy of Fallot: Comparison with cardiovascular magnetic resonance imaging. Am Heart J 147:165–172, 2004.
12. Bogaert J, Dymarkowski S, Taylor AM: Clinical Cardiac MRI. Heidelberg, Germany, Springer-Verlag, 2005.
13. Stark J, Bull C, Stajevic M, et al: Fate of subpulmonary homograft conduits: Determinants of late homograft failure. J Thorac Cardiovasc Surg 115:506–516, 1998.
14. Davlouros PA, Karatza AA, Gatzoulis MA, Shore DF: Timing and type of surgery for severe pulmonary regurgitation after repair of tetralogy of Fallot. Int J Cardiol 97(Suppl 1):91–101, 2004.
15. Fogelman R, Nykanen D, Smallhorn JF, et al: Endovascular stents in the pulmonary circulation: Clinical impact on management and medium-term follow-up. Circulation 92:881–885, 1995.
16. Nordmeyer J, Khambadkone S, Coats L, et al: Risk stratification, systematic classification, and anticipatory management strategies for stent fracture after percutaneous pulmonary valve implantation. Circulation 115:392–397, 2007.
17. Coats L, Tsang VT, Khambadkone S, et al: The potential impact of percutaneous pulmonary valve stent implantation on right ventricular outflow tract re-intervention. Eur J Cardio-Thorac Surg 27:536–543, 2005.

# Management of Tachyarrhythmia in Tetralogy: Ablation versus Surgery

**Sonya V. Babu-Narayan, Jan Till, and Babulal Sethia**

**Age: 46 years**
**Gender: Male**
**Occupation: Accountant**
**Working diagnosis: Repaired tetralogy of Fallot**

## HISTORY

The patient had a primary repair of TOF when he was 8 years old. Following this he remained well under occasional follow-up for the following 28 years.

He then complained of palpitations at age 36. He was started on sotalol. Echocardiography demonstrated severe pulmonary regurgitation. Though occasional palpitations persisted, these were tolerated well, and no further evaluation was pursued.

Eight years later, at age 44, he presented with atrial reentrant tachycardia requiring direct current cardioversion. Sotalol was discontinued and amiodarone commenced. A workup confirmed his severe pulmonary regurgitation. After case discussion, pulmonary valve replacement was deferred and electrophysiology study with a view to ablation was planned. Mapping confirmed atrial reentrant tachycardia around a scar, and he underwent successful ablation of the likely pathway. He was symptom free for 6 months, but atrial reentrant tachycardia continued to recur despite amiodarone, and repeated direct current cardioversion at his local hospital was required. He presented for further management.

*Comments:* Pulmonary regurgitation is a common finding 20 to 30 years after repair of TOF; it has been associated with an increased risk of both atrial and ventricular arrhythmia, late RV dysfunction, and sudden cardiac death. To address legitimate concerns that untreated pulmonary regurgitation may lead to irreversible RV dysfunction, pulmonary valve implantation needs to be considered. However, these issues must be balanced with both the fact that pulmonary regurgitation in some patients is well tolerated for decades and the fact that currently available bioprosthetic valves have a finite lifespan. The timing of pulmonary valve surgery, therefore, remains a challenging clinical decision.

The onset of arrhythmia in the context of pulmonary regurgitation after repair of TOF is an indication to assess the degree of pulmonary regurgitation and ventricular function. Arrhythmia may be considered as an indication for valve replacement. According to the principles of mechanoelectric interaction, arrhythmias may reflect hemodynamic abnormalities, with both components requiring attention.

## CURRENT SYMPTOMS

Apart from recurrent palpitations, the patient had no symptoms. His self-reported exercise tolerance is good, and he was able to work full time. Palpitations and anxiety caused by fear of palpitations were the main limiting factors from the patient's perspective.

NYHA class: I

## CURRENT MEDICATIONS

Amiodarone 200 mg daily

Warfarin (variable dose to maintain INR 2.0–3.0)

## PHYSICAL EXAMINATION

BP 125/86 mm Hg, HR 64 bpm, oxygen saturation 99%

Height 182 cm, weight 62 kg, BSA 1.77 m$^2$

Surgical scars: Midline sternotomy scar

Neck veins: The JVP was not elevated, and the waveform was normal.

Lungs/chest: Clear to auscultation and percussion

Heart: The heart rate was regular. There was an RV heave. Auscultation revealed a normal first heart sound and an ejection systolic murmur followed by a single second heart sound with absent pulmonary component. There was a short, early diastolic murmur at the right sternal edge. Peripheral pulses were palpable and equal.

Abdomen: No abnormality detected

Extremities: No clubbing or swelling of ankles

*Comments:* This patient had classic features of significant pulmonary regurgitation. The short, early diastolic murmur is in keeping with severe pulmonary regurgitation, as is the RV heave. Bear in mind that the clinician may be surprised that in severe pulmonary regurgitation with no turbulence, the murmur may not be heard at all.

## LABORATORY DATA

| | |
|---|---|
| Hemoglobin | 14.7 g/dL (13.0–17.0) |
| Hematocrit/PCV | 45% (41–51) |
| MCV | 96 fL (83–99) |
| Platelet count | $183 \times 10^9$/L (150–400) |
| Sodium | 138 mmol/L (134–145) |
| Potassium | 3.9 mmol/L (3.5–5.2) |
| Creatinine | 0.8 mg/dL (0.6–1.2) |
| Blood urea nitrogen | 6.3 mmol/L (2.5–6.5) |

### OTHER RELEVANT LAB RESULTS

| | |
|---|---|
| T4 | 15.7 pmol/L (7.5–21) |
| TSH | 2.39 IU/L (0.32–5.0) |
| Calcium (corr) | 2.35 mmol/L (2.20–2.62) |
| Inorganic phosphate | 1.09 mmol/L (0.8–1.40) |
| Magnesium | 0.81 mmol/L (0.7–1.0) |
| INR (on warfarin) | 2.5 |

***Comments:*** It is important to remember thyroid dysfunction both as a cause of arrhythmia and as a consequence of amiodarone therapy. In this case, thyroid function was normal.

## ELECTROCARDIOGRAM

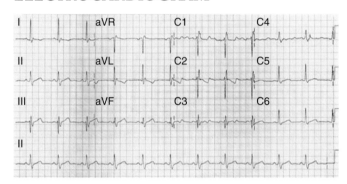

Figure 43-1 Electrocardiogram.

### FINDINGS

Heart rate: 66 bpm

QRS axis: +85°

QRS duration: 144 msec

Sinus rhythm with RBBB. There is voltage evidence for LV hypertrophy (R1 + S3 > 25; raVL > 11 mm).

***Comments:*** RBBB is a typical finding after repair of the TOF, particularly in older adults who had a right ventriculotomy at the time of surgery. The QRS duration in this context may nevertheless additionally change over time reflecting volume dilatation of the right side of the heart. Prolonged QRS duration greater than 180 msec is regarded as a risk factor for sudden cardiac death. Given the history and examination findings one may have expected the QRS duration to have been longer in this patient.

## CHEST X-RAY

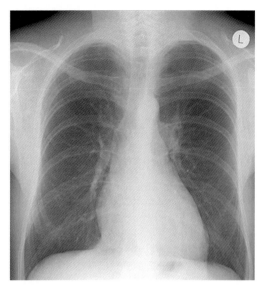

Figure 43-2 Posteroanterior projection.

### FINDINGS
Cardiothoracic ratio: 50%

Borderline cardiomegaly, prominent main and left pulmonary arteries, normal pulmonary vascular markings, no evidence of thoracotomy.

***Comments:*** Despite clinical evidence of significant pulmonary regurgitation, the heart is not significantly enlarged in this patient. This is in keeping with the modest prolongation of QRS duration.

There is no evidence of ascending aortopathy; the aortic knuckle is not enlarged.

## EXERCISE TESTING

| | |
|---|---|
| Exercise protocol: | Modified Bruce |
| Duration (min:sec): | 10:38 |
| Reason for stopping: | Dyspnea |
| ECG changes: | None |

| | Rest | Peak |
|---|---|---|
| Heart rate (bpm): | 64 | 157 |
| Percent of age-predicted max HR: | | 90 |
| O₂ saturation (%): | 99 | 98 |
| Blood pressure (mm Hg): | 125/86 | 140/90 |
| Peak Vo₂ (mL/kg/min): | | 28.5 |
| Percent predicted (%): | | 78 |
| Ve/Vco₂: | | 35 |
| Metabolic equivalents: | | 8.4 |

***Comments:*** Maximal $Vo_2$ and $Ve/Vco_2$ values are abnormal with respect to age and sex-matched controls, but are relatively preserved with respect to other repaired TOF patients with pulmonary regurgitation (see Case 41), though this patient exercised for a shorter duration than average.

# ECHOCARDIOGRAM

## Overall Findings

Normal LV size and systolic function were seen. The RV was moderately dilated with normal systolic function. There was mild tricuspid regurgitation with mild to moderate RA dilatation. Severe pulmonary regurgitation was demonstrated with no functioning pulmonary valve tissue.

There was normal LV size and function. The RVOT was dilated. The aortic root measured 38 mm. A small residual VSD (5 mm) with left-to-right shunt was demonstrated with a gradient of 80 mm Hg.

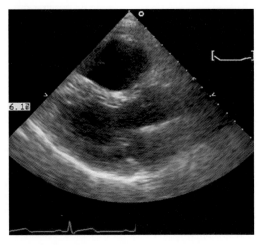

Figure 43-3 Parasternal long-axis view.

***Comments:*** Aortic regurgitation from aortic root dilation must be excluded in any patient with TOF (see Case 45).

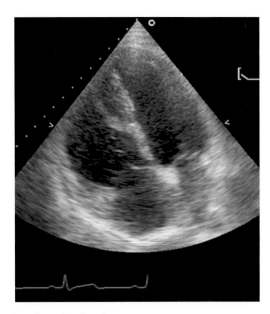

Figure 43-4 Four-chamber view.

## Findings

There was severe dilatation of the RV with normal systolic function. The tricuspid valve was mildly regurgitant with RA enlargement also present.

***Comments:*** Atrial enlargement augments the risk of atrial arrhythmia.

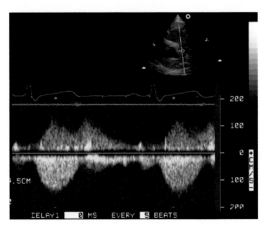

Figure 43-5 Continuous-wave Doppler velocity through the pulmonary valve.

## Findings

There was no residual stenosis through the RVOT. The regurgitation ends well before the completion of diastole, consistent with severe regurgitation.

***Comments:*** Note the antegrade flow in end diastole; the A-wave, suggesting the RV is already filled to capacity in mid diastole such that atrial contraction results in forward flow to the pulmonary artery (PA). This flow pattern tends to be more noticeable in ventricles without severe dilatation (see Case 41), although it can occur in the latter.

For the aortic valve, Doppler traces can be used to calculate a pressure half-time to gauge the severity of regurgitation. No such guidelines have been worked out for pulmonary valve severity, though the general concept is the same. The velocity will fall at a faster rate in the setting of more severe regurgitation, because the pressure difference between the PA and RV will equalize much faster (albeit the pressure difference in diastole between PA and RV is normally much smaller compared to the aorta and the LV).

# MAGNETIC RESONANCE IMAGING

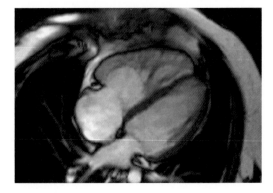

Figure 43-6 Oblique axial plane (four-chamber) steady-state free precession cine.

## FINDINGS

Normal function of the RV and LV was seen. By stroke volume difference the regurgitant fraction was 34%. Mild tricuspid regurgitation and a small residual patch (ventricular septal defect) leak were seen. The aortic root was not significantly dilated, and there was no evidence of branch PA stenosis.

### Ventricular Volume Quantification

|  | LV | (Normal range) | RV | (Normal range) |
|---|---|---|---|---|
| EDV (mL) | 133 | (77–195) | **259** | (88–227) |
| ESV (mL) | 27 | (19–72) | 101 | (23–103) |
| SV (mL) | 106 | (51–133) | **158** | (52–138) |
| EF (%) | 80 | (58–75) | 61 | (52–77) |
| EDVi (mL/m²) | 75 | (64–99) | **146** | (62–108) |
| ESVi (mL/m²) | **15** | (17–38) | **57** | (16–45) |
| SVi (mL/m²) | 60 | (42–66) | **89** | (39–71) |
| Mass index (g/m²) | 61 | (58–91) | **53** | (21–48) |

***Comments:*** The findings are supportive of those of the transthoracic echocardiogram. Preservation of RV function in the setting of severe pulmonary regurgitation is important.

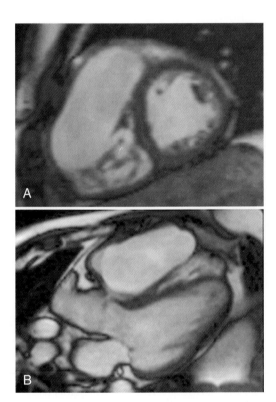

Figure 43-7 **A**, Oblique sagittal plane (short-axis) steady-state free precession (SSFP) cine. **B**, Oblique axial plane left ventricular outflow tract or three-chamber view) SSFP cine.

## FINDINGS

There was a large (50 × 60 mm) akinetic segment of the RV free wall. The aorta was normal in size.

***Comments:*** The dilatation of the outflow region of the RV, namely thinning of the RV free wall, is clearly seen in both views. This akinetic portion is part of the outflow patch placed at the time of initial repair.

It is important to check for aortic root dilatation in all TOF patients (see Case 45).

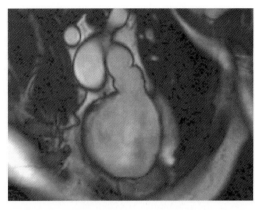

Figure 43-8 Oblique coronal plane (right ventricular outflow tract view) steady-state free precession cine.

## FINDINGS

There was no effective valve tissue in the PA, and the pulmonary regurgitant fraction was calculated as 36% (moderately severe) from non-breath-hold phase contrast velocity mapping.

***Comments:*** Again, the akinetic free wall can be appreciated in this view showing a dilated outflow tract below the PA. In the early days of surgical correction often the surgeon left little or no valve tissue, since the emphasis was on relief of obstruction rather than preservation of valve competency.

## CATHETERIZATION

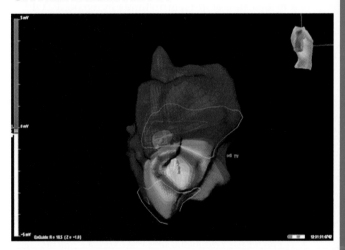

Figure 43-9 Right lateral view showing activation through gap.

## FINDINGS

A macro-reentry circuit was demonstrated by electrophysiological study. The rationale for this test is to perform it to map the clinically relevant atrial arrhythmia and then proceed to ablation. This was done with the aim of improving surgical outcome by dealing with the electrical component of the mechanoelectric combination.

***Comments:*** Using an Ensite balloon, a voltage map was created in sinus rhythm. Two large areas of scar on the lateral wall of the RA were seen. Scar is depicted by the area outlined in white.

A macro-reentry circuit was seen passing between the area of scar and up and around the tip of the RA.

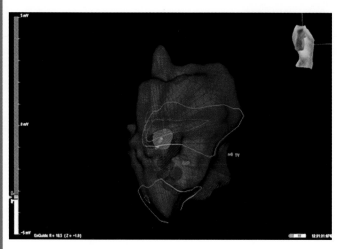

Figure 43-10 Right lateral view showing radiofrequency ablations.

***Comments:*** The areas of scar were therefore joined using an 8-mm tip, and the radiofrequency burns and the reentry circuit were terminated. The brown areas represent the radiofrequency burns.

After the procedure, intra-atrial reentrant tachycardia could no longer be induced.

## FOCUSED CLINICAL QUESTIONS AND DISCUSSION POINTS

1. What is the cause of atrial arrhythmia in repaired TOF?

   *While there is plenty of literature regarding risk factors and causes of ventricular tachycardia in TOF, there has been less attention to atrial arrhythmia in this patient group, although the latter is common. The most usual atrial arrhythmia is atrial macro-reentrant tachycardias or "atrial flutter." These invariably relate to prior atriotomy at the time of surgery and subsequent scar formation and to right atrial dilatation. The presence of RV dilatation, in turn, can worsen tricuspid regurgitation and atrial enlargement.*

2. How does the presence of recurrent atrial arrhythmia alter decisions about timing of pulmonary valve replacement?

   *The most common clinical problem in caring for TOF patients in adult years is timing of pulmonary valve surgery. There are as yet only general principles to guide decision-making, and these have been discussed (see Case 41).*

   *This patient has reasonably preserved exercise function, and palpitations are his only symptom. RV dilatation is only moderate on the TOF spectrum, and RV function is preserved. One may make a reasonable argument to postpone valve replacement further. However, the presence of recurrent atrial arrhythmia must also be considered. A good rule of thumb in this field is that arrhythmia should be considered as a possible sign of unfavorable hemodynamics, which are certainly present here. Addressing the hemodynamic problem usually has a beneficial effect on the arrhythmia, although additional measures to address the latter directly need to be taken.*

3. What is the evidence supporting the use of atrial maze procedures at the time of surgery?

   *Many centers would perform an empiric RA maze procedure in such a patient at the time of pulmonary valve replacement. A recent paper from the Mayo Clinic reported reduction in atrial flutter/fibrillation following a concomitant right-sided maze procedure at the time of intracardiac repair among patients with ACHD and chronic or paroxysmal atrial tachycardia.*

## FINAL DIAGNOSIS

Repaired TOF with moderately severe pulmonary regurgitation

Recurrent atrial reentrant tachycardia

## PLAN OF ACTION

Pulmonary valve replacement with surgical RA maze and VSD closure

## INTERVENTION

Imaging findings were confirmed at surgery.

A surgical maze was performed using cryotherapy confined to the RA.

A large, thin akinetic region of outflow tract was found, within which was a long ventriculotomy scar. The latter was resected and the thin region plicated. A bioprosthetic pulmonary valve was inserted, and the VSD patch leak oversewn.

## OUTCOME

The patient made an uneventful recovery and was discharged from the hospital in 6 days. He remained anticoagulated and on amiodarone for 3 months. One year after his operation he remained free of arrhythmia. The patient reported improved functional capacity and exercise function, although he remained somewhat timid about pushing himself too hard for fear of instigating further arrhythmia.

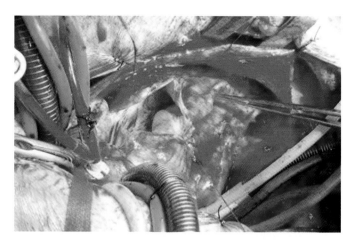

Figure 43-11 Perioperative photograph at the time of pulmonary valve replacement.

***Comments:*** The forceps point to the extensive previous ventriculotomy scar, which was excised.

## Bibliography

Bove EL, Kavey RE, Byrum CJ, et al: Improved right ventricular function following late pulmonary valve replacement for residual pulmonary insufficiency or stenosis. J Thorac Cardiovasc Surg 90:50–55, 1985.

Davlouros PA, Karatza AA, Gatzoulis MA, Shore DF: Timing and type of surgery for severe pulmonary regurgitation after repair of tetralogy of Fallot (Review). Int J Cardiol 97(Suppl 1):91–101, 2004.

Eyskens B, Reybrouck T, Bogaert J, et al: Homograft insertion for pulmonary regurgitation after repair of tetralogy of Fallot improves cardiorespiratory exercise performance. Am J Cardiol 85:221–225, 2000.

Gatzoulis MA, Balaji S, Webber SA, et al: Risk factors for arrhythmia and sudden cardiac death late after repair of tetralogy of Fallot: A multicentre study. Lancet 356:975–981, 2000.

Gengsakul A, Harris L, Bradley TJ, et al: The impact of pulmonary valve replacement after tetralogy of Fallot repair: A matched comparison. Eur J Cardiothorac Surg 32:462–468, 2007.

Harrison DA, Siu SC, Hussain F, et al: Sustained atrial arrhythmias in adults late after repair of tetralogy of Fallot. Am J Cardiol 87:584–588, 2001.

Nollert G, Fischlein T, Bouterwek S, et al: Long-term survival in patients with repair of tetralogy of Fallot: 36-year follow-up of 490 survivors of the first year after surgical repair. J Am Coll Cardiol 30:1374–1383, 1997.

Oosterhof T, van Straten A, Vliegen HW, et al: Preoperative thresholds for pulmonary valve replacement in patients with corrected tetralogy of Fallot using cardiovascular magnetic resonance. Circulation 116:545–551, 2007.

Roos-Hesselink J, Perlroth MG, McGhie J, Spitaels S: Atrial arrhythmias in adults after repair of tetralogy of Fallot. Correlations with clinical, exercise, and echocardiographic findings. Circulation 91:2214–2219, 1995.

Stulak JM, Dearani JA, Puga FJ, et al: Right-sided Maze procedure for atrial tachyarrhythmias in congenital heart disease. Ann Thorac Surg 81:1780–1784, 2006.

Therrien J, Provost Y, Merchant N, et al: Optimal timing for pulmonary valve replacement in adults after tetralogy of Fallot repair. Am J Cardiol 95:779–782, 2005.

Therrien J, Siu SC, Harris L, et al: Impact of pulmonary valve replacement on arrhythmia propensity late after repair of tetralogy of Fallot. Circulation 103:2489–2494, 2001.

Therrien J, Siu SC, McLaughlin PR, et al: Pulmonary valve replacement in adults late after repair of tetralogy of Fallot: Are we operating too late? J Am Coll Cardiol 36:1670–1675, 2000.

Van Huysduynen BH, van Straten A, Swenne CA, et al: Reduction of QRS duration after pulmonary valve replacement in adult Fallot patients is related to reduction of right ventricular volume. Eur Heart J 26:928–932, 2005.

Vliegen HW, van Straten A, de Roos A, et al: Magnetic resonance imaging to assess the hemodynamic effects of pulmonary valve replacement in adults late after repair of tetralogy of Fallot. Circulation 106:1703–1707, 2002.

Warner KG, Anderson JE, Fulton DR, et al: Restoration of the pulmonary valve reduces right ventricular volume overload after previous repair of tetralogy of Fallot. Circulation 88(5 Pt 2):II189–197, 1993.

Yemets IM, Williams WG, Webb GD, et al: Pulmonary valve replacement late after repair of tetralogy of Fallot. Ann Thorac Surg 64:526–530, 1997.

# Consideration for Automatic Implantable Cardioverter-Defibrillator in Tetralogy

Sonya V. Babu-Narayan, Philip J. Kilner, and Darryl F. Shore

**Age: 56 years**
**Gender: Male**
**Occupation: Attorney**
**Working diagnosis: Repaired tetralogy of Fallot**

## HISTORY

At the age of 6 years, this patient had a Brock procedure (1958). Using a transpulmonary approach, Lord Brock resected subpulmonary muscle to relieve the pulmonary stenosis, leaving the patient's VSD untouched.

Three years later, at the age of 9 years, the patient presented with further cyanosis and fainting, and underwent tetralogy repair, also by Lord Brock. The operative note described the following: "Bicuspid pulmonary valve—stretched with an expanding dilator," "the fibro-endocardial tissue constituting the infundibular stenosis was carved away liberally," "the VSD was closed with a pericardial patch." The postoperative notes document a pulmonary diastolic murmur.

A year later the patient experienced an episode of ventricular tachycardia (VT) requiring direct current (DC) cardioversion at a local hospital. Again, at age 14 years, he had a further episode of sustained VT, which apparently occurred following a blow to the chest.[1] This resolved spontaneously. The patient felt well and had no further workup or adverse event.

There was no routine cardiac follow-up until the patient was 44 years old. At that time he complained of palpitations. Although each episode was short lived, he had noted these several times over the previous 9 years.

On reassessment he was found to have moderate to severe pulmonary regurgitation by echocardiography. Both sustained VT and nonsustained VT were also documented on 24-hour Holter ECGs over the following 5 years.

At age 50 his exercise capacity was normal, and his only complaint was of occasional palpitations. His pulmonary regurgitation was reevaluated and found to be severe by echocardiography and cardiac catheterization. He had normal coronary arteriograms.

Because the patient was "asymptomatic" with above-average exercise tolerance, a decision was made to defer pulmonary valve replacement and that there was no current indication for electrophysiologic ablation. Medication for arrhythmia was declined by the patient, who felt that this might treat only the palpitations rather than the underlying cause.

In the years that followed, palpitations were described as either single beats, or short-lived regular and fast heart rhythms relieved by a Valsalva maneuver. His exercise tolerance remained very good.

On the day of presentation, the patient was walking his dog briskly uphill and noted the onset of very fast palpitations and dizziness unrelieved by a Valsalva maneuver. As the rhythm persisted he felt chest pain, diaphoresis, and a feeling like blood was draining from his fingers. He collapsed but did not lose consciousness. A passerby called for help. Paramedics were soon at the scene and gave him aspirin and oxygen. He was taken immediately to a nearby hospital, where the following ECG was obtained.

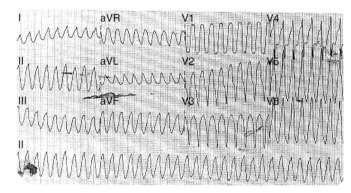

Figure 44-1 Electrocardiogram showing VT at 214 bpm with left bundle branch block pattern and superiorly directed QRS axis.

A DC cardioversion was promptly performed, and sinus rhythm with a stable blood pressure was restored. There were no electrolyte abnormalities, and blood tests did not show any elevation of troponin. He felt well thereafter and was discharged from the local hospital after 24 hours of observation. Follow-up was arranged with a tertiary care center.

The patient was a nonsmoker with no other medical problems. His eldest brother had unspecified congenital heart disease, but there was no history of coronary artery disease in the family.

**Comments:** Historically, pulmonary regurgitation was thought to be a benign lesion. Pulmonary regurgitation is usually the dominant lesion in patients who have had tetralogy repair. A severe degree of pulmonary regurgitation was more likely if a transannular patch was used in the repair (not used in this patient). The diastolic murmur was likely due to pulmonary regurgitation.

The blow to the chest may have resulted in mechanical energy being converted to electrical energy, which resulted in an arrhythmia.[2]

The decision to replace the pulmonary valve after repair of TOF is one of the most commonly discussed and controversial issues in this field. The decision to wait was based on his normal RV function, very good exercise tolerance, and absence of symptoms.

The rhythm is VT. The regular, broad complex tachycardia (rate of 214 bpm), with LBBB conduction pattern and superiorly directed QRS axis is consistent with VT.

## CURRENT SYMPTOMS

Prior to his tachycardia, he had been swimming regularly and walking his dog each day, always without physical limitation. He had palpitations as described above, but they were always short lived and not associated with other symptoms.

NYHA class: 1

## PHYSICAL EXAMINATION

BP 120/60 mm Hg, HR 60 bpm, oxygen saturation (right hand) 100%

Height 188 cm, weight 70 kg, BSA 1.91 m²

Surgical scars: Midline sternotomy scar

Neck veins: JVP was not elevated, and the waveform was normal.

Lungs/chest: Chest was clear to auscultation.

Heart: The heart rhythm was regular. There was an RV heave. Auscultation revealed a normal first heart sound, an ejection systolic murmur followed by a single second heart sound, and a low-pitched early diastolic murmur at the left sternal edge, which was accentuated by inspiration. Peripheral pulses were palpable and equal. Additionally, a high-pitched early diastolic murmur at the right sternal edge was heard, felt to reflect aortic regurgitation.

Abdomen: No abnormality detected

Extremities: There was no clubbing or dependent edema.

***Comments:*** Significant JVP elevation in a patient with repaired tetralogy usually reflects problems requiring reoperation. The absence of an abnormal V-wave suggests there is not substantial tricuspid regurgitation. When tricuspid regurgitation occurs in such patients, it is usually because of RV systolic dysfunction.

An RV heave in such a patient without RVOT obstruction indicates that pulmonary regurgitation is moderate to severe. The absence of such a lift may reflect mild hemodynamic problems or be due to physical factors or lack of discernment on the part of the examiner.

## LABORATORY DATA

| Hemoglobin | 14.7 g/dL (13.0–17.0) |
| Hematocrit/PCV | 46% (41–51) |
| MCV | 93 fL (83–99) |
| Platelet count | 156 × 10⁹/L (150–400) |
| Sodium | 137 mmol/L (134–145) |
| Potassium | 4.4 mmol/L (3.5–5.2) |
| Creatinine | 0.7 mg/dL (0.6–1.2) |
| Blood urea nitrogen | 3.4 mmol/L (2.5–6.5) |

***Comments:*** No abnormalities present.

## ELECTROCARDIOGRAM

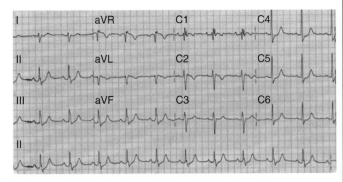

Figure 44-2 Electrocardiogram.

### FINDINGS
Heart rate: 66 bpm

QRS axis: +115°

QRS duration: 137 msec

Sinus rhythm with an RBBB. QRS axis: Initial forces are at +115°, with a terminal RBBB. Six months previously the QRS duration had been 160 msec, and a decade prior it had been 120 msec.

***Comments:*** RBBB was typical in patients with tetralogy repair due to the right ventriculotomy or the placement of the VSD patch. More recently, RBBB is somewhat less common in patients having surgery because a transatrial and transpulmonary approach is now used. QRS duration usually lengthens with time, reflecting increasing RV volume. Increase in QRS duration over time is a marker predictive of sudden cardiac death and may be more sensitive than absolute values.[3]

## CHEST X-RAY

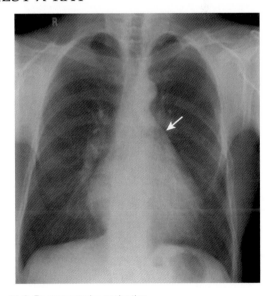

Figure 44-3 Posteroanterior projection.

### FINDINGS
Cardiothoracic ratio: 49%

Upper normal heart size with prominent main pulmonary artery (PA) and RVOT. The lung markings are normal, and there is evidence of a prior sternotomy. RA prominence. Left aortic arch.

***Comments:*** There is a bulging area (*arrow*) of the left cardiac silhouette that corresponds to a dilated main PA and RVOT.

## EXERCISE TESTING

|  | Current Study | 4 Years Prior |
|---|---|---|
| Exercise protocol: | Modified Bruce | Modified Bruce |
| Duration (min:sec): | 13:08 | 15:35 |
| Reason for stopping: | Fatigue | Fatigue |
| ECG changes: | None | None |

|  | Rest | Peak | Peak |
|---|---|---|---|
| Heart rate (bpm): | 60 | 150 | 155 |
| Percent of age-predicted max HR: |  | 91 | 92 |
| O$_2$ saturation (%): | 100 | 100 | 100 |
| Blood pressure (mm Hg): | 120/60 | 160/80 | 165/80 |
| Peak Vo$_2$ (mL/kg/min): |  | 30 | 39 |
| Percent predicted (%): |  | 75 | 124 |
| Ve/Vco$_2$: |  | 24.7 | 22.1 |
| Metabolic equivalents: |  | 9.6 |  |

***Comments:*** Serial cardiopulmonary exercise testing may provide objective evidence of a change in exercise tolerance before the onset of symptoms. It is important that similar methods are used if the tests are to have comparative value.

In this patient, with seemingly good exercise tolerance who is above average for our repaired tetralogy population (see Case 41), there is nevertheless a deterioration seen over the 4-year period.

The patient was not aware of a decrease in his exercise capacity.

## ECHOCARDIOGRAM

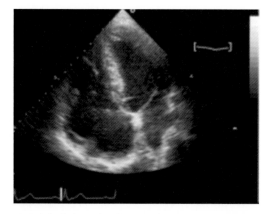

Figure 44-4 Apical four-chamber projection 2D echocardiographic acquisition.

### FINDINGS

The RV was large with respect to the LV, and moderately dilated by measured diameter (RV inflow dimension = 56 mm, LV inflow = 52 mm). RV function was normal.

There was normal LV size and function. There was moderate RA enlargement with a normal LA. There was a normal aortic valve, dilated aortic root (48 mm), no aortic stenosis, mild aortic regurgitation, and no residual VSD.

### M-Mode/2D Measurements and Calculations

IVSD: 11 mm

LVIDD: 50 mm

LVIDS: 34 mm

LVPWD: 12 mm

FS: 31%

EF (Teicholz method): 59%

***Comments:*** RV enlargement is typical in TOF patients with important pulmonary valve regurgitation.

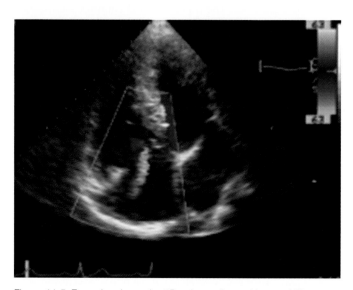

Figure 44-5 Four-chamber color 2D echocardiographic acquisition.

### FINDINGS

A jet of mild tricuspid regurgitation was demonstrated with color Doppler.

***Comments:*** While not present here, new onset or worsening of tricuspid regurgitation in the setting of repaired TOF with pulmonary regurgitation is usually a marker of progressive RV dilatation, as well as potential systolic dysfunction due to pulmonary regurgitation.

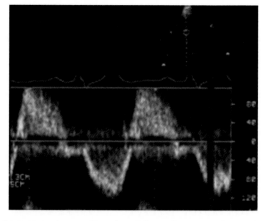

Figure 44-6 Pulsed-wave Doppler of the pulmonary artery echocardiographic acquisition.

### FINDINGS

There is evidence on Doppler of significant pulmonary regurgitation with retrograde flow toward the transducer in most but not all diastole. There is no significant RVOT obstruction.

***Comments:*** Severe regurgitation is confirmed. Note the regurgitation jet ends before end diastole.

# MAGNETIC RESONANCE IMAGING

## Ventricular Volume Quantification

|  | LV | (Normal range) | RV | (Normal range) |
|---|---|---|---|---|
| EDV (mL) | 194 | (77–195) | 336 | (88–227) |
| ESV (mL) | 95 | (19–72) | 179 | (23–103) |
| SV (mL) | 99 | (51–133) | 157 | (52–138) |
| EF (%) | 51 | (58–76) | 47 | (53–79) |
| EDVi (mL/m²) | 101 | (62–97) | 176 | (59–105) |
| ESVi (mL/m²) | 50 | (15–37) | 94 | (13–42) |
| SVi (mL/m²) | 52 | (41–65) | 82 | (38–70) |

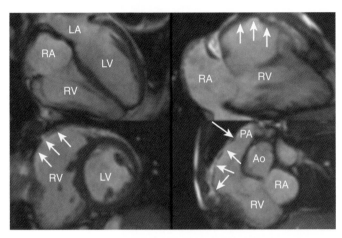

Figure 44-7 *Top left*, four-chamber view; *top right*, two-chamber view; *bottom left*, short-axis view of both ventricles; *bottom right*, oblique RV view.

## FINDINGS

The RV was moderately to severely dilated, and twice the size of the LV. A large (>50-mm length) akinetic area was seen in the RVOT extending down into the body of the RV on both long-axis views of the RVOT and short-axis views (*arrows*). The RV ejection fraction was mildly reduced. There was free pulmonary regurgitation. The *longer arrow* shows the expected level of the pulmonary valve annulus. The origin of the left PA was noted to be angulated without significant stenosis.

***Comments:*** It is notable how deceiving a four-chamber view would be if one were to assess RV dilation on this view alone in this patient.

We do not know whether the akinetic area has progressively dilated with time or whether it has been static from the time of surgery. In terms of RV systolic function, it is difficult to quantify the separate contributions of the muscular and akinetic areas in any robust, reproducible, and validated way. The reason there may be interest in doing so is that the negative impact of akinetic areas on global RV function may mask subtle changes in the contractility of the muscular part of the RV. Regardless, it seems that akinetic RVOT areas are detrimental with respect to function and prognosis and therefore should be taken into account in the overall assessment of RV function. Such areas may also be relevant in terms of electrical circuitry and risk of VT, although this has yet to be studied.

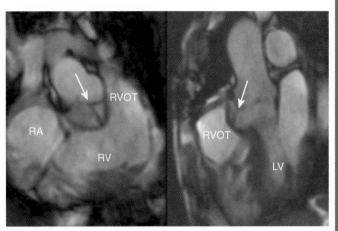

Figure 44-8 RV oblique-type view (*left*), aligned to show diastolic jet. LVOT-type view (*right*) where the same jet is arrowed. Both show that the jet is directed toward the VSD patch (*arrows*).

## FINDINGS

Aortic regurgitation through a perforated right coronary cusp (*arrows*), resulting in a narrow diastolic jet directed at the VSD patch, was shown. The aortic root measured 41 mm at valve level and the ascending aorta measured 30 mm.

***Comments:*** The more common reason for aortic regurgitation late after repair of TOF is aortic root dilatation, which affects a subset of patients.[4] This process seems to be at least in part due to cystic medial necrosis (see Case 45) and appears to carry a risk of dissection, albeit the cutoff point for elective valve replacement in this setting remains unknown. Nevertheless, when the aortic root is severely dilated (in excess of 50 mm), with more than mild aortic regurgitation, and there are grounds for pulmonary valve replacement (PVR), double-valve replacement surgery should be considered.

In this case, however, the narrow diastolic jet appears to be through a cusp perforation that may date from the time of surgery, and the degree of aortic root dilatation is mild.

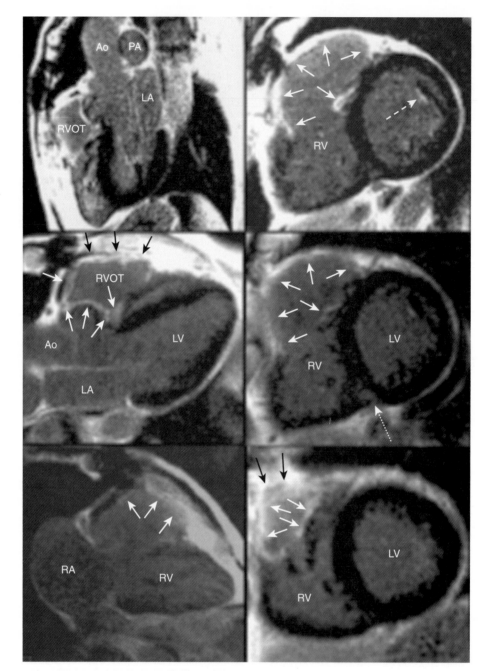

Figure 44-9 *Top left*, LVOT-type view; *top right*, short-axis view of both ventricles at the papillary muscle level; *middle left*, left ventricular outflow tract view; *middle right*, short-axis view 10 mm below the top right image; *bottom left*, two-chamber RA-RV view; *bottom right*, short-axis view 20 mm more apical than the middle right image. All these images are 2D segmented fast low-angle shot inversion recovery sequences acquired after intravenous injection of gadolinium-DTPA.

## FINDINGS

The patient had evidence of RV fibrosis, as suggested by late enhancement after administration of gadolinium-DTPA, in the RVOT, at the site of the VSD patch and at the inferior RV insertion point (*dotted arrow*). This was particularly extensive in the RV. The LV papillary muscle enhancement is less commonly seen in repaired TOF patients. Normal myocardium appears black in these images, and areas of late gadolinium enhancement appear white (*see arrows*). These areas suggest that there is fibrosis or scarring present.

**Comments:** Late gadolinium enhancement CMR was carried out as part of an ongoing and prospective research protocol.[5] More extensive late gadolinium enhancement is associated with older age, arrhythmia, decreased exercise tolerance, increased neurohormones, increased RV volumes, decreased RV systolic function, LV late gadolinium, and restrictive RV physiology on echo Doppler. This larger degree of fibrosis may be the substrate for the clinical ventricular arrhythmia.

# CATHETERIZATION

## HEMODYNAMICS

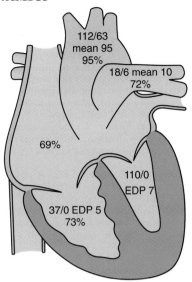

112/63
mean 95
95%

18/6 mean 10
72%

69%

110/0
EDP 7

37/0 EDP 5
73%

Figure 44-10 Diagram showing pressures and saturations at cardiac catheterization.

**Calculations**

| | |
|---|---|
| Qp (L/min) | 4.21 |
| Qs (L/min) | 4.21 |
| Cardiac index (L/min/m$^2$) | 2.20 |
| Qp/Qs | 1.00 |
| PVR (Wood units) | 0.71 |
| SVR (Wood units) | 21.36 |

## FINDINGS

There was mild global impairment of LV function. Aortic regurgitation jet was seen through the aortic valve cusp. Pulmonary regurgitation was severe. There was no proximal left PA or right PA stenosis. Normal caliber distal vessels were seen. There was right coronary dominance with normal origins and no stenoses.

**Comments:** Catheterization was performed, in the context of symptomatic arrhythmia in an older patient, to rule out acquired heart disease and ischemia as the potential cause of arrhythmia. In a younger patient, CMR images would have been regarded as sufficient documentation of branch PA anatomy and biventricular function prior to redo surgery.

### FOCUSED CLINICAL QUESTIONS AND DISCUSSION POINTS

1. Should this patient undergo PVR?

*There is no consensus regarding the exact timing of PVR for this condition, but there is a widespread view that in many cases surgery is often offered too late (see Case 41). The indications for PVR based mainly on retrospective studies include:*
1. *Severe RV dilation (e.g., RVEDV index > 170 mL/m$^2$)*
2. *Attributable exercise intolerance, particularly with interval change*
3. *The onset of sustained atrial flutter, atrial fibrillation, VT, or cardiac arrest*
*This patient has repaired TOF with severe pulmonary regurgitation and severe RV dilatation with mild tricuspid regurgitation. The dilatation is in part attributable to a large akinetic,*

thin-walled area in the RVOT that may be a focus of arrhythmia propagation and certainly results in a reduction of RV ejection fraction. There is preserved, maybe mildly impaired RV systolic function and a modest decrease in objective exercise tolerance (MVo$_2$). The patient has had life-threatening VT requiring cardioversion.

PVR was the chosen strategy in this case.

As a general rule, sustained arrhythmia in the context of complex ACHD requires treatment of both the arrhythmia and the hemodynamic abnormalities underlying them. Prognostically, it was felt that PVR would help prevent longer-term ventricular dysfunction. Partial resection of the aneurysmal area beneath the pulmonary valve may benefit his ventricular function and modify the risk of arrhythmia, albeit to an uncertain degree.

Patients with repaired TOF should be referred to tertiary centers for periodic evaluation.

2. Should his cardiac catheterization from 7 years previously be repeated?

*A decision was made to repeat diagnostic coronary catheterization as 7 years had elapsed since the previous cardiac catheterization. Within this period there had been a new episode of life-threatening arrhythmia. This was to rule out coronary artery disease in this 56-year-old patient, although given his lack of other risk factors, the index of suspicion was relatively low.*

3. Should an electrophysiology study and ablation of the VT focus also be planned?

*The case can certainly be made for determining whether VT is still inducible after PVR and remodeling of the RVOT. In some centers, a mapping and ablation would be undertaken either at the time of redo surgery or soon after it. It may be preferable to have an ICD functioning as an insurance policy, rather than waiting for risk justification with an electrophysiology study after PVR, as arguably arrhythmic risk may persist during a period of remodeling.*

*VT ablation might also be considered for appropriate shock once the device is in situ to reduce the need for appropriate shock. Although this is life-saving it may be unpleasant for patients. Atrial tachycardia might also merit ablation, in particular if associated with inappropriate shock.*

*A recent CMR study using late gadolinium enhancement imaging indicated that extensive fibrosis may prove to be an important determinant in identifying patients at particular risk of VT or sudden cardiac death.[5] This patient's pre-ICD imaging suggested a relatively high scar burden, as illustrated previously.*

## FINAL DIAGNOSIS

Severe pulmonary regurgitation with associated sustained VT

## PLAN OF ACTION

Repeat cardiac catheterization, followed by ICD insertion and PVR

## INTERVENTION

The patient underwent uneventful PVR with placement of an ICD.

## OUTCOME

In the first postoperative month and while the patient was rehabilitating from uneventful PVR he noticed palpitations and lightheadedness, which triggered his defibrillator appropriately. Interrogation of the ICD revealed a fast VT of 230 bpm timely terminated by a single shock, which in turn aborted a life-threatening arrhythmia (Fig. 44-11).

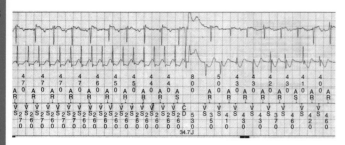

Figure 44-11 Rhythm strip obtained from device interrogation after the patient reported direct current shock. The device has recorded appropriate shock for VT.

## FINDINGS

The strip shown contains atrial activity (*first line*) and ventricular activity (*second line*). There is a rapid ventricular arrhythmia, with clear atrioventricular dysynchrony.

The strip demonstrated that the defibrillation had been triggered by VT in the ventricular fibrillation range (the rate was 230 bpm). The settings were therefore considered appropriate and not adjusted.

***Comments:*** This confirmed that the decision to place an ICD had been a good one.

## Selected References

1. Bove EL, Kavey RE, Byrum CJ, Sondheimer HM, et al: Improved right ventricular function following late pulmonary valve replacement for residual pulmonary insufficiency or stenosis. J Thorac Cardiovasc Surg 90:50–55, 1985.
2. Madias C, Maron BJ, Weinstock J, Estes NA III: Commotio cordis—sudden cardiac death with chest wall impact. J Cardiovasc Electrophysiol 18:115–122, 2007.
3. Gatzoulis MA, Balaji S, Webber SA, et al: Risk factors for arrhythmia and sudden cardiac death late after repair of tetralogy of Fallot: A multicentre study. Lancet 356:975–981, 2000.
4. Niwa K, Siu SC, Webb GD, Gatzoulis MA: Progressive aortic root dilatation in adults late after repair of tetralogy of Fallot. Circulation 106:1374–1378, 2002.
5. Babu-Narayan SV, Kilner PJ, Li W, et al: Ventricular fibrosis suggested by cardiovascular magnetic resonance in adults with

repaired tetralogy of Fallot and its relationship to adverse markers of clinical outcome. Circulation 113:405–413, 2006.

## Bibliography

Davlouros PA, Karatza AA, Gatzoulis MA, Shore DF: Timing and type of surgery for severe pulmonary regurgitation after repair of tetralogy of Fallot (Review). Int J Cardiol 97(Suppl 1):91–101, 2004.

Davlouros PA, Kilner PJ, Hornung TS, et al: Right ventricular function in adults with repaired tetralogy of Fallot assessed with cardiovascular magnetic resonance imaging: Detrimental role of right ventricular outflow aneurysms or akinesia and adverse right-to-left ventricular interaction. J Am Coll Cardiol 40:2044–2052, 2002.

Eyskens B, Reybrouck T, Bogaert J, et al: Homograft insertion for pulmonary regurgitation after repair of tetralogy of Fallot improves cardiorespiratory exercise performance. Am J Cardiol 85:221–225, 2000.

Hazekamp MG, Kurvers MM, Schoof PH, et al: Pulmonary valve insertion late after repair of Fallot's tetralogy. Eur J Cardiothorac Surg 19:667–670, 2001.

Nollert G, Fischlein T, Bouterwek S, et al: Long-term survival in patients with repair of tetralogy of Fallot: 36-year follow-up of 490 survivors of the first year after surgical repair. J Am Coll Cardiol 30:1374–1383, 1997.

Oosterhof T, van Straten A, Vliegen HW, et al: Preoperative thresholds for pulmonary valve replacement in patients with corrected tetralogy of Fallot using cardiovascular magnetic resonance. Circulation 116:545–551, 2007.

Shinebourne EA, Babu-Narayan SV, Carvalho JS: Tetralogy of Fallot—from fetus to adult. Heart 92:1353–1359, 2006.

Therrien J, Provost Y, Merchant N, et al: Optimal timing for pulmonary valve replacement in adults after tetralogy of Fallot repair. Am J Cardiol 95:779–782, 2005.

Therrien J, Siu SC, McLaughlin PR, et al: Pulmonary valve replacement in adults late after repair of tetralogy of Fallot: Are we operating too late? J Am Coll Cardiol 36:1670–1675, 2000.

Van Huysduynen BH, van Straten A, Swenne CA, et al: Reduction of QRS duration after pulmonary valve replacement in adult Fallot patients is related to reduction of right ventricular volume. Eur Heart J 26:928–932, 2005.

Vliegen HW, van Straten A, de Roos A, et al: Magnetic resonance imaging to assess the hemodynamic effects of pulmonary valve replacement in adults late after repair of tetralogy of Fallot. Circulation 106:1703–1707, 2002.

Warner KG, Anderson JE, Fulton DR, et al: Restoration of the pulmonary valve reduces right ventricular volume overload after previous repair of tetralogy of Fallot. Circulation 88(5 Pt 2):II189–197, 1993.

Yemets IM, Williams WG, Webb GD, et al: Pulmonary valve replacement late after repair of tetralogy of Fallot. Ann Thorac Surg 64:526–530, 1997.

# Aortopathy in Tetralogy of Fallot

**Koichiro Niwa**

**Age: 37 years**
**Gender: Male**
**Occupation: Renal perfusionist**
**Working diagnosis: Tetralogy of Fallot**

## HISTORY

Soon after birth a murmur was heard and the patient had cyanotic spells; the diagnosis of TOF was made. He did quite well during childhood and adolescence. Later, at age 20, he underwent repair, including closure of a VSD, resection of the RVOT obstruction and pulmonary valvotomy. A transannular RVOT patch was placed to relieve the obstruction. He recovered fully and led a normal life. He completed his education and became a medical engineer.

He was well until 1 year ago when he felt a rapid heartbeat on some occasions and shortness of breath when climbing stairs. His body weight gradually increased (10 kg over 6 months) with pretibial pitting edema. He visited a local internist and was prescribed diuretics. He was subsequently referred for further evaluation.

He is a nonsmoker.

***Comments:*** In ACHD cases, the importance of obtaining and reading the operative notes cannot be overemphasized.

Patients with repaired TOF without significant residua (residual VSD or pulmonary stenosis) are usually well without symptoms.

The patient has developed shortness of breath, palpitations, and edema. Severe pulmonary regurgitation is not uncommon after TOF repair and can be associated with RV dysfunction, diminished exercise capacity, atrial and ventricular tachyarrhythmias (VTs) and sudden cardiac death. The VT usually originates from the RVOT and can be fatal. Atrial flutter may be observed in patients with tricuspid regurgitation. In some cases, aortic regurgitation with aortic root dilatation may be observed.

## CURRENT SYMPTOMS

The patient could walk several blocks "on the flat" without difficulty but had shortness of breath and palpitations after climbing one flight of stairs. He slept well lying flat without dyspnea.

NYHA class: II

***Comments:*** His symptoms had become worse just over the last several months, suggesting clinical deterioration.

## CURRENT MEDICATIONS

Lasix 20 mg orally twice daily

Aldactone 25 mg orally twice daily

Digoxin 250 µg orally once daily

Enalapril 5 mg orally twice daily

***Comments:*** ACE inhibitors are often used in patients with aortic regurgitation to prevent progression, even though there is no clinical trial evidence supporting this practice. Likewise, there are no data to support the use of ACE inhibitors or any other agent in preventing the consequences of severe pulmonary regurgitation.

## PHYSICAL EXAMINATION

BP 103/40 mm Hg, HR 89 bpm, oxygen saturation 98% in room air

Height 182 cm, weight 72 kg, BSA 1.91 m$^2$

Surgical scars: Median sternotomy scar

Neck veins: Normal A-waves, elevated V-waves were observed

Lungs/chest: Chest was clear.

Heart: The first heart sound was normal. The second heart sound was widely split. A grade 3/6 midsystolic murmur was present at the third intercostal space near the left sternal border. A grade 3/6 blowing early diastolic murmur was present at the fourth intercostal space near the left sternal border.

Abdomen: Moderate hepatomegaly

Extremities: Moderate dependent edema

Face: No facial features suggestive of velocardiofacial syndrome (DiGeorge syndrome)

***Comments:*** The low diastolic blood pressure and wide pulse pressure suggest there may be important aortic regurgitation.

An elevated V-wave is indicative of tricuspid regurgitation.

A widely split second heart sound with a systolic and diastolic murmur is commonly observed in patients with repaired TOF. The delayed pulmonary component reflects delayed pulmonary valve closure often due to a right bundle branch block. The systolic murmur is typically due to residual pulmonary stenosis (or RVOT turbulence due to a large stroke volume). A diastolic murmur is often caused by pulmonary regurgitation, though not always. In this instance, the high-pitched nature of the diastolic murmur indicates that this is caused by aortic regurgitation.

There is a 10% to 15% incidence of chromosome 22q11 microdeletion in TOF patients, and those with the anomaly usually show special facial appearance (velocardiofacial syndrome, or DiGeorge syndrome; see Case 28).

## LABORATORY DATA

| | |
|---|---|
| Hemoglobin | 14.9 g/dL (13.0–17.0) |
| Hematocrit | 43% (41–51) |
| Sodium | 140 mmol/L (134–145) |
| Potassium | 4.0 mmol/L (3.5–5.2) |
| Creatinine | 0.6 mg/dL (0.6–1.2) |
| Blood urea nitrogen | 13 mg/dL (6–24) |
| BNP | **167 pg/mL** |
| ANP | **170 pg/mL** |

***Comments:*** Brain natriuretic peptide (BNP) and atrial natriuretic peptide (ANP) were grossly elevated in this patient, compatible with cardiac failure and/or biventricular enlargement, though there is still much to be learned about the significance of these markers in this patient population.

Other laboratory data were within normal limits.

## ELECTROCARDIOGRAM

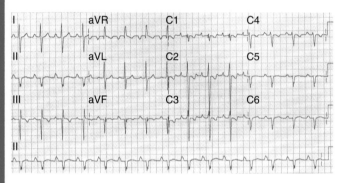

Figure 45-1 Electrocardiogram.

### FINDINGS
Heart rate: 89 bpm

PR interval: 200 msec

QRS axis: −100°

QRS duration: 110 msec

Sinus rhythm with RA overload (peaked P-waves in V2–3). T-wave inversion in V1–4. Poor precordial R-wave progression. No classical evidence of RV hypertrophy.

***Comments:*** While this case seems to be an exception, after TOF repair an RBBB is nearly universal because of the location of the bundle relative to the VSD. Left anterior hemiblock and/or bifascicular block are also common. Bifascicular block was once thought to be one of the predictors of complete AV block and sudden cardiac death in patients with TOF repair. However, this has not been confirmed in more recent studies. Instead, monomorphic VT combined with RV dilatation and pulmonary regurgitation is the major cause of sudden cardiac death in TOF after repair.[1] QRS prolongation over time suggests RV conduction delay, which is related to both the risk of sus-

tained VT and sudden cardiac death. In patients with prolonged QRS, further examination such as an exercise ECG, late potentials, and/or catheterization with electrophysiological study may be considered for refining the risk of VT and sudden cardiac death.

## CHEST X-RAY

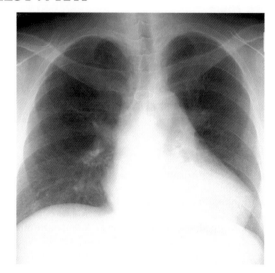

Figure 45-2 Posteroanterior projection.

### FINDINGS
Cardiothoracic ratio: 62%

The cardiac silhouette was grossly enlarged with calcification in the RVOT. There was dilatation of the pulmonary arteries and ascending aorta. The RV and LV were also dilated.

***Comments:*** Patients with repaired TOF often have dilatation of the RV, main pulmonary artery, and right pulmonary artery. RV dilatation is better seen on a lateral view. The left pulmonary artery may be hypoplastic due to pulmonary branch stenosis.

The ascending aorta in patients with TOF (even after repair) may be enlarged due to increased systemic flow and cystic medial necrosis in the aortic wall. Enlargement of the RA may be associated with tricuspid regurgitation.

The arch is left-sided in this case. Right-sided aortic arch is more commonly associated with enlargement of the aortic root.[1]

## EXERCISE TESTING

A cardiopulmonary test was not performed.

## ECHOCARDIOGRAM

### OVERALL FINDINGS
The LVEDd was 56 mm. LV systolic function was normal. The RV cavity was enlarged, and systolic function was decreased. There was severe pulmonary regurgitation and moderate tricuspid regurgitation. The estimated RV pressure was 45 mm Hg. The estimated pressure gradient across the RVOT was 35 mm Hg.

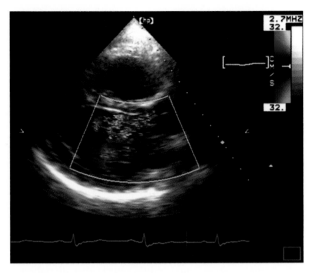

Figure 45-3 Parasternal long-axis view, 2D color Doppler.

## FINDINGS

Echocardiography revealed no residual VSD. There was ascending aortic root dilatation (root diameter of 46 mm) with moderate aortic regurgitation.

*Comments:* Measurement of RV/LV size and assessment of RV/LV function by echo and change over time may be the best guide to optimal timing of intervention. This patient was diagnosed as having biventricular volume overload and RV dysfunction due to a combination of pulmonary regurgitation and aortic regurgitation with a dilated aortic root.

In our opinion, moderate aortic regurgitation with a dilated aorta and/or RV failure together with pulmonary regurgitation warrants consideration of surgery with aortic valve replacement and/or aortic repair. The leaflets themselves appear normal, and therefore the cause of regurgitation is most likely the dilated root.

## MAGNETIC RESONANCE IMAGING

### OVERALL FINDINGS

Both ventricles were dilated. The function of the RV was mildly impaired, as was the LV. The left aortic arch and dilated ascending aorta were abscribed in the systolic phase. No residual VSD was seen.

The study also showed moderate tricuspid regurgitation and trivial mitral regurgitation. In the four-chamber view, the RA was moderately dilated. By phase-contrast velocity flow mapping, the regurgitant fraction of the pulmonary valve was 55%, and of the aortic valve was 52%.

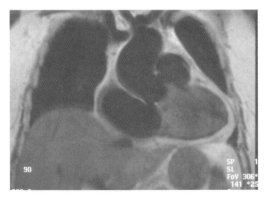

Figure 45-4 Coronal plane spin echo (black blood) imaging.

### Ventricular Volume Quantification

|  | LV | (Normal range) | RV | (Normal range) |
|---|---|---|---|---|
| EDV (mL) | 195 | (77–195) | 255 | (88–227) |
| ESV (mL) | 95 | (19–72) | 130 | (23–103) |
| SV (mL) | 100 | (51–133) | 125 | (52–138) |
| EF (%) | 51 | (57–75) | 49 | (50–76) |
| EDVi (mL/m²) | 102 | (66–101) | 134 | (65–111) |
| ESVi (mL/m²) | 50 | (18–39) | 68 | (18–47) |
| SVi (mL/m²) | 80 | (43–67) | 55 | (39–71) |

## FINDINGS

The ascending aorta measured 51 mm in diameter.

*Comments:* MRI is a very useful imaging modality for assessing RV function, pulmonary regurgitation and/or stenosis, as well as aortic root dilatation. When these lesions coexist, it is necessary to use phase contrast velocity mapping to quantify regurgitant flow, rather than compare the stroke volumes. The presence of tricuspid regurgitation also increases the RV stroke volume.

This MRI confirmed the presence of not only RV dilatation with severe pulmonary regurgitation (see Case 41) but also a dilated ascending aorta with moderate aortic regurgitation. Risk factors for aortic root dilatation in repaired TOF are older age at repair, male sex, longer interval after placement of a palliative shunt, and right aortic arch.[1]

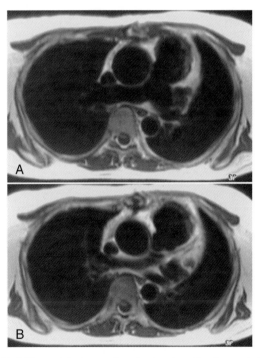

Figure 45-5 Transaxial plane, spin echo imaging. Great vessels level, in end-systolic phase (**A**) and end-diastolic plase (**B**).

## FINDINGS

There was a dilated ascending aorta and a dilated main pulmonary artery.

*Comments:* Measurement of the aorta will vary depending on both the level and the imaging plane used to measure. When serial measurements are performed, they should be done at the same level in the same plane. The coronal plane is convenient because the curvature of the aorta is easily seen and can be accounted for. However, the entire aorta is not visible (e.g., the aortic root is not seen in this particular plane). The axial images are routinely acquired, and the pulmonary artery bifurcation is a convenient landmark on which to reference serial measurements.

## CATHETERIZATION (PREOPERATIVE)

### HEMODYNAMICS

Heart rate   85 bpm

|  | Pressure | Saturation (%) |
|---|---|---|
| SVC | mean 12 | 68 |
| IVC | mean 11 | 71 |
| RA | mean 12 |  |
| RV | 50/10 |  |
| PA | 28/10 mean 17 | 69 |
| PCWP | mean 12 |  |
| LV | 108/11 |  |
| Aorta | 113/39 mean 69 | 98 |

Gradient (pullback) from PA to RV: 28 mm Hg

| Calculations | |
|---|---|
| Qp (L/min) | 4.23 |
| Qs (L/min) | 4.19 |
| Cardiac index (L/min/m²) | **2.20** |
| Qp/Qs | 1.01 |
| PVR (Wood units) | 1.42 |
| SVR (Wood units) | 13.60 |

### FINDINGS

Residual pulmonary stenosis was present, but this was mild. Cardiac output was decreased.

**Comments:** The low cardiac index is concerning. The stroke volume of both ventricles is high, as calculated by MRI, but the relatively low mixed venous saturations indicate that oxygen tissue delivery is compromised. The wide pulse pressure is consistent with significant aortic regurgitation.

### ANGIOGRAPHY

Not performed

### FOCUSED CLINICAL QUESTIONS AND DISCUSSION POINTS

1. Is aortic dilatation an unexpected finding in this patient?

   *The finding of aortic root dilatation is not surprising. Although TOF is considered mainly a lesion involving the RV and pulmonary valve, aortic root dilatation is a well-recognized feature. Aortic root dilatation, defined as a ratio of observed/expected aortic root size by standard nomogram greater than 1.5, was found in 15% of adults with TOF late after repair.[2] Factors associated with this finding included male gender, pulmonary atresia, right aortic arch, a longer shunt-to-repair interval, moderate to severe aortic regurgitation, aortic valve replacement, a larger cardiothoracic ratio, and increased left ventricular end-diastolic dimensions. The association of chromosome 22q11 deletion (DiGeorge syndrome, see Case 28) has also been proposed to be a risk factor for aortic root dilatation.*

   *Although the aortic root and the ascending aorta are often dilated in patients after tetralogy repair, aortic regurgitation is seldom more than moderate.[3,4]*

   *The ascending aorta may often dilate out of proportion to hemodynamic or morphogenetic expectations in a variety of con-*

genital heart defects. These include bicuspid aortic valve and/or coarctation, single ventricle, truncus arteriosus, and transposition of the great arteries, as well as TOF.

2. What is the cause of aortic root dilatation and aortic regurgitation?

   *There are two possible reasons for the aortic dilatation seen in TOF and other congenital abnormalities. One is high flow through the aorta, as seen in pulmonary atresia or with palliative aortopulmonary shunts. The second is a histological abnormality of the tunica media, incorrectly called "cystic medial necrosis," leading to gradual weakening of the muscular wall. The process is particularly well recognized in Marfan syndrome, annuloaortic ectasia or Turner syndrome, as well as conditions such as systemic hypertension, pregnancy, and normal aging. The cause-effect relationship between cystic medial necrosis and aortopathy, however, requires further study.*

   *Usually, there is no abnormality of the aortic valve leaflets themselves, unless there has been some iatrogenic damage at the time of repair or postendocarditis. Aortic root dilatation may eventually lead to aortic regurgitation. There are rare cases of aortic dissection in patients with previous tetralogy repair (and aortic root dilatation), albeit in patients with additional risk factors (such as systemic hypertension).*

3. Should this patient undergo surgical repair of the aortic root and/or replacement of the aortic valve?

   *Mild aortic regurgitation is reported in 15% to 18% of patients with repaired TOF, and aortic valve or aortic root replacement is required in a small percentage of these patients.*

   *It would seem prudent that decisions about the need for and timing of aortic root surgery are made similarly to decisions concerning other forms of acquired aortic root/valve disease. Hence, the size of the aortic root, the degree of aortic insufficiency, the size and function of the LV, and so forth, are all important.*

   *This approach, however, is somewhat controversial, and not all centers would view root enlargement after repair of TOF in the same way. Reports of rupture of the ascending aorta in conotruncal abnormalities are exceptionally rare at present, hence the speculation that the natural history of aortic dilatation in these patients may be different. It is also possible that, because root dilatation seems to be related to the timing of initial repair, this late complication may be less common as infants with tetralogy are repaired earlier in life. However, this is speculative, and vigilance on the aortic root size is warranted both for the older patients and for more contemporary cohorts of tetralogy undergoing earlier repair.*

   *In our opinion, this patient has moderate aortic regurgitation with an enlarged, mildly dysfunctional LV and low cardiac output with concomitant significant pulmonary regurgitation; thus elective aortic surgery at the time of pulmonary valve implantation was recommended. It may be possible to spare the aortic valve after repairing the dilated root.*

4. Should the patient have surgery for his pulmonary regurgitation?

   *The decision to replace the pulmonary valve after repair of TOF is a common dilemma, and factors to consider in making such a decision are discussed elsewhere (see Case 41). Here, our patient has severe pulmonary regurgitation; and established RV dysfunction and symptoms, so that all criteria for pulmonary valve implantation are met.*

## FINAL DIAGNOSIS

TOF (repaired), moderate to severe pulmonary regurgitation with RV dysfunction

Moderate aortic regurgitation, aortic root dilatation

## PLAN OF ACTION

Surgical aortic valve/root replacement and implantation of a stented porcine valve in the pulmonary position

## INTERVENTION

The ascending aorta was dilated to 50 mm. The wall of the ascending aorta was fairly thick. The aortic cusps were slightly thickened and elongated. Aortic valve replacement with a 25-mm St. Jude Medical device was performed. The RV was also dilated. The original pulmonary valve was thickened and bicuspid. A stented porcine valve was implanted in the area of the pulmonary annulus with concomitant reconstruction of the RVOT.

## OUTCOME

The postsurgical course was uncomplicated, and the patient made a complete recovery. He was maintained on furosemide, beta-blockers, and warfarin.

Catheterization was performed 1 year after reintervention, as is our unit's policy. There was no residual gradient between the RV and PA, nor was there any residual pulmonary regurgitation or aortic regurgitation. Angiographic volumes suggested reduction in RV and LV size with preserved systolic function. The cardiac index had improved.

A VT stimulation electrophysiological protocol at the time was negative.

Diuretics were discontinued at that point in time, but he was advised to continue with warfarin and beta-blockers indefinitely.

The patient's exercise capacity was subjectively better 2 years after his operation, and the patient remained arrhythmia free and asymptomatic.

## Selected References

1. Gatzoulis MA, Till JA, Sommerville J, et al: Mechanoelectrical interaction in tetralogy of Fallot. QRS prolongation relates to right ventricular size and predicts malignant ventricular arrhythmias and sudden death. Circulation 92:231–237, 1995.
2. Niwa K, Siu S, Webb G, et al: Progressive aortic root dilatation in adults late after repair of tetralogy of Fallot. Circulation 106:1374–1378, 2002.
3. Capelli H, Ross D, Somerville J: Aortic regurgitation in tetrad of Fallot and pulmonary atresia. Am J Cardiol 49:1979–1983, 1982.
4. Dodds GA, III, Warnes CA, Danielson GK: Aortic valve replacement after repair of pulmonary atresia and ventricular septal defect or tetralogy of Fallot. J Thorac Cardiovasc Surg 113:736–741, 1997.

## Bibliography

Bashore TM: Adult congenital heart disease: Right ventricular outflow tract lesions. Circulation 115:1933–1947, 2007.

Cheung YF, Wong SJ: Central and peripheral arterial stiffness in patients after surgical repair of tetralogy of Fallot: Implication for aortic root dilatation. Heart 92:1827–1830, 2006.

Kim WH, Seo JW, Kim SJ, et al: Aortic dissection late after repair of tetralogy of Fallot. Int J Cardiol 101:515–516, 2005.

Marelli AJ, Perloff JK, Child JS, et al: Pulmonary atresia with ventricular septal defect in adults. Circulation 89:243–251, 1994.

Niwa K, Perloff JK, Bhuta SM, et al: Structural abnormalities of great arterial walls in congenital heart disease: Light and electron microscopic analyses. Circulation 103:393–400, 2001.

Niwa K, Perloff JK, Kaplan S, et al: Eisenmenger syndrome in adults; ventricular septal defect, truncus arteriosus and univentricular hearts. J Am Coll Cardiol 34:223–232, 1999.

Rathi VK, Doyle M, Williams RB, et al: Massive aortic aneurysm and dissection in repaired tetralogy of Fallot; diagnosis by cardiovascular magnetic resonance imaging. Int J Cardiol 101:169–170,2005.

Rieker RP, Berman MA, Stansel HC, Jr: Postoperative studies in patients with tetralogy of Fallot. Ann Thorac Surg 19:17–25, 1975.

Roberts CS, Roberts WC: Dissection of the aorta associated with congenital malformation of the aortic valve. J Am Coll Cardiol 17:712–716, 1991.

Senzaki H, Iwamoto Y, Ishido H, et al: Arterial haemodynamics in patients after repair of tetralogy of Fallot: Influence on left ventricular after load and aortic dilatation. Heart 94:70–74, 2008.

Tan JL, Davlouros PA, McCarthy KP, et al: Intrinsic histological abnormalities of the aortic root and ascending aorta in tetralogy of Fallot: Evidence of causative mechanism to aortic dilatation and aortopathy. Circulation 112:961–968, 2005.

Therrien J, Gatzoulis M, Graham T, et al: CCS Consensus Conference 2001 update: Recommendations for the management of adults with congenital heart disease—Part II. Can J Cardiol 17:1029–1050, 2001.

# Pulmonary Atresia

# Pulmonary Atresia with Intact Ventricular Septum

**Arif Anis Khan, Piers E.F. Daubeney, and Craig S. Broberg**

**Age: 15 years**
**Gender: Male**
**Occupation: Student**
**Working diagnosis: Pulmonary atresia with intact ventricular septum**

## HISTORY

The patient was found to be cyanosed after birth and diagnosed with pulmonary atresia with an intact ventricular septum. A balloon atrial septostomy was performed at one day of age and a left modified BT shunt on day 2. At 2 years of age, a total cavopulmonary (lateral tunnel) Fontan connection with takedown of his BT shunt was performed. A fenestrated intra-atrial baffle with a 19-mm Impra tube (a graft made of synthetic material) was placed, with the RA free wall serving as the other border of the atrial pathway. The operation was successful, and the boy's recovery was unremarkable.

The patient was well until 13 years of age, when he started to experience mild exercise intolerance. He was a very active boy and played badminton regularly, but felt his physical condition was deteriorating. He was reviewed as an outpatient.

**Comments:** Pulmonary atresia with intact ventricular septum is a rare congenital cardiac malformation with considerable morphological heterogeneity.[1-5] There is complete atresia of the pulmonary valve in conjunction with a variable degree of hypoplasia of the tricuspid valve and RV cavity. Ebstein malformation coexists in 10% of patients.[5] The hypoplastic and hypertensive RV can be associated with right ventricular-to coronary communications termed fistulae, present in approximately 50% of patients at birth.[5-8] At the worst end of the spectrum, such fistulae may be associated with coronary artery ectasia, stenoses, or even interruption; this latter situation is known as an RV-dependent circulation for reasons to be discussed subsequently.

In those cases where a biventricular repair is not deemed possible, a univentricular route is embarked on. A balloon atrial septostomy is initially performed to enable right-to-left atrial shunting and so preserve cardiac output. A systemic-to-pulmonary shunt is then performed to increase pulmonary blood flow and thus oxygenation. At 3 to 12 months a bidirectional superior cavopulmonary (Glenn) anastomosis is constructed followed by a total cavopulmonary connection (modified Fontan), usually at 2 to 5 years of age. Most often, these procedures are performed separately, unlike the case described here, where they were performed as a single procedure.

In the Fontan circulation all the systemic venous return is directly to the lungs without the need for a subpulmonary ventricle. This does require high venous pressures to drive the blood across the pulmonary bed. In some cases, a fenestration is performed at the time of the Fontan. This is a small atrial defect created in the lateral tunnel that allows deoxygenated blood to flow into the left heart (by way of right-to-left shunting), reducing the venous pressures and maintaining cardiac output at the expense of mild systemic desaturation. Fenestration of the Fontan circulation has improved operative survival rates among high-risk patients.[9]

## CURRENT SYMPTOMS

The patient was still able to play sports although not with the intensity with which he had previously competed. He did not have any other cardiovascular symptoms such as palpitations, dizziness, or chest pain.

NYHA class: I

**Comments:** The application of the Fontan procedure in one of its several modifications has allowed many patients excellent univentricular palliation. However, patients doing well after a Fontan procedure should be seen at least yearly. The risk of cardiac failure and late death increases progressively. Overall survival is approximately 86% at 5 years and 74% at 10 years.

Intracardiac thrombus formation is not an uncommon sequela after the Fontan operation. Oral anticoagulation therapy is prescribed in many centers, although there is no consensus at present for routine use in all patients.[10] The incidence of thromboembolic events after the Fontan operation is 10% to 20%, and depends on the age of the patient and the size of the RA for patients with an atriopulmonary type of Fontan.[11]

## CURRENT MEDICATIONS

Warfarin (target INR 2–3)

# PHYSICAL EXAMINATION

BP 108/68 mm Hg, HR 72 bpm, oxygen saturation at rest 91%, after climbing four flights of stairs, 78%

Height 190 cm, weight 66 kg, BSA 1.87 m$^2$

Surgical scars: Medial sternotomy and a left thoracotomy scar

Neck veins: Visible 4 cm above the sternal angle with a prominent A-wave

Lungs/chest: Normal on auscultation

Heart: There was a diffuse cardiac impulse. The heart sounds were regular, with a normal first and a single second heart sound with a soft pansystolic murmur and a prolonged diastolic murmur.

Abdomen: Normal with no ascites present

Extremities: Normal with no cyanosis or clubbing

**Comments:** Most Fontan patients without atrial fenestration have a transcutaneous oxygen saturation at the lower end of normal. If oxygen saturations are less than 90%, one should determine the etiology of the hypoxemia. Apart from fenestration, other causes of hypoxemia after a Fontan include:

Residual intra-atrial communication(s)

Systemic-to-pulmonary venous collateralization with right-to-left shunting

Pulmonary arteriovenous malformation

Connection of hepatic veins to the coronary sinus or LA (i.e., excluded from the total cavopulmonary circulation pathway)

Reopening of levoatrial cardinal vein allowing systemic venous blood to enter the LA

Shunting via thebesian veins

Intrinsic pulmonary pathology

Diaphragmatic (phrenic nerve) palsy

Hepatopulmonary syndrome

Murmurs are uncommon in Fontan patients.

A systolic murmur suggests AV valve regurgitation (in this case tricuspid regurgitation from the high-pressure RV), dehiscence of a surgical patch leading to left-to-right ventricular shunting, forward flow through an incompletely ligated main pulmonary trunk, or the development of a restrictive, subaortic VSD (bulboventricular foramen).

Diastolic murmurs may be due to aortic or pulmonary regurgitation. Continuous murmurs may be due to fistulous communications, systemic-to-pulmonary collateral arteries, or incompletely ligated systemic-to-pulmonary shunts.

# LABORATORY DATA

| | |
|---|---|
| Hemoglobin | 16.9 g/dL (13.0–17.0) |
| Hematocrit/PCV | 48% (41–51) |
| MCV | 88 fL (83–99) |
| Platelet count | 163 × 10$^9$/L (150–400) |
| Sodium | 138 mmol/L (134–145) |
| Potassium | 4.2 mmol/L (3.5–5.2) |
| Creatinine | 0.68 mg/dL (0.6–1.2) |
| Blood urea nitrogen | **7.4 mmol/L (2.5–6.5)** |

## OTHER RELEVANT LAB RESULTS

| | |
|---|---|
| ALP | 19 IU/L (8–40) |
| ALT | 24 IU/L (16–41) |
| Total protein | 6.9 g/dL (6.2–8.2) |
| Albumin | 4.4 g/dL (3.7–5.3) |
| Ca | 2.49 mmol/L (2.20–2.62) |
| CRP | 8 mg/L (0–10) |
| PT | 13 sec (10.2–13.2) |
| APTT | 33 sec (26–36) |

**Comments:** An increased hemoglobin and secondary erythrocytosis are the physiologic response to oxygen desaturation in this patient. In fact, the patient may be iron deficient (the normal MCV does not exclude iron deficiency), and if his transferrin saturations are low, he should be supplemented with iron.[12]

Fontan patients should periodically have liver function and protein/albumin testing. The presence of hepatic dysfunction, hypoalbuminemia, or hypoproteinemia may suggest protein-losing enteropathy and should prompt investigations to identify treatable causes of Fontan "failure."

# ELECTROCARDIOGRAM

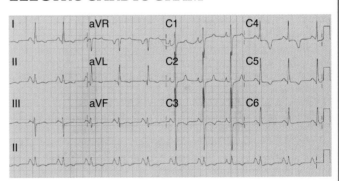

Figure 46-1 Electrocardiogram.

## FINDINGS

Heart rate: 72 bpm

QRS axis: Normal

QRS duration: 105 msec

Sinus rhythm

**Comments:** Biatrial overload is present. There is borderline voltage evidence for LV hypertrophy (R in aVL > 11 mm, RI + S3 > 25 mm). Nonspecific T-wave inversion is also seen.

Atrial rhythm disturbances are common after any type of Fontan operation. The annual incidence of new arrhythmias in Fontan patients ranges from 0.4% to 3.9% with a mean of 2.0% per year.[13]

# CHEST X-RAY

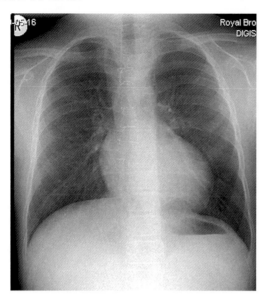

Figure 46-2 Posteroanterior projection.

## FINDINGS

Cardiothoracic ratio: 57%

Situs solitus, levocardia, and left aortic arch. RA prominence. The pulmonary trunk is not seen. The lung fields are clear, and pulmonary blood flow is probably normal.

**Comments:** Cardiomegaly may indicate the presence of significant AV valve regurgitation, myocardial dysfunction, or pericardial effusion, or may be the sequela of prolonged atrial or ventricular tachyarrhythmia.

## EXERCISE TESTING

| Exercise protocol: | Modified Bruce |
|---|---|
| Duration (min:sec): | 12:33 |
| Reason for stopping: | Dyspnea |
| ECG changes: | None |

|  | Rest | Peak |
|---|---|---|
| Heart rate (bpm): | 72 | 153 |
| Percent of age-predicted max HR: |  | 75 |
| O$_2$ saturation (%): | 91 | 82 |
| Blood pressure (mm Hg): | 110/65 | 150/85 |
| Peak Vo$_2$ (mL/kg/min): |  | 30 |
| Percent predicted (%): |  | 66 |
| Ve/Vco$_2$: |  | 31 |
| Metabolic equivalents: |  | 7.9 |

**Comments:** Maximal exercise tolerance in patients after Fontan/total cavopulmonary circulation is subnormal or at best reaches the lower limit of normal. In addition, systemic blood pressure usually does not increase normally during exercise in patients with a Fontan circulation. The main mechanism to increase cardiac output during exercise is through increasing heart rate.

The lower oxygen saturation during exercise here reflects a right-to-left shunt (presumably through the fenestration in the lateral tunnel).

Overall peak oxygen consumption, however, in this young and well-conditioned patient is very good relative to most patients with Fontan physiology.

The absence of angina and/or ischemic changes on exercise is reassuring in a patient with pulmonary atresia with intact septum, a disease in which RV-to-coronary artery communications and coronary stenoses are prevalent. If present, the latter would normally manifest themselves much earlier on in life.

# ECHOCARDIOGRAM

## OVERALL FINDINGS

Enlarged LV with maintained systolic function. There is a smaller right hypertrophied ventricle with a small tricuspid valve.

A lateral tunnel Fontan communication was present with no visible obstruction or thrombus in it, or anywhere else in the heart.

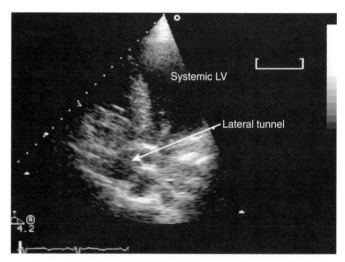

Figure 46-3 Apical four-chamber echocardiogram showing lateral tunnel.

**Comments:** The sonographer should look carefully for any evidence of flow obstruction within the lateral tunnel, even though imaging this area can be difficult. In a patient with pulmonary atresia with intact ventricular septum, evidence of RV-to-coronary artery communications should also be sought.

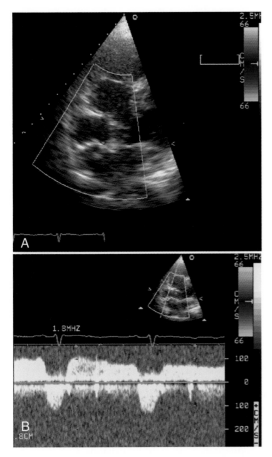

Figure 46-4 Apical four-chamber view. Two-dimensional Doppler color flow through the fenestration (**A**) and pulsed-wave Doppler (**B**).

***Comments:*** Although the actual fenestration can be difficult to see, Doppler is sensitive to flow and facilitates detection. This is likely to be the main source of desaturation. The velocity waveform can give some indication of the amount of flow through the defect and the relative pressure gradient.

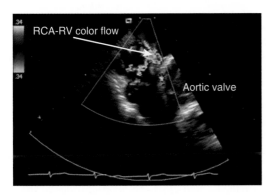

Figure 46-5 Transesophageal echocardiogram, short-axis view.

## FINDINGS

There is a fistula between the right coronary artery and the RV.

***Comments:*** Patients with pulmonary atresia and intact ventricular septum often have fistulous communications between the coronary arteries and the RV cavity.

A major difference between pulmonary atresia with intact septum and pulmonary atresia with VSD is the presence of these fistulous communications in the former, and aortopulmo-

nary collaterals in the latter. Furthermore, right ventricular hypoplasia is common in pulmonary atresia with intact ventricular septum, whereas patients with pulmonary atresia and VSD (and collaterals, some call this entity TOF with pulmonary atresia) almost always have a well-formed RV, albeit hypertrophied. What may preclude a biventricular repair for this latter group is the common coexistence of major abnormalities of the central pulmonary arteries, such as hypoplasia and nonconfluence.

At times the coronary fistulous communications can be a major source of coronary blood flow (RV-dependent circulation). They can also be associated with coronary stenoses and interruptions, ultimately leading to myocardial ischemia and a poor outcome early in life. In our case, the RV-to-coronary artery fistulous communication appeared to be inconsequential at the present time.

## MAGNETIC RESONANCE IMAGING

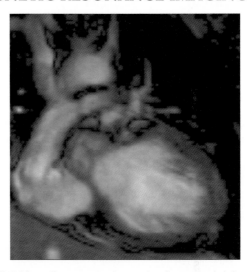

Figure 46-6 Magnetic resonance image showing systemic left ventricle in oblique coronal view.

## FINDINGS

Unobstructed total cavopulmonary circulation lateral tunnel, with a mildly dilated LV.

***Comments:*** MRI usually offers excellent evaluation of the Fontan circuit, and allows quantification of flow and velocity throughout the heart. The findings here were reassuring in that no obstruction was present at the anastomosis with the right pulmonary artery.

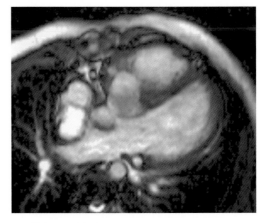

Figure 46-7 Oblique axial plane.

## FINDINGS

Rudimentary anterior RV. The LV has maintained systolic function.

***Comments:*** In pulmonary atresia with intact septum, the RVOT is blind ending (atretic). There is significant mural hypertrophy and a variable degree of RV cavity hypoplasia (moderate in this case). The only exit from the RV is via the coronary fistulae or tricuspid regurgitation—neither directly contributing to cardiac output.

# CATHETERIZATION

## HEMODYNAMICS

Heart rate   72 bpm

|       | Pressure        | Saturation (%) |
|-------|-----------------|----------------|
| SVC   | mean 12         | 64             |
| IVC   | mean 11         | 72             |
| PA    | mean 11         | 76             |
| LV    | 73/9            |                |
| Aorta | 78/39 mean 53   | 92             |

***Comments:*** The pressures are normal for a Fontan circulation. As expected, there is elevation of the venous pressure that drives transpulmonary flow (in the absence of a subpulmonary ventricle in the circuit). The pulmonary artery pressures are reassuringly low, and there is no evidence of significant obstruction to the cavopulmonary pathway.

Desaturation may be due to the right-to-left shunt arising from the baffle fenestration or systemic to pulmonary venous collaterals (as listed previously in this case). The cause would usually be obvious from angiography.

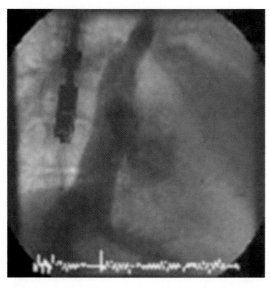

Figure 46-8 Cine in anteroposterior view showing lateral tunnel angiogram and fenestration before device closure.

## FINDINGS

Angiography confirms a right-to-left shunt from the lateral tunnel through the fenestration into the LA. Note the TEE probe.

***Comments:*** Right-to-left shunting has been confirmed through the fenestration. There is good, uninterrupted flow through the lateral tunnel with no evidence of thrombus formation.

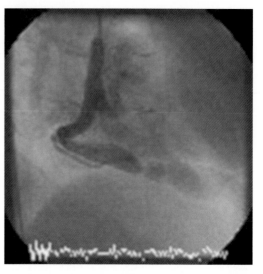

Figure 46-9 Cine in right anterior oblique view showing right coronary artery fistula.

## FINDINGS

The right coronary artery has aneurysmal dilatation (ectasia) and the suggestion of stenoses. There is also a fistulous communication between the left coronary system and RV cavity.

***Comments:*** In this patient there are significant fistulous communications between the RV and coronary system, perhaps even creating an RV-dependent coronary circulation. He has fared extremely well, however, demonstrating that the chosen neonatal management of a univentricular, rather than a biventricular, palliation may have effectively neutralized what, in the past, has been a risk factor for poor outcome.

### FOCUSED CLINICAL QUESTIONS AND DISCUSSION POINTS

1. **Should this patient be offered closure of his fenestration?**

   *Despite the patient's complaint of mildly decreasing exercise tolerance, his measured exercise function is at the upper range for patients with Fontan circulation. He is a young and well-conditioned physically fit individual, which is also relevant. The fenestration is undoubtedly contributing to his mild resting desaturation, which is more severe during exercise and has in turn led to secondary erythrocytosis and perhaps some iron deficiency.[12] Otherwise, there is no evidence of pathology as is sometimes seen (e.g., Fontan obstruction, thrombosis, or significant ventricular dysfunction).*

   *Fenestrations are not always created when a Fontan is performed. When they are, consideration is usually given to their closure some time after the Fontan operation. This is to achieve complete separation of the systemic and pulmonary circuits in Fontan patients with effectively univentricular hearts. Patients with patent fenestrations are usually mildly cyanosed but clinically well. Unless there are problems with the Fontan circuit, elective closure is usually undertaken within 6 to 12 months of the Fontan procedure.*

   *The potential hazards of a fenestration closure are that it may elevate systemic venous pressure and reduce cardiac output, albeit while increasing oxygen saturations. All the systemic venous return is committed to traveling through the lungs, and if the pulmonary vascular resistance is elevated then cardiac output will drop and effective systemic oxygen delivery may fall despite the increase in saturations. Balloon test occlusion of the fenestration is often performed prior to occlusion for patients with a borderline Fontan circulation. If systemic output and venous pressures are not adversely affected with balloon occlusion, then closure is undertaken. In those circumstances fenestration closure will lead to improved saturations and oxygen tissue delivery, and prevent the risk of paradoxical embolus from this source.*

*In our case, early fenestration closure after Fontan completion was deemed unnecessary because the patient was very well. One can be criticized for this decision. However, now the patient is complaining of decreasing exercise tolerance with evidence of desaturation during exercise and absence of other physiological impairment, so elective closure of the fenestration seemed reasonable.*

2. What is the physiologic significance of the right coronary artery-to-RV fistula?

*In pulmonary atresia with intact ventricular septum there is a range of morphology from those with near normal RVs and membranous atresia to those with severely hypoplastic RVs and muscular infundibular atresia.[5] As discussed, there may be fistulous communications between the RV and the coronary arteries. In just under 10% of patients[5] the coronary arteries may be ectatic, stenosed, or interrupted with a significant portion of the myocardium dependent on desaturated blood from the RV rather than antegrade coronary flow from the aorta—the so-called RV-dependent coronary circulation. Myocardium proximal to the stenosis is perfused by the aortic diastolic pressure, while distal myocardium is perfused by the RV systolic pressure. In those circumstances, decompression of the RV by performing an RVOT procedure would lead to infarction of the distal myocardium and often death.*

*In this patient there is an ectatic coronary artery with probable RV dependence to the distal coronary artery territory. As a consequence, a biventricular repair might have led to his demise in the neonatal period.*

*The significance of the RV-to-coronary artery communication at this juncture is unclear. It is known that there can be ongoing coronary artery damage from fistulae,[5] but in this case there does not appear to be any ill effect from its presence—certainly no evident ischemia on exercise testing. It would be wise, therefore, to leave it alone, until there is more evidence to intervene.*

## FINAL DIAGNOSIS

Pulmonary atresia with intact ventricular septum

Satisfactory total cavopulmonary circulation (lateral tunnel Fontan) physiology

Fenestration with right-to-left shunt, and right coronary artery-to-RV fistula

## PLAN OF ACTION

Transluminal percutaneous closure of the Fontan fenestration

## INTERVENTION

At the time of diagnostic catheterization, a STARFlex PFO device was successfully deployed across the fenestration. Sizing and placement were performed with TEE guidance. There was no significant increase in venous pressure after the procedure.

## OUTCOME

The patient was discharged home the following day. At the 2-month clinic visit he reported more enjoyment from his bad-

minton games, more energy, and better general well-being. Repeat exercise testing demonstrated a peak Vo₂ of 38.4% (previously 30), and his oxygen saturations were 95% at the end of the test (previously 82%).

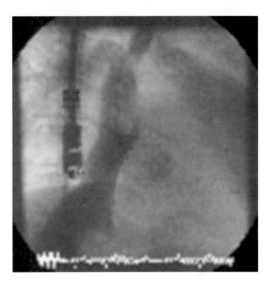

Figure 46-10 Cine in anteroposterior view showing lateral tunnel angiogram and after device closure of fenestration.

***Comments:*** STARFlex PFO device in optimal position, with trivial right-to-left shunting immediately after device deployment.

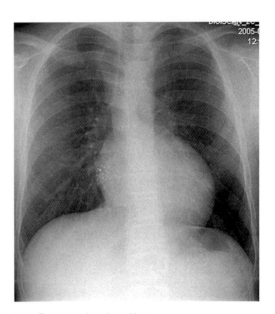

Figure 46-11 Postoperative chest X-ray.

### FINDINGS

The 3-mm STARFlex PFO device was successfully deployed to close the Fontan fenestration (seen in the middle right area of the cardiac silhouette, close to the heart border).

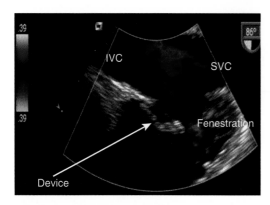

Figure 46-12   Transesophageal long-axis view showing fenestration device closure.

## FINDINGS

TEE during the procedure demonstrated the device deployed in optimal position.

**Comments:** It is imperative to use TEE to size the defect properly, confirm its position, and assess the adequacy of the procedure immediately after deployment.

## Selected References

1. Hjortdal VE, Emmertsen K, Stenbog E, et al: Effects of exercise and respiration on blood flow in total cavopulmonary connection: A real-time magnetic resonance flow study. Circulation 108: 1227–1231, 2003.
2. Lloyd TR, Rydberg A, Ludomirsky A, et al: Late fenestration closure in the hypoplastic left heart syndrome: Comparison of hemodynamic changes. Am Heart J 136:302–306, 1998.
3. Mavroudis C, Zales VR, Backer CL, et al: Fenestrated Fontan with delayed catheter closure. Effects of volume loading and baffle fenestration on cardiac index and oxygen delivery. Circulation 86(5 Suppl):II85–92, 1992.
4. Balling G, Vogt M, Kaemmerer H, et al: Intracardiac thrombus formation after the Fontan operation. J Thorac Cardiovasc Surg 119(4 Pt 1):745–752, 2000.
5. Dyamenahalli U, McCrindle BW, McDonald C, et al: Pulmonary atresia with intact ventricular septum: Management of, and outcomes for, a cohort of 210 consecutive patients. Cardiol Young 14:299–308, 2004.
6. Daubeney PE, Wang D, Delany DJ, et al: UK and Ireland Collaborative Study of Pulmonary Atresia with Intact Ventricular Septum. Pulmonary atresia with intact ventricular septum: Predictors of early and medium-term outcome in a population-based study. J Thorac Cardiovasc Surg 130:1071, 2005.
7. Daubeney PE, Sharland GK, Cook AC, et al: Pulmonary atresia with intact ventricular septum: Impact of fetal echocardiography on incidence at birth and postnatal outcome. UK and Eire Collaborative Study of Pulmonary Atresia with Intact Ventricular Septum. Circulation 98:562–566, 1998.
8. Daubeney PE, Delany DJ, Anderson RH, et al: United Kingdom and Ireland: Collaborative Study of Pulmonary Atresia with Intact Ventricular Septum. Pulmonary atresia with intact ventricular septum: Range of morphology in a population-based study. J Am Coll Cardiol 39:1670–1679, 2002.
9. Bridges ND, Lock JE, Castaneda AR: Baffle fenestration with subsequent transcatheter closure. Modification of the Fontan operation for patients at increased risk. Circulation 82:1681–1689, 1990.
10. Walker HA, Gatzoulis MA: Prophylactic anticoagulation following the Fontan operation. Heart 91:854–856, 2005.
11. Tsang W, Johansson B, Salehian O, et al: Intracardiac thrombus in Fontan patients: Treatment and clinical outcome. Cardiol Young 17:646–651, 2007.
12. Spence MS, Balaratnam MS, Gatzoulis MA: Clinical update: Cyanotic adult congenital heart disease. Lancet 370:1530–1532, 2007.
13. Gewillig M, Wyse RK, de Leval MR, Deanfield JE: Early and late arrhythmias after the Fontan operation: Predisposing factors and clinical consequences. Br Heart J 67:72–79, 1992.

# Multiple Aortopulmonary Collaterals: Too Many or Too Few

**Mark S. Spence**

**Age: 30 years**
**Gender: Female**
**Occupation: Unemployed**
**Working diagnosis: Tricuspid atresia, pulmonary atresia, functionally single ventricle**

## HISTORY

The patient's cardiac status became known when she was admitted to the hospital at 6 weeks of age with cyanosis and failure to thrive. A catheterization confirmed the absence of a right AV connection, a hypoplastic RV, and a single great artery.

At 6 months a Waterston shunt operation was performed. She recovered uneventfully. However, this became inadequate, as evidenced by worsening cyanosis. Consideration was given to the feasibility of a Fontan-type operation. However, the native pulmonary arteries were judged to be too hypoplastic and the pulmonary circulation was too dependent on collateral arteries to permit a Fontan approach. Subsequently, at age 7 years a left BT shunt was placed to improve pulmonary blood flow.

The remainder of her childhood was uneventful, though she remained cyanotic and was frequently treated with venesection.

When she was 20 years old, the patient had a spontaneous abortion (around 6 weeks of gestation) following an unplanned pregnancy.

She reattended the clinic after several years of being lost to follow-up and asked if anything could be done to improve her restricted physical capacity. She partially attributed her nonattendance to a fear of needles that developed in her teens from frequent venesection.

*Comments:* The patient has a form of univentricular heart of LV type with pulmonary atresia and cyanosis. The degree of cyanosis in patients with pulmonary atresia is determined by the amount of pulmonary flow, which may be supplied by the arterial duct, multiple aortopulmonary collaterals, and/or the bronchial circulation.

The rationale for considering a Fontan-style palliation is that it allows separation of the systemic and pulmonary circulations in patients with a functionally single ventricle, thus avoiding the potentially deleterious effects of long-standing ventricular volume overload and cyanosis. However, this requires a pulmonary vascular bed of adequate size with low resistance.

Venesection, or therapeutic phlebotomy, was commonly performed in the past on the assumption that the practice reduced the risk of stroke and improved the patient's symptoms. Recent data, however, challenge both these alleged benefits, and venesections have now been limited to very few selected patients and indications.[1]

The risk of fetal death increases with the degree of maternal cyanosis (see Case 75). Counseling and education of all women with ACHD is a vital component of their management so that they can make informed and planned choices about having children.

Although many patients with ACHD face major employment and psychosocial challenges they generally have quality-of-life scores that are remarkably comparable to those of the general population. Nevertheless, those with persistent cyanosis do have a poorer perception of their physical health.[2]

Unfortunately, it is not uncommon for patients with complex congenital heart disease to be lost to clinical follow-up from adolescence to adulthood, and to reappear when problems develop. It is important that strenuous efforts are made to maintain good lines of communication between the patient, his or her family doctor, and the congenital heart specialist, and that the need for lifelong follow-up is emphasized to patients and their families from a young age.

## CURRENT SYMPTOMS

The patient now has shortness of breath on minimal exertion. She has noted progressive deterioration in her exercise capacity over several years. She has not had hemoptysis, palpitations, syncope, or gout.

NYHA class: III

*Comments:* The patient's functional status was assessed using the NYHA classification although some leaders in the field have recommended using functional classifications specifically designed for patients with congenital heart disease, such as the Warnes-Somerville Ability Index.[3]

Patients with cyanotic ACHD have a substantially greater increase in ventilation during exercise than do normal subjects, and dyspnea is often a prominent symptom. Some of the stimuli for this include hypoxemia, metabolic acidosis, and shunting of carbon dioxide into the systemic arterial circulation.[4,5]

This patient reports a severe and progressive decline in functional capacity. It is imperative to thoroughly investigate the causes for this decline.

## CURRENT MEDICATIONS

None

# PHYSICAL EXAMINATION

BP 92/60 mm Hg (right arm), HR 80 bpm (regular), oxygen saturation (finger) 71%

Height 159 cm, weight 54 kg, BSA 1.54 m²

Surgical scars: Right and left thoracotomy scars were present.

Neck veins: JVP was not elevated.

Lungs/chest: Breath sounds were within normal limits.

Heart: The apical impulse was displaced leftward. There was a normal first heart sound and single second heart sound. A continuous murmur was audible over the anterior and posterior aspect of the thorax (mainly in the midline and to the right).

Abdomen: Normal

Extremities: There were weak left radial and brachial pulses and normal femoral and pedal pulses bilaterally. She was cyanosed with marked clubbing of the fingers and toes. There was no peripheral edema.

***Comments:*** In patients with ACHD cyanosis is a manifestation of either right-to-left shunting or inadequate pulmonary blood flow.[6] In this case, it reflects both.

The patient is cachectic, which is common in cyanotic heart disease.[7]

A single second heart sound is often a feature of pulmonary stenosis or atresia. A continuous murmur in this patient could be due to the Waterston shunt, the BT shunt, MAPCAs, or all of the above. The observation that the murmur is not heard on the left side of the chest raises the suspicion that the left BT shunt is occluded and that, perhaps, MAPCAs may be supplying the left lung.

There is reduced arterial flow ipsilateral to a classic BT shunt (with end-to-side anastomoses of the subclavian and branch pulmonary arteries) as manifest by weak or absent upper limb pulses.

Finger clubbing is a manifestation of chronic cyanotic heart disease. It is postulated that platelet-derived growth factor is released from clumps of platelets and megakaryocytes (shunted from right to left) as they impact in the capillary beds of the digits and periosteum, causing increased capillary permeability, fibroblastic activity, and arterial smooth muscle hyperplasia.[8]

# LABORATORY DATA

| | |
|---|---|
| Hemoglobin | **22.5 g/dL** (11.5–15.0) |
| Hematocrit/PCV | **63%** (36–46) |
| MCV | 89 fL (83–99) |
| Platelet count | 161 × 10⁹/L (150–400) |
| Sodium | 140 mmol/L (134–145) |
| Potassium | 5.1 mmol/L (3.5–5.2) |
| Creatinine | 0.9 mg/dL (0.6–1.2) |
| Blood urea nitrogen | **8.4 mmol/L** (2.5–6.5) |
| Total bilirubin | **28 µmol/L** (3–24) |
| ALP | 64 U/L (38–126) |
| ALT | 10 IU/L (8–40) |
| Total protein | 82 g/L (62–82) |
| Albumin | 43 g/L (37–53) |
| Uric acid | **656 µmol/L** (210–440) |

| | |
|---|---|
| Iron | **7.8 µmol/L** (12.6–26) |
| Ferritin | **11 µg/L** (20–186) |
| Total iron binding capacity | 65 µmol/L (50–80) |
| Transferrin | 2.6 g/L (2.0–3.2) |
| Transferrin saturation | **12%** (20–45) |
| Vitamin B₁₂ | **151 ng/L** (180–914) |
| Folate | 4.0 µg/L (2.5–20) |

***Comments:*** There is evidence of iron depletion. This reduces systemic oxygen transport and may contribute to poorer exercise function.[1] Iron supplementation—and not venesection—is advised here (see Case 72). There is also deficiency of vitamin B₁₂, which requires investigation and replacement. Even though her hemoglobin is severely elevated, it may not be high enough for her severe cyanosis.

The erythrocytosis results in an increase in unconjugated bilirubin and places these patients at greater risk of calcium bilirubinate (pigment) gallstones.

The elevated uric acid level is typical of chronic cyanosis and is due to inappropriately low renal fractional uric acid excretion[9] rather than overproduction.

# ELECTROCARDIOGRAM

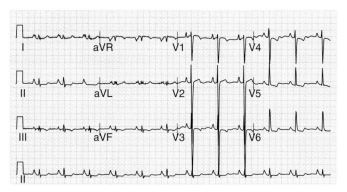

Figure 47-1 Electrocardiogram.

## FINDINGS

Heart rate: 71 bpm

QRS axis: +26°

QRS duration: 100 msec

Sinus rhythm, RA and LA overload, and voltage evidence of LV hypertrophy with nonspecific repolarization abnormalities.

***Comments:*** This ECG is recorded at standard calibration of 10 mm/mV, although half-standard would have separated the overlapping R- and S-waves in the precordial leads.

A marked increase in R- and S-wave voltages in both the limb and precordial leads is typical of univentricular hearts of the LV type. In this case the limb leads did not show this pattern.

The patient is in sinus rhythm, importantly, since the development of arrhythmias (atrial flutter/fibrillation or occasionally ventricular tachycardia) is a common cause of deterioration in these patients.[10]

## CHEST X-RAY

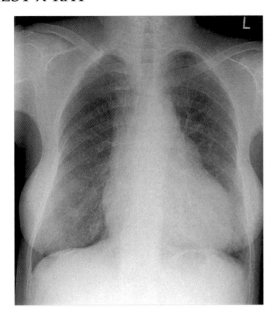

Figure 47-2 Posteroanterior projection.

### FINDINGS
Cardiothoracic ratio: 60%

Situs solitus, levocardia with a left aortic arch. Enlarged cardiac silhouette, with a prominent bulge from the left heart border. Large RA. Pulmonary vascular markings are at the lower limit of normal. There was disruption of the right-sided and, to a lesser extent, the left-sided ribs suggesting prior thoracotomies.

*Comments:* Cardiomegaly reflects the volume loading of the heart in a single-ventricle type of circulation, further exaggerated by the surgical aortopulmonary shunts and potentially large multiple aortopulmonary collateral arteries, when the latter are present (here, there is no such evidence for the latter in the chest radiograph, i.e., there is no rib notching, differential/segmental pulmonary vascular markings, etc).

The bulge from the left heart border is unlikely due to the pulmonary artery, as there is pulmonary atresia and hypoplastic native pulmonary arteries. It seems likely to be due to enlargement of the LA appendage, which is clearly appreciated on the MRI images.

Rib disruption on an adult's CXR provides evidence of thoracotomy in childhood, as there is continued somatic growth while the ribs are healing. Unilateral rib notching may be seen in patients who have had a classic BT shunt.

## EXERCISE TESTING

Type of protocol: 6-minute walk test (6MWT)

No supplemental oxygen

|  | Baseline | End |
|---|---|---|
| Heart rate | 60 | 90 |
| Dyspnea | 2 | 8 (Borg Scale) |
| Fatigue | 1 | 7 (Borg Scale) |
| Saturation | 67% | 45% |

6MWT distance: 170 m

No stopping or pause before 6 minutes

Other: Felt well throughout test except for tingling in her toes

*Comments:* The 6MWT is an established functional walk test that is simple to administer, well tolerated, and reflective of activities of daily living. Optimal reference equations from healthy population-based samples using standardized 6MWT methods are not yet available. In one study, the median 6MWT distance was approximately 580 m for healthy men and 500 m for healthy women.[11] The Borg scale is a 0–10 point scale of dyspnea and work effort, scored by the patient. It is used in conjunction with the 6MWT and reported by the patient at baseline (for the dyspnea component) and at the end of the 6MWT (0 = no dyspnea or fatigue to 10 = maximum dyspnea or extremely hard effort and fatigue).

This patient only managed 170 m, which indicates severe limitation in exertion. For comparison, a recent study of patients with severe functional impairment and Eisenmenger physiology had a mean 6MWT distance of 249 m.[12] This patient had significant desaturation. Still, most individuals with an oxygen saturation of 67% would be unconscious, whereas she was able to complete the test without stopping. Her erythrocytosis is obviously a vital compensation for such severe hypoxemia.

## ECHOCARDIOGRAM

### OVERALL FINDINGS
There was an enlarged, single ventricle of LV morphology with a hypoplastic RV. Both the LA and RA were markedly enlarged.

There was an imperforate right AV connection with a rudimentary RV. Both atria were dilated. The LV diastolic dimension was 67 mm and the systolic dimension 51 mm. Ventricular function was moderately impaired. Color Doppler revealed a trace of mitral regurgitation.

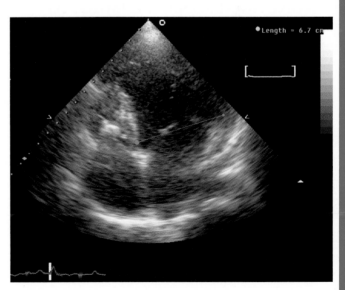

Figure 47-3 Apical four-chamber view, 2D end-diastolic image.

*Comments:* The absence of significant mitral regurgitation is important, as AV valve regurgitation is particularly poorly tolerated by patients with a functionally single ventricle. The ASD is not well visualized on this image but must be present in patients with tricuspid atresia to allow an exit from the RA to the LA.

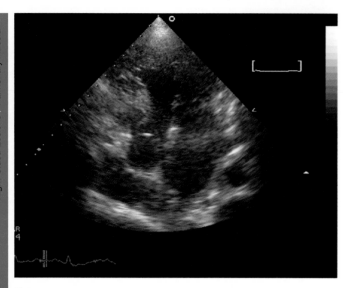

Figure 47-4 Apical long-axis view, 2D end-diastolic image.

## FINDINGS

The LA was dilated. The LV was dilated and hypertrophied. The aorta was dilated. Color flow Doppler demonstrated no aortic stenosis or regurgitation.

**Comments:** This image demonstrates important morphological features that allow identification of the systemic ventricle. A normal ventricle has three components: an inlet, apical, and outlet.

All three components are seen in this image. There is continuity between the inlet (anterior leaflet of the mitral valve) and the outlet (aortic valve). The apical portion is finely trabeculated. These features are morphologic hallmarks of an LV.

## MAGNETIC RESONANCE IMAGING

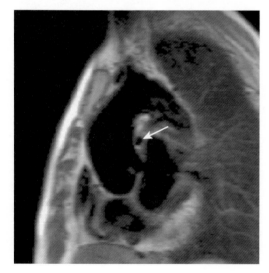

Figure 47-5 "Black blood" spin image sequence in sagittal plane.

## FINDINGS

The aorta was dilated, with a diameter of 55 mm in the ascending aorta. The hypoplastic right pulmonary artery was seen between the ascending aorta and LA, imaged through its short axis in this plane (*arrow*). It was extremely small. There was also a residual stump of an aortopulmonary collateral arising from the undersurface of the descending aorta.

**Comments:** There is dramatic disparity between the pulmonary artery and aortic dimensions.

The ascending aorta is often quite large in patients with pulmonary atresia and a VSD.[13]

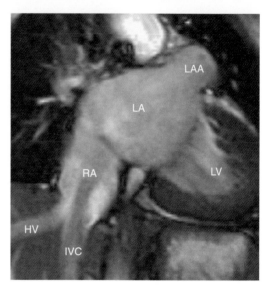

Figure 47-6 Magnetic resonance image using a gradient echo steady-state free precession sequence in a coronal plane. HV, hepatic vein.

## FINDINGS

This imaging plane showed the hepatic veins and IVC entering the RA. There was a 12 mm secundum ASD. The LA was enlarged and has a prominent appendage. The mitral valve and LV were clearly seen. The LV was both dilated and hypertrophied.

**Comments:** The prominent LA appendage correlates with the bulge from the left heart border seen on CXR.

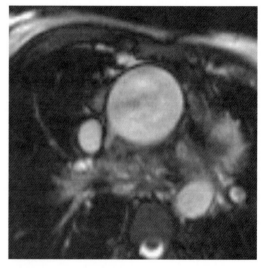

Figure 47-7 Magnetic resonance image using a gradient echo stady-state free precession sequence, transaxial view.

## FINDINGS

The Waterston shunt was seen arising from the right posterior aspect of the ascending aorta and was stenotic as it entered the hypoplastic native right pulmonary artery (both on the left-hand side of the screen). At its maximum, the right pulmonary artery measured 4 mm in diameter.

**Comments:** The Waterston shunt is still patent even though the patient required augmentation of pulmonary blood flow with a left BT shunt (which has now blocked, see Fig. 47-8). The Waterston shunt is now the main source of pulmonary blood flow and is clearly inadequate given the degree of cyanosis.

Waterston shunts are associated with many different complications. If too large they can cause pulmonary vascular disease. They can also cause kinking and distortion of the pulmonary artery and preferential flow to the right pulmonary artery.

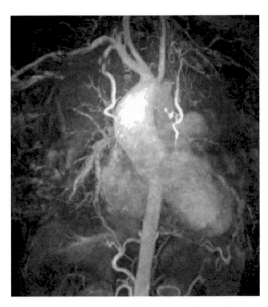

Figure 47-8 Magnetic resonance angiography (with gadolinium enhancement), coronal plane maximum intensity projection.

## FINDINGS

A hypoplastic right pulmonary artery was seen but no left pulmonary artery. The left subclavian artery was occluded just after its origin with no flow to a pulmonary artery. The left and right internal mammary arteries were prominent. There are small vessels arising from the celiac axis, internal mammary arteries, and the pleura that may be providing some pulmonary collateral blood supply.

**Comments:** This demonstrates the paucity of pulmonary blood flow, which explains the degree of cyanosis. The left BT shunt has completely blocked. Although it is impossible to know when this occurred the deterioration in symptoms may be related to this event.

The small systemic-to-pulmonary collaterals seen arising from a multitude of sites including the celiac axis, internal mammary arteries, and the pleura are a major bleeding hazard for any surgical intervention.

## CATHETERIZATION

### HEMODYNAMICS
Patient self-ventilating on 60% oxygen

Heart rate     78 bpm

| | Pressure | Saturation (%) |
|---|---|---|
| LV | 92/13 | |
| Aorta | 92/52 mean 70 | 75 |

## FINDINGS
The LV end-diastolic pressure gives indirect information about ventricular compliance. In this case it was mildly elevated (normal < 12 mm Hg).

It had been hoped to measure the pulmonary artery pressure via the Waterston shunt, but it was so narrowed that a reliable pressure measurement could not be obtained.

**Comments:** The angiographic and hemodynamic data from this diagnostic catheterization provided limited information in planning therapy. The primary objective was to better define the sources of pulmonary blood supply and assess pulmonary vascular resistance.

Cardiac catheterization should be undertaken in such patients only after careful consideration, in particular because, increasingly, decisions can be made using other noninvasive imaging such as MRI.[14] It should be performed in an institution and by an operator experienced in the catheterization of patients with complex ACHD. It is important that patients remain well hydrated throughout and catheter angiography is limited to the lowest contrast load necessary to complement the noninvasive data and to avoid renal failure.

The use of oxygen saturation data to calculate shunts and flows via the Fick principle was technically impossible because the operators could not enter the pulmonary artery. But it was also unnecessary because the dominant hemodynamic problem was inadequate pulmonary blood flow.

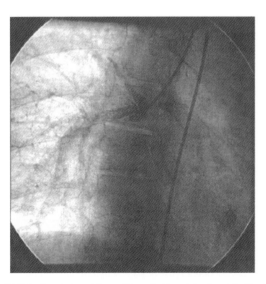

Figure 47-9 Left anterior oblique 30 projection. Injection into the Waterston shunt arising from the ascending aorta.

## FINDINGS
The right pulmonary artery was hypoplastic and filled very poorly through this shunt. There was no opacification of the left pulmonary artery.

**Comments:** This is corroborative of the MRI data that there was very limited pulmonary blood flow via the Waterston shunt because the native right pulmonary artery was hypoplastic and the shunt was stenotic.

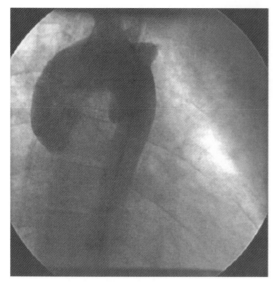

Figure 47-10 Lateral projection. Contrast injection through a pigtail catheter positioned in the arch of the aorta.

## FINDINGS

The aorta was dilated. There was minimal aortic regurgitation. The stump of the PDA or a MAPCA was seen arising from the undersurface of the descending aorta. The left subclavian artery was occluded close to its origin.

**Comments:** Two important sources of pulmonary blood flow have occluded: the left BT shunt (to the left lung) and perhaps a PDA or MAPCA.

### FOCUSED CLINICAL QUESTIONS AND DISCUSSION POINTS

1. What is the anatomy and pathophysiology?

*The patient has a single AV connection. The imperforate right AV connection (tricuspid atresia) means that all systemic venous return exits the RA via an ASD into the left atrium. Consequently there is admixture of systemic and pulmonary venous blood at atrial level resulting in systemic cyanosis. Blood exits the left atrium via the normal mitral valve. The aorta is normally related to the LV. The RV is rudimentary and there is pulmonary atresia. Therefore, the heart is functionally single or "univentricular."*

*The degree of cyanosis is determined by the amount of pulmonary blood flow. In patients with tricuspid atresia the ventriculoarterial connections are usually concordant (roughly 70% of cases). Usually there is a large VSD and pulmonary stenosis or subpulmonary stenosis. This case is an exception since there is also pulmonary atresia; the native pulmonary arteries are hypoplastic and the pulmonary blood supply at birth was from the arterial duct and from MAPCAs. Now it is almost exclusively via a stenotic Waterston shunt and only small remaining collaterals.*

*In the minority of tricuspid atresia patients with discordant ventriculoarterial connections (roughly 30%) pulmonary stenosis is common. The aorta arises from the small/hypoplastic RV. If the VSD is small, there may be obstruction to the aortic flow. Less commonly there is also aortic coarctation or interrupted aortic arch, which tends to be associated with uninterrupted pulmonary blood flow.*

2. What is the physiologic significance of MAPCAs?

*MAPCAs are large distinct muscular arteries with variable morphology and clinical phenotype. They may arise from head*

and neck vessels, the aorta via bronchial arteries, or rarely the coronaries. They may communicate with the native pulmonary tree or supply lung parenchyma directly. They are common in patients with pulmonary atresia and a VSD, but uncommon in patients with pulmonary atresia who do not have a VSD (see Case 46).

*There are three separate clinical presentations in which the consideration of MAPCAs is clinically important:*

1. *Profound cyanosis early in infancy developing after closure of the arterial duct as occurred with this patient, where a lack of adequate MAPCAs delivering blood flow necessitated a surgically created aortopulmonary shunt (in this case a Waterston shunt initially and a BT shunt thereafter).*
2. *Later presentation in childhood with milder and slowly progressive cyanosis, when pulmonary blood supply via MAPCAs is adequate initially. However, MAPCAs tend to become tortuous and stenotic with time, and can develop intravascular thrombosis, which ultimately limits pulmonary blood flow, and thus exaggerates cyanosis.*
3. *Patients with large MAPCAs from birth and unrestricted, excessive pulmonary blood flow who present early in life with exertional dyspnea and failure to thrive and are risk of developing pulmonary vascular disease (often segmental). Left untreated these patients may develop pulmonary hypertension and Eisenmenger physiology.*

*Patients with MAPCAs manifest a wide spectrum of pulmonary vascular morphology and physiology, ranging from patients on the favorable end with normally arborizing, true pulmonary arteries with the collaterals simply contributing systemic flow into the pulmonary vasculature, to patients on the unfavorable end with completely absent, native pulmonary arteries and all of the pulmonary blood supply from collaterals.*

*The management of patients with MAPCAs is complex and must be individualized according to their anatomy and clinical situation. In this patient's case augmenting pulmonary blood flow via Waterston and BT shunts in childhood was necessary to improve cyanosis. It was also done to facilitate sufficient growth of the hypoplastic native pulmonary arteries in the hope of facilitating a later Fontan-type palliation. However, this was not achieved; the native pulmonary arteries were too hypoplastic. It is nevertheless important to bear in mind that there is not a proven survival benefit for patients with a Fontan-type palliation versus aortopulmonary shunt palliation for naturally selected patients with "balanced" circulations.[10]*

3. What are the causes of her worsening symptoms and cyanosis?

*There is inadequate pulmonary blood flow. The patient is almost completely dependent on flow through a stenotic Waterston shunt into a hypoplastic, native right pulmonary artery with no flow in the native left pulmonary artery. The left BT shunt is occluded.*

*Her functional deterioration may be due to any combination of:*
*Increasing stenosis of the insertion of the Waterston shunt*
*Recent occlusion of the left BT shunt and native left pulmonary artery, although the timing of this is uncertain*
*Occlusion of MAPCAs due to stenosis of their origin, which can be part of their natural history*

4. What are the management options?

*Initially, correction of her slightly inappropriately low hemoglobin with careful iron and $B_{12}$ replacement may improve her oxygenation. This is a simple measure that should not be overlooked amid the complexity of problems patients with cyanotic heart disease face. The more challenging problem is how to augment the pulmonary blood supply.*

*One option is the creation of a further surgical interposition aortopulmonary shunt. Such an operation would carry consider-*

able risks given the severe cyanosis, previous surgery, and risk of bleeding from collaterals, and the only target for such a shunt is the hypoplastic native right pulmonary artery. In this situation, even if the patient survives surgery, there is a risk that there would be little improvement in saturation.

Another option is alleviation of the stenotic Waterston shunt. To achieve this surgically carries the risks as outlined above and more, as it is technically even more challenging.

Transcatheter percutaneous balloon dilatation with or without stenting is an alternative approach. There have been small series published reporting improvements in saturation and exercise tolerance at medium-term follow-up after stenting of aortopulmonary shunts.[15,16]

Heart-lung transplantation may need to be considered if other management options are unsuccessful in ameliorating the progressive decline in cardiopulmonary function. Experienced centers have reported that survival rates for heart-lung transplantation for adults with congenital heart disease are comparable to those for adults receiving heart-lung transplantation for other reasons (1-month survival 74%, 1-year survival 58%, and 3-year survival 47%).[17]

## FINAL DIAGNOSIS

Tricuspid atresia

Functionally single ventricle of LV morphology

Rudimentary RV

Pulmonary atresia, hypoplastic native right pulmonary artery supplied by a stenotic Waterston shunt

Occluded left BT shunt

Small MAPCAs

Severe cyanosis

## PLAN OF ACTION

Balloon dilatation and provisional stenting of the Waterston shunt anastomosis

## OUTCOME

Balloon dilatation of the Waterston shunt was attempted unsuccessfully. It proved to be impossible to pass a wire through the stenosis due to its tortuosity.

The patient was then evaluated for heart-lung transplantation. Unfortunately she died suddenly at home 3 months later, while on the active transplant waiting list. The family refused a postmortem examination. Sudden cardiac death, presumably arrhythmic, is the commonest mode of death in these patients.[10] More work in risk stratification and risk modification for sus-

tained arrhythmia and sudden cardiac death in this complex area is clearly required.

## Selected References

1. Broberg CS, Bax BE, Okonko DO, et al: Blood viscosity and its relationship to iron deficiency, symptoms, and exercise capacity in adults with cyanotic congenital heart disease. J Am Coll Cardiol 48:356–365, 2006.
2. Saliba Z, Butera G, Bonnet D, et al: Quality of life and perceived health status in surviving adults with univentricular heart. Heart 86:69–73, 2001.
3. Warnes CA, Somerville J: Tricuspid atresia in adolescents and adults: Current state and late complications. Br Heart J 56:535–543, 1986.
4. Perloff JK: Congenital heart disease in adults. In Braunwald E (ed): Heart Disease: A Textbook of Cardiovascular Medicine. Philadelphia, WB Saunders, 1997, pp 963–987.
5. Dimopoulos K, Okonko DO, Diller GP, et al: Abnormal ventilatory response to exercise in adults with congenital heart disease relates to cyanosis and predicts survival. Circulation 113:2796–2802, 2006.
6. Gatzoulis MA, Swan L, Therrien J, Pantely CA: Care of the cyanosed patient. In Adult Congenital Heart Disease: A Practical Guide. Oxford, Blackwell, 2005, pp 209–212.
7. Vonder Muhll I, Cholet A, Stehr K, et al: Evidence of neurohormonal and cytokine activation in cachectic adult patients with congenital heart disease. Can J Cardiol 20(Suppl D):113D, 2004; Circulation 110(17 Suppl III):III–496, 2004.
8. Dickinson CJ: The aetiology of clubbing and hypertrophic osteoarthropathy. Eur J Clin Invest 23:330–338, 1993.
9. Ross EA, Perloff JK, Danovitch GM, et al: Renal function and urate metabolism in late survivors with cyanotic congenital heart disease. Circulation 73:396–400, 1986.
10. Gatzoulis MA, Munk MD, Williams WG, Webb GD: Definitive palliation with cavopulmonary or aortopulmonary shunts for adults with single ventricle physiology. Heart 83:51–57, 2000.
11. ATS Committee on Proficiency Standards for Clinical Pulmonary Function Laboratories. ATS statement: Guidelines for the six-minute walk test. Am J Respir Crit Care Med 166:111–117, 2002.
12. Gatzoulis MA, Rogers P, Li W, et al: Safety and tolerability of bosentan in adults with Eisenmenger physiology. Int J Cardiol 98:147–151, 2005.
13. Niwa K, Siu SC, Webb GD, Gatzoulis MA: Progressive aortic root dilatation in adults late after repair of tetralogy of Fallot. Circulation 106:1374–1378, 2002.
14. Prasad SK, Soukias N, Hornung T, et al: Role of magnetic resonance angiography in the diagnosis of major aortopulmonary collateral arteries and partial anomalous pulmonary venous drainage. Circulation 109:207–214, 2004.
15. Bader R, Somerville J, Redington A: Use of self expanding stents in stenotic aortopulmonary shunts in adults with complex cyanotic heart disease. Heart 82:27–29, 1999.
16. Redington AN, Somerville J: Stenting of aortopulmonary collaterals in complex pulmonary atresia. Circulation 94:2479–2484, 1996.
17. Pigula FA, Gandhi SK, Ristich J, et al: Cardiopulmonary transplantation for congenital heart disease in the adult. J Heart Lung Transplant 20:297–303, 2001.

# Pacemaker Infection in a Cyanotic Patient

**Per Lunde**

**Age: 26 years**
**Gender: Female**
**Occupation: Laboratory technician**
**Working diagnosis: Pulmonary atresia with ventricular septal defect**

## HISTORY

The patient was born with a diagnosis of pulmonary atresia, large subaortic VSD, overriding aorta, large aortopulmonary collateral arteries, and distal right pulmonary artery stenosis. A modified left BT shunt was performed at the age of 3 to increase her pulmonary blood flow.

Two years later she was found to have intermittent complete heart block with a junctional escape rhythm at a rate of 60 bpm. However, she remained asymptomatic and was followed. She had no clinical problems. For various reasons she was not felt suitable for more definitive repair of her congenital heart lesion.

By the age of 22 years, the patient had gradually developed fatigue, exertional dyspnea, and a low working capacity. A 24-hour ECG recording at the time showed a complete heart block, with atrial rates up to 115 bpm and a narrow complex escape rhythm with a rate of 30 to 45 bpm.

Four years later at age 26 the patient participated in an exercise study as part of her clinical follow-up. Her heart rate response was blunted, the exercise capacity was only 36% of predicted, and she desaturated to 47% at peak exercise. A DDD pacemaker was implanted with epicardial leads placed via a subxiphisternal incision and tunneled to an abdominal pocket. A 5-day course of antibiotics was given. The wire thresholds were low (1.4 and 1.3 volts, respectively).

Five days later ventricular capture was not obtained even at maximal output. At the removal of the system, the ventricular lead seemed not to be properly secured. A new ventricular lead was tunneled to the site of the old pacing box. Appropriate doses of flucloxacillin and amoxicillin were given pre- and postoperatively.

Shortly thereafter, pacing thresholds had greatly increased. After 3 weeks the pacemaker did not work. Blood and pus from the abdominal scar appeared, and the patient was admitted to the hospital.

*Comments:* Patients with pulmonary atresia and VSD usually have a normal sinus node. The AV node occupies its normal position, and the bundle of His is closely related to the posterior rim of the membranous defect. Complete heart block is therefore not a common complication, particularly in patients who have not had intracardiac repair. The etiology of the heart block in this patient is, therefore, unknown. A pacemaker would not necessarily be required in the absence of symptoms.

Epicardial pacing is often preferred in children and adolescents with complex congenital defects and limited vascular access. Yet, compared to endocardial pacing, epicardial leads

have traditionally had higher thresholds and thus shorter longevity. In the presence of an intracardiac (especially right-to-left) shunt, as in this patient, there is also the potential for systemic thromboembolism (see Case 64). The risk may be small but has been consistently reported in recent studies even among patients with simple septal defects.[1,2] Another rationale for using epicardial leads in this patient population is to preserve venous access for later use, as patients with early onset of block require lifelong pacing.[3]

Pacemaker revisions are identified as predictors of infection. Patients undergoing pacemaker replacements are 2.5 times more likely to have a pacemaker infection compared to those undergoing a primary implantation.[4]

In our case, placement of another epicardial pacing system would seem unlikely to be successful. Previous surgical procedures combined with healed infection will create some degree of damage to the epicardial wall, resulting in more fibrosis, scarring, and adhesions, which all carry the risk of higher ventricular thresholds and early battery depletion.

## CURRENT SYMPTOMS

The patient currently complains of mild shortness of breath with exertion and loss of energy and appetite. She has had intermittent fevers and shivers for the past 5 days. She has not experienced palpitations or syncope, and does not have a cough.

NYHA class: II

*Comments:* Fever and shivers in a patient with a permanent pacemaker should alert the physician to the possibility of pacemaker infection.

## CURRENT MEDICATIONS

Perindopril 2 mg once daily

*Comments:* An ACE inhibitor was started for mild biventricular dysfunction several years previously.

## PHYSICAL EXAMINATION

BP 89/56 mm Hg, HR 55 bpm, oxygen saturation 69%, temperature 36.5° C

Height 169 cm, weight 33 kg, BSA 1.24 m$^2$

Surgical scars: There was an old left thoracotomy scar and a transverse abdominal incision. From the left end of the abdominal incision there was some discharge noted.

Neck veins: Mildly elevated with visible cannon waves

Lungs/chest: Chest was clear to auscultation. A continuous murmur from the aortopulmonary collateral(s) was best heard on the dorsal aspect of the chest.

Heart: There was an RV lift with a normal first heart sound, a loud single second heart sound, and a 2/6 ejection murmur at the upper right sternal edge with no diastolic murmur.

Abdomen: Tenderness around the pulse generator pocket was evident and again some discharge was noted. The liver was not enlarged.

Extremities: There was no peripheral edema. Digital clubbing was seen in both hands and feet.

**Comments:** The patient is very small for a mature adult, which is not uncommon in patients with severe cyanosis. The very low oxygen saturations here imply inadequate overall pulmonary blood flow from her collaterals and the BT shunt.

Signs at the pacemaker pocket site on admission suggested infection. Local symptoms at the site of pacemaker implantation often mirror an infective process involving the entire pacing system even though the infection seems to be local.[5]

## LABORATORY DATA

| | |
|---|---|
| Hemoglobin | **15.8 g/dL** (11.5–15.0) |
| Hematocrit/PCV | **49%** (36–46) |
| WBC | **12.8 × 10⁹/L** (3.5–10.8) |
| Neutrophils | 83% |
| MCV | 97 fL (83–99) |
| Platelet count | 279 × 10⁹/L (150–400) |
| Sodium | 135 mmol/L (134–145) |
| Potassium | 3.9 mmol/L (3.5–5.2) |
| Creatinine | 72 mg/dL (60–120) |
| Blood urea nitrogen | 5.5 mmol/L (2.5–6.5) |

### OTHER RELEVANT LAB RESULTS

| | |
|---|---|
| CRP | **90 g/L** (0–10) |
| Albumin | **31 g/L** (37–53) |
| Total protein | **61 g/L** (62–82) |
| Total bilirubin | **32 μmol/L** (3–24) |
| INR | 1.7 |

### PERTINENT NEGATIVES

Wound swab cultures were negative.
   Swabs from epicardial pacing box were negative.
   Blood cultures were negative.

**Comments:** The patient was relatively anemic despite her raised hemoglobin. With an oxygen saturation of 69% one would have expected the hemoglobin to be over 20 g/dL. Explanations for the low hemoglobin need to be sought, but may be related to infection. The MCV is high, though this does not necessarily exclude iron deficiency.[6]

The abnormal liver function test may reflect the abnormal hemodynamics of this patient, but may also relate to her nutrition and chronic ill health.

When a lead is infected, the whole length of the lead is usually involved.[5] The absence of positive cultures does not exclude active infection.

## ELECTROCARDIOGRAM

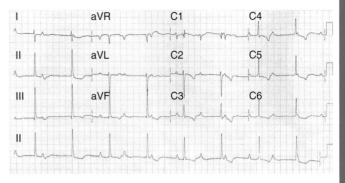

Figure 48-1 Electrocardiogram.

### FINDINGS
Heart rate: 55 bpm

QRS axis: +100°

QRS duration: 108 msec

Complete AV block with a junctional escape rhythm. There is RA overload and nonspecific repolarization abnormalities.

**Comments:** The atrial rate is about 75 bpm. Although the ventricular rate is currently acceptable, it can contribute to exertional intolerance and poses a risk of syncope. Pacemaker therapy is recommended even for symptom-free adults,[7] and would seem all the more appropriate in someone with ACHD.

## CHEST X-RAY

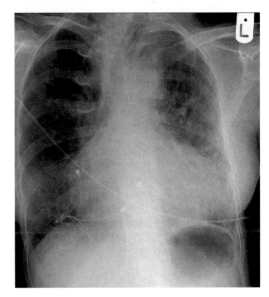

Figure 48-2 Posteroanterior projection.

### FINDINGS
Cardiothoracic ratio: 71%

The cardiac silhouette was markedly enlarged. There was a basal shadowing on the left side. The prominent bulging at the right cardiac border indicated RA enlargement. The epicardial leads were clearly seen without evidence of fractures or malposition. Enlargement of the aortic arch, seen here, is common in pulmonary atresia.[8] There was also mild scoliosis with lung asymmetry.

**Comments:** The cardiac apex is prominent and somewhat upturned suggesting RV hypertrophy. However, the most typical finding is the concavity in the area of the main pulmonary artery (the so-called empty pulmonary artery bay), suggesting hypoplasia or absence of the pulmonary trunk.

## EXERCISE TESTING

Cardiopulmonary exercise testing was not performed.

## ECHOCARDIOGRAM

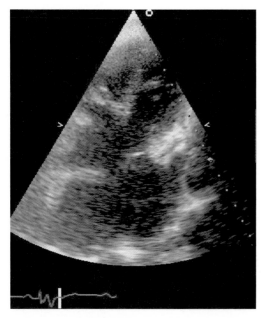

Figure 48-3 Four-chamber view.

### OVERALL FINDINGS

The patient had a normal-sized RV with normal systolic function, and a large VSD with right-to-left shunt. There was also a normal-sized LV, again with overall maintained systolic function. Dilated RA and LA were seen.

Also of note were the RV (*left*) with prominent moderator band and the large and nonrestrictive VSD.

Relative chamber sizes were shown.

**Comments:** The echocardiogram was done prior to placement of the pacing system. Further echocardiography would not likely demonstrate infection as the leads are epicardial.

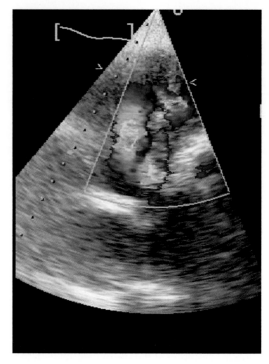

Figure 48-4 Four-chamber 2D Doppler.

### FINDINGS

There was unrestricted flow across the VSD at the bottom of the image. There seemed to be a second muscular VSD superiorly.

**Comments:** As the VSD is the only flow outlet for the RV, it is important that the defect is unrestricted. A VSD can be a nidus for infective endocarditis, although this is usually in the setting of a small and restrictive VSD with turbulent flow (clearly not the case here). No vegetations are seen.

## COMPUTED TOMOGRAPHY

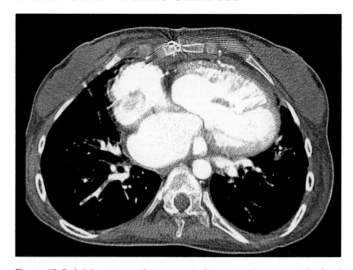

Figure 48-5 Axial cross-section computed tomography scan at the level of the subaortic ventricular septal defect.

## FINDINGS

This CT showed the large subaortic VSD. There was also dilatation of the coronary sinus. The RV was heavily trabeculated, reflecting its exposure to aortic pressures.

***Comments:*** CT scanning is not without the risks of radiation exposure, which must be carefully considered, especially in a young woman. However, this imaging modality can show the patient's anatomy and the collateral vessels in great detail and with none of the risks associated with invasive cardiac catheterization (namely thrombosis, bleeding, and risks related to sedation, when used). MRI was not an option here because of the patient's pacemaker (not visible in these selected views).

The dilatation of the coronary sinus in this patient is due to a persistent left superior caval vein draining into the coronary sinus.

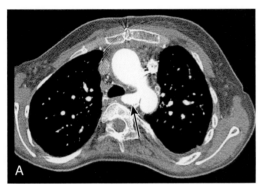
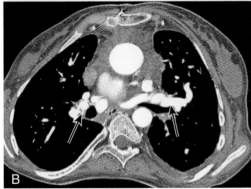

Figure 48-6 Axial cross-section computed tomography scan showing large aortopulmonary collateral arteries.

## FINDINGS

The CT showed aortopulmonary collateral arteries.

A large collateral artery arose off the distal aortic arch to the left of the spine (*arrow* in *A*). Further caudal, two large collaterals were seen coursing to the right and left lungs (*arrows* in *B*).

***Comments:*** In pulmonary atresia with VSD, MAPCAs are the usual source of pulmonary arterial supply. The aortopulmonary collaterals usually arise from the descending aorta and the underside of the aortic arch and occasionally from the subclavian, mammary, and/or coronary arteries. They may communicate with the native pulmonary arterial tree ("dual supply"), or supply areas of lung parenchyma directly. The collaterals may vary in size and number (see Case 47).

In contrast, patients with pulmonary atresia and an intact ventricular septum are not usually born with MAPCAs,

although they may develop collateral vessels later on in life, if severe cyanosis persists (see Case 46).

This patient had not had a definitive repair. Thus, her pulmonary blood flow is entirely dependent on MAPCAs and the surgically created left BT shunt. Her low resting oxygen saturation reflects her low pulmonary blood flow and intracardiac mixing (see Case 47).

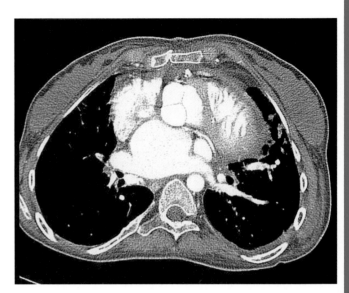

Figure 48-7 Thoracic computed tomography at the level of the aortic root.

## FINDINGS

The dilated aortic valve with its three leaflets was seen in cross section anteriorly and behind the sternum (where normally the pulmonary trunk runs). The LA and the pulmonary veins were easily appreciated behind the aorta.

***Comments:*** The pulmonary artery would normally be visible to the left and anteriorly to the aortic valve in this view. Instead, one sees only the RV infundibulum, and the persistent left SVC coursing along the left lateral aspect of the LA.

## CATHETERIZATION

Not performed

### FOCUSED CLINICAL QUESTIONS AND DISCUSSION POINTS

1. **How should one confirm the diagnosis of pacemaker infection?**

*Infection of the pacemaker pocket or lead is a potential complication after any permanent pacemaker implantation. Rates between 0.5% and 7.0% have been reported in both retrospective and prospective studies.[9] The lack of a precise definition of pacing system–related infection may explain this wide variation.*

*Infections are generally due to local bacterial contamination acquired at the time of implantation.[5] Microorganisms migrate from the insertion site along the surface lead, colonizing the distal part of the lead with the potential for bacteremia and endocarditis in patients with endocardial pacing systems.* **Staphylococcus aureus** *and* **Staphylococcus epidermidis** *are the prevailing microorganisms.[10] Infections may also occur after seeding of* microorganisms through a hematogenous route. Finally, skin erosion may be the mechanism by which local infection occurs.

Morbidity and mortality associated with pacemaker infection are high, particularly in complex cyanotic patients, and therefore an early diagnosis is mandatory to initiate appropriate therapy.

Clinical evidence of pacemaker infection includes local erythema, tenderness, erosion, or fluctuation at the generator site. Infection is microbiologically confirmed when cultures from the generator pocket or electrode lead are positive.

2. How should the pacemaker infection be treated?

Appropriate management of pacemaker-related infection should involve the prompt and complete removal of the generator and leads, regardless of the extent and location of the infection. Delayed or partial removal of the pacing system increases morbidity and mortality and increases the risk of recurrent infection. The removal should be followed by tailored antibiotic therapy, temporary pacing if necessary, and reimplantation at a new site following treatment of the infection. Temporary pacing through a transjugular sheath may be necessary before a new permanent system can be reimplanted without undue risk of further infection. There is no consensus on the duration of antibiotic therapy in patients with pacemaker infection. Two weeks of intravenous therapy followed by 4 weeks of orally administered antibiotic therapy has been suggested.[5] There is also no consensus on how long one should wait before reimplantation of a new system, though the longer the better in terms of reinfection. The answer is tailored to the individual patient and relates to the bacterial burden of the initial infection, the underlying rhythm, and the safety of a temporary transvenous system.

3. Should this patient have a new epicardial pacing system or a transvenous system?

Two attempts have been made at placing an epicardial pacing system, and both failed. The drawbacks of an endocardial pacing system include the potential for thromboembolism in a cyanotic patient such as this, a risk that has been well documented. However, there are also clear advantages. One is that it would save the patient the need for another thoracotomy under general anesthesia. Another is that the bacterial infection at this point involves only the epicardial spaces, not endocardial, and, at least in theory, a new endocardial pacing system may not be as prone to reinfection. Third, poor capture from the epicardial system could be eliminated by placement of a fixed transvenous pacing lead. Fourth, newer developments and research have suggested that the thromboembolic potential from endocardial leads may not be as high as previously believed (see Case 64).

For all of the above reasons, the patient was considered for a transvenous system as an alternative.

4. What other therapy should be considered to improve the patient's exercise intolerance?

Clearly, this patient has other impairments contributing to her symptoms besides simply complete heart block. Her poor pulmonary blood flow resulting in very low oxygen saturation and an inappropriately low hemoglobin all need to be addressed. It may not be possible to offer her a more definitive repair, such as an RV-PA conduit to a large enough pulmonary artery. This is speculative, however, and a thorough assessment of the size and confluence of her central pulmonary arteries and of all individual sources of pulmonary artery supply would be warranted, once infection is eradicated. Short of this, other attempts at improving pulmonary blood flow are difficult and success cannot be guaranteed. The principles guiding such decisions have been discussed elsewhere (see Case 47). For this patient, the physicians involved opted to deal with the pacing and infection issues alone.

## FINAL DIAGNOSIS

Pulmonary atresia with VSD

MAPCAs

Complete AV block

Pacemaker infection

## PLAN OF ACTION

Explantation of existing system including epicardial leads, intravenous antibiotics, followed by reimplantation of a permanent transvenous system

## INTERVENTION

Elective transvenous DDDR pacemaker via right subclavian route was fitted 2 months later following appropriate antibiotic therapy, normalization of C-reactive protein, and multiple negative repeat blood cultures.

## OUTCOME

Blood cultures and multiple swabs from the abdominal scar were taken and intravenous antibiotics started. Culture of the pacing lead grew S. epidermidis. Intravenous piperacillin with tazobactam (Tazocin) and teicoplanin were started to cover staphylococci and presumed hospital-acquired infection. Six days later the entire pacing system was removed. The delay was felt best to allow antibiotics to decrease the bacterial burden and reduce the chance of spreading infection further with surgery.

After 14 days of intravenous antibiotic therapy there was no longer any evidence of local or systemic infection, and antibiotic therapy was stopped. After only 2 weeks, this patient was successfully treated. Obviously, the decision about the length of therapy must be individualized.

Thereafter the patient's C-reactive protein and white blood cell count gradually normalized. During this period she was clinically and hemodynamically stable in complete heart block with a heart rate of 44 to 65 bpm, though continuously watched as an inpatient during the initial period on intravenous antibiotics. She was eventually discharged home.

Two months later a transvenous DDDR pacing system was fitted. Because of concern about the development of venous thrombosis and the potential for systemic thromboembolism, anticoagulation therapy was initiated at the time when the transvenous system was implanted.

After receiving the new pacing device the patient felt fine. Clinically, her working capacity improved substantially and there was less effort dyspnea and fatigue. The pacemaker was functioning normally with low thresholds. After 1 year there has been no recurrent infection or systemic thromboembolism. Her present medications are warfarin, perindopril, and oral iron supplementation.

The patient was not interested in reparative surgery; hence she had no further assessment of her pulmonary arteries. She was referred to our pregnancy and heart disease clinic for advice on contraception and pregnancy risks.[11]

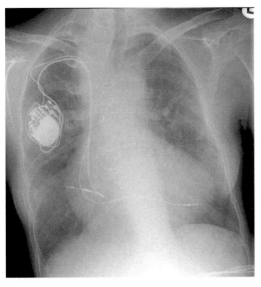

Figure 48-8 Posteroanterior projection chest X-ray following implantation of a transvenous dual-chamber pacing system.

## FINDINGS

The left-sided basal shadowing had cleared and the left vascular markings were less prominent, although still present. The heart was still markedly enlarged.

***Comments:*** The RA lead has a lateral position because the lead could not be properly secured in the RA appendage. The ventricular lead is at the right ventricular apex. Both leads were placed by active fixation, as can be seen by the visible screws at the lead tips.

## Selected References

1. Silka MJ, Rice MJ: Paradoxic embolism due to altered hemodynamic sequencing following transvenous pacing. Pace 14:499–503, 1991.
2. Khairy P, Landzberg MJ, Gatzoulis MA, et al: Transvenous pacing leads and systemic thromboemboli in patients with congenital heart disease and intracardiac shunts: A multicenter study. Circulation 113:2391–2397, 2006.
3. Noiseux N, Khairy P, Fourier A, et al: Thirty years of experience with epicardial pacing in children. Cardiol Young 14:512–519, 2004.
4. Cohen MI, Bush DM, Gaynor JW, et al: Pediatric pacemaker infections: Twenty years of experience. J Thorac Cardiovasc Surg 124:821–827, 2000.
5. Klug D, Wallet F, Kacet S, et al: Detailed bacteriologic tests to identify the origin of transvenous pacing system infections indicate a high prevalence of multiple organisms. Am Heart J 149: 322–328, 2005.
6. Spence MS, Balaratnam MS, Gatzoulis MA: Clinical update: Cyanotic adult congenital heart disease. Lancet 370:1530–1532, 2007.
7. Michaelsson M, Jonzon A, Riesenfeld R: Isolated congenital complete atrioventricular block in adult life: A prospective study. Circulation 92:442–449, 1995.
8. Tan JL, Davlouros PA, McCarthy KP, et al: Intrinsic histological abnormalities of the aortic root and ascending aorta in tetralogy of Fallot: Evidence of causative mechanism to aortic dilatation and aortopathy. Circulation 112:961–968, 2005.
9. Chuna JD, Wilkoff BL, Lee I, et al: Diagnosis and management of infections involving implantable electrophysiologic cardiac devices. Ann Intern Med 133:604–608, 2000.
10. Da Costa A, Lelievre H, Kirkorian G, et al: Role of the preaxillary flora in pacemaker infections: A prospective study. Circulation 97:1791–1795, 1998.
11. Uebing A, Steer PJ, Yentis SM, Gatzoulis MA: Pregnancy and congenital heart disease. BMJ 332:401–406, 2006.

# Complex Congenital Heart Conditions

## Part I

# Transposition of the Great Arteries

Case 49

# Catheter Intervention for Baffle Leak or Venous Obstruction

**Vaikom S. Mahadevan, Peter R. McLaughlin, and Lee N. Benson**

**Age: 33 years**
**Gender: Male**
**Occupation: Musician**
**Working diagnosis: Transposition of the great arteries**

## HISTORY

The patient was diagnosed with D-TGA at birth and underwent an atrial septostomy. Subsequently, a Mustard atrial redirection procedure was performed, and the patient did well.

Three years ago he was noted to have a junctional rhythm with bradycardia. He was not willing to consider insertion of a permanent pacemaker. Soon afterward he was found to have episodes of intra-atrial reentrant tachycardia (atypical atrial flutter) and junctional bradycardia. Beta-blockers to treat the tachyarrhythmia were contraindicated due to bradycardia. In view of this, the issue of insertion of a permanent pacemaker was again raised, and the patient consented to it.

**Comments:** Sinus node dysfunction is common in patients with transposition of the great arteries and prior atrial redirection surgery. The risk is due to a combination of both extensive atrial surgical scar formation and associated hemodynamic abnormalities.

## CURRENT SYMPTOMS

The patient described no symptoms other than palpitations. He had not experienced syncope or presyncope. He could climb two flights of stairs without dyspnea, and in general had no limitations of his daily activities.

NYHA class: I

## CURRENT MEDICATIONS

Warfarin (target INR 2–3)

**Comments:** Warfarin was prescribed as anticoagulation for atrial flutter.

## PHYSICAL EXAMINATION

Pink

BP 100/80 mm Hg, HR 72 bpm, oxygen saturation 97%

Height 173 cm, weight 64 kg, BSA 1.75 m²

Surgical scars: Median sternotomy scar

Neck veins: V-waves seen 3 cm above the sternal angle

Lungs/chest: Clear to auscultation

Heart: The rhythm was irregular. There were no palpable thrills. There was a normal first heart sound and a single second heart sound. A grade 1 systolic murmur was heard at the lower left sternal edge.

Abdomen: The liver was not palpable; there was no ascites.

Extremities: No edema was present, and the skin was warm.

### PERTINENT NEGATIVES

There were no signs of SVC obstruction such as facial puffiness, swelling of the arms, or dilation of veins over the upper thorax.

**Comments:** The single second heart sound is due to the anterior position of the aortic valve, which is audible, whereas the more posteriorly located pulmonic valve is often not.

Patients with prior atrial redirection surgery are at risk of obstruction of the venous pathways. Fullness of the face and fluid retention, such as ascites or edema of the upper or lower extremities, may be evidence of obstruction, but its absence does not exclude the problem.

## LABORATORY DATA

| | |
|---|---|
| Hemoglobin | 16.1 g/dL (13.0–17.0) |
| Hematocrit/PCV | 48% (41–51) |
| MCV | 89 fL (83–99) |
| Platelet count | $169 \times 10^9$/L (150–400) |
| Sodium | 142 mmol/L (134–145) |
| Potassium | 4.3 mmol/L (3.5–5.2) |
| Creatinine | 0.9 mg/dL (0.6–1.2) |

**Comments:** The hemoglobin is at the upper limit of normal.

## ELECTROCARDIOGRAM

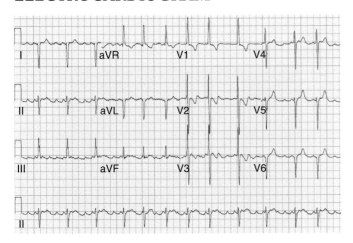

Figure 49-1   Electrocardiogram.

### FINDINGS
Heart rate: ~75 bpm

QRS axis: +165°

QRS duration: 106 msec

Atrial flutter at a rate of ~250 bpm with a controlled ventricular response

Marked RV hypertrophy with right-axis deviation

**Comments:** RV hypertrophy is universal in patients with a Mustard or Senning repair of transposition of the great arteries. This is due to the hypertrophy of the RV in response to systemic arterial pressures. The right-axis deviation is due to the dominant forces produced by the systemic RV. Arrhythmias (especially atrial flutter variants) are common in these patients.

## CHEST X-RAY

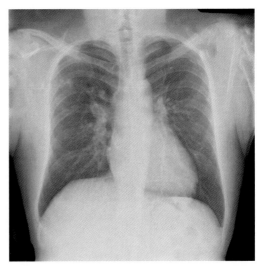

Figure 49-2  Posteroanterior projection.

### FINDINGS
Cardiothoracic ratio: 47%

Normal heart size. There were prominent vascular markings with probably upper lobe distribution flow. There were no Kerley B lines and no clear evidence of interstitial edema.

**Comments:** There is no cardiomegaly and no evidence of overt heart failure in this patient. There is no appreciable dilatation of the azygos vein or SVC to suggest venous pathway obstruction.

## EXERCISE TESTING

| | |
|---|---|
| Exercise protocol: | Bicycle ergometer starting at 12 W and increasing 10 W every min |
| Duration (min:sec): | 11:00 |
| Reason for stopping: | Sense of choking |
| ECG changes: | None |

| | Rest | Peak |
|---|---|---|
| Heart rate (bpm): | 72 | 147 |
| Percent of age-predicted max HR: | | 79 |
| $O_2$ saturation (%): | 97 | 90 |
| Blood pressure (mm Hg): | 100/80 | 120/80 |
| Peak $Vo_2$ (mL/kg/min): | | 24 |
| Percent predicted (%): | | 48 |
| Ve/Vco$_2$: | | 48 |
| Metabolic equivalents: | | 7.0 |

### FINDINGS
His peak $Vo_2$ had been 27.7 mL/kg/min (55% of predicted maximum) 1 year earlier.

**Comments:** Typically, the exercise capacity of a patient with a previous Mustard procedure and a systemic right ventricle will be low. We note the mild reduction in maximum oxygen uptake compared with 1 year earlier. It is important that any serial comparison be made with similar exercise protocols (bicycle, treadmill, etc).

The oxygen saturation dropped to 90% during exercise, which may indicate the presence of a small right-to-left shunt at atrial/baffle level, or the occurrence of exertional pulmonary edema.

# ECHOCARDIOGRAM

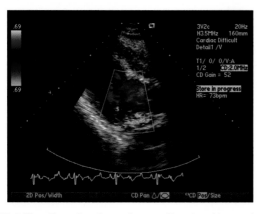

Figure 49-3 Transthoracic echocardiogram. Parasternal long-axis view of the heart.

## FINDINGS

The LV chamber size and function were normal. The morphologic LV was the venous ventricle. The mitral valve, which was the venous AV valve, had trivial regurgitation. The RV cavity size was moderately enlarged, with moderate reduction in systolic function, and this was the systemic ventricle. The tricuspid valve, which was the systemic AV valve, was mildly regurgitant. The baffles were patent with turbulence noted at entry of the systemic venous baffle suggesting stenosis. The SVC baffle velocity was 1.5 m/sec, the baffle velocity was 1.8 m/sec, and the pulmonary venous velocity was 1.5 m/sec.

*Comments:* Baffle stenoses are not uncommon in older patients who have had a Mustard procedure. Baffle leaks, especially small leaks, are difficult to identify with echocardiography. Bubble studies increase the sensitivity of echocardiography. Angiography and MRI may also be helpful.

# MAGNETIC RESONANCE IMAGING

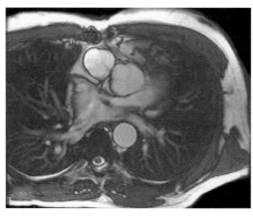

Figure 49-4 Oblique coronal plane showing baffle stenosis.

## Ventricular Volume Quantification

|  | LV | (Normal range) | RV | (Normal range) |
|---|---|---|---|---|
| EDV (mL) | 98 | (77–195) | 182 | (88–227) |
| ESV (mL) | 43 | (19–72) | **112** | (23–103) |
| SV (mL) | 55 | (51–133) | 70 | (52–138) |
| EF (%) | **56** | (57–75) | **38** | (50–76) |
| EDVi (mL/m²) | **56** | (66–101) | 104 | (65–111) |
| ESVi (mL/m²) | 25 | (18–39) | **64** | (18–47) |
| SVi (mL/m²) | **31** | (43–67) | 40 | (39–71) |

## FINDINGS

The aorta arose from the morphologic RV. The RV showed moderate hypertrophy, as expected. The aortic valve was anterior to the pulmonary valve, in keeping with D-transposition of the great vessels. There was moderate global hypokinesis of the systemic RV, and mild tricuspid regurgitation.

*Comments:* The systemic RV is dysfunctional, a common problem in transposition patients. The stroke volumes quantified, taking into account mild tricuspid regurgitation, do not suggest a large shunt.

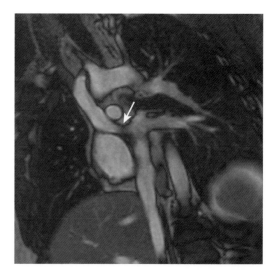

Figure 49-5 Sagittal view of cardiac magnetic resonance.

## FINDINGS

The superior systemic venous baffle was narrowed to 8 mm in its mid and distal extent (*arrow*). Flow in the azygos vein was noted to be retrograde. There was also an unusual outpouching at the cranial aspect of the superior systemic baffle (out of plane). The inferior baffle was patent with no evidence of baffle stenosis. No baffle leak was identified.

*Comments:* Given the common need for placement of a permanent pacemaker, assessment of the venous pathways becomes clinically important. MRI is an excellent noninvasive method to assess patency of the baffles and of the thoracic veins and gives very good anatomical visualization. However, it cannot yet be used in most patients with pacing devices. Baffle leaks may not be visualized on MRI.

# CATHETERIZATION

## HEMODYNAMICS

Heart rate    72

| | Pressure | Saturation (%) |
|---|---|---|
| SVC | Mean 12 | 68 |
| IVC | Mean 9 | 74 |
| RA | Mean 9 | |
| LV (pulmonary ventricle) | 37/14 | |
| PA | 31/8 mean 14 | 73 |
| | | |
| PCWP | | |
| LA | Mean 12 | |
| RV (systemic ventricle) | 100/14 | 97 |
| Aorta | 100/80 mean 92 | 97 |

### Calculations

| | |
|---|---|
| Qp (L/min) | 4.01 |
| Qs (L/min) | 3.64 |
| Cardiac index (L/min/m$^2$) | 2.08 |
| Qp/Qs | 1.10 |
| PVR (Wood units) | 0.75 |
| SVR (Wood units) | 22.77 |

## FINDINGS

Hemodynamic data confirmed a small gradient from the SVC to the systemic venous chamber, and a small resting shunt.

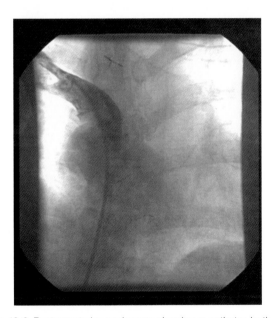

Figure 49-6 Posteroanterior angiogram showing a catheter in the right upper pulmonary vein via baffle leak.

## FINDINGS

The catheter inserted via the IVC entered the pulmonary venous compartment and right upper pulmonary vein.

**Comments:** This catheter placement seen here can only be possible through a hole in the atrial baffle; hence a baffle leak must be present. Catheterization is a useful technique to detect and quantify baffle leaks, which may be missed by other imaging modalities. The clinical clue to this diagnosis was the falling saturation on the exercise test.

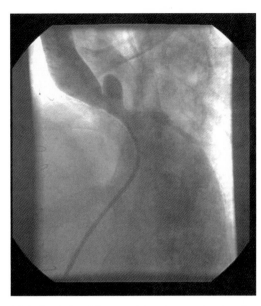

Figure 49-7 Left anterior oblique cranial angiogram showing stenosis with aneurysmal region of superior vena cava baffle.

## FINDINGS

Angiography revealed stenosis in the SVC baffle with a reduction in caliber from 20 mm to a minimum diameter of 8 mm at the narrowest point. There is also an aneurysmal area just before the area of severe stenosis in the SVC baffle.

**Comments:** This confirms the MRI findings, although the small aneurysm was unexpected.

### FOCUSED CLINICAL QUESTIONS AND DISCUSSION POINTS

1. **Should the systemic venous pathway obstruction be dilated and stented?**

    *Systemic venous pathway obstruction is not uncommon in patients with a previous Mustard operation and can occur in up to 15% of patients on follow up[1] and should definitely be treated if symptomatic. Stenosis of the superior limb of the systemic venous baffle is more common than of the inferior limb. Symptoms may include fullness or flushing around the head or arm for SVC obstruction, or ascites/leg edema from an IVC obstruction.*

    *Often, however, the presence of venous runoff through the azygos system will prevent such symptoms from occurring, and thus intervention may be deferred.*

    *In this patient—as in many adult patients with TGA and atrial switch procedures—a fully patent SVC baffle is necessary to enable insertion of transvenous pacing leads, which are often required. This is usually achievable by percutaneous stent placement.[2] Transvenous pacing leads, in turn, are more reliable and last longer than epicardial pacing leads, and are usually easier to place. Stenting of the SVC baffle will hopefully reduce the chance of baffle restenosis or progression to complete occlusion. Still, thrombus formation around the pacing wire is a risk.*

2. **What is the significance of the incidental finding of a baffle leak, and should the leak be closed?**

    *Baffle leaks usually cause a left-to-right shunt and, if large enough, volume overload of the subpulmonary ventricle (the anatomical LV). The hemodynamic significance of a leak can be determined by quantification of the Qp/Qs ratio, as with any other shunt. Sizeable shunts should be closed. This can often be achieved by percutaneous deployment of a closure device. Evi-*

*dence of right-to-left shunting through the baffle may also be an indication for closure.*

*In this patient, because a transvenous pacing system was planned, the baffle leak needed to be closed irrespective of the shunt size to avoid the risk of paradoxical emboli arising from thrombus formation on the pacing leads.[3] The small degree of desaturation with exercise in this patient would probably not, in itself, justify closure.*

## FINAL DIAGNOSIS

D-TGA with a prior Mustard procedure

Stenosis of the SVC venous pathway

Baffle leak

Paroxysmal atrial flutter

Sinus node dysfunction

## PLAN OF ACTION

Transcutaneous balloon dilatation and stenting of SVC baffle stenosis, and transcutaneous closure of baffle leak

## INTERVENTION

Intervention was carried out at the time of the diagnostic catheterization, under local anesthesia and mild sedation, with access obtained via the right femoral artery. After a wire was placed across the obstruction, the stenosis was predilated with a 15-mm balloon and a stent dilated up to 18 mm. Postprocedural venography showed unobstructed flow into the RA with no gradient.

Subsequently, a venous catheter was directed into the left atrium and left upper pulmonary vein via the baffle leak. On balloon sizing the leak had a stretch diameter of 19 mm. A 22-mm Amplatzer septal occluder was deployed across the defect with no residual leak on follow-up angiography. Fluoroscopy confirmed anterior positioning of the device and a pulmonary artery angiogram confirmed unobstructed blood flow of the right pulmonary veins into the LA.

## OUTCOME

The patient tolerated the procedure well without any complications. He was discharged the following day, with instructions to continue aspirin for 6 months along with warfarin.

A permanent AV pacemaker was subsequently implanted followed by successful direct current cardioversion to sinus rhythm. On review at 8 months, the patient was feeling better, free of paroxysmal atrial flutter, and was being maintained on beta-blockers and warfarin.

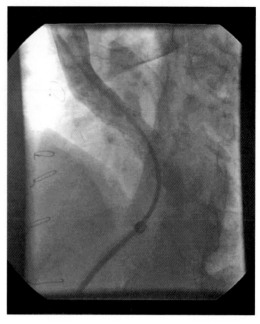

Figure 49-8 Angiogram in the left anterior oblique cranial view, showing the stent across the stenosis of the superior vena cava baffle with free flow of contrast into the right atrium.

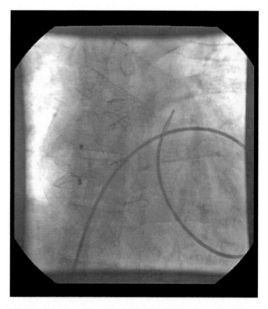

Figure 49-9 Angiogram with catheter in the right pulmonary artery showing the Amplatzer duct occluder in situ across the baffle leak.

### FINDINGS

Imaging in the pulmonary artery view shows position of the stent across the SVC baffle and the Amplatzer septal occluder device across the baffle leak. The balloon-tipped catheter is in the main pulmonary artery.

## Selected References

1. Moons P, Gewillig M, Sluysmans T, et al: Long term outcome up to 30 years after the Mustard or Senning operation: A nationwide multicentre study in Belgium. Heart 90:307–313, 2004.
2. Bu'Lock FA, Tometzki AJ, Kitchiner DJ, et al: Balloon expandable stents for systemic venous pathway stenosis late after Mustard's operation. Heart 79:225–229, 1998.
3. Daehnert I, Hennig B, Wiener M, Rotzsch C: Interventions in leaks and obstructions of the interatrial baffle late after Mustard and Senning correction for transposition of the great arteries. Catheter Cardiovasc Interv 66:400–407, 2005.

## Bibliography

Giardini A, Lovato L, Donti A, et al: A pilot study on the effects of carvedilol on right ventricular remodelling and exercise tolerance in patients with systemic right ventricle. Int J Cardiol 114:241–246, 2007.
Warnes CA: Transposition of the great arteries. Circulation 114: 2699–2709, 2006.

# Transcatheter Options for Atrial Arrhythmia after the Mustard Procedure

Yat-Yin Lam, Joseph Y.S. Chan, and Michael A. Gatzoulis

**Age: 28 years**
**Gender: Female**
**Occupation: Flight attendant**
**Working diagnosis: Transposition of the great arteries and Mustard procedure**

## HISTORY

The patient had transposition of the great arteries, and received a successful atrial switch (Mustard procedure) in early life. Recovery and follow-up were uneventful.

At age 16, the patient had her first episode of palpitations; atrial flutter was diagnosed, which self-terminated. Because of several recurrences, she was started on bisoprolol 5 mg once daily. Apart from occasional palpitations, she felt fine.

She married and wanted to start a family, and thus was referred to an ACHD clinic for prepregnancy advice. She was again in atrial flutter. Baseline imaging studies including a transthoracic echocardiogram, and cardiac MRI revealed patent pulmonary and systemic pathways and good systemic RV function, with no atrial thrombus. Sinus rhythm was restored by direct current cardioversion and maintained with sotalol 80 mg twice daily. She also performed well in cardiopulmonary exercise testing.

She became pregnant 6 months later, and the pregnancy was well tolerated. Warfarin was stopped when pregnancy was confirmed.

She had two episodes of breakthrough atrial flutter with hemodynamic compromise requiring electrical cardioversion, both occurring during the third trimester. Amiodarone was added for the remainder of pregnancy to prevent arrhythmia recurrences. She delivered uneventfully at 38 weeks of gestation.

She had frequent palpitations and dizzy spells in the 6 months after delivery, and returned to the outpatient clinic.

A Holter recording showed paroxysmal sustained atrial flutter with, occasionally, a slow ventricular response of 33 to 50 bpm and sinus pauses (longest was 2.5 seconds). She received a dual-chamber pacemaker implantation for symptomatic bradycardia. She was restarted on amiodarone (in combination with bisoprolol), but this failed to prevent recurrence of symptomatic fast atrial flutter. She was at that point advised to have electrophysiological evaluation of the tachycardia and radiofrequency ablation.

**Comments:** The Mustard procedure redirects blood at the atrial level using a baffle. The systemic venous return is directed to the LV and the pulmonary venous blood is directed to the RV.[1] The surgery achieves physiological correction, but the RV remains the systemic pumping chamber. The overall survival of patients with atrial switch is about 75% at 25 years.[2]

Atrial arrhythmia occurs in 20% of patients by age of 20.[3]

Successful pregnancies have been reported in patients with atrial switch procedures, that is, Mustard or Senning operations.[4] Imaging studies may identify significant baffle obstruction or leakage that should be dealt with before conception (see Case 49). Furthermore, RV function may deteriorate during and after pregnancy, and there is reported maternal mortality, albeit the experience is relatively small.

Our patient should be a relatively low risk subject during pregnancy, as she has a normal functional class and good systemic RV function.[5] She is, however, at high risk for atrial arrhythmia recurrence during pregnancy. Pharmacological or electrical strategy to restore/maintain sinus rhythm before conception may be advisable. Beta-blockers in this respect have a good safety profile for the mother and the fetus.

Warfarin or Coumadin need not always be stopped in a pregnant patient, although concerns about warfarin embryopathy certainly have been discussed.[6] Furthermore, there is an underreported incidence of fetal cerebral bleeding with warfarin therapy, which may be of greater concern (see Case 14 for a more thorough discussion of the options).

If needed, DC cardioversion during pregnancy is a very low risk procedure.[7]

## CURRENT SYMPTOMS

The patient is asymptomatic apart from intermittent palpitations. She describes several distinct episodes of a rapid, regular pulse lasting several hours. However, she can climb two to three flights of stairs without difficulty, and actively participates in horseback riding and swimming.

NYHA class: I

## CURRENT MEDICATIONS

Bisoprolol 5 mg daily

## PHYSICAL EXAMINATION

BP 110/70 mm Hg (right arm), HR 110 bpm, oxygen saturation 98% on room air

Height 160 cm, weight 55 kg, BSA 1.56 m²

Surgical scars: Median sternotomy scar

Neck veins: JVP was visible 3 cm above the sternal angle, with no visible V-wave.

Lungs/chest: Chest was clear.

Heart: She had an irregular rhythm. A marked RV heave was noted. Her first heart sound was normal with a single and loud second heart sound. There was a grade 2/6 pan-systolic murmur best heard at the left lower sternal border compatible with tricuspid regurgitation.

Abdomen: Her abdomen was soft, and no organomegaly was detected.

Extremities: No peripheral edema

***Comments:*** A resting heart rate above 100 bpm in a Mustard (or Senning) patient with previous atrial switch procedures or other surgery for ACHD should not be assumed to be sinus tachycardia (it is more likely to be atrial flutter or atrial reentry tachycardia).

The irregularity of the rapid pulse does not necessarily exclude atrial flutter.

The murmur of tricuspid regurgitation in a Mustard patient would not increase with inspiration since the tricuspid valve is in the systemic rather than the pulmonary circuit.

## LABORATORY DATA

| | |
|---|---|
| Hemoglobin | 13.9 g/dL (11.5–15.0) |
| Hematocrit/PCV | 40% (36–46) |
| MCV | 91 fL (83–99) |
| Platelet count | $199 \times 10^9$/L (150–400) |
| Sodium | 138 mmol/L (134–145) |
| Potassium | 3.9 mmol/L (3.5–5.2) |
| Creatinine | 0.6 mg/dL (0.6–1.2) |
| Blood urea nitrogen | 5.7 mmol/L (2.5–6.5) |

***Comments:*** Blood laboratory results were normal.

## ELECTROCARDIOGRAM

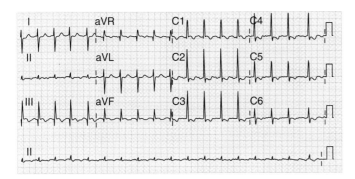

Figure 50-1 Electrocardiogram.

### FINDINGS
Heart rate: 110 bpm

QRS axis: +145°

QRS duration: 93 msec

Atrial flutter, or intra-atrial reentry (see P-waves, best seen in lead V3), with variable ventricular response. RV pressure overload with RV strain.

***Comments:*** RV hypertrophy and right-axis deviation are typical for patients with a Mustard or Senning procedure and a systemic RV.

Atrial arrhythmia in Mustard patients is usually due to intra-atrial reentry or atrial flutter. Atrial flutter is a common result of prior extensive atrial surgery and/or may reflect atrial dilation and stretch due to systemic tricuspid regurgitation or ventricular decompensation. Mustard patients are also prone to sick sinus syndrome and junctional rhythm for the same reasons.

## CHEST X-RAY

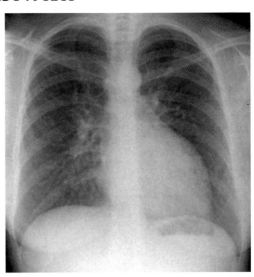

Figure 50-2 Posteroanterior projection.

### FINDINGS
Cardiothoracic ratio: 49%

Situs solitus, levocardia, left aortic arch with borderline cardiomegaly and normal pulmonary vascular markings.

***Comments:*** The vascular pedicle is narrow with an oblong cardiac silhouette ("egg on string"), which is fairly typical for transposition of the great arteries.

## EXERCISE TESTING

| | |
|---|---|
| Exercise protocol: | Modified Bruce |
| Duration (min:sec): | 11:35 |
| Reason for stopping: | Leg fatigue |
| ECG changes: | Junctional rhythm at baseline, sinus rhythm restored at exercise stage 2 |

| | Rest | Peak |
|---|---|---|
| Heart rate (bpm): | 45 | 139 |
| Percent of age-predicted max HR: | | 72 |
| O$_2$ saturation (%): | 98 | 98 |
| Blood pressure (mm Hg): | 110/70 | 170/80 |
| Peak Vo$_2$ (mL/kg/min): | | 26.7 |
| Percent predicted (%): | | 85 |
| Ve/Vco$_2$: | | 40 |
| Metabolic equivalents: | | 7.6 |

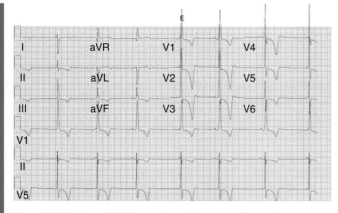

Figure 50-3 Resting ECG shows sinus alternating with junctional escape rhythm.

**Comments:** The patient demonstrated both AV conduction problems and atrial tachycardia. Both are relatively common in patients with prior atrial redirection surgery and may be interrelated with each other (i.e., bradytachycardia syndrome).

## ECHOCARDIOGRAM

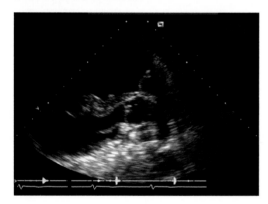

Figure 50-4 Parasternal long-axis view.

### FINDINGS

There was a dilated systemic RV with mildly reduced systolic function. The subpulmonary morphologic LV was banana shaped, small, with normal function. There was ventriculoarterial discordance. The tricuspid valve (systemic AV valve) appeared normal, and there was only mild regurgitation.

**Comments:** The aortic valve, seen superiorly (anteriorly), and the pulmonary valve, seen inferiorly (posteriorly), are seen in parallel, consistent with transposition, as the normally arranged semilunar valves, are in perpendicular planes (crisscross relationship). It is important to assess the function of the tricuspid valve in patients with transposition of the great arteries, as its regurgitation may reflect systemic ventricular dysfunction. Furthermore, the adverse hemodynamic effects of substantial tricuspid regurgitation may be greater than the effects of mitral regurgitation on a systemic LV in concordant hearts.

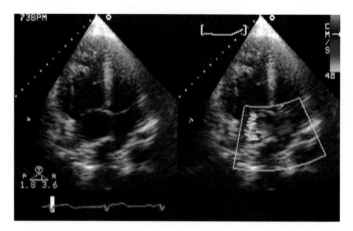

Figure 50-5 Apical four-chamber view.

### FINDINGS

Mildly dilated RV with mildly impaired RV systolic function. Color Doppler showing mild tricuspid regurgitation and patency in both systemic and pulmonary venous pathways.

**Comments:** Mild RV dysfunction and tricuspid valve regurgitation are not uncommon and propagate each other. Ordinarily, dysfunction and valve regurgitation would be expected to cause atrial enlargement and contribute to arrhythmia. It is essentially impossible to gauge the size of the atrial chambers in these patients because the atrial redirection baffle distorts the original anatomy.

## MAGNETIC RESONANCE IMAGING

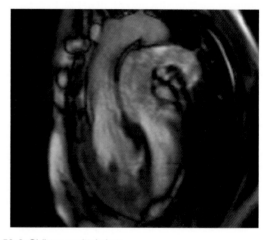

Figure 50-6 Oblique sagittal view.

### FINDINGS

The RV was hypertrophied and mildly dilated, and connected to the aorta. The LV was small by comparison, and connected to the pulmonary artery.

**Comments:** The septum bowed toward the LV, demonstrating that the latter is the lower-pressure ventricle.

### Ventricular Volume Quantification

| | LV | (Normal range) | RV | (Normal range) |
|---|---|---|---|---|
| EDV (mL) | 64 | (52–141) | 128 | (58–154) |
| ESV (mL) | 18 | (13–51) | 77 | (12–68) |
| SV (mL) | 46 | (33–97) | 51 | (35–98) |
| EF (%) | 72 | (56–75) | 40 | (49–73) |
| EDVi (mL/m²) | 41 | (65–99) | 82 | (65–102) |
| ESVi (mL/m²) | 12 | (19–37) | 49 | (20–45) |
| SVi (mL/m²) | 29 | (42–66) | 33 | (39–63) |
| Mass index (g/m²) | 31 | (47–77) | 57 | (22–42) |

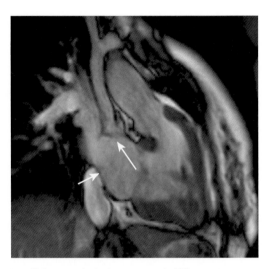

Figure 50-7 Oblique sagittal plane, systemic RV to aorta.

## FINDINGS

The pulmonary venous chamber was patent, as was the systemic venous chamber.

**Comments:** In this view the SVC and IVC are seen and would normally flow to the RA. However, their paths have been redirected out of plane toward the pulmonary LV by surgically placed baffles (*arrows*). Instead, the pulmonary veins (*upper right*) drain now to this atrial chamber that flows through the tricuspid valve to the RV and subsequently the aorta (all visible here).

Mustard patients should be considered at least once for assessment of potential baffle obstruction and/or leak. While baffle obstruction may be detected by a transthoracic echo, an MRI is likely more sensitive. CT and TEE can also be helpful as alternatives to catheterization, which is the gold standard.

### FOCUSED CLINICAL QUESTIONS AND DISCUSSION POINTS

1. What are the types of arrhythmia seen in patients who undergo Mustard repair?

*Patients with Mustard repair, as illustrated by our patient, can have both brady- and tachyarrhythmias. Atrial flutter (intra-atrial reentry) occurs in 20% of atrial switch patients by age 20, whereas sinus node dysfunction and/or junctional bradycardia is seen in half of the patients by that time.[3]*

*A Mustard repair involves reconstructing the atria, with excision of the atrial septum and placement of baffles for redirecting systemic and pulmonary venous return to morphologic LV and RV, respectively. Such extensive atrial surgery performed in early*

infancy often damages the sinoatrial node with progressive loss of sinus node function in long-term follow-up.

*Extensive incisions and suture lines also lead to intra-atrial conduction delay and abnormalities in atrial refractoriness that create the substrate for intra-atrial reentrant tachycardia. Cavotricuspid isthmus-dependent reentry has been found to be the most common type of intra-atrial reentrant tachycardia.[8] Ventricular tachyarrhythmias may also occur in transposition patients as a consequence of a failing systemic RV.[9]*

2. What is the best way to manage atrial arrhythmia during pregnancy?

*Management issues for patients with previous atrial switch procedures during pregnancy include monitoring of RV function, systemic tricuspid regurgitation, rate or rhythm control, and anticoagulation (if applicable). Excluding deterioration of RV function by echocardiogram is important in Mustard patients who develop atrial arrhythmia during pregnancy. Other causes for atrial arrhythmia, if present, should be treated accordingly.*

*Antiarrhythmic therapy is largely empiric in Mustard patients. No drug is completely safe although most appear to be relatively safe for the fetus. Beta-blockers are generally considered safe, but they could potentially affect fetal growth and "mask" or "suppress" signs of fetal distress during labor. Amiodarone usage is commonly associated with transient fetal thyroid dysfunction and has also been reported to cause teratogenicity in a small series.[10] Alternatively, antiarrhythmics could be hazardous to the mother. They can lead to bradycardia—especially in patients with concomitant sinus node dysfunction—and can also be proarrhythmic in patients with poor systemic RV function. The general rules for prescribing antiarrhythmics are to use drugs with good safety records if necessary and to avoid combination therapies. DC cardioversion is safe and effective during pregnancy.[6,7]*

3. Should Mustard patients with atrial arrhythmia during pregnancy be anticoagulated?

*The decision of anticoagulation should be made after risk-benefit analysis. The reported risk of thromboembolism in Mustard patients during pregnancy is 4%, possibly due to clot formation in the baffle as well as atrial arrhythmia.[11,12] However, there is no ideal anticoagulation option during pregnancy. Warfarin crosses the placenta and may cause embryopathy (6.4%)[13] and spontaneous miscarriage, especially when taken during weeks 6 to 12 of gestation at a dosage greater than 5 mg daily.[14] Unfractionated heparin is safe for the fetus but leads to more maternal bleeding and osteoporosis. Low molecular weight heparin has the advantages of easier administration and claimed lower osteoporotic risk,[15] but its safety and efficacy in Mustard patients remain unknown. Low molecular weight heparin was used in our patient during the third trimester because of her paroxysmal atrial flutter, with seemingly good effect. Pregnant patients should be informed about the risks and benefits of thromboprophylaxis, and the final decision should be made by specialized cardiologists and obstetricians on an individual basis and in conjunction with the patient.*

4. What are the indications and technical considerations for pacemaker implantation and electrophysiologic ablation in Mustard patients?

*Indications for pacemaker implantation include symptomatic bradycardia (syncope due to bradycardia and effort intolerance due to chronotropic incompetence)[16] and facilitation of the treatment of tachyarrhythmias.[5] Intracardiac thromboses and hemodynamically significant lesions like baffle leak or obstruction ideally should be treated beforehand.[17] Transvenous pacing leads must traverse the SVC baffle of the atrial switch to enter the morphologic LA appendage and/or LV, and active lead fixation is recommended.[6] The epicardial approach is a good alternative especially when venous access is troublesome or a baffle leak is present. Atrial pacing is preferred for patients without AV nodal disease. Rate responsiveness is preferred in patients with sinus node disease. Antitachycardia devices for overdrive atrial pacing and implantable cardioverters/defibrillators for terminating ventricular arrhythmia have been implanted in selected patients. Cardiac resynchronization therapy for patients with concomitant failing systemic RV is still at the investigational stage.*

*Despite the complexities of the atrial anatomy and venous access, ablation of intra-atrial reentrant tachycardia is feasible.[18,19] Electrophysiologic study is generally reserved for patients with symptomatic arrhythmia following a trial of antiarrhythmic drug therapy, although this can be questioned in the light of recent advances in diagnostic and interventional electrophysiology. The arrhythmia circuit frequently involves the isthmus tissue between the tricuspid valve and IVC orifice, the area of the mouth of the coronary sinus, and the region extending from the mouth to the tricuspid annulus and, as such, is often the site of ablation. As the coronary sinus could drain into either atrium, biatrial involvement of the arrhythmia circuit is possible. Access to the pulmonary venous atrium through either a small baffle leak or the aorta to achieve bidirectional isthmus conduction block therefore may be necessary. Using the above approach, an initial success rate of 60% to 70% by experienced operators has been reported.[20] Other identified focal atrial arrhythmia, most likely atrioventricular nodal reentrant tachycardia, should be treated or ablated accordingly.*

## FINAL DIAGNOSIS

TGA with Mustard procedure

Atrial flutter complicating pregnancy

Drug-refractory atrial arrhythmia

## PLAN OF ACTION

Pacemaker implantation and electrophysiology ablation for managing corresponding brady- and tachyarrhythmia

## INTERVENTION

Cavotricuspid isthmus-dependent type intra-atrial reentrant tachycardia was identified during electrophysiologic study, and radiofrequency catheter ablation was performed successfully.

## OUTCOME

One year after successful delivery of her first child, the patient remained at her prepregnancy functional class I, without palpitations or documented arrhythmia. There was mild RV dysfunction with mild tricuspid regurgitation reported by echo. She had no plans for further pregnancies, and thus a Mirena coil was inserted for effective contraception.[21]

## Selected References

1. Warnes CA: Transposition of the great arteries. Circulation. 114:2699–2709, 2006.
2. Oechslin E, Jenni R: 40 years after the first atrial switch procedure in patients with transposition of the great arteries: Long-term results in Toronto and Zurich. Thorac Cardiovasc Surg 48:233–237, 2000.
3. Flinn CJ, Wolff GS, Dick M, et al: Cardiac rhythm after the Mustard operation for complete transposition of the great arteries. N Engl J Med 310:1635–1638, 1984.
4. Uebing A, Gatzoulis MA: Right heart lesion. In Steer PJ, Gatzoulis MA, Baker P (eds): Heart Disease and Pregnancy. London, RCOG, 2006, pp 191–210.
5. Gatzoulis M, Webb G, Daubeney P (eds): Chapters 13 and 41, Diagnosis and Management of Adult Congenital Heart Disease. Churchill Livingstone, 2003.
6. Therrien J, Gatzoulis M, Graham T, et al: Canadian Cardiovascular Society Consensus Conference 2001 update: Recommendations for the management of adults with congenital heart disease—Part III. Can J Cardiol 17:1135–1158, 2001.
7. Barnes E, Eben F, Patterson D: Direct current cardioversion during pregnancy should be performed with facilities available for fetal monitoring and emergency caesarean section. BJOG 109:1406–1407, 2002.
8. Puley G, Siu S, Connelly M, et al: Arrhythmia and survival in patients > 18 years of age after the Mustard procedure for complete transposition of the great arteries. Am J Cardiol 83:1080–1084, 1999.
9. Kammeraad JA, van Deurzen CH, Sreeram N, et al: Predictors of sudden cardiac death after Mustard or Senning repair for transposition of the great arteries. J Am Coll Cardiol 44:1095–1102, 2004.
10. Joglar JA, Page RL: Antiarrhythmic drugs in pregnancy. Curr Opin Cardiol 16:40–45, 2001.
11. Drenthen W, Pieper PG, Ploeg M, et al: Risk of complications during pregnancy after Senning or Mustard (atrial) repair of complete transposition of the great arteries. Eur Heart J 26:2588–2595, 2005.
12. Siu SC, Sermer M, Coleman JM, et al: Prospective multicenter study of pregnancy outcomes in women with heart disease. Circulation 104:515–521, 2001.
13. Chan WS, Anand S, Ginsberg JS: Anticoagulation of pregnant women with mechanical heart valves: A systematic review of the literature. Arch Intern Med 160:191–196, 2000.
14. Vitale N, De Feo M, De Santo LS, et al: Dose-dependent fetal complications of warfarin in pregnant women with mechanical heart valves. J Am Coll Cardiol 33:1637–1641, 1999.
15. Bates SM, Greer IA, Hirsh J, et al: Use of antithrombotic agents during pregnancy. The Seventh ACCP Conference on Antithrombotic and Thrombolytic Therapy. Chest 126:627S–644S, 2004.
16. Diller G-P, Okonko DO, Uebing A, et al: Impaired heart rate response to exercise in adult patients with a systemic right ventricle or univentricular circulation: Prevalence, relation to exercise and potential therapeutic implications. Int J Cardiol 2008; [Epub ahead of print].
17. Khairy P, Landzberg MJ, Gatzoulis MA, et al: Transvenous pacing leads and systemic thromboemboli in patients with congenital heart disease and intracardiac shunts: A multicenter study. Circulation 113:2391–2397, 2006.
18. Kanter RJ, Papagiannis J, Carboi MP, et al: Radiofrequency catheter ablation of supraventricular tachycardia substrates after Mustard and Senning operations for D-transposition of the great arteries. J Am Coll Cardiol 35:428–441, 2000.
19. Van Hare GE, Lesh MD, Ross BA, et al: Mapping and radiofrequency ablation of intraatrial re-entrant tachycardia after the Senning or Mustard procedure for transposition of the great arteries. Am J Cardiol 77:985–991, 1996.
20. Delacretaz E, Ganz LI, Soejima K, et al: Multiple atrial macro-reentry circuits in adults with repaired congenital heart disease: Entrainment mapping combined with three-dimensional electroanatomic mapping. J Am Coll Cardiol 37:1665–1676, 2001.
21. Dhanjal MK: Contraception in women with heart disease. In Steer PJ, Gatzoulis MA, Baker P (eds): Heart Disease and Pregnancy. London, RCOG, 2006, pp 9–26.

# Considerations for Tricuspid Valve Replacement in Patients with a Systemic Right Ventricle

**Candice K. Silversides and Gary D. Webb**

**Age: 29 years**
**Gender: Male**
**Occupation: College instructor**
**Working diagnosis: Mustard repair of transposition of the great arteries**

## HISTORY

The diagnosis of TGA was made postnatally, and the patient underwent a balloon atrial septostomy (Rashkind procedure) followed by a Mustard operation at 2 years of age. He did well after the procedure and had a normal childhood.

He had been well until 6 months prior to his presentation (29 years old) when he developed a rapid and significant decline in his functional status. Exertional dyspnea prevented him from walking more than a block on flat ground, and he was not able to climb a flight of steps.

He was seen and started on diuretics. Soon the patient was able to return to his usual activities. He then underwent further evaluation.

***Comments:*** The atrial redirection, or "switch," operations, as described by Mustard[1] and Senning[2] were the first definitive operations for TGA. These operations involved redirecting blood flow at the atrial level. However, these operations leave the RV and the tricuspid valve in the systemic (subaortic) position. They have now been largely replaced by the arterial switch operation.[3]

## CURRENT SYMPTOMS

On diuretics, he was able to walk up several flights of stairs and felt that he had no functional limitation. His main recreational activity was dancing, which he had resumed.

NYHA class: I

***Comments:*** After an atrial switch operation, potential cardiovascular causes of functional decline include systemic ventricular dysfunction, AV valve regurgitation, sustained arrhythmias, baffle obstruction and leaks, and pulmonary hypertension.

## CURRENT MEDICATIONS

Furosemide 40 mg once daily

## PHYSICAL EXAMINATION

BP 110/75 mm Hg, HR 70 bpm, oxygen saturation 99% on room air

Height 176 cm, weight 76 kg, BSA 1.93 m$^2$

Surgical scars: Midline sternotomy scar

Neck veins: JVP was normal.

Lungs/chest: Lungs were clear to auscultation.

Heart: There was no cyanosis or clubbing. There was a thrill at the left sternal border. The first heart sound was normal, and the second heart sound was loud and single. There was a grade 4/6 pan-systolic murmur heard best at the lower left sternal border.

Abdomen: No clinical hepatosplenomegaly

Extremities: No peripheral edema, and the peripheral pulses were normal.

***Comments:*** Normal arterial saturations indicate that there is no significant right-to-left shunt through a baffle leak, although baffle leaks typically shunt left to right like other ASDs.

In atrial switch patients, the JVP reflects filling of the LV through the mitral valve.

The second heart sound is usually single in patients with TGA. This is because the aortic valve is located anteriorly, and the softer pulmonary sound is more posterior and less audible. Splitting of the second heart sound may indicate the development of pulmonary hypertension, when the normally soft posteriorly placed pulmonary closure sound becomes accentuated and thus audible.

The presence of a loud pan-systolic murmur suggests significant tricuspid regurgitation in this context. If this patient had a VSD, the murmur intensity would not be in the usual location since the shunt would be from RV to LV. Dynamic LVOT obstruction can also result in a systolic ejection murmur, but this was a not present in this patient.

# LABORATORY DATA

| | |
|---|---|
| Hemoglobin | 13.3 g/dL (13.0–17.0) |
| MCV | 92.2 fL (83–99) |
| Platelet count | $163 \times 10^9$/L (150–400) |
| Sodium | 140 mmol/L (134–145) |
| Potassium | 4.2 mmol/L (3.5–5.2) |
| Creatinine | 0.91 mg/dL (0.6–1.2) |

# ELECTROCARDIOGRAM

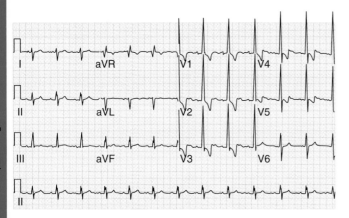

Figure 51-1 Electrocardiogram.

## FINDINGS

Heart rate: 75 bpm

QRS axis: +140°

QRS duration: 122 msec

Normal sinus rhythm, normal P-wave morphology, right-axis deviation, and voltage criteria for RV hypertrophy with RV strain or repolarization abnormalities.

24-hour Holter ECG monitor: There was sinus rhythm throughout the study with an average heart rate of 75 bpm. There were rare, isolated ventricular and atrial premature complexes.

**Comments:** There is mandatory hypertrophy of the systemic RV, which is almost always obvious on the ECG.

Arrhythmias are common in patients after an atrial switch operation, and loss of sinus rhythm may precipitate functional deterioration. Arrhythmias that may develop include bradyarrhythmias, especially sinus bradycardia with junctional escape rhythms; intra-atrial reentry tachyarrhythmias (mainly atrial flutter variants); ventricular tachycardia; and sudden death. Arrhythmias are associated with cardiac morbidity and mortality.[4]

# CHEST X-RAY

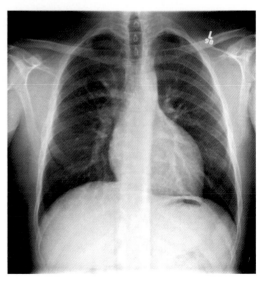

Figure 51-2 Posteroanterior projection.

## FINDINGS

Cardiothoracic ratio: 47%

The cardiac silhouette is at the upper limits of normal. There was a narrow vascular pedicle, with absence of the main pulmonary artery along the left heart border. There was no evidence of pulmonary venous hypertension or pulmonary edema. Sternal wires were present.

**Comments:** The narrow vascular pedicle is often (but not always) seen in TGA because of the parallel anteroposterior or side-by-side (as opposed to the normal crossed) relationship of the great vessels. The cardiac silhouette should be normal in size unless there is atrial or ventricular dilation.

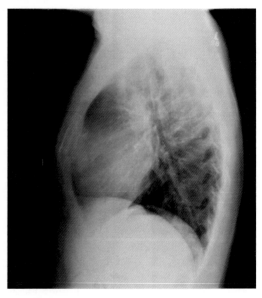

Figure 51-3 Lateral view.

## FINDINGS

There is evidence of a prior sternotomy. There seems to be filling of the retrosternal space.

**Comments:** Retrosternal filling on a lateral CXR may be due to RV prominence, TGA (aorta anterior to pulmonary artery), ascending aortic aneurysms, and anterior mediastinal masses (most notably teratoma, thymoma, and thyroid masses).

## EXERCISE TESTING

Not performed

## ECHOCARDIOGRAM

### OVERALL FINDINGS

The morphologic RV is the systemic ventricle. There was moderate dilation of the systemic ventricle with mild global hypokinesis. The subpulmonary morphologic LV was mildly decreased in size with normal systolic function. There was systolic and diastolic flattening of the interventricular septum reflecting the pressure overload of the systemic RV. Flow in the pulmonary venous atrium and SVC and IVC was unobstructed with normal Doppler profiles.

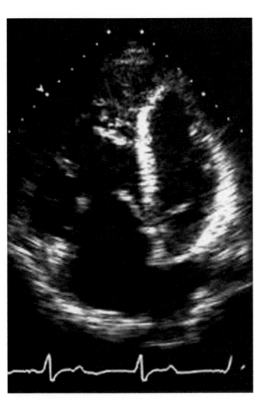

Figure 51-4 Apical four-chamber view.

### FINDINGS

The RV was considerably larger than the LV, and there was mild systolic dysfunction.

**Comments:** In the context of an atrial switch for TGA, the echocardiogram is useful to identify the morphology of the ventricles. It is good at assessing the severity of tricuspid regurgitation (if present), and can detect baffle stenosis (turbulence and/or increased Doppler velocities ≥ 1.5 m/sec) or baffle leaks. Saline contrast injections may provide additional information regarding baffle leaks. The LVOT should be assessed for fixed and dynamic obstruction. The LV systolic pressure should be measured. The atrial septum is removed at surgery to permit placement of the baffles. Systemic and pulmonary venous flow passes through what were originally parts of both atria.

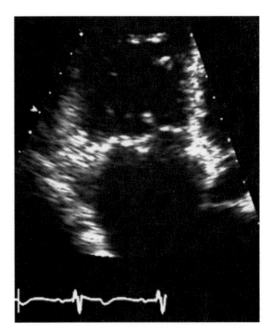

Figure 51-5 Apical four-chamber view, tricuspid valve focus.

### FINDINGS

There was tricuspid valve prolapse along with a partial flail segment.

**Comments:** Tricuspid regurgitation after atrial switch operations is almost always "functional," that is, secondary to systemic RV systolic dysfunction and displaced septal chordal attachments. When this is the cause of severe tricuspid regurgitation in a Mustard or Senning patient, surgery is seldom advised or wise. In occasional patients such as this patient, the tricuspid regurgitation is instead due to primary tricuspid valve disease, and there may be a clear indication for surgery if RV function is preserved.

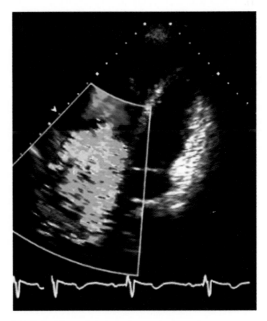

Figure 51-6 Apical four-chamber view, color Doppler.

## FINDINGS

There was severe tricuspid regurgitation.

***Comments:*** This echocardiogram shows a large jet area indicating severe tricuspid regurgitation.

## MAGNETIC RESONANCE IMAGING

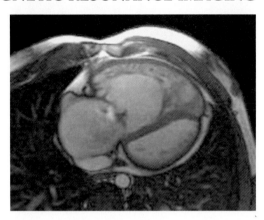

Figure 51-7 Steady-state free precession cine, oblique axial plane, four-chamber view.

### Ventricular Volume Quantification

|  | LV | (Normal range) | RV | (Normal range) |
|---|---|---|---|---|
| EDV (mL) | 101 | (77–195) | **344** | (88–227) |
| ESV (mL) | 34 | (19–72) | **187** | (23–103) |
| SV (mL) | 67 | (51–133) | **157** | (52–138) |
| EF (%) | 66 | (57–74) | **46** | (48–74) |
| EDVi (mL/m²) | **52** | (68–103) | **178** | (68–114) |
| ESVi (mL/m²) | **18** | (19–41) | **97** | (21–50) |
| SVi (mL/m²) | **35** | (44–68) | **81** | (40–72) |
| Mass index (g/m²) | **33** | (59–93) | **65** | (23–50) |

## FINDINGS

There was moderate hypertrophy of the systemic RV (as expected). There was a severely dilated systemic RV and mild systolic dysfunction. There was dilation of the atrium. A jet of tricuspid insufficiency was seen in the atrium. The subpulmonary morphologic LV was of normal size and had normal systolic function. There was no stenosis in the superior or inferior baffle. No baffle leak was detected. The main pulmonary artery was dilated (47 mm).

***Comments:*** CMR is useful to accurately assess the size and function of the systemic RV and has become the gold standard for these measurements. MRI is also useful to assess the patency of the baffles and to assess the pulmonary vasculature.

The RV ejection fraction of 46% is low considering the presence of severe AV valve regurgitation. One should anticipate a somewhat lower postoperative RV ejection fraction if the tricuspid valve were replaced.

The dilation of the main pulmonary artery is unexplained, but anecdotally not uncommonly noted in patients with transposition.

## FOCUSED CLINICAL QUESTIONS AND DISCUSSION POINTS

1. **What is the cause of the patient's heart failure symptoms?**

   *The clinician should consider several potential causes of heart failure in any patient with an atrial switch operation. These include systemic ventricular dysfunction, severe AV valve regurgitation, sustained atrial or ventricular arrhythmias, baffle obstructions and/or leaks, and pulmonary hypertension.[5]*

   *Therefore, the most important issue in assessing a patient with a "failed Mustard" is to verify the diagnosis with both clinical findings and imaging. These should focus on determining the systolic function of the systemic ventricle (see Case 56), the degree of AV valve regurgitation, and patency of the venous flow systems. This can be difficult using echocardiography alone but is particularly important, as an obstruction or leak in the baffle is potentially reversible (see Case 49).*

   *In this case, the patient most likely developed heart failure secondary to severe tricuspid regurgitation. As a rule, severe tricuspid regurgitation in a Mustard or Senning patient is a sequela of severe systemic RV dysfunction and subsequent dilation. The valve leaflets themselves are normal. This patient is atypical. His severe tricuspid regurgitation was due to a partially flail tricuspid valve leaflet in the setting of preserved RV function.*

2. **Should this patient have his tricuspid valve repaired/replaced?**

   *As a rule, Mustard or Senning patients with severe tricuspid regurgitation are not candidates for tricuspid valve replacement or repair because most have severe systemic RV dysfunction. This patient is an exception, and tricuspid valve surgery could potentially protect his functional capacity and his systemic ventricular function.*

3. **What other treatment options are available to patients with a failing Mustard or Senning repair?**

   *If there is pulmonary venous congestion secondary to significant systemic RV dysfunction, treatment options include standard heart failure treatment; resynchronization therapy; and heart transplantation or switch conversion surgery (from an atrial switch to an arterial switch). Conversion of an atrial switch operation to an arterial switch is a complex procedure and usually requires subpulmonary LV "retraining" with pulmonary artery banding. This can result in LV failure.[6] In some patients, pulmonary artery banding with a resultant rise in subpulmonary LV pressure may improve the ventricular septal geometry and improve the tricuspid regurgitation. Once sufficient LV hypertrophy has developed (e.g., 6–12 months), the atrial baffle can be taken down and an arterial switch performed. Alternatively, pulmonary artery banding can be a "definitive palliation."*

   *The switch conversion strategy is a controversial one in adult patients, and some experts will not perform this after adolescence. These patients have few good options, and sorting out the best strategy requires recruiting the most experienced and best possible consultants plus a measure of good fortune to turn such problems around. Identifying hemodynamic problems—even "minor" ones—early and addressing them appropriately in a proactive fashion before patients decompensate are equally important.*

## FINAL DIAGNOSIS

Mustard operation for complete TGA, severe systemic AV valve regurgitation secondary to a partially flail tricuspid valve leaflet

## PLAN OF ACTION

The patient was referred for replacement of the tricuspid valve with a mechanical tricuspid valve prosthesis.

## INTERVENTION

The patient underwent a tricuspid valve replacement. At the time of surgery, there was mild thickening of the tricuspid valve leaflets and severe prolapse of the tricuspid valve. A 33-mm diameter St. Jude's mechanical bileaflet valve was inserted uneventfully.

## OUTCOME

Postoperatively, the patient transiently developed a junctional rhythm that converted to sinus rhythm prior to hospital discharge. The postoperative echocardiogram showed a normally functioning bileaflet mechanical tricuspid valve with moderately enlarged systemic ventricular size and mildly reduced systolic function.

One year after surgery, the patient has done well and remains in NYHA class I. An MRI has not been repeated to evaluate the response of the RV to the surgery, although one is planned. The patient is on Coumadin and an ACE inhibitor (although there is no clinical trial evidence indicating efficacy in the setting of a systemic RV).

## Selected References

1. Mustard WT: Successful two-stage correction of transposition of the great vessels. Surgery 55:469–472, 1964.
2. Senning A: Surgical correction of transposition of the great vessels. Surgery 45:966–980, 1959.
3. Jatene AD, Fontes VF, Paulista PP, et al: Anatomic correction of transposition of the great vessels. J Thorac Cardiovasc Surg 72:364–370, 1976.
4. Puley G, Siu S, Connelly M, et al: Arrhythmia and survival in patients > 18 years of age after the Mustard procedure for complete transposition of the great arteries. Am J Cardiol 83:1080–1084, 1999.
5. Oechslin E, Jenni R: Forty years after the first atrial switch procedure in patients with transposition of the great arteries: Long-term results in Toronto and Zurich. Thorac Cardiovasc Surg 48:233–237, 2000.
6. Mee RB: Severe right ventricular failure after Mustard or Senning operation. Two-stage repair: Pulmonary artery banding and switch. J Thorac Cardiovasc Surg 92:385–390, 1986.

# Late Complications after the Arterial Switch Operation

**Arif Anis Khan, Craig Broberg, and Elisabeth Bédard**

**Age:** 15 years
**Gender:** Female
**Occupation:** Student
**Working diagnosis:** D-transposition of the great arteries

## HISTORY

The diagnosis of D-TGA was made in utero. Postnatally, the infant had a good-sized ASD, and she underwent arterial switch operation (ASO) at day 6 of life uneventfully. Aortopulmonary collaterals were detected several days later, and these were successfully ligated.

At age 1, the patient had a follow-up echocardiogram demonstrating a high gradient through the RVOT. Catheterization confirmed the presence of supravalvular pulmonary stenosis, and a catheter balloon dilatation was performed with resolution of the pressure gradient. Five years later, however, restenosis above the pulmonary valve was noted and this was again treated with catheter balloon dilatation.

At age 10, she had no significant complaints during follow-up, but echocardiography demonstrated recurrent supravalvular pulmonary stenosis. Given the prior two attempts at balloon dilatation, it was decided to repair the area surgically. She underwent relief of the supravalvar pulmonary stenosis with placement of a T-shaped patch of bovine pericardium and closure of a residual ASD. The operation was uncomplicated, and the patient was discharged home within a week.

Over the past few years she noted progressive shortness of breath compared to her peers and mentioned this during her routine follow-up visit at the tertiary cardiac center.

***Comments:*** Whereas most patients with D-TGA in today's adult cardiology clinics will have been repaired with an atrial switch procedure (i.e., Mustard or Senning repair), those treated with an arterial switch are just now reaching adulthood. The successful anatomic correction for TGA was first described in 1975 by Jatene and colleagues in Brazil. The procedure involves the transection of the aorta and pulmonary artery (PA) at a level above the sinuses of the semilunar valves and reimplantation in their normal position. The coronary arteries are detached from the aorta with a surrounding "button" of aortic wall and reimplanted into the neoaorta. The procedure is usually performed within the first 2 weeks of life and should be undertaken within the first 4 to 6 weeks of life at the latest, while the LV is still capable of sustaining the systemic load.

Although the very long-term outcomes of patients with an ASO are unknown, complications of ASO are now known to include endocarditis, RVOT obstruction (as with our patient), and coronary artery disease/obstruction.

## CURRENT SYMPTOMS

The patient is breathless when climbing stairs at school. Her parents are convinced that she is more breathless than others on light exertion and that she has slowed down recently. She has occasional short-lived palpitations without any history of dizziness or syncope.

NYHA class: I–II

***Comments:*** Patients tend to underestimate their own symptoms, although occasionally parents may be unduly concerned about signs or symptoms. Objective assessment with exercise testing, for example, is often necessary and recommended as a real tool for assessing functional capacity and cardiac output.

## CURRENT MEDICATIONS

None

## PHYSICAL EXAMINATION

BP 110/62 mm Hg, HR 74 bpm, oxygen saturation at rest 99%

Height 172 cm, weight 56 kg, BSA 1.64 m$^2$

Surgical scars: Midline sternotomy

Neck veins: 1 cm above the sternal angle, with a normal waveform

Lungs/chest: Normal on examination

Heart: Regular sinus rhythm. There was a mild parasternal lift, normal first and second heart sounds, and a grade 3/6 ejection systolic heart murmur heard maximally at the second left intercostal space.

Abdomen: Normal

Extremities: Normal. No edema seen, and the skin was warm. There was no cyanosis or clubbing.

***Comments:*** Examination in patients with arterial switch repair should focus on signs of PA stenosis and neoaortic valve stenosis or regurgitation. The murmur heard here is consistent with further stenosis of either outflow tract.

## LABORATORY DATA

| | |
|---|---|
| Hemoglobin | 11.9 g/dL (11.5–15.0) |
| Hematocrit/PCV | 36% (36–46) |
| MCV | 83 fL (83–99) |
| Platelet count | $321 \times 10^9$/L (150–400) |
| Sodium | 137 mmol/L (134–145) |
| Potassium | 3.6 mmol/L (3.5–5.2) |
| Creatinine | 0.6 mg/dL (0.6–1.2) |
| Blood urea nitrogen | 5 mmol/L (2.5–6.5) |

### OTHER RELEVANT LAB RESULTS

| | |
|---|---|
| Albumin | 4.3 g/dL |

## ELECTROCARDIOGRAM

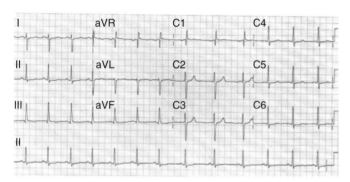

Figure 52-1 Electrocardiogram.

### FINDINGS

Heart rate: 79 bpm

QRS axis: +119°

QRS duration: 94 msec

Normal sinus rhythm, right-axis deviation, nonspecific ST segment changes in the inferior leads. Prominent R-wave in V1.

***Comments:*** It is important to exclude signs of myocardial ischemia in a patient with prior arterial switch, as the coronary arteries and ostia were reimplanted. Right-axis deviation and the tall R in V1 are not unexpected. RV hypertrophy would suggest RVOT obstruction.

## CHEST X-RAY

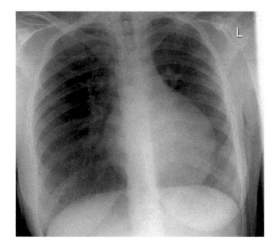

Figure 52-2 Posteroanterior projection showing globular heart.

### FINDINGS

Cardiothoracic ratio: 58%

The cardiac size is mildly enlarged. The cardiac apex is elevated suggesting RV overload, in keeping with the ECG. Sternal wires are noted. The lungs and pleural spaces are clear.

***Comments:*** Patients with TGA have a narrow mediastinal shadowing due to the parallel anteroposterior relationship of the great arteries. Ordinarily, the cardiothoracic ratio is normal in D-TGA patients without ventricular dilatation, and pulmonary vascular markings should be normal in the absence of PAH.

## EXERCISE TESTING

| | |
|---|---|
| Exercise protocol: | Bruce |
| Duration (min : sec): | 12 : 57 |
| Reason for stopping: | Dyspnea |
| ECG changes: | None |

| | Rest | Peak |
|---|---|---|
| Heart rate (bpm): | 74 | 203 |
| Percent of age-predicted max HR: | | 99 |
| $O_2$ saturation (%): | 99 | 98 |
| Blood pressure (mm Hg): | 110/62 | 140/50 |
| Peak $Vo_2$ (mL/kg/min): | | 36 |
| Percent predicted (%): | | 75 |
| $Ve/Vco_2$: | | 24 |
| Metabolic equivalents: | | 10.3 |

***Comments:*** Exercise testing is useful in recognizing or confirming changes in the clinical status of the individual patient. In patients in which there is suspicion of coronary artery disease exercise testing should be performed together with appropriate myocardial perfusion imaging; this is often relevant in patients with prior arterial switch.

The patient's exercise tolerance here is below expected for gender and age, although still fairly robust compared to many congenital heart patients.

## ECHOCARDIOGRAM

### OVERALL FINDINGS

Concordant AV and ventriculoarterial (now) connections. Function of the LV was normal. There was neither LVOT obstruction nor significant aortic regurgitation. The RV was dilated and hypertrophied.

Preserved LV systolic function was seen.

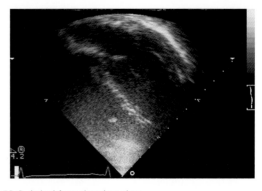

Figure 52-3 Apical four-chamber view.

*Comments:* Normal function of the LV is important, as it implies (though does not prove) the absence of myocardial ischemia. Because the right AV valve can sometimes be abnormal in transposition (see Case 58), its function should also be specifically assessed.

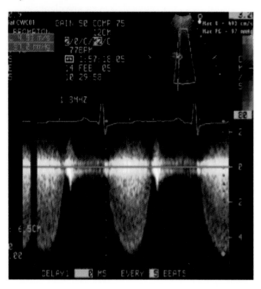

Figure 52-4 Parasternal short-axis view with continuous-wave Doppler across the right ventricular outflow tract.

## FINDINGS

From the parasternal short-axis view, RVOT continuous-wave Doppler peak velocity was 4.9 m/sec, suggestive of significant RVOT obstruction.

*Comments:* Routine echocardiography should specifically look for neoaortic valve regurgitation and LV dysfunction. The study should also try to exclude supravalvular and branch PA stenosis, although these structures can be difficult to see in an adult, and were not well visualized in this case. As the history and physical examination suggested in this patient, there is residual or recurrent stenosis of the RVOT. Differentiation between supravalvular, valvar, and subvalvular stenosis is important but can be difficult if echocardiographic windows are limited. MRI is often helpful in these circumstances.

# MAGNETIC RESONANCE IMAGING

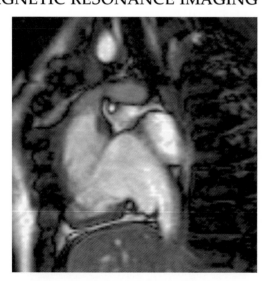

Figure 52-5 Oblique sagittal plane steady-state free precession cine (right ventricular outflow tract view).

## FINDINGS

There was PA stenosis at the suture line 10 mm distal to the valve and 15 mm proximal to the bifurcation. The peak velocity was 5 m/sec.

The left pulmonary artery was hypoplastic measuring 8 mm in diameter. The RV was hypertrophied.

### Ventricular Volume Quantification

|  | LV | (Normal range) | RV | (Normal range) |
|---|---|---|---|---|
| EDV (mL) | 95 | (52–141) | 82 | (58–154) |
| ESV (mL) | 43 | (13–51) | 36 | (12–68) |
| SV (mL) | 52 | (33–97) | 46 | (35–98) |
| EF (%) | **55** | (56–75) | 56 | (49–73) |
| EDVi (mL/m²) | **58** | (65–99) | **50** | (65–102) |
| ESVi (mL/m²) | 26 | (19–37) | 22 | (20–45) |
| SVi (mL/m²) | **32** | (42–66) | **28** | (39–63) |

*Comments:* One reason for the recurrent stenosis is the abrupt angle (nearly 90°) between the RVOT and the PA, which reflects the strained repositioning of the PA at the time of the arterial switch.

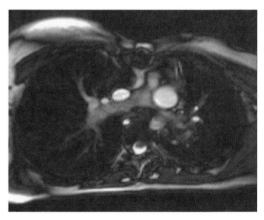

Figure 52-6 Axial steady-state free precession cine.

## FINDINGS

The PA bifurcation is shown with evidence of left pulmonary artery narrowing.

*Comments:* Note that the PA bifurcation lies to the right of the ascending aorta, with the left pulmonary artery coursing posterior to the aorta.

Because of the abnormal position of the PA relative to the aorta at birth, the surgical correction requires that the main PA be pulled anteriorly and rightward to anastomose with the RVOT. This distortion can lead to the recurrent stenosis as in this case, and perhaps contribute to the origin stenosis of the left pulmonary artery.

# CATHETERIZATION

Heart rate   63 bpm

*Preangioplasty*

| | Pressure | Saturation (%) |
|---|---|---|
| SVC | 8/6 mean 7 | 66 |
| IVC | | 72 |
| RA | 6/7 mean 6 | 77 |
| RV | 65/7 | |
| PA | 25/15 mean 18 | 80 |
| LPA | 23/15 mean 19 | |
| PCWP | | |
| LA | | |
| LV | 110/8 | 99 |
| Aorta | 104/59 mean 73 | 98 |

### Calculations

| | |
|---|---|
| Qp (L/min) | 6.73 |
| Qs (L/min) | 4.04 |
| Cardiac index (L/min/m²) | 2.47 |
| Qp/Qs | 1.67 |
| PVR (Wood units) | 1.49 |
| SVR (Wood units) | 16.58 |

## FINDINGS

Catheterization was done to carefully measure the RVOT gradient and to assess its impact on global hemodynamics.

There was a significant pressure gradient across the RVOT as expected. Furthermore, there seemed to be a step-up in saturations at the RA level suggestive of an atrial communication with left-to-right shunting. Otherwise there were no unexpected findings. There were no significant gradients between the main and the branch pulmonary arteries.

There was no obstruction or origin stenoses of the coronary arteries on selective angiography.

***Comments:*** The RV-PA peak-to-peak gradient was 40 mm Hg, which is less than anticipated from the Doppler and MR flow velocity findings. Such discrepancies are not uncommon, however, and reflect in part the differences between peak-to-peak and peak instantaneous gradients, as well as the effects of general anesthesia that might be used, particularly in younger patients.

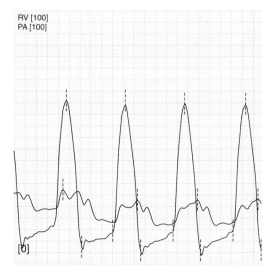

Figure 52-7 Right ventricle and pulmonary artery pressure waveforms showing peak-to-peak gradient.

## FINDINGS

The RV-PA pressures measured simultaneously. The gradient is 45 mm Hg.

***Comments:*** Note the abnormal waveform of the PA tracing, showing a dip in pressure at peak RV systole. It has the appearance of a dynamic outflow obstruction, although the stenosis is supravalvular.

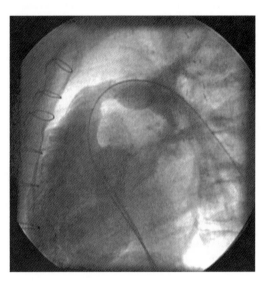

Figure 52-8 Lateral pulmonary angiography.

## FINDINGS

Angiography confirmed the presence of complex stenosis of the main PA distal to the pulmonary valve. The narrowest portion had a diameter of 9 mm and was 15 mm in length. The left PA was relatively small as it coursed posterior to the aorta (and anteriorly to the right PA).

***Comments:*** The RVOT flow vector turns almost 90 degrees from a predominantly inferosuperior direction to an anteroposterior direction just at the site of the supravalvular stenosis, whereas in the normal anatomical relationship this curve is much more gentle. This angle likely contributes to the turbulence and high velocity found at this location, though it is a by-product of the arterial switch procedure.

### FOCUSED CLINICAL QUESTIONS AND DISCUSSION POINTS

1. What are common long-term complications after an ASO?

*Since Jatene and coworkers performed and reported the first successful ASO in a patient with TGA and VSD in 1975, this has become the procedure of choice[1] since the early 1980s. The main rationale for this approach over the atrial switch procedure is the use of the morphologic LV as the systemic ventricle, which long term should convey obvious advantages in terms of function and longevity.*

*The most commonly observed complication after the ASO is supravalvular PA stenosis, which occurs with an incidence of about 24%.[2-4] Our case here typifies the reasons for this, namely the often obligatory distortion of the PA and outflow tract to make the arterial anastomosis. A modification of the arterial switch procedure, the LeCompte maneuver, involves moving the left PA to the left of the aorta, such that the neoaortic valve lies between the left PA and right PA. This causes less distortion of the pulmonary arteries.*

*Another important complication is stenosis of the coronary ostia. Coronary reimplantation at the time of the arterial switch requires the coronaries to be deviated from their normal position anteriorly in the mediastinum to be brought back to the aorta. As surgical techniques have evolved, this has been less of a problem, but must still be considered by a vigilant physician. Long term, it remains to be seen how often problems with the coronary circulation will occur and have an impact on outcome.*

2. What is the optimal management strategy for this patient?

*There is a hemodynamically significant RVOT obstruction. The stenosis here is likely to contribute to her reduced exercise tolerance, even though her capacity was quite good relative to other patients. Waiting for more symptoms or clinical decompensation would be inappropriate and may compromise the chances for complete RV reverse remodeling.*

*Percutaneous intervention with balloon angioplasty and stenting is an option. Although the patient has already been through two balloon angioplasty procedures, neither of them included stent implantation.*

*Balloon angioplasty of PA stenosis after ASO has a relatively high failure rate, with most series reporting a success rate of 50% or less. Primary stent implantation appears to have higher initial success rates. However, stent implantation is more challenging technically than balloon angioplasty, since stent positioning must be precise to avoid pulmonary regurgitation. Still, technical experience has grown and stent deployment has been increasingly employed in this population with good results. In this case, this seemed to present the best first-line treatment option for this patient under the current conditions.*

## FINAL DIAGNOSIS

D-TGA

Arterial switch repair

Recurrent supravalvular pulmonary stenosis

## PLAN OF ACTION

Angioplasty and stenting of the main PA stenosis

## INTERVENTION

The stent was very carefully positioned angiographically and deployed during apnea and fast ventricular pacing to reduce cardiac output. The stent was postdilated using a 15-mm balloon.

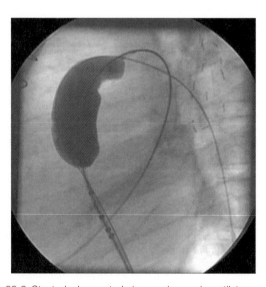

Figure 52-9 Stent deployment during pacing and ventilator-controlled apnea.

***Comments:*** The indentation of the balloon demonstrates the location of the stenosis.

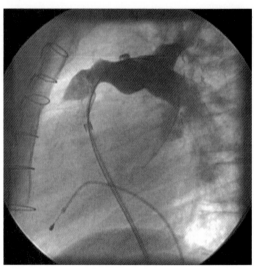

Figure 52-10 Cine lateral view showing pulmonary artery angiogram after stenting of the pulmonary artery.

## FINDINGS

The area of main PA stenosis was directly stented using a 17-mm Genesis stent initially mounted on a 12-mm balloon.

***Comments:*** The angiographic result was satisfactory, although there was little visible change and still residual stenosis. Follow-up hemodynamics showed an improved pressure gradient across the RVOT.

*Postangioplasty*

|  | **Pressure** |
|---|---|
| RV | 35 /11 mean 23 |
| PA | 21/11 mean 15 |
| Aorta | 105/60 mean 75 |

One year later the patient reported improved functional capacity and no exercise intolerance or arrhythmia.

## Selected References

1. Losay J, Touchot A, Serraf A, et al: Late outcome after arterial switch operation for transposition of the great arteries. Circulation 104(Suppl 1):I-121–I-126, 2001.
2. Hutter PA, Kreb DL, Mantel SF, et al: Twenty-five years' experience with the arterial switch operation. J Thorac Cardiovasc Surg 124:790–797, 2002.
3. Nogi S, McCrindle BW, Boutin C, et al: Fate of the neopulmonary valve after the arterial switch operation in neonates. J Thorac Cardiovasc Surg 115:557–562, 1998.
4. Zeevi B, Keane JF, Perry SB, Lock JE: Balloon dilation of postoperative right ventricular outflow tract obstructions. J Am Coll Cardiol 14:401–408, 1990.

# Long-Term Outcome after Rastelli Repair

**Aikaterini Chamaidi, Massimo Griselli, and Filippos Triposkiadis**

**Age:** 38 years
**Gender:** Female
**Occupation:** Hotel manager
**Working diagnosis:** Transposition of the great arteries/ventricular septal defect/pulmonary stenosis

## HISTORY

The patient had bilateral BT shunts early in life. She had a Rastelli operation 31 years ago (at age 7) for TGA/VSD/PS. The aorta was tunneled to the LV with a Dacron patch. At the time, a 20-mm Hancock valved conduit connected the RV to the pulmonary artery (PA).

At the age of 15 years, she was found to have her original valvular and subvalvular pulmonary stenosis (as expected) with a small residual VSD. No intervention was necessary.

Ten years later, at age 25, she developed *Streptococcus sanguis* endocarditis that responded well to intravenous and oral penicillin.

Three months later, she was readmitted into the hospital with a decline in her exercise tolerance, shortness of breath on modest exertion, and difficulty climbing stairs. A series of investigations were undertaken (echocardiogram, cardiac catheterization, MRI), which revealed severe conduit obstruction with small residual VSD and moderate subaortic stenosis with preserved LV and RV function.

She underwent surgical replacement of the RV-PA conduit with a cryopreserved homograft. The VSD was enlarged by wedge resection of the infundibular septum, and the VSD baffle was augmented with a Gore-Tex patch. She had an excellent postoperative course.

At age 33 she conceived. During her pregnancy, she was given diuretics for mild right heart failure but delivered a healthy baby successfully. Following her pregnancy and delivery, she became more symptomatic, with breathlessness on exertion as well as orthopnea. She noted short, nonsustained palpitations. She had a follow-up MRI scan showing mild-to-moderate narrowing of the RV-PA conduit. A ventilation/perfusion scan done at the same time excluded the possibility of recent pulmonary embolism. She was treated with diuretics and angiotensin-II receptor antagonists, and improved.

Two years later, her exercise tolerance and palpitations deteriorated. Echocardiography showed RV hypertrophy, mild LV outflow obstruction, and mild aortic regurgitation, but could not adequately assess the RV-PA conduit. She underwent cardiac catheterization that revealed a 40 mm Hg gradient across the conduit. Medical therapy was further optimized; candesartan was stopped, spironolactone was added, and sotalol was started to control what was felt to be recurrent supraventricular tachycardia, though 24-hour ECG monitoring failed to capture any significant arrhythmias. Warfarin was introduced as well.

Despite these changes, symptoms progressed further over several more years, and she felt it increasingly difficult to keep up with the demands of work and caring for her child.

*Comments:* The clinical presentation of patients with TGA/VSD/PS is varied and depends both on the severity and site of pulmonary stenosis and on the size and location of the VSD. If the cyanosis is severe, a systemic-to-PA shunt, combined with atrial septectomy, is often required in early life. Occasionally, patients are well balanced, as with our case here, allowing for a more definitive repair later on in life.

The Rastelli operation is the preferred surgical route for patients with TGA/VSD/PS.[1] The VSD is used to make the LVOT; the Rastelli procedure includes placement of a VSD baffle (Dacron or Gore-Tex), directing blood from the LV to the aorta via the VSD. Surgical enlargement of the VSD may be necessary. The pulmonary trunk is often transected, and the pulmonary valve or the root of the pulmonary trunk is oversewn. A conduit is inserted from an incision made in the RV to the distal part of the pulmonary trunk. This operation was first described in 1969 and advantageously leaves the morphologic LV as the systemic ventricle. The aortic valve overrides the ventricular septum. This feature and the pulmonary stenosis relate to the posterior deviation of the outlet septum. Pulmonary stenosis, in turn, with a malaligned VSD maintains LV pressure equivalent to the RV that supports the systemic circulation. Morphologically speaking, this malformation is to some extent analogous to TOF in the setting of discordant ventriculoarterial connection. Late complications of the Rastelli procedure include conduit obstruction/regurgitation, LVOT obstruction, and arrhythmias.

Prosthetic valve endocarditis (PVE) is an endovascular infection occurring on parts of a prosthetic valve or on reconstructed native heart valves. It has a low but increasing frequency ranging from 0.1% to 2.3% per patient year. PVE occurs either perioperatively (early PVE) or more than a year after surgery as community-acquired (late PVE). These two forms usually involve different microorganisms. Infective endocarditis accounts for 4% of admissions to a specialized ACHD unit. Reparative surgery does not prevent endocarditis except for closure of a VSD and a patent ductus arteriosus. LVOT lesions are most commonly involved.[2]

Conduit stenosis after the Rastelli procedure is very common. Most patients will require multiple conduit replacements, as the longevity of currently used conduits is often only a few years in children and perhaps 10 to 20 years in older patients. Because of homograft unavailability and problems with early homograft preservation, the use of Hancock bioprosthetic valved conduits was favored before the 1980s. They consist of a standard unstented porcine aortic valve, sutured into the center of a woven fabric conduit (Dacron). Later cryopreservation improved the preservation of homografts, which then became the conduit of choice in some centers,[3] while heterograft valved conduits continued to be preferred in other centers.

Substantial hemodynamic changes occur during pregnancy, and pregnancy may unmask previously asymptomatic problems. The 30% to 50% increase in cardiac output may result in maternal arrhythmia and/or heart failure, as well as potential fetal problems. The high-risk group includes women with prosthetic valves, conduits, and obstructive cardiac lesions, as may be seen after the Rastelli operation.[4]

Nearly all homografts eventually require replacement. Factors that adversely affect graft longevity include a higher systolic gradient immediately after placement, younger age, longer donor ischemic time, smaller homograft size, extracardiac location, or the use of an aortic homograft in an older patient.[5]

Echocardiography often has difficulty evaluating such valved conduits, and other modalities, such as MRI or heart catheterization, may be needed.

Arrhythmia is the most common reason for the hospitalization of adults with congenital heart disease. There is a high incidence of late arrhythmias, both supraventricular and ventricular, which are generally felt to be associated with chamber dilatation, hypertrophy, and/or ventricular dysfunction. Scar tissue, complex tunnel repair, and severely stenosed conduits are additional risk factors. Correction of residual hemodynamic abnormalities may be the most important tool in the treatment of arrhythmia.[6]

## CURRENT SYMPTOMS

The patient complained primarily of exertional dyspnea and fatigue, noted after walking for 100 m on flat ground, and on climbing a few stairs. Occasionally she felt dizziness and palpitations at rest, but these episodes were self-limited. She denied chest pain or syncope.

NYHA class: III

***Comments:*** Dyspnea in a patient with complex congenital heart disease can be secondary to many factors, some of which are mechanical and/or reversible and should be investigated. Beyond these, it is becoming increasingly recognized that late ventricular dysfunction is a common cause of dyspnea.

## CURRENT MEDICATIONS

Warfarin 6 mg once daily

Sotalol 80 mg twice daily

Furosemide 20 mg once daily

Sertraline 100 mg once daily

Spironolactone 50 mg twice daily

## PHYSICAL EXAMINATION

BP 110/70 mm Hg, HR 46 bpm, oxygen saturation 97% on room air

Height 178 cm, weight 95.5 kg, BSA 2.17 m²

Surgical scars: Midline sternotomy and bilateral thoracotomy scars were visible.

Neck veins: JVP was 8 cm above the sternal angle and had a normal contour.

Lungs/chest: Chest was clear.

Heart: There was a right ventricular lift. The first heart sound was normal, the second heart sound was single and loud. There was a grade 5/6 long ejection systolic murmur at the left upper sternal edge and an early diastolic (pulmonary, augmented on inspiration) murmur.

Abdomen: The abdomen was normal. There was no hepatomegaly.

Extremities: There was no clubbing or peripheral edema. Peripheral pulses were not palpable in either arm.

***Comments:*** The parasternal lift reflects the raised RV pressure. The second heart sound is single because only the substernal aortic component can be heard. The long systolic murmur is related to severe conduit obstruction. The diastolic murmur reflects prosthetic conduit regurgitation.

## LABORATORY DATA

| | |
|---|---|
| Hemoglobin | 14.6 g/dL (11.5–15.0) |
| Hematocrit/PCV | 46% (36–46) |
| MCV | 96 fL (83–99) |
| Platelet count | $180 \times 10^9$/L (150–400) |
| Sodium | 135 mmol/L (134–145) |
| Potassium | 4.8 mmol/L (3.5–5.2) |
| Creatinine | 0.76 mg/dL (0.6–1.2) |
| Blood urea nitrogen | 4.8 mmol/L (2.5–6.5) |

## ELECTROCARDIOGRAM

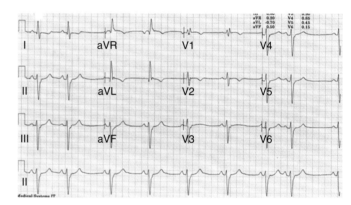

Figure 53-1 Electrocardiogram.

### FINDINGS

Heart rate: 46 bpm

PR interval: 182 msec

QRS axis: −87°

QRS duration: 162 msec

Sinus bradycardia with sinus arrhythmia or premature atrial contractions. Left-axis deviation with RBBB. Bifascicular block. No atrial overload pattern.

***Comments:*** Patients after the Rastelli operation commonly have an RBBB pattern because of the incision in the RVOT and baffle suturing on the septum. They are also at a risk of developing complete heart block. The sinus bradycardia presumably relates to her sotalol use.

## CHEST X-RAY

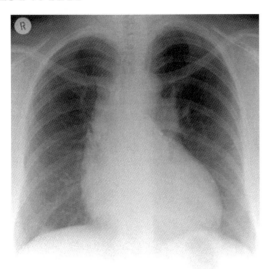

Figure 53-2 Posteroanterior projection.

### FINDINGS
Cardiothoracic ratio: 67%

The cardiac silhouette is enlarged. There is dilatation of the left pulmonary artery. The bulging at the right cardiac border reflects in part RA enlargement. The aortic arch is prominent. The pulmonary vascular markings are normal.

*Comments:* The CXR findings suggest right heart dilatation, but there is a homograft and that will alter the appearance somewhat unpredictably. Vascular markings are not attenuated and there is no evidence of pulmonary hypertension.

## EXERCISE TESTING

| Exercise protocol: | Modified Bruce |
| Duration (min:sec): | 6:20 |
| Reason for stopping: | Chest tightness |
| ECG changes: | None |

| | Rest | Peak |
| --- | --- | --- |
| Heart rate (bpm): | 46 | 92 |
| Percent of age-predicted max HR: | | 51 |
| O₂ saturation (%): | 97 | 96 |
| Blood pressure (mm Hg): | 110/70 | 130/70 |
| Peak Vo₂ (mL/kg/min): | | 12.4 |
| Percent predicted (%): | | 40 |
| Ve/Vco₂: | | 32 |
| Metabolic equivalents: | | 5.8 |

*Comments:* Peak $Vo_2$ was quite severely impaired. There are several factors potentially responsible for this limitation.

The patient obtained a very low heart rate at peak exercise, despite reaching a respiratory quotient of 1.1 implying adequate effort. The patient had a resting heart rate of 46 bpm (taking

sotalol). Still, chronotropic incompetence is a major limiting factor in the ACHD population.[7]

Blood pressure response to exercise was also suboptimal, suggesting perhaps an inability to increase stroke volume and cardiac output.

Finally, FEV1 and FVC, sometimes measured at rest before exercise testing, were also abnormal, suggesting that exercise intolerance could be partly due to pulmonary abnormalities. These could include scarring from previous operations and aggravated by increased weight.[8]

In addition to the above factors, ventricular dysfunction or further conduit obstruction will need to be considered as possible contributors to her exercise intolerance.

## ECHOCARDIOGRAM

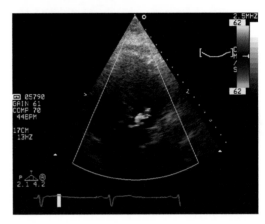

Figure 53-3 Apical five-chamber view, 2D color Doppler, with poor echo window.

### FINDINGS
The LV was normal in size and systolic function. The aortic root was mildly dilated with mild aortic regurgitation. From the LV to the aorta a 2.2 m/sec jet was seen arising from the region of the VSD suggesting slight narrowing of the LV-to-aorta pathway. The RV was hypertrophied with mildly to moderately impaired long-axis function. The anterior RV-PA conduit could not be visualized. There was mild tricuspid valve regurgitation with mild RA dilation.

A systolic jet of turbulence was visible from the LV to the aorta. The maximal velocity of 2.2 m/sec across the LVOT corresponds to a peak systolic gradient of 20 mm Hg, indicative of mild stenosis.

*Comments:* The poor echo windows did not allow imaging of the RV-PA conduit, which can often be challenging to image due to its anterior position and prior surgeries.

The findings are suggestive of mildly to moderately impaired RV systolic function. The RV hypertrophy is consistent with chronic pressure overload. There was also a mild aortic regurgitation, not shown in the previous studies.

The presence of maintained LV function with mild LVOT stenosis suggests that the deteriorating symptoms are not related to the intracardiac baffle but to the RV-PA conduit narrowing. The intracardiac tunnel had already been revised following the initial Rastelli procedure with a further resection of the outlet septum and patch enlargement of the baffle.

# MAGNETIC RESONANCE IMAGING

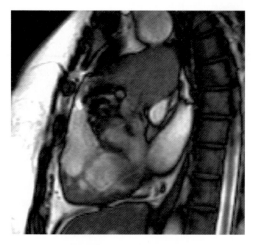

Figure 53-4 Right ventricular outflow tract plane, oblique sagittal plane steady-state free precession cine.

## FINDINGS

The RV was hypertrophied and mildly dilated. Its systolic function was moderately impaired mainly due to a large akinetic region in the reconstructed RVOT. The RV-PA conduit was stenosed at valve level, with a peak velocity of 3.5 m/sec (gradient 50 mm Hg). There was mild regurgitation of the homograft valve. The thin-walled portion of the RVOT lay immediately behind the sternum.

The RA was dilated. The tricuspid valve functioned normally. The main PA was unremarkable. The right PA was of normal caliber (17 mm) but was angled more acutely than is normally expected. The left PA was dilated (36 mm).

**Comments:** MRI provides an accurate noninvasive assessment of the size and function of the RV and shows the extent and degree of outflow tract obstruction. It is also helpful in presurgical planning as well as during follow-up.[9] At times, signal loss artifact from sternal wires can make imaging of structures in the anterior mediastinum, such as a conduit, more difficult. The study showed a moderate-to-severe RV-PA conduit obstruction.

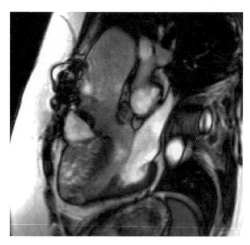

Figure 53-5 Left ventricular outflow tract plane, oblique sagittal plane steady-state free precession cine.

## FINDINGS

The LV was normal in size and systolic function. The LA was small. The mitral valve was normal. The LVOT was mildly stenosed due to a mild subaortic restriction, with a peak velocity of 3 m/sec. The aortic valve was unremarkable. The ascending aorta was mildly dilated. The arch and descending aorta were unremarkable.

**Comments:** The MRI confirmed the echo findings of preserved LV function and mildly stenosed LVOT, and gave further valuable information about the conduit.

# CATHETERIZATION

## HEMODYNAMICS

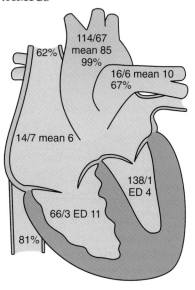

Figure 53-6 Hemodynamic data.

**Calculations**

| | |
|---|---|
| Qp (L/min) | 3.09 |
| Qs (L/min) | 2.97 |
| Cardiac index (L/min/m$^2$) | 1.37 |
| Qp/Qs | 1.04 |
| PVR (Wood units) | 1.94 |
| SVR (Wood units) | 26.60 |

| | Peak Gradient | Mean Gradient | Area |
|---|---|---|---|
| RVOT | 50 | 27 | 0.54 cm$^2$ |
| LVOT | 31 | 23 | 0.83 cm$^2$ |

## FINDINGS

Cardiac catheterization was performed to confirm the severity of outflow obstruction by recording pressure withdrawal gradients across the respective outflow tracts and to determine suitability for repair. Coronary angiography was also performed.

The study demonstrated moderate-to-severe obstruction of the RVOT with a peak-to-peak pull-back systolic pressure gradient of 50 mm Hg. The end diastolic pressure in the RV was mildly elevated, although that may also reflect RV hypertrophy. The LVOT systolic pressure gradient was 24 mm Hg suggesting mild obstruction. The end diastolic pressure in the LV was normal. PA pressure and pulmonary vascular resistance were normal.

**Comments:** Though several lesions are present, namely the aortic regurgitation, LVOT obstruction, RV dysfunction, and conduit obstruction, the latter appears to be the most significant. Indeed, poor RV function (if present) may cause the RV-PA gradient to be lower than it would be from a normally functioning ventricle, such as is observed in aortic stenosis with reduced LV function.

The cardiac output and index were very low, so the gradients are underestimated.

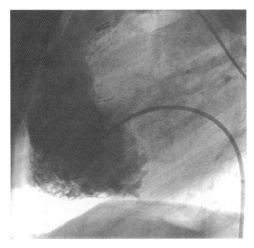

Figure 53-7 Lateral projection angiogram.

## FINDINGS

The conduit was stenosed. It was also remarkably close to the sternum, which presents an obstacle to the surgeon in any future sternotomy.

**Comments:** Conduit failure is inevitable, and replacement has become a very common procedure. The attributes of the "ideal" conduit include long-term patency, availability in a range of sizes, excellent handling characteristics, growth potential, low cost, low infectious potential, and nonthrombogenicity. A conduit that possesses all of these characteristics has not yet been developed.

While the cryopreserved homografts, regarding the handling characteristics, offer a clear advantage over heterografts, the late results comparing heterograft and homograft conduit survival are probably comparable.

Other surgical options that address the durability limitations of both the homograft and the heterograft conduits are available. These include the stentless valved heterografts that have not shown a superiority to homografts, the valved bovine jugular vein conduit that is currently in trials with promising early results (Contegra), the fresh autologous, pericardial valved conduit with limited experience, and the tissue engineering techniques that hold long-term promise.[3]

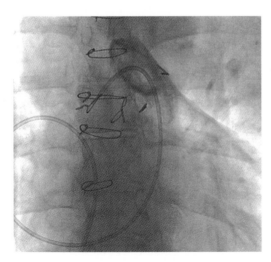

Figure 53-8 Anteroposterior angiogram, right ventricular outflow tract calcification.

## FINDINGS

There was extensive calcification of the homograft RV-PA conduit.

**Comments:** Calcification and degeneration are the main reasons for conduit revision and replacement. The superiority of pulmonary homografts as RV-PA conduit over aortic homografts is controversial, particularly regarding the immunological reaction after surgery.

The reported lower survival in reoperative homografts is probably attributed to technical factors caused by adhesions and calcification.[10]

### FOCUSED CLINICAL QUESTIONS AND DISCUSSION POINTS

1. **What is the cause of this patient's deteriorating exertional function?**

   *Several cases in this book demonstrate the pitfalls of jumping to conclusions about a single etiologic factor causing symptoms. The investigations performed in this patient have identified several possible reasons for the patient's progressive symptoms, all of which must be considered and addressed.*

   *To begin, she has chronotropic incompetence, which may be primarily related to her beta-blocker therapy. She seems to have a tendency to nonsustained arrhythmia and is at risk for complete heart block, though neither has been documented.*

   *In addition, she has several possible hemodynamic problems, namely conduit obstruction, RV systolic dysfunction, LVOT obstruction, and aortic insufficiency. The RV-PA conduit obstruction of course seems the most likely reason for her symptoms, though all should be considered together. In her case, however, the RV systolic dysfunction, though present, did not manifest itself with signs or symptoms of right heart failure. Relief of outflow obstruction would be expected to improve function by reducing afterload. Importantly, significant tricuspid regurgitation was not present. The left-sided problems were mild and unlikely to contribute to her current situation. Thus, the most likely culprits are the 13-year-old conduit and the beta-blockers.*

2. **What are the therapeutic options for this patient?**

   *Medical treatment of ventricular dysfunction has been already optimized, and a further increase in medications does not seem warranted. Discontinuation of sotalol may improve chronotropic response to exercise yet exacerbate bothersome tachyarrhythmias. If documented, such arrhythmias might be ablated.*

   *Catheter-based interventions with implantation of stents or even a pulmonary valve are possible alternatives, although their implementation in this case is not recommended due to severe calcification of the conduit, which may cause problems during the ballooning phase.[11] The remaining alternative is surgical replacement of her conduit.*

3. **What are the indications and contraindications for replacement of an RV-PA conduit?**

   *Generally, patients should be considered for conduit replacement when their symptomatic status deteriorates in association with substantial conduit obstruction/regurgitation, especially if there is objective evidence of right heart dysfunction including the onset of tricuspid insufficiency or ventricular or supraventricular arrhythmias.*

   *RVOT obstruction is the main indication for reoperation in this group of patients. An RV pressure higher than two thirds of the LV systolic pressure or a pressure gradient of more than 50 mm Hg across the RVOT can be considered a threshold for reoperation. In a large series of long-term follow-up, late mortality was predicted by older age at time of operation and increased gradient postoperatively.[12]*

*However, reoperating on these patients carries some risks: The thin-walled portion of the RVOT, often degenerated and calcified, lies immediately behind and is probably attached to the sternum. This makes resternotomy risky for the surgeon, and institution of cardiopulmonary bypass using femoral vessels would be required. These reoperations are normally very long and increase the risk of serious bleeding. RV dysfunction will make the immediate postoperative recovery more difficult. Some patients may need several conduit replacements serially, each more difficult and taxing on the ventricle than the one before.*

*Despite the risks, this patient should undergo further surgery for three main reasons: First, she has symptoms with modest effort, and these symptoms have progressed over the last 5 years, precipitated by her pregnancy. She is in NYHA class III, and is unable to cope with her daily life. Second, fairly severe RVOT obstruction is clearly present by two imaging modalities, and this has worsened over the last 2 years. The gradient across the RVOT at cardiac catheterization is now 50 mm Hg, which, in the presence of symptoms, is an important indication. Third, the presence of moderate RV impairment already will only worsen over time if the obstruction is not relieved.*

# FINAL DIAGNOSIS

TGA/VSD/PS

Previous Rastelli procedure with conduit replacement

RV-PA conduit restenosis

# PLAN OF ACTION

RV-PA conduit replacement

# INTERVENTION

At first, the femoral artery and vein were exposed (as a backup for cannulation) before sternal division (resternotomy). However, the sternum was divided without major bleeding or laceration to the structures behind the bone, and therefore femoral-femoral bypass was not necessary in this case. After dissection needed for surgical maneuvers, cardiopulmonary bypass was commenced in a standard fashion. Under cardiac arrest, the previous homograft and all the calcified tissues related to the conduit were removed entirely. On the RV side, some muscle bands were divided so as to make the RVOT as unobstructed as possible. A new aortic homograft (23 mm in size) was interposed between the RV and the PA. A piece of bovine pericardium was used to supplement the connection between the RV incision and the proximal end of the homograft. Coming off bypass was uneventful. With stable cardiac rhythm and hemodynamics, the chest was closed.

The femoral vessels should be prepared for potential femoral-femoral cardiopulmonary bypass in patients with conduits or with the ascending aorta very close (or stuck) to the sternum, because of the risk of injury to the structures behind the sternum and massive bleeding. The aorta needs attention when the ascending aorta is significantly dilated, or is anteriorly located such as in TGA or some forms of double-outlet RV. The sternum could not be divided without making a hole in a calcified conduit had it previously been placed onto the medial part of the RV. Such risk assessment should be performed preoperatively, and MRI, CT scanning, and/or lateral angiographic views can be particularly helpful.

Right heart surgery could be performed with a beating heart when there is no intracardiac communication present. If there is any suspicion of a ventricular or atrial communication, no matter how small, the heart should be stopped. Otherwise, air bubbles may cross to the LV because of active sucking by the beating LV, potentially ejecting air bubbles into the ascending aorta with catastrophic consequences (e.g., brain injury, etc.). The same thing could happen when the right heart is opened during division of the sternum on femoral-femoral cardiopulmonary bypass, when an intracardiac communication is present. Deep hypothermic circulatory arrest would be needed in such circumstances. Further attention is required when a patient has significant aortic regurgitation. When the heart gets fibrillated during the course of cooling, aortic regurgitation may cause left ventricular distention; this, in turn, may adversely impact postoperative ventricular function and recovery.

# OUTCOME

The patient made an uneventful hospital recovery after surgery and was discharged in 6 days. Rehabilitation continued at home over the ensuing weeks. After 2 months she felt well enough to return to work.

Two years later she remains well functionally and has not had a recurrence of her arrhythmia. She continues to take a beta-blocker.

# Selected References

1. Kreutzer C, De Vive J, Oppido G, et al: Twenty-five-year experience with the Rastelli repair for transposition of the great arteries. J Thorac Cardiovasc Surg 120:211–223, 2000.
2. Li W, Somerville J: Infective endocarditis in the grown-up congenital heart population. Eur Heart J 19:166–173, 1998.
3. Forbess JM: Conduit selection for right ventricular outflow tract reconstruction: Contemporary options and outcomes. Semin Thorac Cardiovasc Surg Pediatric Card Surg Ann 7:115–124, 2004.
4. Siu S, Chitayat D, Webb G: Pregnancy in woman with congenital heart defects: What are the risks? Heart 81:225–226, 1999.
5. Tweddell JS, Pelech AN, Frommelt PC, et al: Factors affecting longevity of homograft valves used in right ventricular outflow reconstruction for congenital heart disease. Circulation 102(Suppl III):III130–III135, 2000.
6. Deanfield J, Thaulow E, Warnes C, et al: Management of grown up congenital heart disease. The Task Force on the management of grown-up congenital heart disease of the European Society of Cardiology. Eur Heart J 24:1035–1084, 2003.
7. Diller GP, Dimopoulos K, Okonko D, et al: Exercise intolerance in adult congenital heart disease: Comparative severity, correlates, and prognostic implication. Circulation 112:828–835, 2005.
8. Glaser S, Opitz CF, Bauer U, et al: Assessment of symptoms and exercise capacity in cyanotic patients with congenital heart disease. Chest 125:368–376, 2004.
9. Boxt LM: Magnetic resonance and computed tomography evaluation of congenital heart disease. J Magn Reson Imaging 19:827–847, 2004.
10. Bielefeld MR, Bishop DA, Campbell DN, et al: Reoperative homograft right ventricular outflow tract reconstruction. Ann Thorac Surg 71:482–488, 2002.
11. Khambadkone S, Coats L, Taylor A, et al: Percutaneous pulmonary valve implantation in humans. Circulation 112:1189–1197, 2005.
12. Dearani JA, Danielson GK, Puga FJ, et al: Late follow-up of 1905 patients undergoing operation for complex congenital heart disease utilizing pulmonary ventricle to pulmonary artery conduits. Ann Thorac Surg 75:399–411, 2003.

# Pregnancy and the Systemic Right Ventricle

**Deborah R. Gersony and Marlon S. Rosenbaum**

**Age: 27 years**
**Gender: Female**
**Occupation: Teacher**
**Working diagnosis: Pregnancy in a patient with a systemic right ventricle**

## HISTORY

The patient was cyanotic at birth due to D-TGA (simple transposition). She underwent balloon septostomy in infancy and Mustard repair at 11 months of age.

She required reoperation at 12 years of age for a residual atrial septal defect and pulmonary venous obstruction. She recovered fully and had no further problems throughout adolescence.

At age 26, sinus node dysfunction was noted and required placement of a dual-chamber permanent pacemaker.

At age 27, she expressed a desire to become pregnant. She reported occasional palpitations but no shortness of breath or sustained arrhythmias. An exercise treadmill test demonstrated normal exercise capacity for age. She completed 9.5 minutes on a standard Bruce protocol with a peak heart rate of 182 (93% maximum predicted heart rate), an appropriate blood pressure response, and no arrhythmias. Her echo showed a moderately hypertrophied systemic RV with mildly reduced systolic function (see Fig. 54-4). Mild-to-moderate tricuspid regurgitation was present (systemic AV valve). The SVC and IVC limbs of the atrial baffle were unobstructed as was the pulmonary venous to tricuspid valve connection. Cardiac catheterization was performed to determine whether any intervention might be required prior to pregnancy. The study demonstrated no baffle obstruction or residual ASD. Systemic RV systolic function was preserved with mild tricuspid regurgitation.

After a discussion of potential risks of pregnancy, she decided to proceed. During the first trimester, she had two short episodes of supraventricular tachycardia that were terminated with the Valsalva maneuver.

She had no further cardiac complaints until the 35th week of pregnancy when she developed orthopnea. She found it difficult to climb one flight of stairs without stopping and required two pillows to sleep. An echocardiogram demonstrated worsening tricuspid regurgitation. Her symptoms responded to diuretic therapy. She had an uncomplicated cesarian section for obstetrical indications but 1 week later developed worsening dyspnea and bilateral pedal edema treated with diuretics and an ACE inhibitor. Symptoms of heart failure persisted. Two months later, she developed sustained tachycardia, which was treated with radiofrequency ablation. Repeat cardiac catheterization was planned for three months post ablation.

**Comments:** D-TGA, or ventriculoarterial discordance with AV concordance, is a form of cyanotic heart disease that typically presents during the first week of life. If untreated, it carries a greater than 90% mortality in the first year. Balloon septostomy (the Rashkind procedure) is performed when necessary to improve intracardiac mixing in preparation for subsequent cardiac repair. In the 1960s, the atrial switch operations (Senning and Mustard repair) were introduced, wherein systemic venous blood is baffled across the atrial septum after which it passes through the mitral valve and morphologic LV and into the pulmonary artery. Pulmonary venous blood is directed across the tricuspid valve through the RV and into the aorta.

While the medium-term results are generally good, significant late complications following the atrial switch have been observed including failure of the systemic RV, systemic AV valve regurgitation (tricuspid valve), atrial flutter/fibrillation, sinus node dysfunction, baffle obstruction, and sudden death.[1] Some reports suggest less baffle obstruction with the Senning repair,[2] although overall morbidity and mortality are similar.

Most women with a systemic RV after atrial switch repair are now of reproductive age. Although there are no large studies evaluating the pregnancy risks in women after atrial switch procedures, several small retrospective series have reported successful outcomes in the majority of patients, although a significant number experienced deterioration in functional class. A recent retrospective study of 28 pregnancies in 16 patients reported a good clinical outcome; however, a reduction in systemic RV function was seen in 25% of cases that persisted for a mean follow-up of 2 years.[3,4]

When considering medical therapy of arrhythmias in pregnancy, proarrhythmia and other potential adverse effects to the mother and fetus must be considered. It is probably best to avoid antiarrhythmic drugs as much as possible during the first weeks of gestation when the risk of developing congenital malformations is greatest. However, if needed, some drugs are considered safe. Beta-blockers are often used despite their reported association with small gestational size. Digoxin is safe during pregnancy. It crosses the placenta freely and is used to treat fetal supraventricular tachycardia.[5]

## CURRENT SYMPTOMS

The patient felt moderately short of breath with minimal exertion, such as walking up a slight incline or climbing a few stairs. She had notable orthopnea. She denied significant palpitations, lightheadedness, or dizziness.

NYHA class: III

## CURRENT MEDICATIONS

Digoxin 0.25 mg orally daily

Furosemide 40 mg orally daily

K-dur 20 mEq orally daily (potassium supplement)

Lisinopril 5 mg orally daily

**Comments:** Diuretics are initial therapy in patients with a failing systemic RV and congestive symptoms. Although there is evidence that ACE-inhibitor therapy reduces mortality, hospitalizations, and recurrent cardiac events in adult patients with congestive heart failure unrelated to congenital heart disease,[6] its use in patients with a systemic RV and Mustard or Senning repair has not been rigorously investigated.[7] Small studies have not shown an improvement in exercise capacity or ventricular function after short-term ACE-inhibitor therapy.[8–10] However, given the limitations of these small nonrandomized studies, no absolute conclusions regarding the cardioprotective benefit of ACE-inhibitor therapy in this population can be drawn.

During pregnancy, ACE inhibitors are contraindicated. Hydralazine, nitrates, and/or beta-blockers may be used as alternatives if required.

Digoxin has been extensively used without documented adverse effects to the mother or the fetus.

## PHYSICAL EXAMINATION

BP 105/65 mm Hg, HR 80 bpm, oxygen saturation 98%

Height 168 cm, weight 86 kg, BSA 2.00 m²

Surgical scars: Healed sternotomy scar

Neck veins: JVP was mildly elevated.

Lungs/chest: Clear lung sounds were heard in all fields.

Heart: An RV heave was present. S1 was normal. S2 was single and accentuated. A grade 2–3/4 holosystolic murmur was present at the lower left sternal border. No third heart sound was heard.

Abdomen: No hepatosplenomegaly was appreciated, and the liver was not pulsatile.

Extremities: Pedal edema was present; there was no cyanosis.

**Comments:** This patient had a prominent RV heave typical of patients with D-TGA and Mustard repair, which is related to the presence of the systemic RV. The loud aortic component of S2 is due to the anteriorly positioned aorta.

A pulsatile liver would not be expected, as tricuspid regurgitation is related to the systemic ventricle.

The elevated JVP and dependent edema attest to the presence of heart failure.

## LABORATORY DATA

| Hemoglobin | 13.2 g/dL (11.5–15.0) |
|---|---|
| Hematocrit/PCV | 41.2% (36–46) |
| MCV | **77.7 fL** (83–99) |
| Platelet count | 173 × 10⁹/L (150–400) |
| Sodium | 136 mmol/L (134–145) |
| Potassium | 4.0 mmol/L (3.5–5.2) |
| Creatinine | 0.7 mg/dL (0.6–1.2) |
| Blood urea nitrogen | **9 mmol/L** (2.5–6.5) |

## ELECTROCARDIOGRAM

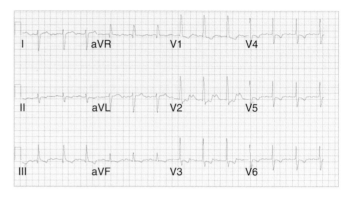

Figure 54-1 Electrocardiogram.

### FINDINGS

Heart rate: 77 bpm

QRS axis: +153°

QRS duration: 122 msec

Sinus rhythm with first-degree AV block and RV hypertrophy (marked right-axis deviation of initial QRS forces and R' of 17 mm in V1).

**Comments:** RV hypertrophy is an expected finding in patients with D-TGA after Mustard or Senning repair, reflecting systemic RV pressure.

Simus node dysfunction and junctional rhythms are common in patients with D-TGA status after the Mustard procedure, although this is not seen in this ECG.

## CHEST X-RAY

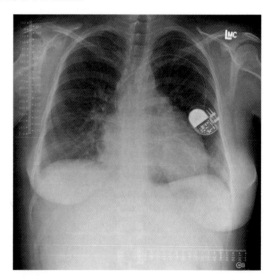

Figure 54-2 Anteroposterior projection.

## FINDINGS

Cardiothoracic ratio: 58%

There was evidence of cardiac enlargement with pulmonary vascular congestion. A permanent pacemaker was in place. There were no pleural effusions.

**Comments:** Note the position of the ventricular pacemaker lead, which courses through the systemic venous pathway to the LV apex.

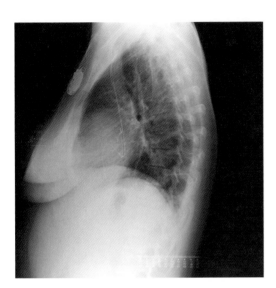

Figure 54-3 Lateral view.

**Comments:** The lateral view also demonstrates transvenous pacing leads in the anatomic LA and LV consistent with a patient who has undergone an atrial switch operation for D-TGA.

## EXERCISE TESTING

### Cardiopulmonary Exercise Stress Test Performed 5 Months Postpartum

| Exercise protocol: | Modified Bruce |
| Duration (min:sec): | 13:50 |
| Reason for stopping: | Fatigue |
| ECG changes: | None |

| | Rest | Peak |
|---|---|---|
| Heart rate (bpm): | 80 | 158 |
| Percent of age-predicted max HR: | | 82 |
| $O_2$ saturation (%): | 98 | 97 |
| Blood pressure (mm Hg): | 96/60 | 104/60 |
| Peak $Vo_2$ (mL/kg/min): | | 13.6 |
| Percent predicted (%): | | 48 |
| RER: | | 0.95 |
| $Ve/Vco_2$: | | 37 |

**Comments:** The peak oxygen consumption of 13.6 demonstrates moderate-to-severe functional impairment. The respiratory quotient was less than 1.0, suggesting submaximal effort.

Prior to conception she exercised 9 minutes on a full Bruce protocol. The protocol here is slightly different, and thus comparisons would be inappropriate.

## ECHOCARDIOGRAM

### OVERALL FINDINGS

The TTE performed 3 months prior to pregnancy demonstrated D-TGA status post atrial switch repair. The systemic RV was moderately dilated and hypertrophied with mildly reduced ventricular function. Mild-to-moderate tricuspid regurgitation was seen. The pulmonary ventricle (morphologic LV) was normal. There was no evidence of intra-atrial baffle obstruction or pulmonary venous obstruction.

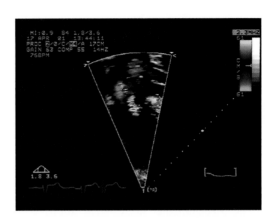

Figure 54-4 Transesophageal apical four-chamber view with color flow Doppler across the tricuspid valve (prepregnancy).

### FINDINGS

There was mild-to-moderate tricuspid regurgitation. Systemic RV function was reduced.

**Comments:** Assessment of systemic RV function can be subjective, and robust means of quantifying function with echo have not been well established. Currently, cardiac MRI is the preferred imaging modality to evaluate the systolic function of the systemic RV. This patient was not a cardiac MRI candidate because of the presence of a pacemaker.

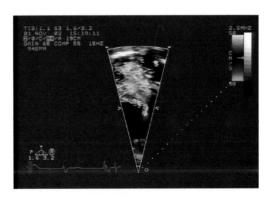

Figure 54-5 Transthoracic apical four-chamber view with color flow Doppler across the tricuspid valve (3 months postpartum).

### FINDINGS

This postpartum TTE demonstrated a moderately to severely dilated systemic RV with moderately reduced systolic function. Severe tricuspid regurgitation was seen. The rest of the study was unchanged.

**Comments:** Severe tricuspid regurgitation (systemic AV valve) with moderate RV systolic dysfunction has developed during her pregnancy, leading to heart failure symptoms and reduced exercise tolerance.

# CATHETERIZATION

## HEMODYNAMICS

Heart rate    80 bpm

|            | Pressure          | Saturation (%) |
|------------|-------------------|----------------|
| SVC        | 11                | 66             |
| IVC        | 12                | 74             |
| RA         | 10                | 53             |
| LV (anat)  | 46/10             | 65             |
| PA         | 42/18 (30)        | 65             |
| PCWP       | a 24 v 17 **mean 16** |            |
| RV (anat)  | 100/**16**        | 95             |
| Ao         | 105/60 (82)       | 97             |

**Calculations**

| | |
|---|---|
| Cardiac output | 4.65/L |
| Cardiac index (L/min/m²) | 2.4 |
| Qp/Qs | 1.0 |
| PVR (Wood units) | 3.0 |
| SVR (Wood units) | 15.3 |

***Comments:*** Cardiac catheterization was performed 6 months postpartum to determine whether the patient was a candidate for tricuspid valve replacement and to better assess the function of the systemic ventricle. The study also provided information about the pulmonary artery pressure and any potential gradients across the systemic or pulmonary venous pathways.

## FINDINGS

The hemodynamic data showed no gradients across the SVC and IVC limbs of the systemic venous baffle. In addition, there was no significant gradient between the RV end-diastolic pressure and the pulmonary capillary wedge pressure (PCWP) indicating no pulmonary venous obstruction. The RV end-diastolic pressure was mildly elevated at 16 mm Hg consistent with RV dysfunction, and there was mild pulmonary hypertension and mildly elevated RA pressure. Mixed venous saturation was mildly reduced indicating a reduced resting cardiac output. No shunts were demonstrated.

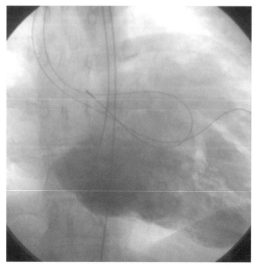

Figure 54-6 Right ventriculogram in right anterior oblique projection.

## FINDINGS

There was an enlarged and heavily trabeculated RV with moderately reduced systolic function. There was mild-to-moderate tricuspid regurgitation.

***Comments:*** Ventriculography can be an important imaging modality for qualitative assessment of RV function, particularly in patients who have limited echocardiographic windows and a contraindication to CMR.

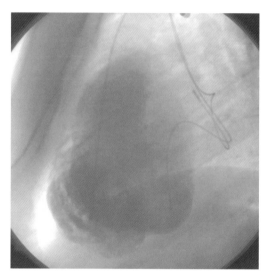

Figure 54-7 Right ventriculogram, lateral projection.

## FINDINGS

There was marked RV dilatation with moderately reduced systolic function. Transvenous pacing leads are seen in the anatomic LA and posterior ventricle.

***Comments:*** The right ventriculogram confirmed significant impairment of the systemic ventricle. The degree of tricuspid regurgitation was judged to be mild to moderate, and significantly less than was seen by echocardiographic studies at that time. This discrepancy was likely due to angiographic underestimation. This is not unusual in adult patients and is related to both filming techniques and dilution of contrast in patients with large ventricles.

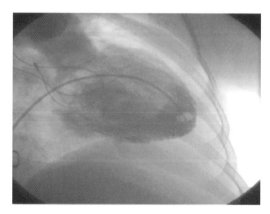

Figure 54-8 Right anterior oblique left ventriculogram of the pulmonary ventricle.

## FINDINGS

The left ventriculogram showed preserved function of the pulmonary ventricle without mitral regurgitation.

**Comments:** The catheter is seen entering the LV via the IVC limb of the systemic venous portion of the baffle.

## FOCUSED CLINICAL QUESTIONS AND DISCUSSION POINTS

1. What should the recommendations be to women with Mustard repairs who would like to become pregnant?

*Patients with Mustard or Senning repairs who are asymptomatic with good exercise capacity, preserved function of the systemic RV, and mild tricuspid regurgitation will likely tolerate pregnancy well. Nonetheless, women should be counseled about the cardiac risks of pregnancy including arrhythmia, heart failure, and change in functional class. Women who have significant depression of systemic RV function or moderate or severe tricuspid regurgitation should be counseled about the increased likelihood for adverse outcome during and/or after pregnancy. The most difficult cases are the asymptomatic patients in whom there is modest reduction in RV function with moderate tricuspid regurgitation. Although many of these patients will be able to tolerate pregnancy, it is difficult to predict who will be left with persistent heart failure that may culminate in the need for cardiac transplantation.*

2. Why did this patient decompensate in the peripartum period?

*The systemic RV may not have the same cardiac reserve as a morphologic LV. Pregnancy poses an additional hemodynamic burden on the systemic RV. The normal hemodynamics of pregnancy include a 40% to 50% increase in blood volume, an increase in heart rate by 10 to 20 bpm, and a decrease in systemic vascular resistance. These changes result in a significant increase in cardiac output (30%–50%) that peaks at approximately 32 weeks gestation.[11] Older patients with a Mustard repair may have reduced exercise performance due to failure to adequately increase cardiac output.[12] This finding has been attributed to chronotropic incompetence and abnormal right ventricular contractility.[13–15]*

*Although this patient was asymptomatic and performed adequately on an exercise treadmill test prior to pregnancy, she was likely at increased cardiac risk because of a combination of a moderately dilated systemic RV with reduced ejection fraction, and tricuspid regurgitation. Several months of progressive volume overload from pregnancy likely worsened systemic AV valve regurgitation and led to RV dysfunction and cardiac decompensation. Further deterioration postpartum was related to an acute increase in systemic vascular resistance and intravascular volume, as well as the development of recurrent atrial tachycardia.*

3. What is the prognosis for this patient? Should the tricuspid valve be replaced? What are her options at this point?

*Although this patient had significant deterioration in functional class early postpartum, some degree of clinical improvement was anticipated with restoration of her prepregnancy volume status. The cardiac catheterization was performed 6 months postpartum because the patient continued to deteriorate and there was concern that tricuspid valve surgery would need to be performed expeditiously. When the angiogram showed significant RV impairment with somewhat less-than-expected tricuspid regurgitation, the potential benefits of tricuspid valve surgery became less clear and the decision was made to continue medical management.*

*Although there are occasional Mustard patients with moderate-to-severe tricuspid regurgitation and relatively preserved RV function who may benefit from tricuspid valve surgery, the experience with tricuspid valve replacement in Mustard patients with advanced RV dysfunction is appropriately very limited.*

*In the pediatric population, selected Mustard patients with failing RVs and preserved LV function have undergone Mustard takedown with arterial switch repair that results in anatomic correction of this lesion. In these patients, banding of the pulmonary artery is usually required prior to arterial switch repair to "prepare" the LV for systemic pressure by increasing ventricular mass. Unfortunately, the outcome of this procedure, when performed in adults, has been poor.[16]*

## FINAL DIAGNOSIS

D-TGA, status post Mustard repair

Postpartum congestive heart failure

Worsening tricuspid valve regurgitation (systemic AV valve)

Recurrent atrial tachycardia

## PLAN OF ACTION

Medical therapy

## INTERVENTION

None

## OUTCOME

Two months postpartum, the patient was admitted with sustained atrial tachycardia at a rate of 200 bpm. She underwent an electrophysiologic study with electroanatomic mapping of the arrhythmia. The tachycardia was mapped to the pulmonary venous atrium. Application of radiofrequency energy in this region terminated the tachycardia. Symptoms of congestive heart failure persisted, and an echo continued to show severe tricuspid regurgitation with depressed RV function.

One month later, she had recurrent atrial tachycardia. Repeat mapping demonstrated another form of atrial tachycardia that was eliminated with radiofrequency ablations from both a retrograde aortic approach into the pulmonary venous atrium and an IVC approach in the systemic venous limb of the baffle. Despite restoration of sinus rhythm, an echocardiogram 2 months later continued to show severe tricuspid regurgitation with moderately severe RV dysfunction.

The patient was further treated medically for significant tricuspid regurgitation with depressed RV function. Medications included sotalol 80 mg twice daily to suppress short runs of symptomatic nonsustained atrial tachycardia, digoxin 0.125 mg daily, and aspirin 81 mg daily. An ACE inhibitor was discontinued because of a cough, and losartan was stopped after the development of a rash.

Her symptoms improved progressively, and diuretics were discontinued. An echocardiogram 18 months postpartum showed severely reduced RV systolic function with only mild tricuspid regurgitation. The degree of tricuspid regurgitation had returned to prepregnancy levels; however, RV function remained impaired. The patient was in NYHA class II. It is anticipated that the patient will eventually require heart transplantation.

## Selected References

1. Sarkar D, Bull C, Yates R, et al: Comparison of long-term outcomes of atrial repair of simple transposition with implications for a late arterial switch strategy. Circulation 100(Suppl 19): II176–II181, 1999.
2. Moons P, Gewillig M, Sluysmans T, et al: Long-term outcome up to 30 years after the Mustard or Senning operation: A nationwide multicentre study in Belgium. Heart 9:307–313, 2004.

3. Guedes AG, Mercier LA, Leduc L, et al: Impact of pregnancy on the systemic right ventricle after a Mustard operation for transposition of the great arteries. J Am Coll Cardiol 44:433–437, 2004.

4. Canobbio MM, Morris CD, Graham TP, Landzberg MJ: Pregnancy outcomes after atrial repair for transposition of the great arteries. Am J Cardiol 98:668–672, 2006.

5. Joglar JA, Page RL: Antiarrhythmic drugs in pregnancy. Curr Opin Cardiol 16:40–45, 2001.

6. SOLVD Investigators: Effect of enalapril on survival in patients with reduced left ventricular ejection fraction and congestive heart failure. N Engl J Med 325:293–295, 1991.

7. Vonder Muhll I, Liu P, Webb G: Applying standard therapies to new targets: The use of ACE inhibitors and B-blockers for heart failure in adults with congenital heart disease. Int J Cardiology 97(Suppl 1):25–33, 2004.

8. Robinson B, Heise CT, Moore JW, et al: Afterload reduction therapy in patients following intraatrial baffle operation for transposition of the great arteries. Pediatr Cardiol 23:618–623, 2002.

9. Hechter SJ, Fredriksen PM, Liu P, et al: Angiotensin-converting enzyme inhibitors in adults after the Mustard procedure. Am J Cardiol 87:660–663, A11, 2001.

10. Dore A, Houde C, Chan KL, et al: Angiotensin receptor blockade and exercise capacity in adults with systemic right ventricles: A multicenter, randomized, placebo-controlled clinical trial. Circulation 112:2411–2416, 2005.

11. Cole PL, Sutton MS: Normal cardiopulmonary adjustments to pregnancy: Cardiovascular evaluation. Cardiovasc Clin 19:37–56, 1989.

12. Ohuchi H, Hiraumi Y, Tasato H, et al: Comparison of the right and left ventricle as a systemic ventricle during exercise in patients with congenital heart disease. Am Heart J 137:1185–1194, 1999.

13. Derrick GP, Narang I, White PA, et al: Failure of stroke volume augmentation during exercise and dobutamine stress is unrelated to load-independent indexes of right ventricular performance after the Mustard operation. Circulation 102(Suppl 3):III154–III159, 2000.

14. Ebenroth ES, Hurwitz RA: Functional outcome of patients operated for d-transposition of the great arteries with the Mustard procedure. Am J Cardiol 20:49–56, 2002.

15. Meijboom F, Szatmari A, Deckers JW, et al: Long-term follow-up (10 to 17 years) after Mustard repair for transposition of the great arteries. J Thorac Cardiovasc Surg 111:1158–1168, 1996.

16. Benzaquen BS, Webb GD, Colman JM, et al: Arterial switch operation after Mustard procedures in adult patients with transposition of the great arteries: Is it time to revise our strategy? Am Heart J 147:E8, 2004.

# Palliative Mustard for Transposition and Ventricular Septal Defect

Daniele Prati, Craig S. Broberg, and Antonia Pijuan-Domenech

**Age:** 26 years
**Gender:** Male
**Occupation:** Unemployed
**Working diagnosis:** D-transposition of the great arteries with ventricular septal defect with Eisenmenger syndrome

## HISTORY

The patient was blue at birth, and the diagnosis of TGA with ventricular communication was suspected. At 2 months of age he underwent catheterization, and the diagnosis of TGA with a VSD was confirmed. Pulmonary vascular disease was already present. Therefore, no corrective surgery was performed.

At the age of 11 he again underwent cardiac catheterization that showed severely elevated pulmonary artery pressure (equal to systemic arterial pressures).

Since the age of 20 he has undergone multiple routine venesections. One venesection was performed when he presented with a hemoglobin of 14 g/dL.

*Comments:* Complete TGA is fatal unless there is a communication and thus mixing between the venous and arterial circulations, in this case a large VSD. Thus the only oxygenated blood that will reach the aorta must be shunted across the VSD.

Patients with complete TGA are predisposed to developing PAH, especially in the presence of a nonrestrictive VSD.[1] Vasoconstriction of pulmonary arterioles is induced by hypoxemic blood carried in systemic arterial collaterals, accelerating the pulmonary vascular disease. Moreover, hypoxemia provokes a fall in systemic vascular resistance and an increase in the volume of unsaturated blood in the systemic vascular bed.

A therapeutic phlebotomy when the hemoglobin was only 14 was misguided, since this would worsen systemic oxygen transport and make symptoms worse.

Thrombocytopenia and clotting factor deficiencies have been described in patients with cyanotic ACHD[2] and predispose to bleeding.

## CURRENT SYMPTOMS

The patient has shortness of breath on exertion. He cannot climb stairs and is limited to walking only 200 to 300 m on flat ground. He frequently complains of headaches, especially with exertion. He denies any orthopnea, palpitations, chest pains, or hemoptysis.

NYHA class: III

*Comments:* Exertional breathlessness and headaches are very common in cyanotic patients with ACHD. Headache may be a manifestation of hyperviscosity, but usually only when the hematocrit is greater than 65%. It can also be due to inadequate hemoglobin and low oxygen tissue delivery. Many cyanotic patients complain of headaches after exertion as their oxygen saturation falls, which tend to resolve relatively quickly with rest.

## CURRENT MEDICATIONS

Ranitidine 20 mg orally daily

## PHYSICAL EXAMINATION

BP 100/60 mm Hg, HR 70 bpm, oxygen saturation on room air 60%

Height 180 cm, weight 60 kg, BSA 1.73 m$^2$

Neck veins: JVP was 3 cm above the sternal angle (A-wave higher than V-wave).

Lungs/chest: Chest was clear.

Heart: Regular rhythm. There was a palpable RV impulse and a systolic thrill over the upper left sternal edge. Normal first heart sound, loud second heart sound with a loud pulmonary component. There was a 4/6 coarse ejection systolic murmur in the pulmonary area.

Peripheral pulses: Normal

Abdomen: No organomegaly

Extremities: Marked clubbing of fingers and toes, minimal ankle swelling

*Comments:* An oxygen saturation of 60% is extremely low even within the spectrum of cyanotic ACHD. This in itself implies a very poor prognosis.

The dominant A-wave reflects ventricular hypertrophy.

The heart exam suggests some degree of pulmonary stenosis.

## LABORATORY DATA

| | |
|---|---|
| Hemoglobin | **17.0 g/dL** (11.5–15.0) |
| Hematocrit/PCV | **51%** (36–46) |
| MCV | 84 fL (83–99) |
| Platelet count | **87 × 10⁹/L** (150–400) |
| White blood cells | 5.3 × 10⁹/L (4.0–10.0) |
| Sodium | 137 mmol/L (134–145) |
| Potassium | 4.6 mmol/L (3.5–5.2) |
| Creatinine | 0.81 mg/dL (0.6–1.2) |
| Blood urea nitrogen | 5.8 mmol/L (2.5–6.5) |

### OTHER RELEVANT LAB RESULTS

| | |
|---|---|
| Total protein | 7.2 g/dL (6.2–8.2) |
| Albumin | 3.7 g/dL (3.7–5.3) |
| Bilirubin | **38 mmol/L** (3–24) |
| Alk phos | **128 U/L** (38–126) |
| INR | 1.1 |
| Iron | 13 μmol/L (12.6–26.0) |
| Ferritin | **16 μg/L** (32–284) |
| Transferrin sat | **18%** (20–45) |

**Comments:** There is mild erythrocytosis. The hemoglobin is much lower than expected for the patient's oxygen saturation levels, and he would probably feel better at a higher hemoglobin level. The hemoglobin tends to rise proportionally to the fall in oxygen saturation. Iron deficiency anemia is frequent in Eisenmenger patients, the etiology of which may be multifactorial (see Case 72). Iron supplementation is warranted. Even though the MCV is not low, iron deficiency may still be present.[3]

Thrombocytopenia is a common finding in patients with Eisenmenger syndrome. It may be secondary to shortened platelet survival due to a peripheral consumption or destruction.

## ELECTROCARDIOGRAM

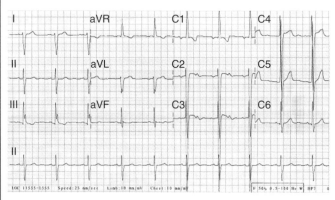

Figure 55-1 Electrocardiogram.

### FINDINGS

Heart rate: 61 bpm

PR interval: 204 msec

QRS axis: +168°

QRS duration: 128 msec

Sinus rhythm, first-degree AV block, RBBB, RV hypertrophy

**Comments:** RV hypertrophy is manifested by marked right-axis deviation, the very tall R-waves in lead V1, and the deep S-waves in leads V4–5.

RV hypertrophy is the expected finding in transposition, since the RV is the systemic ventricle.

## CHEST X-RAY

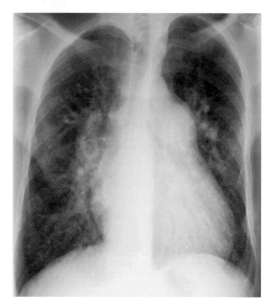

Figure 55-2 Posteroanterior projection.

### FINDINGS

Cardiothoracic ratio: 60%

There is marked cardiomegaly. There is enlargement of the pulmonary trunk and central pulmonary arteries with peripheral "pruning." The pleural spaces are clear.

**Comments:** The large central pulmonary arteries suggest pulmonary hypertension and/or high circulating volume through the pulmonary circulation. The "pruning" reflects high pulmonary vascular resistance.

## EXERCISE TESTING

| | |
|---|---|
| Exercise protocol: | Modified Bruce |
| Duration (min:sec): | 1:30 |
| Reason for stopping: | Dyspnea |
| ECG changes: | None |

| | Rest | Peak |
|---|---|---|
| Heart rate (bpm): | 70 | 142 |
| Percent of age-predicted max HR: | | 73 |
| O₂ saturation (%): | 60 | 41 |
| Blood pressure (mm Hg): | 100/55 | 138/50 |

**Comments:** The patient was only able to exercise on a modified Bruce protocol for 90 seconds, which is very low for a 26-year-old, and low even for a patient with cyanotic heart disease and pulmonary hypertension. His low baseline oxygen saturation combined with the relatively low hemoglobin makes this result credible. Although formal cardiopulmonary measurements were not made, the severity of exercise limitation is indisputable.

# ECHOCARDIOGRAM

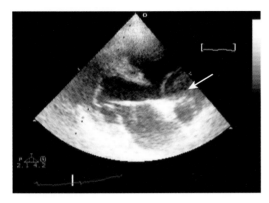

Figure 55-3 Modified short-axis view.

## FINDINGS

The echocardiogram was of poor quality. The RV (anteriorly located) was severely hypertrophied. There was an unrestricted outlet VSD. The aortic valve (*arrow*) arose from the RV.

**Comments:** For a variety of reasons echocardiography at times can be a challenging modality both to obtain clear images and to demonstrate complex anatomy. Here, the echocardiogram shows the VSD, but it was difficult to demonstrate clearly the ventriculoarterial relationship. Other modalities can often be helpful in such situations.

# MAGNETIC RESONANCE IMAGING

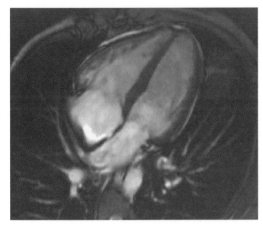

Figure 55-4 Oblique axial plane four-chamber view (steady-state free precession).

## FINDINGS

Both the RV and LV were normal in size and had normal function. The RV mass was increased, consistent with hypertrophy. The atria were normal in size. There was no significant mitral or tricuspid valve regurgitation. The atrial septum was intact.

**Comments:** This view does not show the VSD, which is in the outlet septum. RV (systemic) hypertrophy is be expected when the RV supports high pressures, and in the presence of a nonrestrictive VSD. The calculated volumes tell us about the relative amounts of pulmonary and systemic circulation, but not about the amount of bidirectional shunt across the VSD.

**Ventricular Volume Quantification**

|  | LV | (Normal range) | RV | (Normal range) |
|---|---|---|---|---|
| EDV (mL) | 155 | (77–195) | 106 | (88–227) |
| ESV (mL) | 48 | (19–72) | 49 | (23–103) |
| SV (mL) | 107 | (51–133) | 57 | (52–138) |
| EF (%) | 69 | (57–74) | 54 | (48–74) |
| EDVi (mL/m$^2$) | 89 | (68–103) | **61** | (68–114) |
| ESVi (mL/m$^2$) | 28 | (19–41) | 28 | (21–50) |
| SVi (mL/m$^2$) | 62 | (44–68) | **33** | (40–72) |
| Mass index (g/m$^2$) | **58** | (59–93) | **57** | (23–50) |

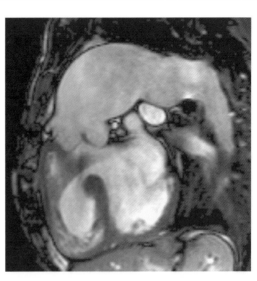

Figure 55-5 Oblique coronal section. Left ventricular outflow to the pulmonary artery.

## FINDINGS

The subpulmonary VSD measured 19 mm and was not restrictive.

The great vessels were parallel (not shown in Fig. 55-5). The pulmonary artery was very dilated.

**Comments:** Oxygenated blood returning from the pulmonary veins must cross the VSD to reach the aorta and systemic circulation. The fact that resistance in the pulmonary arteries is high will actually favor shunting of blood across this septal defect, without which survival would not be possible.

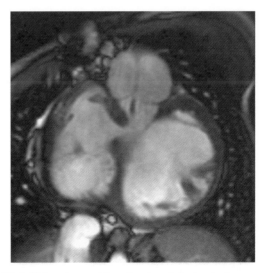

Figure 55-6 Oblique transaxial section, basal short-axis view.

## FINDINGS

The LV was subpulmonary. The VSD was also visible, measuring 1.0 cm in this dimension.

***Comments:*** Essentially all blood that flows from the LV through to the pulmonary artery is the left-to-right shunt volume, whereas blood flowing through the right (systemic) ventricle to the aorta is the right-to-left shunt volume. Instead, the amount of blood that shunts across the defect is the true effective circulation, meaning the amount of blood that travels from the systemic capillary bed to the pulmonary vascular bed. Bidirectional shunting across the VSD is critically important in allowing for both systemic oxygenation and pulmonary $CO_2$ delivery.

In this case the Qp/Qs ratio is misleading because it only shows the relative volumes in the pulmonary versus systemic circulation and does not reflect the net flow across the VSD.

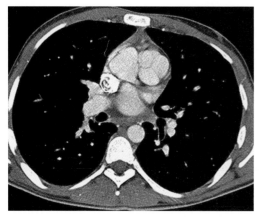

Figure 55-7 Transverse section, short-axis view of the great arteries.

## FINDINGS

D-TGA anatomy, right-sided aorta, and dilated pulmonary arteries. There was no pulmonary artery thrombosis.

***Comments:*** CT pulmonary angiography is often used to determine the presence of thrombi in the pulmonary arteries, which are common in patients with Eisenmenger physiology (see Case 74), and harder to detect with MRI.[4] Although CT can be used to quantify ventricular volume and function and clarify anatomical relationships, MRI would be preferred for this because it produces no ionizing radiation exposure.

The CT shows nicely the side-by-side relationship of the two semilunar valves. The aortic valve is more anterior than usual, and leaflets can be seen in both valves, whereas usually the semilunar valve planes are perpendicular to each other.

## CATHETERIZATION

### HEMODYNAMICS

Heart rate     70 bpm

|  | Pressure | Saturation (%) |
|---|---|---|
| SVC |  | 35 |
| IVC |  | 47 |
| RA | mean 4 | 38 |
| RV | 114/8 | 62 |
| PA | 115/39 mean 73 | 87 |
| LV | 100/7 | 94 |
| Aorta | 105/66 mean 81 | 61 |

### Calculations

| | |
|---|---|
| Qp (L/min) | 8.66 |
| Qs (L/min) | 4.14 |
| Cardiac index (L/min/m²) | 2.39 |
| Qp/Qs | 2.09 |
| PVR (Wood units) | 6.12 |
| SVR (Wood units) | 18.60 |
| | |
| Effective blood flow | 2.00 L/min |
| Right-to-left shunt volume | 2.26 L/min |
| Left-to-right shunt volume | 6.92 L/min |

After 10 minutes of 6 L/min oxygen, pulmonary artery saturation increased to 94%, while aortic saturation stayed at 61%.

## FINDINGS

Coronary arteriography showed right coronary dominance and no stenoses. Aortography showed the anteriorly situated aorta, which was right-sided. No aortic regurgitation. Ventriculography confirmed ventriculoatrial discordance, with a subpulmonary VSD. Good LV and RV function.

***Comments:*** Cardiac catheterization was performed primarily to measure the oxygen saturation in the aorta and pulmonary artery.

The data show systemic pulmonary artery pressures with much higher arterial oxygen saturation in the pulmonary artery than in the aorta. The aortic saturation is 26 percentage points lower than the saturation in the pulmonary artery. These numbers clearly demonstrate transposition physiology.

The data confirm the estimated flows by MRI, but only catheterization allows one to measure right-to-left and left-to-right shunt volumes. The Qp/Qs is misleading since ordinarily a ratio of 2 implies left-to-right shunt without cyanosis (such as with an ASD; see Case 2).

In this case, the high left-to-right shunt is not the volume shunted across the VSD, but the volume perpetually circulating from LV to pulmonary artery (PA) and back to LV. The effective blood flow (Qef), defined as the amount of blood flowing from the systemic capillary bed to the pulmonary capillary bed, is essentially the volume shunted through the VSD from RV to PA. It is calculated as the oxygen consumption divided by the difference in oxygen content between the PA and the RA.

### FOCUSED CLINICAL QUESTIONS AND DISCUSSION POINTS

1. Should the VSD be closed?

   *Any patient with pulmonary vascular disease due to chronic left-to-right shunt at systemic level pressure should not have a closure of the shunt. If anything, one should ensure that the shunt is not restrictive and that it can allow flow between the systemic and pulmonary circulations to pass through unhindered.*

2. Should this patient undergo a palliative atrial switch?

   *Any procedure to allow more oxygenated blood to reach the systemic circulation should in theory be beneficial. The procedure that has been performed is a palliative atrial switch (Mustard or Senning procedure), meaning creation of an ASD with redirection of atrial blood flow from right to left and vice versa via an atrial baffle, without closure of the VSD (see Fig. 55-8).[5–8]*

   *Outcomes from the palliative Mustard operation have been studied in patients with transposition physiology (usually defined as a pulmonary artery saturation at least 8% greater than aortic saturation).[9,10] It has been shown to be beneficial for patients with*

TGA or other complex lesions with VSD who show higher arterial oxygen saturation in the pulmonary artery than in the aorta. It may not be feasible if severe pulmonary vascular resistance is present, which may occur after years of cyanosis. Here the pulmonary vascular resistance of under 6 Wood units is not prohibitive, as long as the VSD is not closed.

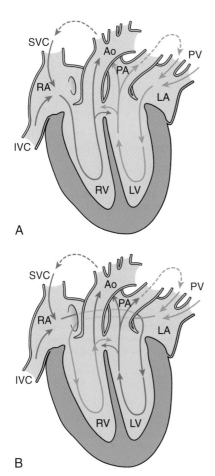

Figure 55-8 **A,** Anatomy and physiology of transposition of the great arteries with a sizeable ventricular septal defect (VSD): The desaturated systemic blood (*blue arrows*) predominantly supplies the aorta whereas the more saturated blood (*red arrows*) predominantly supplies the pulmonary artery. Mixing occurs at the level of the VSD and is the only source of oxygenated blood in the systemic circulation. **B,** Hemodynamic effect of a palliative atrial switch procedure in such a patient: after rerouting the systemic and pulmonary venous flow at the atrial level via a baffle, the amount of saturated blood substantially increases in the aorta (*red arrows*), and flow across the VSD becomes relatively inconsequential. (Adapted from Burkhart HM, Dearani JA, Williams WG, et al: Late results of palliative atrial switch for transposition, ventricular septal defect, and pulmonary vascular obstructive disease. Ann Thorac Surg 77:464–468, 2004.)

3. **Would an arterial switch procedure be more advantageous?**

*An arterial switch, with reimplantation of the coronary arteries, is felt to be the best repair in patients with transposition when done early in life. The advantages are fewer problems with atrial arrhythmias than with the atrial switch operation (see Case 52),*

*and utilization of the morphologic LV as the systemic ventricle. The long-term complications include stenoses at the coronary ostia, and outflow tract obstruction (see Case 52).*

*A palliative arterial switch operation would carry a very high operative risk, whereas a palliative atrial switch can be conducted fairly safely.*

## FINAL DIAGNOSIS

D-TGA with a nonrestrictive VSD

Pulmonary vascular disease

Suboptimal hemoglobin

## PLAN OF ACTION

Palliative atrial switch (Senning operation)

## INTERVENTION

In anticipation of surgery, the venesections were abandoned and the patient was started on oral iron therapy.[4,11] Within several weeks the hemoglobin climbed to 21 g/dL. The operation was planned soon thereafter.

After sternotomy and cardiac bypass, an atrial incision was made and a baffle created using pericardium (Senning). The VSD was not closed. The oxygen saturations after cardiopulmonary bypass circulation was stopped were in the 90s with satisfactory hemodynamics.

## OUTCOME

In the days and months following the operation the patient experienced recurrent paroxysms of atrial flutter and required cardioversion on two occasions. For this reason he was started on anticoagulation with warfarin (therapeutic goal of INR 2.0–3.0). He was also started on amiodarone, which controlled his rhythm abnormality.

Two years after cardiac surgery he presented with melena and hematemesis. He required transfusion of 23 units of red blood cells, 6 units of colloid, and 11 units of fresh frozen plasma, but remained hemodynamically stable. An esophagogastroduodenoscopy showed gastritis. Because of persistent bleeding despite a normalized INR he underwent a mesenteric angiogram. This showed a bleeding mesenteric vessel that was embolized with gel foam and coil.

After this event anticoagulation therapy was not restarted.

Now 9 years after the palliative Mustard procedure the patient's oxygen saturation ranges between 89% and 92% on room air. Exercise testing was repeated. He completed 10 minutes of the modified Bruce protocol and reached a peak of oxygen consumption of 20.6 mL/kg/min (54% of predicted). This reflected a substantial improvement in his exercise capacity. He was able to hold a full-time job and generally felt well.

He was recently hospitalized again for an episode of atrial tachycardia requiring cardioversion. The problems with atrial arrhythmia in Mustard/Senning patients are well recognized (see Case 50). As part of that workup, elevation of PA pressure was found, with a calculated pulmonary vascular resistance of 8.4 Wood units. The late development of further pulmonary vascular disease is not surprising, since the palliative procedure did not correct the VSD.

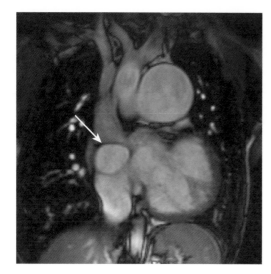

Figure 55-9 Oblique coronal steady-state free precession.

## Findings

By employment of the surgical baffle (*arrow*), the SVC and IVC flow entering the RA has been directed toward the LV (the subpulmonary ventricle). Pulmonary venous flow is directed anteriorly (toward the viewer in this plane) to the systemic RV.

**Comments:** Note marked dilatation of the pulmonary trunk, due to PAH. PAH-targeted therapy may be considered, should clinical deterioration ensue.[12]

## Selected References

1. Bando K, Turrentine MW, Sharp TG, et al: Pulmonary hypertension after operations for congenital heart disease: Analysis of risk factors and management. J Thorac Cardiovasc Surg 112:1600–1607, 1996.
2. Henriksson P, Varendh G, Lundstrom NR: Haemostatic defects in cyanotic congenital heart disease. Br Heart J 41:23–27, 1979.
3. Kaemmerer H, Fratz S, Braun SL, et al: Erythrocyte indexes, iron metabolism, and hyperhomocysteinemia in adults with cyanotic congenital cardiac disease. Am J Cardiol 94:825–828, 2004.
4. Broberg CS, Bax BE, Rampling MW, et al: Blood viscosity and its relation to iron deficiency, symptoms, and exercise capacity in adults with cyanotic congenital heart disease. J Am Coll Cardiol 48:356–365, 2006.
5. Mustard WT, Keith JD, Trusler GA, et al: The surgical management of transposition of the great vessels. J Thorac Cardiovasc Surg 48:953–958, 1964.
6. Lindesmith GG, Stiles QR, Tucker BL, et al: The Mustard operation as a palliative procedure. J Thorac Cardiovasc Surg 63:75–78, 1972.
7. Mair DD, Ritter DG, Danielson GK, et al: The palliative Mustard operation: Rationale and results. Am J Cardiol 37:762–768, 1976.
8. Humes RA, Driscoll DJ, Mair DD, et al: Palliative transposition of venous return: Long-term follow-up. J Thorac Cardiovasc Surg 96:364–367, 1988.
9. Dhasmana JP, Stark J, de Leval M, et al. Long-term results of the "palliative" Mustard operation. J Am Coll Cardiol 6:1138–1141, 1985.
10. Burkhart HM, Dearani JA, Williams WG, et al: Late results of palliative atrial switch for transposition, ventricular septal defect, and pulmonary vascular obstructive disease. Ann Thorac Surg 77:464–468, 2004.
11. Spence MS, Balaratnam MS, Gatzoulis MA: Clinical update: Cyanotic adult congenital heart disease. Lancet 370:1530–1532, 2007.
12. Diller G-P, Gatzoulis MA: Pulmonary vascular disease in adults with congenital heart disease. Circulation 115:1039–1050, 2007.

# Part II

# Congenitally Corrected Transposition

# Assessment of Systemic Right Ventricle Function

**Henryk Kafka**

**Age: 29 years**
**Gender: Male**
**Occupation: Chef**
**Working diagnosis: Congenitally corrected transposition of the great arteries**

## HISTORY

A childhood murmur brought the patient to attention at a young age, and echocardiograms showed congenitally corrected TGA. At age 9, cardiac catheterization had documented his CCTGA, secundum ASD (shunt ratio of 1.5:1), mild subvalvular pulmonary stenosis with moderate pulmonary regurgitation, and a very dilated main pulmonary artery (PA).

Investigation of exertional dyspnea at age 16 revealed AV conduction abnormalities and resulted in placement of an endocardial DDD pacemaker.

At age 19, he was admitted with congestive heart failure (CHF) and was found to have severe impairment of the systemic RV. There was still only a small gradient across the pulmonary valve. He was started on captopril and improved clinically. Warfarin was also started.

Three years later, at age 22, he was admitted with worsening dyspnea and fatigue. There was further worsening of his systemic RV function. He had several episodes of atrial fibrillation and was started on amiodarone. Cardiac catheterization revealed a large increase in his ASD shunt with ratio of 3.5:1. He was referred for consideration of heart transplantation. He responded to intensification of his ongoing medical therapy, and it was decided to not yet pursue transplantation.

Over the subsequent 6 years, he had gradual worsening of dyspnea and fatigue with increasing abdominal girth and discomfort, despite escalation of his medical therapy. At age 29, he was referred to the ACHD clinic for consideration of other interventions, notably closure of the ASD and/or possible use of cardiac resynchronization therapy (CRT).

**_Comments:_** CCTGA is an uncommon defect accounting for only about 0.5% of all congenital heart disease. It is defined by AV discordance and ventriculoarterial discordance, so that the pulmonary and systemic circuits are correctly in series but the morphologic RV becomes the systemic ventricle and the LV is in the subpulmonary position. Although extracardiac anomalies are infrequent, associated cardiac anomalies are very common,[1] as exemplified by this patient's anatomy. The most common defects include VSD (60%–80%) and pulmonary

outflow tract obstruction (30%–50%). Systemic tricuspid valve dysplasia, including Ebstein anomaly, is frequently noted at autopsy.[2] These intrinsic tricuspid valve anomalies, in conjunction with systemic RV dysfunction, are responsible for the tricuspid regurgitation incidence of up to 80% in CCTGA. Despite being called "congenitally corrected" TGA, it must be recognized for its common late complications and need for regular follow-up.[3]

ASDs are uncommonly seen and will overload the pulmonary ventricle rather than the systemic ventricle. Although an ASD will result in right-sided volume overload with dilatation of the atria and the subpulmonary ventricle, the size of the shunt in this case would not have been expected, in the presence of subpulmonary stenosis, to give rise to significant chamber enlargement and certainly not to the marked dilatation of the PA.

In CCTGA, the AV node is positioned more anteriorly in the RA (near the junction of the right AV valve and the pulmonary valve), and the bundle of His follows a long course anteriorly across the infundibular septum to reach the bundle branches.[1] This results in a high rate of complete heart block (about 2% per year), especially in patients who have had VSD or tricuspid valve surgery.

The presence of an endocardial pacemaker has been shown to be a significant risk factor for thromboembolism,[4] which may cause arterial embolization in the setting of an intracardiac shunt. A recent long-term follow-up study reported more thromboembolic complications associated with endocardial leads versus epicardial leads in patients with an intracardiac shunt.[5] Although there are no published studies regarding the routine use of anticoagulants in such individuals, the use of warfarin seems prudent, but in this particular study, warfarin was not protective. Other recent studies have not reached similar conclusions about endocardial leads in Fontan patients (see Case 64). Alternatively, epicardial leads have a higher failure rate than endocardial leads, and hence a balance of risk must be considered in each patient.

ACE inhibitors are frequently used for medical therapy for systemic RV failure,[1] although there are not yet good data for their elective, prophylactic application in this setting.[6]

The increase in the size of the left-to-right shunt across the ASD is not surprising in the face of worsening systemic ventricular function with rising LA pressures and consequently higher driving forces across the atrial septum from left to right.

## CURRENT SYMPTOMS

The patient complains of marked exertional dyspnea and fatigue, as well as paroxysmal nocturnal dyspnea and orthopnea. He has noted increased abdominal girth but no ankle edema. He denies palpitations.

NYHA class: III–IV

## CURRENT MEDICATIONS

Warfarin as directed

Amiodarone 100 mg daily

Bisoprolol 2.5 mg daily

Digoxin 125 µg daily

Lisinopril 20 mg daily

Furosemide 160 mg daily

Amiloride 5 mg daily

Metolazone 2.5 mg daily

Spironolactone 25 mg daily but only three times a week

Slow K 2 tabs three times daily

*Comments:* Warfarin is indicated for the prevention of thromboembolism in the presence of atrial fibrillation. The amiodarone is being used to keep the patient out of atrial fibrillation, since patients with CCTGA tend to tolerate atrial arrhythmias poorly.[1]

Spironolactone can be symptomatically beneficial in patients with elevated venous pressure and hepatic congestion. Caution against hyperkalemia is especially important in patients with compromised renal function. This patient has developed gynecomastia and therefore is taking the spironolactone only three times a week.

## PHYSICAL EXAMINATION

BP 90/60 mm Hg, HR 76 bpm, oxygen saturation 97%

Height 176 cm, weight 69 kg, BSA 1.84 m$^2$

Surgical scars: None

Neck veins: 5 cm above the sternal angle

Lungs/chest: No deformity of the chest wall; the chest was clear.

Heart: Heart rate was 76 bpm and regular. The first heart sound was normal with fixed splitting of the second heart sound. There was a pan-systolic murmur along both sternal borders followed by a low-pitched diastolic murmur. Carotid upstroke was normal with normal peripheral pulses.

Abdomen: The abdomen was soft with normal bowel sounds. There was epigastric tenderness, and the liver edge was palpable 2 cm below the costal margin and was slightly tender.

Extremities: There was no peripheral edema. No clubbing was seen.

*Comments:* One expects to hear fixed splitting of S2 in the presence of a large ASD because of delayed pulmonary valve closure throughout the respiratory cycle. However, the pacemaker in the pulmonary ventricle would be expected to cause delayed aortic valve closure, thereby narrowing the S2 split. The pan-systolic murmur is likely due to the systemic tricuspid valve regurgitation. Its unusual location is probably due to the unusual position of the heart itself, as is obvious in the CXR and CT scans. The diastolic murmur may be secondary to pulmonary regurgitation or represent an inflow rumble associated with the ASD.

## LABORATORY DATA

| | |
|---|---|
| Hemoglobin | 11.**8 g/dL** (13.0–17.0) |
| Hematocrit/PCV | **34%** (41–51) |
| MCV | 92 fL (83–99) |
| Platelet count | $191 \times 10^9$/L (150–400) |
| Sodium | **133 mmol/L** (134–145) |
| Potassium | 4.0 mmol/L (3.5–5.2) |
| Creatinine | **2.8 mg/dL** (0.6–1.2) |
| Blood urea nitrogen | **51 mg/dL** (7–18.2) |
| INR | **3** |

*Comments:* The cause of the anemia may not be directly linked to the congenital cardiac defect. There is no evidence of intravascular hemolysis, and the indices do not support the diagnosis of iron deficiency. The anemia may be associated with chronic Coumadin use, although one would expect iron deficiency if that were true. Alternately, anemia is nearly always present in patients with subacute infective endocarditis,[7] and endocarditis must always be considered in any congenital heart patient presenting with anemia and nonspecific systemic symptoms. A thorough assessment of his anemia will be necessary.

Renal dysfunction is likely due to overtreatment of his CHF against a background of chronically low cardiac output. This is commonly seen in patients with systemic LV failure therapy. He is on four diuretics and lisinopril.

Special attention needs to be paid to his digoxin dose. It should be determined whether there is sufficient benefit from the digoxin to continue its use in the face of renal insufficiency.

## ELECTROCARDIOGRAM

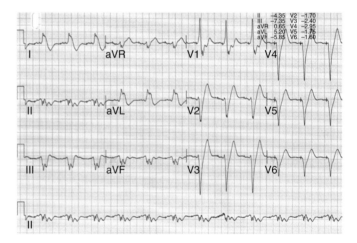

Figure 56-1 Electrocardiogram.

### FINDINGS
Heart rate: 72 bpm

QRS axis: −30°

QRS duration: 200 msec

This shows a paced atrial and ventricular rhythm with a very wide QRS complex. The P-waves are very prolonged and notched, suggesting LA overload. We are also reminded that amiodarone tends to prolong cardiac electrical activity.

***Comments:*** This very wide QRS complex indicates delays in depolarization that can form the basis for discoordinate ventricular contraction. In patients with morphologic RV pacing, such pacing-induced electromechanical dissynchrony has been associated with a higher incidence of LV dysfunction.[8] In a similar fashion, pacing of the subpulmonary LV may contribute to systemic RV desynchronization and consequent RV dysfunction.[9]

The common ECG features of CCTGA are not present in this case because of the paced rhythm. Commonly one sees a QS or QR pattern in V1, with absence of Q-waves in V5 and V6. This is because the septal depolarization occurs from right to left due to the ventricular inversion.[10] There may be enlarged P-waves as a result of atrial dilatation linked to systemic AV valve regurgitation. First-degree AV block may be present in up to 50% and complete heart block may occur in up to 50% of patients with CCTGA. Delta waves may be present, since Wolff-Parkinson-White syndrome is found in 2% to 4% of patients.

## CHEST X-RAY

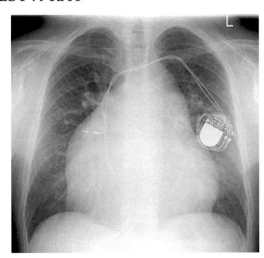

Figure 56-2 Posteroanterior projection.

### FINDINGS
Cardiothoracic ratio: 70%

Marked enlargement of the cardiac silhouette with a very prominent right heart border and PA enlargement. The atrial pacing lead was in the RA and the ventricular lead was sitting in the apex of the morphologic LV that was to the right of the midline. There was some pulmonary plethora noted but no evidence of pulmonary edema.

***Comments:*** In CCTGA, the prominent upper left heart border is due to the side-by-side configuration of the ascending aorta and the PA. This is evident on the coronal slice of the CT scan (see Fig. 56-5). In this case, the upper left border is further accentuated by the enlarged PA, and the prominent right heart border is actually due to the enlarged subpulmonary LV that sits to the right of the midline.

## EXERCISE TESTING

| | | | |
|---|---|---|---|
| Exercise protocol: | Modified Bruce | | |
| Duration (min:sec): | 4:22 | | |
| Reason for stopping: | Fatigue and dyspnea | | |
| ECG changes: | Paced | | |

| | Rest | Peak |
|---|---|---|
| Heart rate (bpm): | 76 | 103 |
| Percent of age-predicted max HR: | | 54% |
| $O_2$ saturation (%): | 95 | 98 |
| Blood pressure (mm Hg): | 90/60 | 106/80 |
| Peak $Vo_2$ (mL/kg/min): | | 10.6 |
| Percent predicted (%): | | 26 |
| $Ve/Vco_2$: | | 51 |
| Metabolic equivalents: | | 3.1 |

***Comments:*** The exercise test demonstrated very poor exercise tolerance for a man of his age. Peak $Vo_2$ has been used to assess prognosis in heart failure patients with acquired disease. Recently, there has been evidence of the ability of peak $Vo_2$ to predict hospitalization or death in adults with congenital heart disease. Patients with peak $Vo_2$ less than 15.5 mL/kg/min were five times more likely to die over the subsequent year and three times more likely to be hospitalized.[11]

This patient's symptomatic state (class III–IV) and the results of his peak $Vo_2$ clearly indicate a poor prognosis in the short term.

The patient shows no evidence of desaturation with exercise despite the known intracardiac shunt. This suggests that the pulmonary vascular resistance is probably not elevated.

## ECHOCARDIOGRAM

### OVERALL FINDINGS
Function of the systemic RV was significantly impaired with an ejection fraction of 30%. The subpulmonary LV was enlarged, measuring 80 mm in diameter, but with good overall systolic function (ejection fraction was 50%). Both atria were enlarged. There was a large secundum ASD. The main PA was markedly enlarged. The Doppler study revealed moderate to severe systemic tricuspid regurgitation.

The systemic RV was enlarged and heavily trabeculated.

There was apical Ebstein-like displacement of the septal tricuspid leaflet toward the apex. The pacer wires were seen in the RA and in the subpulmonary LV.

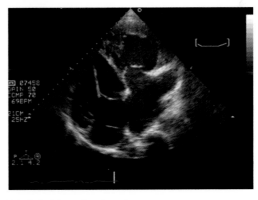

Figure 56-3 Apical four-chamber view.

***Comments:*** This view demonstrates the AV discordance and the apically displaced tricuspid valve that is commonly seen in CCTGA. Accurate assessment of ventricular function is difficult in the presence of AV valve regurgitation because of off-loading during systole through the regurgitant jet. This may provide a falsely optimistic assessment of ventricular function.

The presence of endocardial pacemaker leads in the subpulmonary LV and the RA in close proximity to a large ASD reinforce the rationale for anticoagulation in such patients.

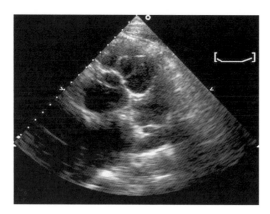

Figure 56-4 Two dimensional short-axis view of the great vessels.

## FINDINGS

Doppler study revealed no significant valvar pulmonary stenosis, but there was mild subpulmonary stenosis with mild pulmonary valve regurgitation. There was no aortic stenosis, but mild aortic regurgitation was present on the Doppler study.

*Comments:* This demonstrates the typical side-by-side configuration of the semilunar valves with the aorta to the left and anterior. There is mild enlargement of the PA at this level.

## COMPUTED TOMOGRAPHY

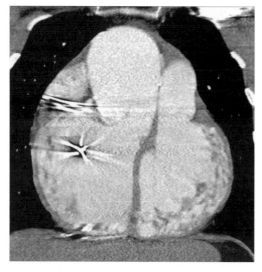

Figure 56-5 Coronal plane reconstruction.

## FINDINGS

The heavily trabeculated ventricle on the patient's left is the systemic RV from which the aorta originates. The smooth-walled dilated ventricle on the patient's right is the subpulmonary LV, which gives rise to a dilated PA. Note the side-by-side configuration of the course of the great vessels. Bright artifacts on the left of the image correspond to pacer wires in the RA and in the subpulmonary LV.

*Comments:* This CT image helps explain the appearance of the posteroanterior chest film in Figure 56-2. The subpulmonary LV makes up a great deal of the right heart border. The septum runs in an anterior-posterior direction with both ventricular apices essentially facing forward. It is the combination of the parallel course of the PA and the aorta, as well as the dilated PA, that accounts for the prominence of the upper left heart border on the CXR.

A retrospectively gated multichannel CT scanner can allow for quantification of ventricular volumes, but this was not the case for this scan. No doubt quantification would have only confirmed the RV enlargement and dysfunction already seen on echocardiography.

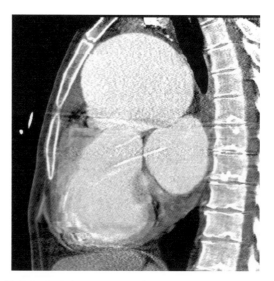

Figure 56-6 Sagittal plane reconstruction.

## FINDINGS

There was a markedly dilated main PA occupying the superior aspect of the mediastinum. The PA originated from the smooth-walled subpulmonary LV. The dilated LA was seen posteriorly.

*Comments:* Aneurysmal dilatation of the PA is not a feature of CCTGA. In fact, such PA dilatation in a patient without pulmonary hypertension or valvular pulmonary stenosis or marked pulmonary regurgitation is quite rare. PA aneurysm rupture has occurred in the presence of pulmonary hypertension or connective tissue disorders. The risk of rupture in the absence of these factors, even with a PA as dilated as this one, is very small. Aneurysm size in itself is not an indication for surgery.[12]

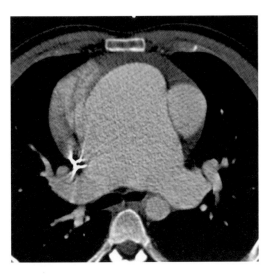

Figure 56-7 Axial plane scan.

## FINDINGS

The markedly dilated PA was again well seen. The main PA measures 100 mm in anterior-posterior diameter, with the left PA measuring 30 mm in cross-sectional diameter and the right PA measuring 25 mm. The ascending aorta was on the patient's left.

***Comments:*** The aneurysmal main PA leads to dilated left PA and main PA branches. This would add to the challenge of cardiac transplantation surgery.

## CATHETERIZATION

### HEMODYNAMICS

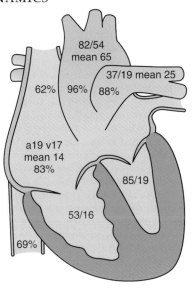

Figure 56-8 Hemodynamic data.

### Calculations

| | |
|---|---|
| Qp (L/min) | 14.67 |
| Qs (L/min) | 4.55 |
| Cardiac index (L/min/m²) | 2.48 |
| Qp/Qs | 3.23 |
| PVR (Wood units) | 0.41 |
| SVR (Wood units) | 11.22 |

## FINDINGS

There was a large left-to-right shunt at the atrial level. There was no significant pulmonary hypertension, and the pulmonary vascular resistance was not increased. There was only mild pulmonary stenosis. Both the RV and LV demonstrated impaired hemodynamics with elevation of diastolic pressures.

***Comments:*** The cardiac catheterization was done to assess PA pressure and the diastolic pressures of both ventricles as a prelude to transplant consideration.

The markedly dilated PA occurred despite the normal pulmonary pressures, normal pulmonary vascular resistance, and only mild pulmonary regurgitation.

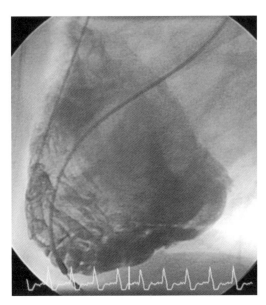

Figure 56-9 Left lateral projection of the right ventriculogram.

## FINDINGS

The systemic RV has been entered in a retrograde fashion through the anteriorly placed aorta. The systemic RV was dilated and poorly contractile.

***Comments:*** The appearance of the compromised systemic RV function was similar to that noted on echocardiography and CT. Although it was appropriate to undertake cardiac catheterization to obtain important hemodynamic data, this RV ventriculogram has not really added to the understanding of RV function and could have been omitted. The other radio-opaque structure in this frame is the pacer wire in the apex of the subpulmonary LV.

### FOCUSED CLINICAL QUESTIONS AND DISCUSSION POINTS

1. **What is the cause of systemic RV systolic dysfunction in patients with CCTGA?**

   *Systemic RV failure is common in patients with CCTGA, with increasing incidence as the patient ages. Although there have been reports of unoperated individuals with CCTGA presenting late in life, this is uncommon. The presence of associated defects in most of these patients (VSD and AV valve regurgitation) adds to the volume load on the systemic ventricle and contributes to its failure. Two thirds of patients with associated defects will have developed CHF by age 45, and 25% of patients with minimal or no associated lesions develop CHF by age 45.[2]*

*It is generally believed that the RV is structurally inadequate to cope with the pressure load of the systemic circulation, and that its poor geometric adaptation fails to cope with the increased demand. There have been reports of myocardial perfusion defects in these patients, and the extent of those defects has correlated inversely with RV performance.[13] The presence of scarring in the systemic RV probably contributes to RV dysfunction. This scarring may be due to an RV blood supply inadequate to meet the needs of a hypertrophied systemic RV.[14]*

*Because conduction defects are common, many of these CCTGA patients become pacemaker dependent. Recently, there has been speculation that pacing the subpulmonary ventricle may add to the deterioration in function of the systemic RV.[9]*

## 2. What is the best way to assess function of the systemic RV?

*The complex anatomy of the RV makes assessment of RV function challenging. Geometric assumptions that are used in the calculation of LV volume and function do not apply to the RV.*

*There is no doubt that CMR is the established method for RV volume and function assessments[15] with good interstudy reproducibility. But many patients with CCTGA, such as this patient, have a pacemaker, and CMR is, at least at the time of writing, contraindicated.*

*Angiographic assessment of RV function by ventriculography has been traditionally used, but the same confounding geometric challenges apply and the assessment is largely subjective. It has generally been replaced by other noninvasive means. Cardiac catheterization may still be necessary in certain cases to assess hemodynamics but not to assess RV volume.*

*Nuclear assessment of systemic LV function is commonly used in adult cardiology, but RV assessment has been a problem. In cases where MR cannot be done, equilibrium radionuclide ventriculography can be considered. It has been shown to have acceptable agreement with CMR,[1] but interpretation of these images requires an understanding of the abnormal anatomy and should be done in departments experienced with ACHD.*

*Although universally available, safe, and relatively inexpensive, echocardiography can still be a challenge when used to assess RV volumes, both because of the irregular RV shape and limitations of the acoustic windows. Advances in 3D echo have shown good results in RV assessment for children,[16] but there are concerns about the application of this method in adults with a larger RV and less accessible windows, the situation found in the typical adult patient with a systemic RV.*

*The Doppler-derived myocardial performance index (MPI) (or Tei index) to assess RV function is independent of geometry. Systemic RV function as assessed by RV MPI (calculated from the equation: $(a - b)/b$ where $a$ = aortic outflow ejection time obtained in the left parasternal short-axis view and $b$ = left AV regurgitation jet time obtained in the apical four-chamber view) was recently compared to the CMR assessment of RV function[17] and found to correlate well. The MPI has been used successfully to estimate RV ejection fraction ($RVEF = 64.5 - [44.8 \times MPI]$). Although the RV MPI may become a useful tool to measure RV function, it does not provide any information about RV volumes.*

*Multisector fast cardiac CT may play a more important role in the future for patients unsuitable for CMR. It can view the RV in multiple planes and use Simpson's rule much in the same way as CMR. However, the radiation dose is substantial and it requires the use of a contrast agent. As a result, it really cannot be used for regular serial studies. There has been recent work comparing 16 slice cardiac CT and CMR assessment of RV size and function in patients with ACHD.[18] The analysis showed good agreement between the methods in the estimates of systolic and diastolic volumes, as well as ejection fraction. It should be remembered that CT is typically performed at held-inspiration, whereas CMR is performed at held end-expiration, and small*

*differences may result. We await further comparative studies, but in the interim, cardiac CT probably offers the best alternative to CMR for evaluation of RV size and function in the patient who cannot undergo CMR.*

## 3. What treatment options should be considered for worsening exercise function in CCTGA?

***Tricuspid Valve Surgery:*** *In CCTGA, tricuspid regurgitation occurs as a result of the valvular anatomic abnormalities, as well as the higher pressure load of the systemic circulation on the tricuspid valve. The tricuspid regurgitation, in turn, places additional volume load on the systemic RV leading to RV dilatation and greater tricuspid valve dysfunction. Patients with CCTGA should be followed for tricuspid regurgitation and considered for tricuspid valve replacement (repair is rarely possible) at an early stage before further worsening of RV function. Better outcomes of tricuspid valve replacement have been noted in patients with a preoperative ejection fraction higher than 44%.[19] In this patient's case, tricuspid valve replacement was not being considered because of his already severe RV dysfunction. Poor preoperative ejection fraction has been associated with the postoperative need for heart transplant in CCTGA patients.[20]*

***ASD Closure:*** *In general, an ASD places excess volume load on the pulmonary ventricle. Early closure of a significant ASD is advocated in an effort to prevent atrial enlargement and dysfunction of the pulmonary ventricle. In this patient's case, closure of the ASD will not improve systemic RV failure. In fact, the presence of the ASD in this case has a protective feature in that it reduces the volume delivered to the systemic ventricle. Closure of the ASD would only add to the volume load of the systemic RV and would worsen the clinical situation.*

***CRT:*** *Increasingly, CRT is applied to systemic LV failure in acquired heart disease. In selected patients, CRT has been shown to improve symptoms and to reduce the mortality rate by 50%.[21] Experience with CRT in patients with systemic RV failure is limited. CRT has demonstrated a beneficial reduction of functional MR when used in LV failure, but there has not been a similar reduction of tricuspid regurgitation in patients with systemic RV failure.[9]*

***Cardiac Transplantation:*** *ACHD patients account for less than 2% of all patients undergoing orthotopic heart transplantation, but this percentage is increasing as the number of adults with congestive heart disease increases. There are special challenges. These patients have often had previous surgeries, and have complex anatomy. This patient has the special challenge of the PA aneurysm. Extra care will be needed to avoid direct entry into that aneurysm at the time of sternotomy, and it will be necessary for the donor heart to have the entire length of the PA and bifurcation available for the eventual anastomosis to the right and left branches. Transplant recipients with ACHD have a higher perioperative mortality as well as a lower 5-year (68%) and 8-year (62%) survival when compared to patients receiving transplant for acquired heart disease. Recent data have clarified that the excess mortality occurs in the first year. Three-year survival (95%) among first-year survivors was no worse than for patients who had been transplanted for ischemic heart disease or cardiomyopathy (88%). Risk factors for increased first-year mortality included prolonged ischemic time during the surgery because of the increased complexity of the surgery, as well as elevated right atrial pressures in keeping with poorer RV function in these patients.[22] Even with these concerns, cardiac transplant surgery offers this patient his best therapeutic option.*

*This young man has all the indicators of poor prognosis in the short term. He is failing medical therapy and has class III–IV symptoms. ASD closure will be of no benefit, and his systemic RV function is too poor to consider TVR at this late stage. CRT is of unproven benefit in patients with failing systemic RV and would be technically challenging. Although not without its own challenges, cardiac transplantation is known to be of long-term benefit and is the best therapeutic option for this patient.*

## FINAL DIAGNOSIS

CCTGA with systemic RV failure despite aggressive medical therapy

## PLAN OF ACTION

Referral for transplantation

## OUTCOME

After considerable discussion with the patient and his family, and multidisciplinary panels, he was referred for transplantation. He was admitted for complete pretransplant assessment and medication adjustment but subsequently left the hospital against medical advice. He did not return for medical follow-up and 2 weeks later was found dead at home. No autopsy was undertaken.

The tragedy of this case is unfortunately not a rare occurrence in CHD, and a humbling reminder of the frailty of many of these patients. The published literature shows that the long-term survival in CCTGA is lower than the general population (75% survival to 20 years).[23] Mortality is worse when coexisting lesions exist. Unexpected patient deaths are a strong reminder of the need for dedicated research in the field.

This young man's deteriorating course points out the limitations in the available therapies for patients with complicated CCTGA. His decision to leave the hospital rather than pursue a course to cardiac transplantation may have been related to his frustration of having been a lifelong patient and not being prepared to face not only major surgery, but also the ongoing morbidities of heart transplantation.[24] As an adult, he has the right to make therapeutic decisions but the clinician has the responsibility to ensure that any decision is made on the basis of an informed choice and that the patient is aware of implications of his or her choice.

## Selected References

1. Hornung TS, Derrick GP, Deanfield JE, Redington AN: Transposition complexes in the adult: A changing perspective. Cardiology Clinics 20:405–420, 2002.
2. Graham TP, Bernard YD, Mellen BG, et al: Long term outcome in congenitally corrected transposition of the great arteries: A multi-institutional study. J Am Coll Cardiol 36:255–261, 2000.
3. Connelly MS, Liu PP, Williams WG, et al: Congenitally corrected transposition of the great arteries in the adult: Functional status and complications. J Am Coll Cardiol 27:1238–1243, 1996.
4. Heit JA. Risk factors for venous thromboembolism. Clin Chest Med 24:1–12, 2003.
5. Khairy P, Landzberg MJ, Gatzoulis MA, et al, for the Epicardial Versus ENdocardial pacing and Thromboembolic events (EVENT) Investigators: Transvenous pacing leads and systemic thromboemboli in patients with intracardiac shunts: A multicenter study. Circulation 113:2391–2397, 2006.
6. Hechter SJ, Fredriksen PM, Merchant N, et al: Angiotensin converting enzyme inhibitors in adults with the Mustard procedure. Am J Cardiol 87:660–663, 2001.
7. Bayer AS, Scheld WM: Endocarditis and intravascular infections. In Mandell GL, Bennett JE, Dolin R (eds): Principles and Practice of Infectious Diseases, 5th ed. Philadelphia, Churchill Livingstone, 2000.
8. Wilkoff BL, Cook JR, Epstein AE, et al: Dual-chamber pacing or ventricular backup pacing in patients with an implantable defibrillator: The Dual Chamber and VVI Implantable Defibrillator (DAVID) Trial. JAMA 288:3115–3123, 2002.
9. Janousek J, Tomek V, Chaloupecky V, et al: Cardiac resynchronization therapy: A novel adjunct to the treatment and prevention of systemic right ventricular failure. J Am Coll Cardiol 44:1927–1931, 2004.
10. Webb GD, Smallhorn JF, Therrien J, Redington AN: Congenital heart disease. In Zipes DP, Libby P, Bonow RO, Braunwald E (eds): Braunwald's Heart Disease, 7th ed. Philadelphia, Elsevier Saunders, 2005.
11. Diller GP, Dimopoulos K, Okonko D, et al: Exercise intolerance in adult congenital heart disease. Comparative severity, correlates, and prognostic implication. Circulation 112:828–835, 2005.
12. Veldtman GR, Dearani JA, Warnes CA: Low pressure giant pulmonary artery aneurysms in the adult: Natural history and management strategies. Heart 89:1067–1070, 2003.
13. Hornung TS, Bernard EJ, Celermajer DS, et al: Right ventricular dysfunction in congenitally corrected transposition of the great arteries. Am J Cardiol 84:1116–1119, A10, 1999.
14. Babu-Narayan SV, Goktekin O, Moon JC, et al: Late gadolinium enhancement cardiovascular magnetic resonance of the systemic right ventricle in adults with previous atrial redirection surgery for transposition of the great arteries. Circulation 111:2091–2098, 2005.
15. Grothues F, Moon JC, Bellenger NG, et al: Interstudy reproducibility of right ventricular volumes, function and mass with cardiovascular magnetic resonance. Am Heart J 147:218–223, 2004.
16. Papavassiliou DP, Parks WJ, Hopkins KL, Fyfe DA: Three-dimensional echocardiographic measurement of right ventricular volume in children with congenital heart disease validated by magnetic resonance imaging. J Am Soc Echocardiogr 11:770–777, 1998.
17. Salehian O, Schwerzmann M, Merchant N, et al: Assessment of systemic right ventricular function in patients with transposition of the great arteries using the myocardial performance index. Comparison with cardiac magnetic resonance imaging. Circulation 110:3229–3233, 2004.
18. Raman SV, Cook SC, McCarthy B, Ferketich AK: Usefulness of multidetector row computed tomography to quantify right ventricular size and function in adults with either tetralogy of Fallot or transposition of the great arteries. Am J Cardiol 95:683–686, 2005.
19. Van Son JAM, Danielson GK, Huhta JC, et al: Late results of systemic atrioventricular valve replacement in corrected transposition. J Thorac Cardiovasc Surg 109:642–653, 1995.
20. Beauchesne LM, Warnes CA, Connolly HM, et al: Outcome of the unoperated adult who presents with congenitally corrected transposition of the great arteries. J Am Coll Cardiol 40:285–290, 2002.
21. Cleland JG, Daubert JC, Erdmann E, et al; Cardiac Resynchronization-Heart Failure (CARE-HF) Study Investigators: The effect of cardiac resynchronization on morbidity and mortality in heart failure. N Engl J Med 352:1539–1549, 2005.
22. Clemson BS, Kirklin JK, Canter CE, et al: Late outcomes after heart transplantation in adults with congenital heart disease: A multiinstitutional analysis (Abstract). J Heart Lung Transplantation 23:S168–S169, 2004.
23. Rutledge JM, Nihill MR, Fraser CD, et al: Outcome of 121 patients with congenitally corrected transposition of the great arteries. Pediatr Cardiol 23:137–145, 2002.
24. Horner T, Liberthson R, Jellinek MS: Psychosocial profile of adults with complex congenital heart disease. Mayo Clin Proc 75:31–36, 2000.

# Management of Systemic Ventricular Failure

**Judith Therrien**

Age: 28 years
Gender: Male
Occupation: Travel guide
Working diagnosis: Congenitally corrected transposition of the great arteries

## HISTORY

The presence of a murmur at birth led to an echocardiogram, and the patient remembered being told by his parents that he had reversed heart chambers. However, he had never undergone any surgical interventions.

Recently, during routine evaluation, he was told he may need valve surgery and sought a second opinion.

**Comments:** TGA means that there is a discordant ventriculoarterial connection. The term *congenitally corrected* means there is also a discordant AV connection, which hemodynamically "corrects" the abnormal ventriculoarterial connection. Thus, systemic venous blood enters the RA, empties into the LV, and is pumped to the pulmonary artery (PA). Hence, blood travels through the two circulatory beds in the normal sequence (in the absence of septal defects), but the RV is the systemic ventricle. Unless there are associated anomalies, the patients are not cyanotic and no intervention is needed in childhood or early adulthood. Common associated lesions are pulmonary stenosis and VSD. The expected consequences of CCTGA itself are systemic ventricular dysfunction, systemic tricuspid regurgitation (often associated with an Ebsteinoid malformation of the tricuspid valve), and complete heart block. Complete heart block is most likely related to the abnormal course of the conduction bundle (more anterosuperior and longer than seen in the normal heart).

## CURRENT SYMPTOMS

The patient was completely asymptomatic. He denied any shortness of breath on exertion and could run for 45 minutes without any problems. He had no orthopnea or nocturnal dyspnea. He also denied any palpitations, dizziness or syncope, chest pain, or leg swelling.

NYHA class: I

**Comments:** Patients even with mild to moderate systemic RV dysfunction will often be asymptomatic. Established moderate ventricular dysfunction will often precede the development of symptoms. Thus, when symptoms do develop, the patient's mortality is much higher (47% after 15 years, compared to only 5% in asymptomatic patients).[1]

## CURRENT MEDICATIONS

Perindopril 4 mg daily

**Comments:** Although there is little evidence proving the benefit of ACE inhibitor in patients with systemic right ventricular dysfunction,[2,3] data from studies of ACE inhibitors on systemic LV dysfunction in other forms of heart disease have been extrapolated to adults with systemic RVs. As a consequence, many adults with a systemic RV are empirically treated with such drugs, even without symptoms, unless contraindicated.

## PHYSICAL EXAMINATION

BP 130/80 mm Hg, HR 64 bpm, oxygen saturation at rest 95%

Height 165 cm, weight 55 kg, BSA 1.59 m$^2$

Surgical scars: None

Neck veins: There was a normal waveform visible 3 cm above the sternal angle.

Lungs/chest: Clear to auscultation

Heart: The rhythm was regular. The apex beat was normal (palpable at 10 cm from the midsternal line in the fifth intercostal space). Heart sounds were also normal except for a single S2. No S3 or S4 was heard. There was a grade 3/4 systolic ejection murmur best heard at the second right intercostal space, and a 3/4 holosystolic murmur best heard at the apex radiating toward the left axilla. Peripheral pulses were normal.

Abdomen: There was no hepatosplenomegaly.

Extremities: Normal, no edema present, no clubbing

**Comments:** Unless the patient has severe pulmonary stenosis with a VSD, most patients with CCTGA will be acyanotic on examination.

The S2 is single, made of the A2 component. This is because the aorta is anterior and easily heard, whereas the pulmonary valve is posterior, which makes the P2 inaudible.[4]

The murmur may be due to subpulmonary stenosis.

## LABORATORY DATA

| | |
|---|---|
| Hemoglobin | 14.9 g/dL (11.5–15.0) |
| Hematocrit/PCV | **49%** (36–46) |
| MCV | 88 fL (83–99) |
| Platelet count | 215 × 10$^9$/L (150–400) |
| Sodium | 139 mmol/L (134–145) |
| Potassium | 4.1 mmol/L (3.5–5.2) |
| Creatinine | 0.7 mmol/dL (0.6–1.2) |
| Blood urea nitrogen | 3.1 mmol/L (2.5–6.5) |

# ELECTROCARDIOGRAM

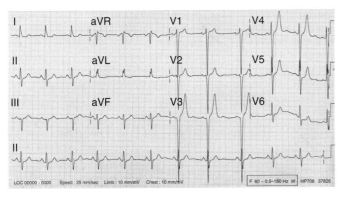

Figure 57-1 Electrocardiogram.

## FINDINGS

Heart rate: 68 bpm

QRS axis: −30°

QRS duration: 100 msec

Sinus rhythm with normal PR interval. The P-waves are broad and possibly notched in lead II. There are Q-waves in V2–3. Deep S-waves in V1–3. Tall peaked T-waves in the precordial leads.

***Comments:*** These are typical ECG findings of a patient with CCTGA. Note the absence of Q-waves laterally in leads V5 and V6 as well as the presence of Q-waves anteriorly, in this case in V2 and V3 but more commonly found in V1 and V2. This pattern is due to ventricular inversion with the septum depolarizing from right to left as opposed to the usual left-to-right depolarization pattern.[4] Note also the presence of probable LA enlargement (P-wave of 0.12 msec in lead II), which may suggest left AV valve regurgitation.

This patient does not have delta waves on his ECG, which should be sought since Wolff-Parkinson-White syndrome (accessory pathway) may be encountered in patients with CCTGA.

# CHEST X-RAY

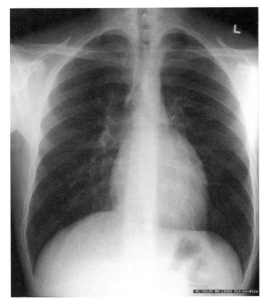

Figure 57-2 Posteroanterior projection.

## FINDINGS

Cardiothoracic ratio: 43%

Situs solitus, levocardia, left-sided aortic arch. The cardiac silhouette was not enlarged, and the lung parenchyma appeared normal.

***Comments:*** Because of the unusual position of the great vessels (a variable left anteroposterior relationship arrangement of the aorta and the pulmonary trunk), the pulmonary trunk is inconspicuous and the pedicle of the heart may be narrow because of the loss of the normal perpendicular relationship of the great vessels.

The patient has normal bronchial anatomy. The left bronchus (measured from the carina to its first branch) is nearly twice as long as the right bronchus. This finding indicates normal thoracic situs (situs solitus). Also, the gastric bubble is on the left, indicating normal abdominal situs. About a third of patients with CCTGA have dextrocardia (apex points to the right with most of the heart being located in the right hemithorax).

# EXERCISE TESTING

| Exercise protocol: | Bruce |
| Duration (min:sec): | 12:00 |
| Reason for stopping: | Leg fatigue |
| ECG changes: | None |

| | Rest | Peak |
| --- | --- | --- |
| Heart rate (bpm): | 64 | 175 |
| Percent of age-predicted max HR: | | 91 |
| O₂ saturation (%): | 97 | 97 |
| Blood pressure (mm Hg): | 130/80 | 155/90 |
| | | |
| Peak Vo₂ (mL/kg/min): | | 34.2 |
| Percent predicted (%): | | 84 |
| Metabolic equivalents: | | 9.6 |

***Comments:*** Often, patients with systemic RVs will consider themselves "asymptomatic" but will perform poorly on an exercise capacity test compared to normal controls.[5,6]

This was not the case for this patient, who performed at 84% of maximum predicted capacity for age, which is reassuring.

There is no evidence of chronotropic incompetence or exercise-induced AV block.

# ECHOCARDIOGRAM

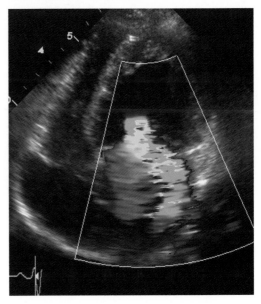

Figure 57-3 Left-sided atrioventricular valve regurgitation.

## FINDINGS

There was discordant AV connection and discordant ventriculoarterial connection, diagnostic of CCTGA. The morphologically right (systemic) ventricle was dilated but appeared to have good systolic function. The morphologically left (subpulmonary) ventricle was relatively small but also functioned normally. The septum deviated toward the pulmonary ventricle. There was moderate-to-severe regurgitation of the systemic AV valve (tricuspid valve). There was LA enlargement (48 mm). There was mild acceleration through the LVOT to the PA

*Comments:* The systemic ventricle (on the left in the four-chamber view; see Fig. 57-3) is a morphologic RV. Clues for this are apical displacement of the systemic AV valve, extensive trabeculations, and the presence of a moderator band in the systemic ventricle.

Significant regurgitation of the systemic (morphologically tricuspid) valve is a common problem in patients with a systemic RV. Many of them have an Ebstein-like anomaly of the tricuspid valve. Furthermore, tricuspid regurgitation may reflect systemic RV dysfunction and annular dilatation resulting in failure of the coaptation of the tricuspid valve leaflets.

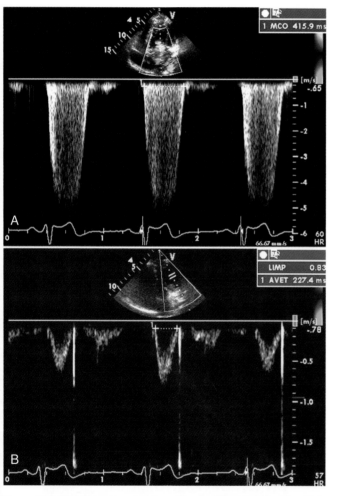

Figure 57-4 Doppler across the tricuspid valve (**A**) and aortic valve (**B**) is used to quantify the myocardial performance index.

## FINDINGS

Systemic RV function as assessed by the RV myocardial performance index (MPI, calculated from the equation: [a – b]/b

where b is aortic outflow ejection time obtained in the left parasternal short-axis view and a is left AV regurgitation jet time obtained in the apical four-chamber view).[7]

*Comments:* There is a good inverse correlation between systemic RV MPI obtained on echocardiography and systemic RV ejection fraction calculated by MRI. RV ejection fraction can be extrapolated from RV MPI using the following equation: EF (%) = 64.5 – (44.8 × MPI).[8]

# MAGNETIC RESONANCE IMAGING

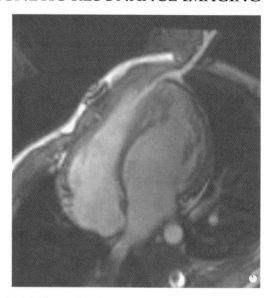

Figure 57-5 Oblique axial plane steady-state free precession cine, four-chamber view in diastole.

## FINDINGS

The study confirmed the anatomical findings of the echocardiogram, including moderate-to-severe systemic AV valve regurgitation and LA enlargement. Function of the systemic RV was mildly reduced, and the ventricle was enlarged.

### Ventricular Volume Quantification

|  | LV | (Normal range) | RV | (Normal range) |
|---|---|---|---|---|
| EDV (mL) | 98 | (77–195) | 215 | (88–227) |
| ESV (mL) | 39 | (19–72) | 117 | (23–103) |
| SV (mL) | 59 | (51–133) | 98 | (52–138) |
| EF (%) | 60 | (57–74) | 46 | (48–74) |
| EDVi (mL/m²) | **64** | (68–103) | **135** | (68–114) |
| ESVi (mL/m²) | 25 | (19–41) | **74** | (21–50) |
| SVi (mL/m²) | **39** | (44–68) | 62 | (40–72) |

*Comments:* MRI is considered the gold standard method to evaluate systemic RV size and function.[9,10] The RV cavity area is manually traced at multiple parallel levels from the base of the heart to the apex, including the RV outflow, in systole and diastole. These areas are summed to determine volume using Simpson's method.

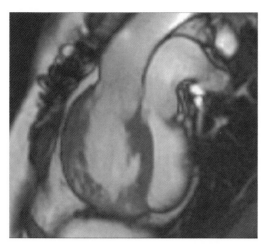

Figure 57-6 Oblique sagittal plane steady-state free precession cine.

## FINDINGS

The great arteries were parallel with the anterior aorta. There was mild dynamic subpulmonary stenosis.

**Comments:** A defining hallmark of transposed great arteries is their parallel relationship, with the aorta located more anteriorly. Note that the aorta and PA lie in a plane directly behind the sternum, which is why a traditional posteroanterior CXR projection often shows a narrow vascular pedicle, as in this patient.

Some degree of dynamic narrowing of the subpulmonary outflow tract is appreciated, though it does not appear severe.

## CATHETERIZATION

### HEMODYNAMICS

Heart rate      64 bpm

|          | Pressure            | Saturation (%) |
|----------|---------------------|----------------|
| SVC      |                     | 71             |
| IVC      |                     | 74             |
| RA       | mean 8              |                |
| LV       | 39/9                |                |
| PA       | 28/12 mean 16       | 72             |
| PCWP     | mean 10 (V-wave 24) | 98             |
| RV       | 108/6               | 98             |
| Aorta    | 105/70 mean 84      | 98             |

**Calculations**

| | |
|---|---|
| Qp (L/min) | 3.74 |
| Qs (L/min) | 3.70 |
| Cardiac index (L/min/m²) | 2.33 |
| Qp/Qs | 1.01 |
| PVR (Wood units) | 2.68 |
| SVR (Wood units) | 20.53 |

### FINDINGS

Gradient across the LV-PA outflow was 11 mm Hg.

**Comments:** Large V-waves reflected the severity of the systemic AV valve regurgitation.

1. How should function of a systemic RV be assessed?

*Functional assessment of the RV has always been a challenge because of its position and irregular geometry. The current gold standard for measuring systemic right ventricular volume and function is CMR.[9,10] CT angiography can provide similar volume data. Other easily obtainable measurements have recently emerged as alternatives. The RV MPI by transthoracic echocardiography is easy to obtain and has been shown to correlate well with RVEF.[8] Radionuclide angiography is also an alternative when MRI is not available or is contraindicated.[11] Three-dimensional echocardiography may emerge as a clinical tool to assess RV function in the adult patient, whether in the pulmonary or systemic position. These quantification methods estimate an ejection fraction, which is still used as the main yardstick for assessment of systemic ventricular function.*

2. Why does this patient have left (systemic) AV valve regurgitation?

*There are two possible reasons for left (systemic tricuspid) AV valve regurgitation in CCTGA patients. One is failed leaflet coaptation from ventricular systolic dysfunction and/or ventricular and annular dilatation. When the morphologic LV produces lower pressure than the morphologic RV, the geometry of the inlet valves can become more unfavorable for the morphologic tricuspid valve.[12] The other is from associated Ebsteinoid deformation of the valve (apical displacement of the septal leaflet, see Cases 30 and 31), which occurs in a significant subset of patients.*

3. When should CCTGA patients with substantial systemic AV valve regurgitation be offered surgery?

*The decision to offer AV valve replacement or repair in a systemic RV is a difficult one. The considerations include the morphology of the valve, the size and function of the systemic RV, and the patient's symptoms. Systemic AV valve repair in this setting is invariably unsuccessful, hence the need for replacement.*

*Poor outcome in patients with CCTGA is associated with severe systemic AV valve regurgitation, as well as with systemic RV dysfunction, or the presence of other associated lesions, namely VSD, pulmonary stenosis, or an Ebsteinoid systemic AV valve (tricuspid valve).[13-15] Therefore, this argues for intervention before dysfunction develops.*

*Given that most patients with CCTGA are asymptomatic despite some degree of systemic ventricular dysfunction, and given that mortality is extremely high once symptoms develop,[1] intervention should be offered before the onset of symptoms. In patients with moderate-to-severe systemic AV valve regurgitation, it is generally accepted that AV valve replacement should be offered before the RV ejection fraction drops below 45%.[16] This reemphasizes the need for a reliable method to determine serial RV ejection fraction.*

*In this patient, his reassuring exercise tolerance and normal ventricular function perhaps argue for waiting. At the same time, the severity of the regurgitation (regurgitant fraction of 43%) is severe enough to warrant intervention even in the absence of symptoms.*

4. Is the subpulmonary stenosis clinically important?

*The appearance of the subpulmonary area (LVOT) by MRI suggests mild dynamic obstruction.*

*When the inlet valve of the systemic ventricle is to be replaced, we do not need to worry about geometry between the morphologic tricuspid and the mitral valves. In other words, the morphologic LV can be pressure-offloaded as much as the RV is in the normal circulation. However, the known abnormal course of the conduc-*

*tion bundle greatly limits incision to musculature of the subpulmonary area. It is virtually impossible, in many cases, to create an effective myectomy without causing heart block for treating obstruction across the LVOT in CCTGA.*

5. Should other surgical alternatives be explored?

*The patient is asymptomatic, and therefore drastic measures are not necessary. In the setting of worsening progressive ventricular failure and severe valve regurgitation, valve replacement may be too risky. Other interventions that might be considered include a double switch operation or heart transplantation.*

*A double switch procedure (atrial redirection using an intra-atrial baffle combined with an arterial switch) can be done after adequate LV retraining (LV undergoing hypertrophic change) with PA banding. This is a theoretical option that has been applied to children. This approach converts an intrinsically abnormal systemic AV valve (with Ebstein anomaly) to a subpulmonary AV valve, and thus obviates the need for systemic AV valve replacement, which is more hazardous in children.[17]*

*The presence of LVOT obstruction represents a relative contraindication or absolute contraindication when the obstruction is fixed, even though the obstruction in theory would help "train" the LV. Thus, a double switch procedure is not recommended for adult patients, as the effects of pulmonary banding on left ventricular retraining are questionable in adults (hypertrophic as opposed to hyperplastic effect).[18]*

*Some may argue that banding of the pulmonary trunk alone, without consideration of the anatomic biventricular repair, could make regurgitation across the systemic inlet valve less. Despite obstruction across the LVOT in this patient, catheterization demonstrated that systolic pressure of the morphologic LV was less than half systemic. With LV pressure raised to a systemic level, the ventricular septum could be flattened and the left-sided AV valve might get a better configuration. However, this palliative procedure, particularly in adults, would possess too much uncertainty to choose.*

*The abnormal anatomy in CCTGA does not disqualify a patient from heart transplantation. CCTGA is often associated with dextrocardia, but transplant can be performed even in this setting, though surgical expertise on the unique anatomy is necessary. This patient's pulmonary vascular resistance is still normal, which would also not disqualify him. Therefore, if and when symptoms and ventricular dysfunction warrant this in the future, transplantation might be an option. However, he does not require this now.*

## FINAL DIAGNOSIS

Asymptomatic CCTGA

Mild systemic RV systolic dysfunction

Moderate-to-severe left AV valve regurgitation

Mild subpulmonary obstruction (dynamic)

## PLAN OF ACTION

Elective systemic AV valve replacement

## INTERVENTION

Through a median sternotomy, the heart was approached. Establishing cardiopulmonary bypass in a standard way, the aorta was cross-clamped. By a trans-septal approach (incising the RA and the atrial septum), the left-sided morphologic tricuspid valve was approached. A bileaflet mechanical valve (size: 31 mm) was placed at a para-annular position. The LVOT was inspected through the right-side morphologic mitral valve.

The outflow tract appeared to be widely open, and there were no resectable tissues present to enlarge the area. After oversewing the atrial septal incision and right atriotomy, coming off bypass was uneventful without heart block.

To maintain a contribution from the tensor apparatus to ventricular contraction, it is recommended to preserve tendinous cord–papillary muscle complexes as often employed in ordinary mitral valve replacement. This can be more relevant in the setting of the RV as a systemic pumping chamber. In terms of choice of prostheses, either a mechanical or a bioprosthetic valve is available. There is no fundamental difference from ordinary mitral valve replacement except for a minor concern that when a bioprosthesis is to be implanted for the tricuspid position, redundant leaflet remnants, if too much is left, might interfere with the function of the artificial leaflets in the longer term.[19]

## OUTCOME

The postoperative recovery was unremarkable, and the patient quickly returned to normal activities in less than a month. He felt well. He had regularly scheduled visits and echocardiography in the first year after surgery.

Three years later he continued to report no limiting symptoms. His prosthetic systemic AV valve was functioning well by echocardiography. His peak $Vo_2$ was 37.8 mL/kg/min, and his RV ejection fraction by MRI was 51%.

## Selected References

1. Piran S, Veldtman G, Siu S, et al: Heart failure and ventricular dysfunction in patients with single or systemic right ventricles. Circulation 105:1189–1194, 2002.
2. Hechter SJ, Fredriksen PM, Merchant N, et al: Angiotensin converting enzyme inhibitors in adults with the Mustard procedure. Am J Cardiol 87:660–663, 2001.
3. Lester SJ, McElhinney DB, Virola E, et al: Effects of losartan in patients with a systemically functioning morphologic right ventricle after atrial repair of transposition of the great arteries. Am J Cardiol 88:1314–1316, 2001.
4. Therrien J, Webb GD: Adult congenital heart disease. In Braunnald E, Zipes DP, Libby P (eds): Heart Disease: A Textbook of Cardiovascular Medicine, 6th ed. Philadelphia: WB Saunders, 2001.
5. Connelly MS, Walters JE, McLaughlin PR, et al: Functional capacity in adult patients with Mustard correction. J Am Coll Cardiol 25:378A, 1995.
6. Fredriksen PM, Chen A, Hechter S, et al: Exercise capacity in adult patients with congenitally corrected transposition of the great arteries. Heart 85:191–195, 2001.
7. Tei C, Ling LH, Hodge DO, et al: New index of combined systolic and diastolic myocardial performance: A simple and reproducible measure of cardiac function—a study in normals and dilated cardiomyopathy. J Cardiol 26:357–366, 1995.
8. Salehian O, Schwerzmann M, Merchant N, et al: Assessment of systemic right ventricular function in patients with transposition of the great arteries using myocardial performance index: Comparison with cardiac magnetic resonance imaging. Circulation 110:3229–3233, 2004.
9. Jauhiainen T, Jarvinen VM, Hekali PE, et al: MR gradient echo volumetric analysis of human cardiac casts: Focus on the right ventricle. J Computer Assisted Tomography 22:899–903, 1998.
10. Heusch A, Koch JA, Krogmann ON, et al: Volumetric analysis of the right and left ventricle in a porcine heart model: Comparison of three-dimensional echocardiography, magnetic resonance imaging and angiocardiography. Eur J Ultrasound 9:245–255, 1999.
11. Hornung TS, Anagnostopoulos C, Bhardwaj P, et al: Comparison of equilibrium radionuclide ventriculography with cardiovascular magnetic resonance for assessing the systemic right ventricle after Mustard or Senning procedures for complete transposition of the great arteries. Am J Cardiol 92:640–643, 2003.
12. Koh M, Yagihara T, Uemura H, et al: Functional biventricular repair using left ventricle-pulmonary artery conduit in patients

with discordant atrioventricular connections and pulmonary outflow tract obstruction: Does conduit obstruction maintain tricuspid valve function? Eur J Cardio-Thorac Surg 26:767–772, 2004.

13. Graham TP, Jr, Bernard YD, Mellen BG, et al: Long-term outcome in congenitally corrected transposition of the great arteries: A multi-institutional study. J Am Coll Cardiol 36:1365–1370, 2000.

14. Voskuil M, Hazekamp MG, Kroft LJ, et al: Postsurgical course of patients with congenitally corrected transposition of the great arteries. Am J Cardiol 83:558–562, 1999.

15. Prieto LR, Hordof AJ, Secic M, et al: Progressive tricuspid valve disease in patients with congenitally corrected transposition of the great arteries. Circulation 98:997–1005, 1998.

16. Van Son JA, Danielson GK, Huhta JC, et al: Late results of systemic atrioventricular valve replacement in corrected transposi-tion. J Thor Cardiovasc Surg 109:642–652, 1995.

17. Yeh T Jr, Connelly MS, Coles JG, et al: Atrioventricular discordance: Results of repair in 127 patients. J Thor Cardiovasc Surg 117:1190–1203, 1999.

18. Benzaquen BS, Webb GD, Colman JM, et al: Arterial switch operation after Mustard procedures in adult patients with transposition of the great arteries: Is it time to revise our strategy? Am Heart J 147:E8, 2004.

19. Kawahira Y, Yagihara T, Uemura H, et al: Replacement of the tricuspid valve in children with congenital cardiac malformations. J Heart Valve Dis 9:636–640, 2000.

# Late Outcome Following Systemic Tricuspid Valve Replacement

**Andrew N. Redington and Khalid Alnajashi**

**Age: 55 years**
**Gender: Female**
**Occupation: Accountant**
**Working diagnosis: Congenitally corrected transposition of the great arteries, ventricular septal defect, pulmonary stenosis**

## HISTORY

The patient was well during her early childhood, only coming to medical attention when a heart murmur was heard at the age of 11 years. She was initially diagnosed (elsewhere, and incorrectly) as having TOF. She remained unoperated and relatively well. She was advised to avoid pregnancy because of her ACHD.

At age 31, she presented with progressive functional deterioration and was referred to an ACHD center. Repeat cardiac catheterization established the diagnosis of situs inversus with mirror-image atrial arrangement, dextrocardia, discordant AV and ventriculoarterial connections (CCTGA), a large VSD, severe pulmonary stenosis, and a single coronary artery from the right coronary sinus.

Soon thereafter she underwent VSD patch closure with placement of a LV-to-pulmonary artery (PA) valved conduit.

The immediate postoperative course was complicated by complete heart block; thus a transvenous permanent pacemaker, VVI mode, was inserted.

The early postoperative period was complicated by recurrent episodes of atrial flutter, ultimately requiring a low dose of amiodarone for control. Thereafter she was well, with a marked improvement in symptoms and functional capacity.

Within 2 years of surgery she had symptoms and signs of pulmonary venous congestion and had developed a new pansystolic murmur. The echocardiogram and cardiac catheter performed at that time showed severe regurgitation of the morphologically tricuspid (systemic AV) valve. Consequently, 3 years after her initial surgery, she underwent tricuspid valve replacement with a 25-mm Bjork-Shiley mechanical prosthesis.

Despite developing paroxysmal atrial flutter for which she was treated with atenolol, she remained very well with excellent functional capacity and only mild symptoms of exercise limitation. She was seen for routine evaluation.

***Comments:*** CCTGA is an uncommon congenital cardiac anomaly. It accounts for less than 0.5% of all congenital heart disease. The most common associated defects are VSD (60%–80%), and pulmonary stenosis, or, more appropriately, LVOT obstruction (30%–50%). Tricuspid valve abnormalities are also common (14%–56%).[1,2] Ebstein malformation, dysplasia of the valve, abnormalities of the subvalve apparatus, and straddling and overriding with respect to the VSD have all been reported.[3,4]

Neither her ACHD nor anticoagulation is an absolute contraindication to pregnancy. The outcomes of pregnancy in 22 women with CCTGA[5] have been reported. There were a total of 60 pregnancies resulting in 50 live births, with no pregnancy-related deaths, and none of the live infants was diagnosed with congenital heart disease.

Patients with CCTGA are at high risk of developing AV block whether operated on or not. The sinus node is normally positioned, but the AV conduction tissue is grossly abnormal. At 20-year follow-up, 45% of unoperated patients will have developed third-degree heart block, slightly higher than the suggested figure of 30%.[6,7] Subsequently, it has been reported that spontaneous complete heart block in this population occurs at a rate of about 2% per year.[8,9] Surgically induced heart block is still common. The anatomy of the AV node was described in 1973 by Bob Anderson.[10] While this knowledge transformed the incidence of complete heart block in those undergoing surgery, it remains a risk.

Several authors have shown that the regular AV node located at the apex of the triangle of Koch rarely gives origin to a penetrating AV conduction bundle. Instead, there is an anterior course of an anomalous AV node and penetrating bundle, which is commonly located beneath the opening of the right atrial appendage at the lateral margin of the area of pulmonary-to-mitral valve continuity. The elongated bundle has a superficial course underneath the right anterior facing leaflet of the pulmonary valve and descends for some distance before branching.[10,11] Histological study often reveals pathologic changes within the bundle, such as fibrosis, even in the absence of abnormal conduction.[12]

The development of new tricuspid regurgitation within 2 years of operation is not surprising in CCTGA after a conventional (classic) repair. Voskuil and colleagues studied the postoperative outcomes of 73 patients with CCTGA and found that RV function and tricuspid valve function both deteriorated with age. These complications developed more frequently after conventional intracardiac operations compared with patients undergoing palliative intervention or no surgery at all.[13] Indeed, several studies have shown that RV dysfunction and tricuspid regurgitation both deteriorate more frequently following intracardiac operation than in patients either unoperated or treated with closed heart procedures.[14,15]

Tricuspid valve function depends on the loading conditions of the ventricles and the secondary effects on septal geometry.

Interventions that increase RV volume or decrease LV pressure induce and worsen tricuspid regurgitation.[16] Graham and colleagues reviewed 182 adult patients from 19 institutions.[17] The strongest risk factors for clinical congestive heart failure and RV dysfunction included tricuspid valve surgery, important tricuspid regurgitation, history of any open-heart surgery, and pacemaker therapy.

Atrial arrhythmia is common. Connelly and associates[18] reported outcomes in 52 patients with CCTGA. During a period of approximately 10 years of follow-up, 25% died and 36% of the survivors had documented atrial fibrillation, atrial flutter, or supraventricular tachycardia.

## CURRENT SYMPTOMS

Now 22 years after valve replacement, the patient is asymptomatic. She works full time and tolerates long walks and occasional vigorous activity.

NYHA class: I

## CURRENT MEDICATIONS

Warfarin (target INR 2.5–3.5)

Aspirin 81 mg once daily

Atenolol 50 mg once daily

**Comments:** Patients with all types of mechanical valves require antithrombotic prophylaxis. Bjork and Iienze in 1975 reported that among patients (without complex ACHD) with the Bjork-Shiley spherical disk valves who received no prophylaxis or prophylaxis with aspirin alone, thromboemboli occurred in 23% per year.[19]

In patients who have mechanical valves and additional risk factors such as atrial fibrillation, myocardial infarction, left atrial enlargement, endocardial damage, and low ejection fraction, the American College of Chest Physicians recommended adding low-dose aspirin, 75 to 100 mg/day.[20,21]

## PHYSICAL EXAMINATION

BP 110/70 mm Hg, HR 75 bpm, oxygen saturation 98%

Height 150 cm, weight 45.4 kg, BSA 1.38 m²

Surgical scars: Bilateral thoracotomy and median sternotomy scars

Neck veins: JVP was 4 cm above the sternal angle.

Lungs/chest: Chest was clear. Apex beat was to the right.

Heart: Normal prosthetic heart sounds. The time between the second heart sound and the opening click of the mechanical valve was wide, indicating relatively normal LA pressures. There was a short, grade 2–3/6 systolic ejection type murmur at the left sternal border. There was no diastolic murmur. Peripheral pulses were palpable and normal in character.

Abdomen: Soft with no organomegaly

Extremities: No peripheral edema

**Comments:** Her clinical examination is in keeping with her underlying diagnosis and good clinical status. The finding of a right-sided apical impulse is seen in about 20% of patients with CCTGA. The atrial situs is inversus (mirror image) in 5% to 8% of patients, and solitus (usual) in 92% to 95%.[22]

At the time of her initial VSD closure and conduit placement, the surgeon elected to expose the heart using two thoracotomy incisions because of, as he described, "an awkward anatomy with situs inversus."

The short ejection systolic murmer implies little LVOT/conduit obstruction.

The absence of a diastolic murmur argues against significant conduit valve regurgitation, especially since the conduit is substernal.

The liver in situs inversus will be left-sided, so one must palpate in the correct area.

## LABORATORY DATA

| | |
|---|---|
| Hemoglobin | 14.0 g/dL (11.5–15.0) |
| Hematocrit/PCV | 43% (36–46) |
| MCV | 94 fL (83–99) |
| Platelet count | $168 \times 10^9$/L (150–400) |
| Sodium | 139 mmol/L (134–145) |
| Potassium | 4.2 mmol/L (3.5–5.2) |
| Creatinine | 0.62 mg/dL (0.6–1.2) |
| Blood urea nitrogen | 2.8 mmol/L (2.5–6.5) |

### OTHER RELEVANT LAB RESULTS
| | |
|---|---|
| PT | 33.1 seconds |
| INR | 3.04 |

**Comments:** The normal hemoglobin and MCV are somewhat remarkable in the context of chronic warfarin therapy.

In patients who have mechanical valves and additional risk factors such as atrial fibrillation, myocardial infarction, LA enlargement, endocardial damage, and low ejection fraction, the American College of Chest Physicians recommended a target INR of 3.0 or a range of 2.5 to 3.5.[20,21]

## ELECTROCARDIOGRAM

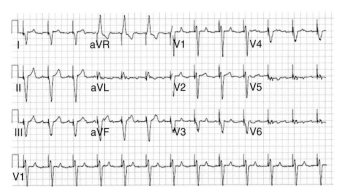

Figure 58-1 Electrocardiogram.

### FINDINGS
Heart rate: 76 bpm (paced)

QRS axis: Extreme right-axis deviation

QRS duration: 172 msec

The ECG showed characteristic loss of precordial voltage in the left chest leads because the patient has dextrocardia.

**Comments:** Patients with CCTGA have a higher incidence of preexcitation; the incidence of left- versus right-sided bypass tracts appears to be equal.[23]

The current ECG (left) shows a paced ventricular rhythm with atypical atrial flutter at 200 bpm and AV dissociation.

The patient is well, but the atrial arrhythmia should be managed and consideration should be given to an AV synchronous pacing mode to maximize function and perhaps prevent deterioration.

# CHEST X-RAY

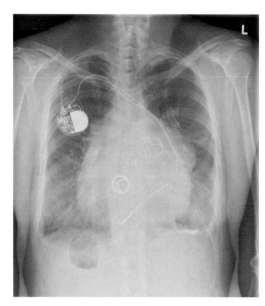

Figure 58-2 Posteroanterior projection.

## FINDINGS

Cardiothoracic ratio: 63%

Atrial and abdominal situs inversus (mirror image) with dextro/mesocardia. There was mild-to-moderate cardiomegaly.

***Comments:*** It is just possible to discern the presence of bronchial situs inversus (long morphologic left mainstem bronchus to the right-sided lung field), which indicates atrial situs inversus. This is supported by the mirror-image visceral situs (stomach bubble to the right, liver shadow to the left), and the course of the pacing wires. Atrial and abdominal situs are expected to concur.

Both valve prostheses can be seen, the tricuspid valve replacement (TVR) is shown centrally, and the frame of the LV-PA tissue valve is seen in the lateral projection.

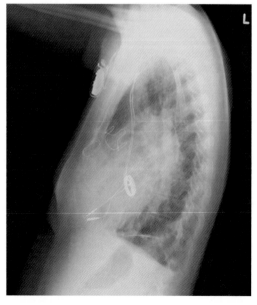

Figure 58-3 Lateral view.

## FINDINGS

As noted in the posteroanterior projection there is calcification of the left diaphragmatic pleura and thickening of the lower left pleural recess. The heart is very close to the posterior border of the sternum.

# EXERCISE TESTING

| Exercise protocol: | Bruce |
| Duration (min:sec): | 12:30 |
| Reason for stopping: | Leg pain |
| ECG changes: | Paced |

|  | Rest | Peak |
| --- | --- | --- |
| Heart rate (bpm): | 75 | 170 |
| Percent of age-predicted max HR: |  | 103 |
| O$_2$ saturation (%): | 98 | 93 |
| Blood pressure (mm Hg): | 110/70 | 150/85 |
|  |  |  |
| Peak Vo$_2$ (mL/kg/min): |  | 28 |
| Percent predicted (%): |  | 60 |
| Metabolic equivalents: |  | 9.4 |

***Comments:*** Aerobic capacity in patients with CCTGA is generally severely diminished, varying from 30% to 50% of the results achieved by healthy subjects. There is very little overlap with the normal range, with none of the CCTGA patients achieving Vo$_2$ values within the lower 15th centile range for normal values in one study.[24]

Furthermore, patients with CCTGA achieved significantly lower values of FVC, FEV1, and heart rate and systolic blood pressure compared to the predicted values, all of which may contribute to the reduced maximal oxygen uptake (Vo$_2$ max) found in these patients. Our patient has done surprisingly well. She is clearly NYHA class I.

# ECHOCARDIOGRAM

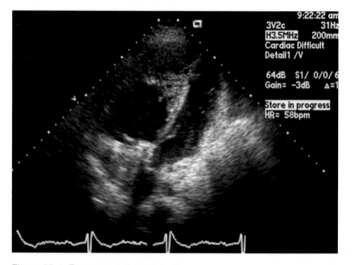

Figure 58-4 Parasternal short-axis view.

## FINDINGS

The prosthetic tricuspid valve was functioning normally with only trace regurgitation, a peak diastolic gradient of 12 mm Hg/mean gradient 5 mm Hg. There was moderate reduction in RV function, with mild enlargement of the RV at end diastole. The mitral valve (venous AV valve) was moderately regurgitant.

The LV (venous ventricle) was normal in size and function. The LV-PA conduit appeared unobstructed and only mildly incompetent. No aortic valve regurgitation was present.

***Comments:*** This patient was originally misdiagnosed on the basis of a cardiac catheterization performed elsewhere, prior to the introduction of cross-sectional echocardiography. Even so, the echo diagnosis of CCTGA relies on careful sequential analysis. In this case, there is mirror-image atrial arrangement and the systemic RV is on the right but connected to the right-sided morphologic LA and aorta.

This case also highlights an issue with nomenclature. This patient does not have L-TGA (a term often used generically to describe patients with CCTGA, or double discordance), as the aorta is anterior and right-sided. This is demonstrated by her CT images, as she had poor echo windows, and her aortic valve is anterior and to the right of the pulmonary valve. Thus, while this patient has discordant AV and ventriculoarterial connections, this is clearly not L-TGA. The substitution of the term L-TGA would be incorrect in this case.

## COMPUTED TOMOGRAPHY

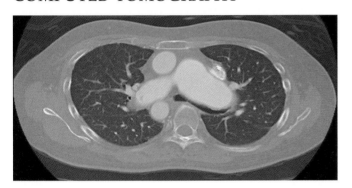

Figure 58-5 Axial view.

### Ventricular Volume Quantification

|  | LV | (Normal range) |
| --- | --- | --- |
| EDV (mL) | 116 | (52–141) |
| ESV (mL) | **63** | (13–51) |
| SV (mL) | 53 | (33–97) |
| EF (%) | **46** | (59–77) |
| EDVi (mL/m²) | 84 | (56–90) |
| ESVi (mL/m²) | **46** | (14–33) |
| SVi (mL/m²) | 39 | (37–62) |

### FINDINGS

Abdominal and cardiac situs inversus. There was AV and ventriculoarterial discordance, with a subaortic morphologic RV and a subpulmonary morphologic LV. A pacing wire was seen running into the (subpulmonary) ventricle. A prosthetic systemic AV valve was also seen (tricuspid position).

The PAs are enlarged (main PA, 31 mm; right PA, 28 mm; left PA, 42 mm), with quick tapering within the lungs. There were four pulmonary veins draining properly to the LA. The pericardium was unremarkable. A right-sided aortic arch was seen, with a mirror-image branching pattern. A left-sided supradiaphragmatic calcified plaque was noted (likely postoperative change).

***Comments:*** Ventricular function assessment revealed moderate dilation and dysfunction of the systemic RV. This is a frequent finding, even in asymptomatic patients with CCTGA.

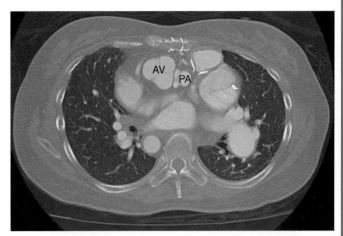

Figure 58-6 Axial view.

### FINDINGS

The aortic valve was anterior and to the right of the hypoplastic native pulmonic valve, but in the same cranio-caudal plane. The native pulmonic valve was bicuspid with a suboptimal opening and connected to a hypoplastic outflow tract and a hypoplastic proximal main PA.

***Comments:*** A ventriculopulmonary conduit was created with a bioprosthetic valve positioned to the left, slightly anteriorly and superiorly in comparison to the native pulmonic valve. The conduit was likely adherent to the chest wall. No stenosis was seen within the conduit. The posterior leaflet opened incompletely, but the opening area was felt to be satisfactory (around 1 cm²).

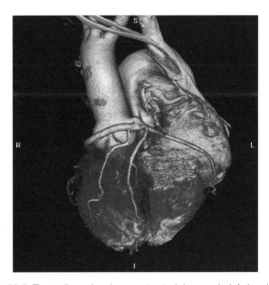

Figure 58-7 Three-dimensional reconstructed image. I, inferior; L, left; R, right; S, superior.

## FINDINGS

There was a single main coronary trunk arising from the left anterolateral coronary sinus that branched into the left and right coronary arteries. The right coronary artery lay just behind the sternum.

The hypoplastic native pulmonary valve/main PA, still in continuity with the PAs, was just behind the main single coronary artery.

**Comments:** (Note: For image clarity the LV-PA conduit had been removed during the 3D reconstruction to see the coronary artery course.) CMR was not possible because of the pacemaker in this patient. While there are some disadvantages to CT scanning (particularly the radiation dosage for repeated studies), this case illustrates the beautiful clarity of anatomic imaging that now can be achieved.

It is not uncommon to find anomalous coronary arteries in complex cases of situs inversus and CCTGA such as this.

## RADIONUCLIDE ANGIOGRAPHY

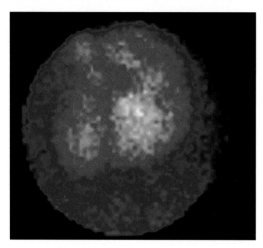

Figure 58-8 Radionuclide angiocardiography is a tool for assessment of the ventricular function during rest and exercise.

## FINDINGS

Decreased RV ejection fraction at rest (39%) and during exercise (46%). The LV ejection fraction at rest was 49% and 47% during exercise.

**Comments:** Fredriksen et al[24] reported a limited exercise-induced increase in systemic ventricular ejection fraction and a decrease in LV contractility in patients with CCTGA. The reduced fractional shortening of the systemic RV (both at rest and during exercise) is demonstrable with all techniques. The relevance of these observations is less well described, however. It is not known whether this represents an adaptive response, or a pathologic one. There are few data that show a correlation between RV shortening and either exercise capacity or outcomes in the absence of coexisting abnormalities such as tricuspid regurgitation. Indeed, RV failure in the absence of significant tricuspid regurgitation is rare in patients with CCTGA.

The explanation for the slight decrease in the subpulmonary LV ejection fraction, also widely reported, is also unclear. The diastolic pressure overload of the morphologic RV may be at the expense of pulmonary LV volume as the septum bulges into the LV. This may result in impaired diastolic filling of the LV, as suggested in previous studies of ventricular interdependence, and a lower ejection fraction on the pulmonary side. This remains speculative.

## CATHETERIZATION

Not performed

### FOCUSED CLINICAL QUESTIONS AND DISCUSSION POINTS

1. **Can the morphologic RV function as the systemic ventricle in the long term?**

*It has been argued that because of several disadvantages, the morphologic RV will inevitably fail in the systemic position.[25] Key factors include the shape of the morphologic RV, the configuration of the tricuspid valve, the disposition of the papillary muscles of the tricuspid valve, and that the RV is a one-coronary artery ventricle whereas the LV is a two-coronary artery ventricle.*

*Nonetheless, there are a number of reports of asymptomatic adults in the sixth, seventh, eighth, and ninth decades of life with CCTGA whose diagnosis was made incidentally. Such patients are used as evidence that the RV can function as the systemic RV for a normal life span.[26–32] The systemic RV in CCTGA patients has been compared to the normal morphologic LV function in healthy adults using MRI dobutamine stress testing.[33] The systemic RV had larger volume, a lower ejection fraction, but an appropriate response to dobutamine stress. The authors also found that values of unoperated patients with CCTGA were closer to normal.*

*Nonetheless, patients with "double discordance" but without any additional associated cardiac anomalies have a high prevalence of reversible and fixed myocardial ischemia, and these defects were associated with impaired wall motion and thickening.[34] Younger patients tended to have a normal RV ejection fraction, while this was likely to be reduced in the older patients.*

*Thus, in the absence of significant associated abnormalities, the function of the systemic RV may remain adequate for decades. It seems reasonable to suggest that it is less well adapted to cope with the secondary effects of cardiac surgery, tricuspid regurgitation and systemic hypertension, for example.*

2. **Can the previously normotensive subpulmonary LV be retrained to be capable of functioning as a systemic ventricle in an adult with CCTGA?**

*Brawn reported that PA banding with the aim of retraining the morphologic LV to allow a double switch to be performed can realign the septum with a higher morphologic LV pressure and can variably decrease the amount of tricuspid valve regurgitation.*

*Their cutoff for successful retraining of the morphologic LV was about 15 years of age in their cohort, and although PA banding can be considered in older patients, they had no success in retraining such a patient.[35]*

*Duncan and Mee reported that retraining the subpulmonary LV should produce (1) normal LV function in adolescents and older patients, with the capability of generating greater than 80% systemic blood pressure and suprasystemic pressure with the administration of isoproterenol, and/or (2) normal LV mass and wall thickness, indexed for weight and age, demonstrated by echocardiography and MRI. LV retraining is said to have failed if there is inadequate hypertrophy, if LV dysfunction develops, or if there is progression of atrial arrhythmias.[36]*

*It is unclear whether these recommendations reflect a physiologic resistance to retraining the "adult" subpulmonary LV, or failure of contemporary techniques to progressively band the ventricle without inducing failure. Benzaquen and colleagues[37] reported in a different population (adult patients with TGA after Mustard procedures) that acute PA banding achieving near-*

systemic subpulmonary LV pressure can rapidly lead to ventricular failure. A more gradual approach to PA banding may be required to achieve a successful outcome. Such a strategy may be easier to achieve with an externally adjustable PA band, currently in development at one or more centers.

At the time of her surgery, there was not the option of anatomic repair ("the double switch") for our patient.

Langley et al[38] reported that certain groups of patients with CCTGA are not suitable for anatomic repair, including older patients who may not respond to PA banding and younger patients with anatomic or morphologic contraindications. The presence of a straddling AV valve or an inlet VSD with no outlet extension, for example, would make it difficult to tunnel the VSD to the aorta without compromising the volume of the RV because of the size of the baffle. They suggested that patients who have well-balanced systemic and pulmonary circulations without marked desaturation, usually in association with a VSD and moderate pulmonary stenosis, are best managed conservatively without surgical intervention until such time as they show symptoms.

Brawn stated in 2005 that the risk of the operation, that is, an atrial switch with a Rastelli operation, the need for conduit change in the future, and the risk of heart block with pacemaker placement may outweigh the advantages of potentially improved quality of life with more stable hemodynamics after an anatomic repair.[39]

Therefore, the role of anatomic (as compared with "classic") repair remains controversial (see subsequent discussion).

3. **What are the indications for and long-term results of TVR in CCTGA?**

Van Son studied 40 patients with CCTGA and systemic AV valve insufficiency who underwent replacement (39 patients) or repair (one patient). The early mortality was 10% (n = 4), and 8 patients died at later follow-up. The principal cause of death in all 12 patients was systemic ventricular failure. Overall survival including early mortality was 78% at 5 years and 61% at 10 years. Survival excluding early mortality was 87% at 5 years and 68% at 10 years. Survivorship correlated with a preoperative systemic ventricular ejection fraction of 44% or more by echocardiography. Two patients underwent reoperations related to the systemic AV valve prosthesis. Follow-up extended to 26 years. To preserve systemic ventricular function, the authors suggested operation be considered at the earliest sign of systemic ventricular dysfunction as assessed by serial clinical evaluation and echocardiography.[40]

In the study of Hraska et al,[41] 20-year freedom from RV dysfunction after an intracardiac procedure was 39%. Significant risk factors for RV dysfunction were Ebstein malformation of the tricuspid valve, the need for TVR, and complete heart block. This finding is consistent with the report of Sano and colleagues,[42] in which 55% of patients had RV dysfunction after a classic intracardiac repair. On the basis of the data, deterioration of systemic RV function was not delayed by TVR. In fact, patients who required TVR at the initial operation or during follow-up had significantly poorer outcomes. Furthermore, the need for TVR was a significant predictor of RV dysfunction.[43]

Yeh et al also performed a meta-analysis of patients who had undergone physiologic or anatomic repair, reported from seven different centers. The age range was wide, varying from neonates until late adulthood, and the follow-up period ranged from a few months to decades, depending on the series. Overall, there were 480 patients who had physiologic repair. There were 61 operative deaths (13%), and the 10-year actuarial survival for these patients was approximately 70%. There were fewer patients who had anatomic repairs. Ten patients had arterial switch and atrial switch, while 48 had Rastelli atrial switch operations. The actuarial 10-year survival is not available because of the recent advent of these operations. The overall mortality (cohort to 1999), however, was 7%.[43]

4. **Should this patient undergo further surgery?**

This patient remains asymptomatic from a cardiac point of view, carrying out her daily activity and work with no limitation, in NYHA class I.

Her systemic RV is moderately reduced in function as seen by echocardiography, radionuclide angiography, and cardiac CT, with a well-functioning systemic mechanical tricuspid valve. The LV-PA conduit is functioning well with minimal stenosis and regurgitation as seen both by the echocardiography and the CT. While conduit replacement is likely to be required at some stage (this patient might also be suitable for transcatheter valve insertion), this is not necessary at present. Yeh et al[43] reported that in one series 15% (4 out of 27) of the patients required redo surgery because of tricuspid valve failure at a mean age of 10 years after the initial surgical repair, and, within 12 years, 49% of the patients required conduit replacement; another 13% of the patients had died before coming to conduit replacement. Therefore, there is no justification for surgery as yet.

## FINAL DIAGNOSIS

CCTGA, pulmonary stenosis, VSD

Prior VSD repair and placement of valved conduit from LV to PA

Prior systemic AV valve replacement

## PLAN OF ACTION

Routine follow-up

## INTERVENTION

None

## OUTCOME

The patient was again educated about the nature of her condition and things to watch for in the future, including worsening exertional breathlessness, palpitations, syncope, or unexplained fevers.

The patient remains well without any evidence of clinical deterioration.

## Selected References

1. Anderson KR, Danielson GK, McGoon DW, Lie JT: Ebstein's anomaly of the left-sided tricuspid valve. Pathological anatomy of the valvular malformation. Circulation 58:87–91, 1978.
2. Allwork SP, Bentall HH, Becker AE: Congenitally corrected transposition of the great arteries. Morphologic study of 32 cases. Am J Cardiol 38:910–912, 1976.
3. Losekoot TG, Becker AE: Discordant atrioventricular connexion and congenitally corrected transposition. In Anderson RH, Macartney FJ, Shinebourne EA, Tynan M (eds): Paediatric Cardiology. Edinburgh, Churchill Livingstone, 1987, pp 867–888.
4. Horvath P, Szufladowicz M, de Leval MR, et al: Tricuspid valve abnormalities in patients with atrioventricular discordance: Surgical implications. Ann Thorac Surg 57: 941–945, 1994.
5. Connelly MS, Liu PP, McLaughlin PR: Congenitally corrected transposition of the great arteries in the adult: Functional status and complications. JACC 27:1238–1243, 1996.
6. Fyler DC: L-transposition. In Nadas' Pediatric Cardiology. St. Louis, MO, Mosby, 1992, pp 701–708.
7. Mullins CE: Ventricular inversion. In Garson A, Jr, Bricker JT, McNamara DG (eds): The Science and Practice of Pediatric Cardiology. Philadelphia, Lea and Febiger, 1990, pp 1233–1245.

8. Huhta JC, Danielson GK, Ritter DG, Ilstru DM: Survival in atrio-ventricular discordance. Pediatr Cardiol 6:57–62, 1985.

9. McGrath LB, Kirklin JW, Blackstone EH, et al: Death and other events after cardiac repair in discordant atrioventricular connection. J Thorac Cardiovasc Surg 90:711–728, 1985.

10. Anderson RH, Arnold R, Wilkinson JL: The conducting system in congenitally corrected transposition. Lancet 1:1286–1288, 1973.

11. Losekoot TG, Anderson RH, Becker AE, et al: Congenitally Corrected Transposition. Edinburgh, Churchill Livingstone, 1983.

12. Anderson RH, Becker AE, Arnold R, Wilkinson JL: The conducting tissues in congenitally corrected transposition. Circulation 50:911–924, 1974.

13. Voskuil M, Hazekamp MG, Kroft LJ, et al: Postsurgical course of patients with congenitally corrected transposition of the great arteries. Am J Cardiol 83:558–562, 1999.

14. Termignon JL, Leca F, Vouhe PR, et al: "Classic" repair of congenitally corrected transposition and ventricular septal defect. Ann Thorac Surg 62:199–206, 1996.

15. Vouhe P, Sidi D: Congenitally corrected transposition of the great arteries: Results of classical surgery. In Redington AN, Brawn WJ, Deanfield JE, Anderson RH (eds): The Right Heart in Congenital Heart Disease. London, Greenwich Medical Media, 1998, pp 231–236.

16. Acar P, Sid D, Bonnet D, et al: Maintaining tricuspid valve competence in double discordance: A challenge for the pediatric cardiologist. Heart 80:479–483, 1998.

17. Graham TP, Bernard YD, Mellen BG, et al: Long-term outcome in congenitally corrected transposition of the great arteries: A multi-institutional study. J Am Coll Cardiol 36:255–261, 2000.

18. Connolly HM, Grogan M, Warnes CA: Pregnancy among women with congenitally corrected transposition of great arteries. J Am Coll Cardiol 33:1692–1695, 1999.

19. Bjork VO, Iienze A: Management of thrombo-embolism after aortic valve replacement with the Bjork-Shiley tilting disc valve: Medicamental prevention with dicumarol in comparison with dipyridamole-acetylsalicylic acid; surgical treatment of prosthetic thrombosis. Scand J Thorac Cardiovasc Surg 9:183–191, 1975.

20. Salem DN, Stein PD, Pauker SG: Antithrombotic therapy in valvular heart disease native and prosthetic: The Seventh ACCP Conference on Antithrombotic and Thrombolytic Therapy. Chest 126(Suppl 3):S457–S482, 2004.

21. Bates SM, Greer IA, Hirsh J, Ginsberg JS: Use of antithrombotic agents during pregnancy: The Seventh ACCP Conference on Antithrombotic and Thrombolytic Therapy. Chest 126(Suppl 3): S627–S644, 2004.

22. Chiu I-S, Wu S-J, Chen S-J, et al: Sequential diagnosis of coronary arterial anatomy in congenitally corrected transposition of the great arteries. Ann Thorac Surg 75:422–429, 2003.

23. Freedom RM: Discordant atrivventricular connections and congenitally corrected transposition. In Anderson RH, Baker EJ, Macartney FJ, et al (eds): Pediatric Cardiology, 2nd ed, vol 2. Philadelphia, Churchill Livingstone, 2002, pp 1339.

24. Fredriksen PM, Chen A, Veldtman G, et al: Exercise capacity in adult patients with congenitally corrected transposition of the great arteries. Heart 85:191–195, 2001.

25. Van Praagh R, Papagiannis J, Grunenfelder J, et al: Pathologic anatomy of corrected transposition of the great arteries: Medical and surgical implications. Am Heart J 135:772–785, 1998.

26. Ikeda U, Furuse M, Suzuki O, et al: Long-term survival in aged patients with corrected transposition of the great arteries. Chest 101:1382–1385, 1992.

27. Sasaki O, Hamada M, Hiasa G, et al: Congenitally corrected transposition of the great arteries in a 65-year-old woman. Jpn Heart 42:645–649, 2001.

28. Dimas AP, Moodie DS, Sterba R, Gill CC: Long-term function of the morphologic right ventricle in adult patients with corrected transposition of the great arteries. Am Heart J 118:526–530, 1989.

29. Cowley CG, Rosenthal A: Congenitally corrected transposition of the great arteries: The systemic right ventricle. Prog Pediatr Cardiol 10:31–35, 1999.

30. Roffi M, de Marchi SF, Seiler C: Congenitally corrected transposition of the great arteries in an 80-year-old woman. Heart 79: 622–662, 1998.

31. Sumner AD, Campbell JA, Sorrell VL: Echocardiographic diagnosis of congenitally corrected transposition of the great arteries in a 76-year-old woman. Am J Geriatr Cardiol 10:162–163, 2001.

32. Yamazaki I, Kondo J, Imoto K, et al: Corrected transposition of the great arteries diagnosed in an 84-year-old woman. J Cardiovasc Surg 42:201–203, 2001.

33. Dodge-Khatami A, Tulevski H, Bennink GB, et al: Comparable systemic ventricular function in healthy adults and patients with unoperated congenitally corrected transposition using MRI dobutamine stress testing. Ann Thorac Surg 73:1759–1764, 2002.

34. Hornung TS, Bernard EJ, Celermajer DS, et al: Right ventricular dysfunction in congenitally corrected transposition of the great arteries. Am J Cardiol 84:1116–1119, 1999.

35. Winlaw DS, McGuirk SP, Brawn WJ: Intention-to-treat analysis of pulmonary artery banding in conditions with a morphological right ventricle in the systemic circulation with a view to anatomic biventricular repair. Circulation 111:405–411, 2005.

36. Duncan BW, Mee RB: Management of the failing systemic right ventricle. Semin Thorac Cardiovasc Surg 17:160–169, 2005.

37. Benzaquen BS, Webb GD, Therrien J: Arterial switch operation after Mustard procedures in adult patients with transposition of the great arteries: Is it time to revise our strategy? Am Heart J 147:E8, 2004.

38. Langley SM, Winlaw DS, Brawn WJ: Midterm results after restoration of the morphologically LV to the systemic circulation in patients with congenitally corrected transposition of the great arteries. J Thorac Cardiovasc Surg 125:1229–1241, 2003.

39. Brawn WJ: The double switch for atrioventricular discordance. Semin Thorac Cardiovasc Surg: Pediatr Card Surg Annu 8:51–56, 2005.

40. Van Son JA, Danielson GK, Huhta JC, et al: Late results of systemic atrioventricular valve replacement in corrected transposition. J Thorac Cardiovasc Surg 109:642–652; discussion 652–653, 1995.

41. Hraska V, Duncan BW, Jonas RA: Long-term outcome of surgically treated patients with corrected transposition of the great arteries. J Thorac Cardiovasc Surg 129:182–191, 2005.

42. Sano T, Riesenfield T, Karl TR, Wilkinson JL: Intermediate-term outcome after intracardiac repair of associated cardiac defects in patients with atrioventricular and ventriculo-arterial discordance. Circulation 92(9 Suppl):11272–11278, 1995.

43. Yeh T, Jr, Connelly MS, Coles JG, et al: Atrioventricular discordance: Result of repair in 127 patients. J Thorac Cardiovasc Surg 117:1190–1203, 1999.

# The Criss-Cross Heart

**Kai Andersen, Antonia Pijuan-Domenech, Henryk Kafka, and Craig S. Broberg**

**Age: 33 years**
**Gender: Male**
**Occupation: Salesman**
**Working diagnosis: Large ventricular septal defect**

## HISTORY

During infancy, the patient was diagnosed with a large VSD and underwent pulmonary artery (PA) banding through a left thoracotomy at the age of 5 months.

At the time of PA banding for this patient, two-dimensional echocardiography and MRI were not yet available, and the complex anatomy could not be detected as easily as it can be today.

When he was 4 years old, he underwent a sternotomy to close the VSD. However, after direct inspection of the anatomic setting, the VSD appeared unsuitable for closure. The chest was, thus, closed without any intracardiac repair.

The possibility of a Fontan circulation was discussed at the age of 16 years, but it was felt better to be postponed at the time.

Over the ensuing years the patient remained well without any particular shortness of breath on exertion and without any report of cyanosis. He returned for routine follow-up.

**Comments:** A large VSD will allow for a pronounced interventricular left-to-right shunt as the pulmonary vascular resistance falls soon after birth. The consequent volume overload of the LV in infancy may then give rise to heart failure. PA banding is performed to decrease pulmonary blood flow, thereby preventing or alleviating ventricular failure and—more importantly—preventing the development of PA occlusive disease.

A Fontan circulation would be an option in which systemic venous return could be directed to the PA without passing through an RV.[1] This would normally involve proximal PA ligation as well. Due to the large interventricular communication, both ventricles would then have acted as a "single" systemic ventricle.

Lack of notable cyanosis in this situation suggests an optimally balanced VSD shunt, namely adequate PA banding without excessive pulmonary flow and without substantial right-to-left shunting, at least at rest. The degree of secondary erythrocytosis in such a patient, when present—provided there is no iron deficiency—indicates indirectly the magnitude of right-to-left shunting at rest and/or during exercise.

## CURRENT SYMPTOMS

The patient remains essentially asymptomatic without any history of exercise-induced dyspnea, cyanosis, or angina. On average he has one or two episodes of palpitations per year, always short lived, with no associated syncope or any other symptoms. He is fit, can climb several flights of stairs, and exercises several times a week.

NYHA class: I

**Comments:** The history suggests the VSD shunt to be appropriately balanced by the PA banding also during exercise, with no symptoms indicating inadequate pulmonary blood flow, significant hypoxemia, or LV dysfunction precipitated by exertion. The episodes of palpitation might represent transient atrial tachyarrhythmia although they also might be explained by ectopic beats.

## CURRENT MEDICATIONS

Digoxin 125 µg orally once daily

**Comments:** The value of the digoxin therapy is doubtful.

## PHYSICAL EXAMINATION

BP 130/80 mm Hg, HR 67 bpm, oxygen saturation 93% on room air

Height 165 cm, weight 70 kg, BSA 1.79 m$^2$

Surgical scars: There was a left thoracotomy and a median sternotomy scar.

Neck veins: JVP was not elevated.

Lungs/chest: Chest was clear.

Heart: There was an RV lift and a faint precordial thrill. Moreover, there was a normal first and a split second heart sound with a soft pulmonary component to it, and a grade 4/6 systolic ejection murmur at the upper left sternal edge, which radiated well to the back.

Abdomen: Soft and normal to palpation

Extremities: There was no evidence of clubbing or peripheral edema.

**Comments:** The scars originated from the PA banding during infancy and the intended VSD closure in childhood, respectively.

The RV heave suggests marked hypertrophy, presumably due to increased intraventricular pressure. Since the large VSD is not restrictive, the pronounced systolic murmur is therefore attributed to the impeded flow through the PA band rather than to the VSD, as is also indicated by its ejection character. This is supported by the radiation to the back, a finding more common in murmurs due to obstruction of intrathoracic vessels than in those of intracardiac origin.

These findings add to the other evidence suggesting no significant interventricular right-to-left shunting or any sign of heart failure.

## LABORATORY DATA

| | |
|---|---|
| Hemoglobin | 16.1 g/dL (13.0–17.0) |
| Hematocrit/PCV | 46% (41–51) |
| MCV | 91 fL (84–98) |
| Platelet count | $205 \times 10^9$/L (136–343) |
| Sodium | 138 mmol/L (134–145) |
| Potassium | 4.0 mmol/L (3.5–5.2) |
| Creatinine | 0.72 mg/dL (0.60–1.2) |
| Blood urea nitrogen | 3.8 mmol/L (2.5–6.5) |
| Ferritin | 237 µg/L (32–284) |
| Transferrin | 2.5 g/L (2.0–3.2) |

***Comments:*** A significantly increased hemoglobin and hematocrit would reflect right-to-left shunting. The opposite is not always true: An apparently normal hemoglobin/hematocrit may be present with cyanosis if the patient has concomitant iron deficiency or other cause of anemia.[2]

In this case, the hemoglobin and hematocrit values are not elevated and there is no evidence of iron deficiency. The laboratory findings therefore indicate that there has been no significant secondary erythrocytosis. This supports the clinical impression of no significant right to left shunting.

## ELECTROCARDIOGRAM

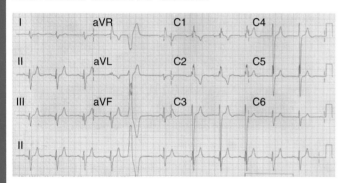

Figure 59-1 Electrocardiogram.

### FINDINGS

Heart rate: 67 bpm

PR interval: 220 msec

QRS axis deviation: +254°

QRS duration: 129 msec

Sinus rhythm with one ventricular ectopic beat, first-degree heart block, extreme axis deviation, RBBB.

***Comments:*** The marked QRS axis deviation is similar to that usually associated with AVSDs or tricuspid atresia, and is not a typical finding in patients with VSD. The depolarization pattern might therefore suggest an unusual topographical arrangement of the ventricular myocardium.

The diagnosis of RV hypertrophy is difficult in the presence of RBBB.

## CHEST X-RAY

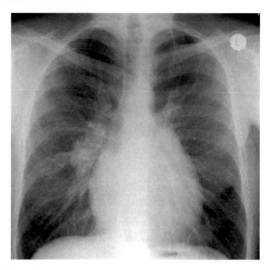

Figure 59-2 Posteroanterior projection.

### FINDINGS

Cardiothoracic ratio: 52%

The cardiac silhouette was mildly enlarged with evidence of RA dilatation. The central pulmonary arteries were dilated while the peripheral vascular markings were not definitely increased.

***Comments:*** Central PA dilation is consistent with PA banding and enlargement of the vessel distal to the narrowing from poststenotic dilatation as well. RV hypertrophy resulting from PA banding may impair ventricular filling, thereby explaining the enlarged atrium. The lack of overtly increased vascular markings suggests there is no hemodynamically important excess pulmonary blood flow.

## EXERCISE TESTING

| | |
|---|---|
| Exercise protocol: | Modified Bruce |
| Duration (min:sec): | 11:13 |
| Reason for stopping: | Dyspnea |
| ECG changes: | None |

| | Rest | Peak |
|---|---|---|
| Heart rate (bpm): | 67 | 125 |
| $O_2$ saturation (%): | 93 | 87 |
| Blood pressure (mm Hg): | 130/80 | 170/90 |
| Double product: | | 21,250 |
| Peak $Vo_2$ (mL/kg/min): | | 22.8 |
| Percent predicted (%): | | 67 |
| Ve/$Vco_2$: | | 68 |
| Metabolic equivalents: | | 4 |

### FINDINGS

Exercise tolerance was fair, with mild desaturation during exercise.

***Comments:*** Despite the unrepaired VSD, the patient has only mild desaturation with exercise. This is generally good and reflects the protection gained from his earlier pulmonary arterial band. Without this, the patient's baseline and exercise oxygen saturations would be much lower.

# ECHOCARDIOGRAM

## OVERALL FINDINGS

There was normal visceral situs. There was a conspicuous AV connection with abnormal ventricular relationships (see below). LV size and function were normal. The RV was hypertrophic with good systolic function. The LA was normal in size while the RA was mildly enlarged. There was no significant valve regurgitation. There was considerable PA obstruction with an estimated peak pressure gradient of 93 mm Hg.

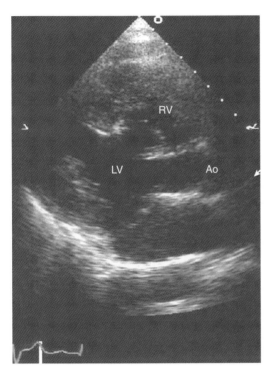

Figure 59-3 Parasternal long-axis view. Ao, aorta.

## FINDINGS

The parasternal long-axis imaging demonstrated a large nonrestrictive VSD 36 mm in diameter with bidirectional flow. Ventriculoarterial concordance was reported.

*Comments:* The relationship between the atria and ventricles and great arteries must be clarified to be certain of the true anatomic diagnosis. Here, the AV and ventriculoatrial relationships seemed to be concordant (i.e., normally related), as shown by the normally related LA, LV, and aorta.

The VSD is large and nonrestrictive, so there is equalization of pressures between the LV and RV. The measured arterial systolic blood pressure is 130 mm Hg, which means the RV systolic pressure is also 130 mm Hg. Given the gradient of 93 to 100 mm Hg between RV and PA, one can estimate the systolic PA pressure to be between 30 and 37 mm Hg. Thus, pulmonary vascular disease is not likely to be present.

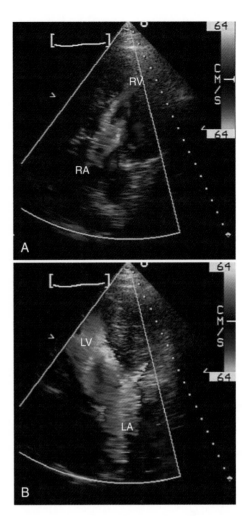

Figure 59-4 Apical four-chamber view, color Doppler imaging.

## FINDINGS

There was midline crossing of the systemic venous blood stream from the RA to the RV, as the latter is abnormally positioned to the left (*A*). Moreover, the pulmonary venous blood stream is shown to cross the midline from the LA to the LV, which is abnormally positioned to the right (*B*).

*Comments:* Although the AV connection seemed to be concordant as determined by segmental analysis, it differs conspicuously from what is usually observed. As opposed to the normally located RA and LA, the RV is positioned to the left while the LV is positioned to the right. The AV connections are therefore crossing each other, as demonstrated by the course of the depicted systemic and pulmonary venous blood streams. This anatomic setting has been denoted as a criss-cross heart.[3]

The essence of the criss-cross heart is a rotational abnormality of the ventricular mass so that the relationships of the ventricular chambers are not as anticipated for the given AV connection.[4] This might be explained by postseptational rotation of the ventricular mass along its long axis during embryogenesis.

One indication of the abnormal relationship is the inability to obtain a traditional four-chamber view, since the atrial septum and ventricular septum do not lie in the same plane. A VSD is a mandatory part of the criss-cross relationship.

# MAGNETIC RESONANCE IMAGING

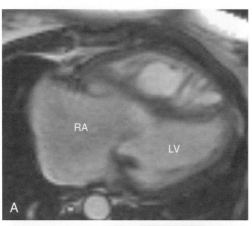

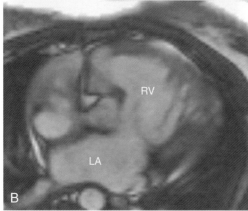

Figure 59-5 Axial steady-state free precession cines.

## FINDINGS

AV discordance with criss-cross connections and ventriculoarterial discordance.

LV and RV systolic function were normal. There was RV hypertrophy. Both mitral and tricuspid valves functioned well apart from mild mitral regurgitation. There was a large VSD.

**Comments:** Both atria and both ventricles were present, but it was not possible to obtain a four-chamber view. The mitral and tricuspid valves were not in the same plane. The mitral valve opened right to left from RA to LV (*A*) and the tricuspid valve opened posteroanteriorly, from LA to RV (*B*).

## Ventricular Volume Quantification

|  | LV | (Normal range) | RV | (Normal range) |
|---|---|---|---|---|
| EDV (mL) | 112 | (77–195) | 86 | (88–227) |
| ESV (mL) | 48 | (19–72) | 32 | (23–103) |
| SV (mL) | 64 | (51–133) | 54 | (52–138) |
| EF (%) | 57 | (57–75) | 63 | (50–76) |
| EDVi (mL/m$^2$) | 63 | (66–101) | 48 | (65–111) |
| ESVi (mL/m$^2$) | 27 | (18–39) | 18 | (18–47) |
| SVi (mL/m$^2$) | 36 | (43–67) | 30 | (39–71) |
| Mass index (g/m$^2$) | 61 | (59–92) | 49 | (22–49) |

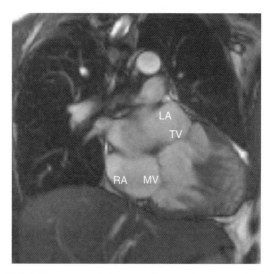

Figure 59-6 Oblique coronal plane steady-state free precession cine.

## FINDINGS

The LA was located superior to the RA. The right upper pulmonary vein was visible entering the LA. The tricuspid and mitral valves did not open in the same plane, their paths of flow being almost perpendicular to one another.

**Comments:** The atrial septum normally lies in a plane that is nearly parallel with the long axis of the body, that is, in a superior-inferior direction. Here the atrial septum is almost horizontal.

Both inlet valves are seen in this view and may appear to enter a common ventricular chamber. Instead, we are actually seeing the interventricular septum *en face*, in a plane almost perpendicular to that of the atrial septum.

As mentioned, one feature of criss-cross anatomy is that it can be impossible to obtain a true four-chamber view, because of the rotation of the ventricular cavities relative to the atria.

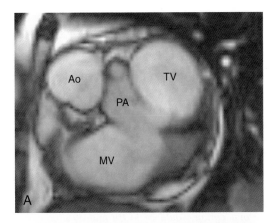

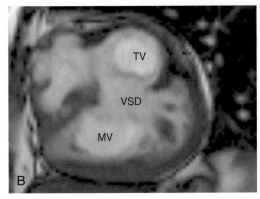

Figure 59-7 Oblique sagittal short-axis view steady-state free precession cine (**A**, basal plane; **B**, subbasal plane).

## FINDINGS

In the upper frame, the relative position of the four valves was visible (clockwise from upper left were the aortic valve, pulmonary valve, tricuspid valve opening to the RV, and mitral valve below opening to the LV). The aortic valve lay anterior to the pulmonary valve, whereas the tricuspid valve lay superior and posterior to the mitral valve.

In the lower frame, taken 1 cm more apically from the base, the open tricuspid (upper right) and mitral (lower left) valves were seen. The ventricular septum between them was interrupted by a large septal defect. Farther toward the apex (not seen), the ventricular septum lies in a more anterior-superior plane.

**Comments:** It is difficult to conceptualize the 3D configuration between the atria and ventricle from 2D images. Knowing the relative location of the valves can be helpful.

Recall that from earlier views, the tricuspid and mitral valves do not truly lie in the same plane as is suggested here, but each deviates slightly toward its respective ventricle, opening at 90-degree angles to each other.

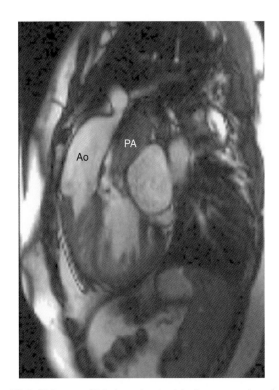

Figure 59-8 Oblique sagittal plane steady-state free precession cine.

## FINDINGS

The great arteries were parallel, with the aorta located anteriorly. There was mild subvalvar pulmonary stenosis and severe valvar pulmonary stenosis (peak velocity > 5 m/sec). The location of the previous band was not obvious. The PA branches appeared relatively normal.

**Comments:** One advantage of MRI is its ability to clearly demonstrate the relative location of the great arteries, which can be hard to see behind the sternum with echocardiography. Here they appear transposed, meaning that the echocardiogram was likely incorrect in its description of ventriculoarterial concordance.

The severe pulmonic stenosis (rather than just a PA band) may have protected the pulmonary vasculature from excessive flow.

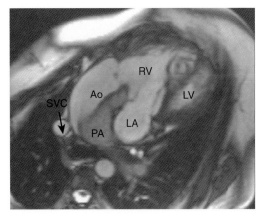

Figure 59-9 Oblique axial plane steady-state free precession cine (right ventricular in-and-out view).

# FINDINGS

The LA drained through the tricuspid valve to the anterior RV, which then ejected to the anteriorly located aorta.

**Comments:** This image illustrates the AV and VA discordance. The PA is located between the RV inlet from the LA and its outlet to the aorta (see Fig. 59-7).

Out of plane, the LV, partially seen posterior to the RV in this view, fills from the RA (inferior to the plane depicted here), and empties to the PA. The SVC is present here in cross section adjacent to the aorta.

# CATHETERIZATION

Not performed

## FOCUSED CLINICAL QUESTIONS AND DISCUSSION POINTS

1. What is the complete anatomic diagnosis?

*The patient has atrial situs solitus, AV discordance, and a criss-cross AV relationship with a large, nonrestrictive VSD and ventriculo-arterial discordance, which may also be known as congenitally corrected transposition of the great arteries, or CCTGA.*

*The criss-cross relationship is not difficult to conceptualize once it is understood that it refers to the relative orientations of the AV valves, and hence the locations of the ventricles relative to the atria, regardless of the atrial situs or the sequence of connections, which can each be normal or abnormal.[5,6] A key to recognizing the criss-cross relationship can be failure to locate a four-chamber plane, the atrial septum and the ventricular septum being almost perpendicular to each other (see Fig. 59-4), as are the two AV flow paths. Associated cardiac anomalies are common, encompassing transposition of the great arteries, double-outlet RV, VSDs, straddling AV valves, and pulmonary outflow tract obstruction.*

2. What is the clinical importance of the criss-cross configuration?

*Criss-cross heart is an infrequently occurring abnormality. Nevertheless, knowledge of this condition is highly important, as the complex anatomy may make the other commonly associated lesions more difficult to manage surgically. This is illustrated by the present history, as the operation embarked on in childhood had to be discontinued when exposure of the heart demonstrated an anatomy considered not suitable for VSD closure.*

3. Why did the echocardiogram and MRI differ in the anatomical interpretation?

*Both modalities identified the main criss-cross relationship and indicated the various locations of each of the four chambers. The key difference was in differentiating the morphologic RV from LV. In identifying the more anterior ventricle as the morphologic RV, the MRI changed the diagnosis from AV and ventriculoarterial concordance (normal relationships), to AV and ventriculo-arterial discordance (or CCTGA).*

*The key means of differentiating the morphologic RV from LV were not readily apparent by the echocardiogram. First, trabeculations usually identify the RV, but both ventricles were fairly similar in their trabeculations given the RV hypertrophy. Second, the moderator band is present in the RV, but a distinct moderator band was not easily seen in the echo. Third, the tricuspid valve, always part of the RV, is usually apically displaced, but both AV valves arose from the same location on the septum in this complex arrangement. Fourth, the RV is typically the more anterior ventricle, as in this case, although typically this is not seen in CCTGA. Hence, the discrepancy between the two studies is easily understood.*

*In this case, the MRI proved unquestionably the double discordance by demonstrating the anterior aorta and parallel great arteries, which indicate transposition. The great arteries can be difficult to visualize with echocardiography.*

4. What surgical options could be entertained?

*There are three surgical options. Usually, the preferred approach is biventricular repair that would involve VSD closure and takedown of the PA band. This would relieve the pressure load on the RV, reducing the risk for heart failure, and would provide adequate pulmonary blood flow. However, the criss-cross configuration would still make this a difficult repair, with a high operative risk markedly exceeding that of a regular VSD repair. Risks would include heart block, incomplete closure, and outflow tract obstruction.*

*A second option would be to try and do a double switch to correct the discordance and leave the patient with a systemic LV. Of uncertain benefit in even the best of circumstances, here again, however, the criss-cross relationship makes this option impossibly complex.*

*The third option is a Fontan palliation. Because of the pulmonary stenosis, the pulmonary pressure and resistance may be normal. Hence, one might still consider surgical cavopulmonary connection. This is predominantly performed in functionally univentricular hearts[7] to eliminate cyanosis and provide adequate pulmonary blood flow.*

*However, as the patient is doing very well and is relatively acyanotic, one might consider him ideally "balanced" (see Case 60). A Fontan circulation would not offer improvement over his hemodynamic situation at the moment, and the long-term results of Fontan connections are still associated with significant mortality and morbidity caused by atrial arrhythmia, venous congestion, protein-losing enteropathy, thromboembolism, and ventricular failure.[7,8] Any surgery, therefore, would not likely improve the patient's current clinical situation.*

5. What is the patient's long-term prognosis?

*Although the patient's clinical situation is currently satisfactory, there might be a need for further intervention over time. The RV has been exposed to systemic intraventricular pressure for many years and there is pronounced RV hypertrophy, though without any evidence of impaired systolic function. However, there is a long-term possibility of right-sided heart failure. There is the risk of paradoxical embolism. Tachyarrhythmias may also occur requiring intervention.*

*The patient has done extremely well thus far and has demonstrated an optimal balance of pulmonary blood flow and little cyanosis or shunt. Typically, this "balanced" physiology is best left alone (see Case 60). The patient's future prospects are uncertain, but a limited life span can be anticipated.*

# FINAL DIAGNOSIS

Criss-cross heart with large VSD and consequent PA banding established during infancy

# PLAN OF ACTION

Yearly follow-up

# INTERVENTION

None

# OUTCOME

Two years later, at his routine follow-up, the patient noted no change in his exertional tolerance and continued to maintain his healthy, active lifestyle.

# Selected References

1. Fontan F, Baudet E: Surgical repair of tricuspid atresia. Thorax 26:240–248, 1971.
2. Oechslin E: Eisenmenger's syndrome. In Gatzoulis MA, Webb GD, Daubeney PEF (eds): Diagnosis and Management of Adult Congenital Heart Disease. Edinburgh, Churchill Livingstone, 2003, pp 363–377.
3. Anderson RH, Shinebourne EA, Gerlis LM: Criss-cross atrioventricular relationships producing paradoxical atrioventricular concordance or discordance. The significance to nomenclature of congenital heart disease. Circulation 50:176–180, 1974.
4. Anderson RH: A question of definition. Criss-cross hearts revisited. Pediatr Cardiol 3:305–313, 1982.
5. Han H-S, Seo JW, Choi JY: Echocardiographic evaluation of hearts with twisted atrioventricular connections (criss-cross heart). Heart Vessels 9:322–326, 1994.
6. Marino M, Sanders SP, Pasquini L, et al: Two-dimensional echocardiography in crisscross heart. Am J Cardiol 58:325–333, 1986.
7. Freedom RF, Li J, Yoo S-J: Late complications following the Fontan operation. In Gatzoulis MA, Webb GD, Daubeney PEF (eds): Diagnosis and Management of Adult Congenital Heart Disease. Edinburgh, Churchill Livingstone, 2003, pp 85–91.
8. Fontan F, Kirklin JW, Fernandez G, et al: Outcome after a "perfect" Fontan operation. Circulation 81:1520–1536, 1990.

# Congenitally Corrected Transposition of the Great Arteries with Pulmonary Stenosis and Ventricular Septal Defect: When to Intervene?

**Igor Knez**

**Age: 30 years**
**Gender: Female**
**Occupation: Student**
**Working diagnosis: Congenitally corrected transposition of the great arteries**

## HISTORY

At age 11, transposition was diagnosed after evaluation of a murmur. The patient was also found to have a VSD and pulmonary stenosis. No intervention was offered.

When the patient was 22 years old, she had an episode of lightheadedness and was found to have second-degree AV block. An epicardial pacemaker was implanted, and 2 years later, it was changed to a transvenous dual-chamber system.

The patient returned for routine follow-up. She reported completing her education, announcing plans for marrying soon, and was making future plans, including possibly starting a family. She wondered whether anything should be done for her to improve her long-term prospects.

*Comments:* CCTGA is an uncommon form of congenital heart disease first described by von Rokitansky in 1875.[1]

It accounts for less than 1% of all forms of congenital heart disease and is characterized by AV and ventriculoarterial discordance. There are two forms of CCTGA, depending on whether situs is normal (situs solitus, L-loop, L-transposition [S, L, L]) or inverted (situs inversus, D-loop, D-transposition [I, D, D]).

Associated abnormalities occur frequently and include VSD (usually a large, nonrestrictive conoventricular defect), LVOT obstruction (valvar and subvalvar pulmonary stenosis), AV conduction abnormalities, and an Ebstein-like left AV valve.[2-5] Therefore, the need for a pacemaker in this patient is somewhat typical.

While these differ from the figures in infants, the relative frequency of associated lesions in adulthood from one study are given below:[6]

Any associated lesion: 50%

VSD: 20%

ASD: 23%

LVOT obstruction: 32%

Ebstein-like systemic AV valve (tricuspid): 27%

3–4+ systemic AV valve (tricuspid) regurgitation: 59%

Dextrocardia: 16%

High-grade AV block: 32%

Permanent pacemaker: 14%

3–4+ pulmonary AV valve (mitral) regurgitation: 7%

3–4+ aortic valve regurgitation: 7%

Transvenous pacing in a patient with an intracardioc shunt carries a risk of systemic thromboembolism (see Case 48).

## CURRENT SYMPTOMS

Generally the patient reported no symptoms. Occasionally, with severe emotional stress, she became acutely dyspneic and blue, although the symptoms usually settled spontaneously within minutes. Her reported exercise capacity was unlimited on flat ground, and she could climb two flights of stairs without stopping. She had no sustained palpitations.

NYHA class: II

## CURRENT MEDICATIONS

Warfarin 6.25 mg per day (target INR 2–3)

Perindopril 2 mg once daily

*Comments:* The patient was put on warfarin because of her transvenous pacing leads (potentially with thrombus formation) in the setting of some right-to-left shunting to reduce the prospect of a paradoxic embolus.

There are few clinical data on the use of ACE inhibitors in patients with a systemic RV. Thus, their use is not evidence-based and not routinely recommended.

## PHYSICAL EXAMINATION

BP 95/60 mm Hg, HR 80 bpm, oxygen saturation 95% on room air

Height 161 cm, weight 54 kg, BSA 1.55 m$^2$

Surgical scars: Present from pacemaker implantations

Neck veins: JVP was not elevated, and waveform was normal.

Lungs/chest: Clear

Heart: The heart rate was regular. There was a left parasternal lift with no apical displacement. There was a palpable thrill in the pulmonary area, a normal first heart sound, and a single second heart sound. A grade 4/6 quite-late-peaking ejection systolic murmur was maximal at the upper left sternal edge. There was no diastolic murmur.

Abdomen: No signs of hepatomegaly

Extremities: Good peripheral pulses, no cyanosis or clubbing, no edema

**Comments:** The patient is not cyanotic at rest, despite the diagnosis of a large VSD. The loud ejection systolic murmur at the upper left sternal edge indicates pulmonary stenosis at one or more levels, which limits excessive pulmonary blood flow and raises the systolic pressure in the pulmonary ventricle. The minimal desaturation fits with a nicely balanced pulmonary stenosis and VSD or a small VSD in the setting of pulmonary stenosis.

## LABORATORY DATA

| | |
|---|---|
| Hemoglobin | 14.0 g/dL (11.5–15.0) |
| Hematocrit/PCV | 40% (36–46) |
| MCV | 94 fL (83–99) |
| Platelet count | $262 \times 10^9$/L (150–400) |
| Sodium | 144 mmol/L (134–145) |
| Potassium | 3.9 mmol/L (3.5–5.2) |
| Creatinine | 0.9 mmol/dL (0.6–1.2) |
| Blood urea nitrogen | 3.1 mmol/L (2.5–6.5) |

**Comments:** No abnormalities were seen. The patient has a normal hemoglobin, which argues that her oxygen saturation stays in a fairly normal range with her usual activities.

## ELECTROCARDIOGRAM

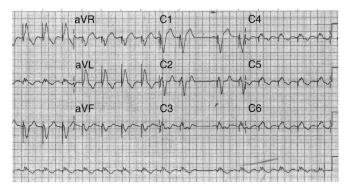

Figure 60-1 Electrocardiogram.

### FINDINGS
Sinus rhythm at 100 bpm. Atrial sensing, ventricular pacing with an LBBB pattern, suggesting RV pacing.

**Comments:** Heart block is common in CCTGA, and this patient has a functioning sinus node. One P-wave seems not to be sensed, and the pacemaker escapes before resuming atrial tracking.

## CHEST X-RAY

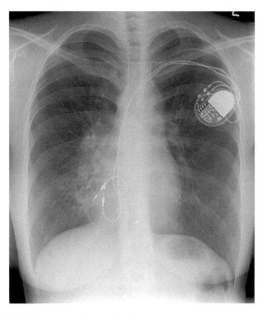

Figure 60-2 Posteroanterior projection.

### FINDINGS
Cardiothoracic ratio: 30%

There is a narrow cardiac silhouette in the center of the chest, with likely mesocardia. A dual-chamber pacemaker is present with leads in the RA and LV (pulmonary ventricle). A third epicardial lead from the former epicardial pacing system is also present. Some excessive vascularity is suggested in the right lower lung field, which may reflect bronchiectasis.

**Comments:** There are no signs of pulmonary vascular congestion or pulmonary hypertension despite the presence of a large VSD (see Fig. 60-3), which emphasizes the balanced nature of the patient's lesions. Pulmonary stenosis (valvular or subvalvular) is preventing excessive pulmonary blood flow and subsequent pulmonary arterial hypertension. Bronchiectasis may be present from abnormal ciliary motility (Kartagener's syndrome), which can accompany various forms of ACHD, including CCTGA and dextrocardia.[7]

Though somewhat semantic in this case, the position of the ventricular apex determines dextro- versus levocardia. Here, the position is somewhat ambiguous. The left hemidiaphragm is lower than the right, which argues in favor of levocardia. However, the position of the LV pacing wire seems to favor dextrocardia. The term *mesocardia* is often employed in such cases.

## EXERCISE TESTING

| | | | |
|---|---|---|---|
| Exercise protocol: | Bruce | | |
| Duration (min:sec): | 11:10 | | |
| Reason for stopping: | Fatigue | | |
| ECG changes: | None | | |

| | Rest | Peak |
|---|---|---|
| Heart rate (bpm): | 80 | 105 |
| Percent of age-predicted max HR: | | 55 |
| O₂ saturation (%): | 95 | 94 |
| Blood pressure (mm Hg): | 110/70 | 150/80 |

**Comments:** Reasons for reduced exercise capacity may include abnormal chronotropic response, ventricular dysfunction, poor lung function, poor effort, poor fitness, or other factors. There is a rate response program in the pacemaker, which should allow the exercise rate to rise further. One cannot be certain that the patient's effort was maximal. The ECGs should be examined.

A notable finding here is that the oxygen saturation did not fall significantly with exercise. Despite having a VSD, the patient maintains very reasonable pulmonary blood flow relative to systemic blood flow, and shunting is minimized. This is enabled by the pulmonary stenosis, which in this patient's case is severe enough to limit excessive left-to-right shunt at rest and protect against pulmonary vascular disease, but not so severe as to limit pulmonary blood flow at the expense of more right-to-left shunting, even during exercise. As above, it is difficult to say whether the patient's effort was maximal, and whether further desaturation would have occurred with more vigorous exercise.

## ECHOGARDIOGRAM

### OVERALL FINDINGS

Atrial situs solitus with AV and ventriculoarterial discordance.

The systemic RV was hypertrophied, but function was normal. There was only trivial/mild tricuspid valve regurgitation. There was a large nonrestrictive, doubly committed VSD (2 cm in diameter).

The pulmonary LV was normal in size with mild-to-moderate left ventricular hypertrophy and normal systolic function with a low-velocity bidirectional shunt. The atria were of normal size.

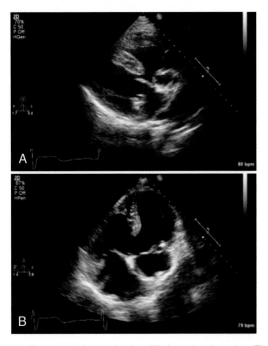

Figure 60-3 Parasternal long-axis view (**A**), four-chamber view (**B**).

**Comments:** A VSD and PS are the most commonly associated lesions with CCTGA.[6] The term doubly committed VSD denotes that the VSD lies below both the pulmonary valve and the aortic valve.

It is also important to note the good function of the systemic AV valve (tricuspid valve), supporting the reportedly good systemic RV function.

## TRANSTHORACIC ECHOCARDIOGRAM

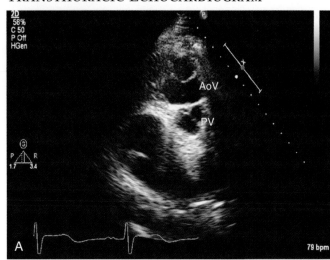

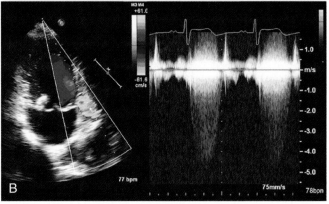

Figure 60-4 Pulmonary valve posterior to the aortic valve (**A**), continuous-wave Doppler sample (**B**).

### FINDINGS

The pulmonary outflow tract was small and stenotic. The pulmonary valve was located posterior to the aortic valve (*A*). Pulmonary flow obstruction was both valvar (bicuspid and stenotic pulmonary valve) and subvalvar with a peak Doppler velocity of 4.9 m/sec (see continuous-wave Doppler sample, *B*). The aortic valve was normal with no stenosis and no regurgitation.

**Comments:** Consistent with the physical exam findings, there is a severe gradient across the pulmonary outflow tract. During systole, the pressure in the LV (pulmonary ventricle) must be at or near systemic level.

## CATHETERIZATION

### HEMODYNAMICS

Heart rate     61 bpm

| | Pressure | Saturation (%) |
|---|---|---|
| SVC | mean 6 | 71 |
| IVC | mean 6 | 78 |
| RA | mean 6 | 77 |
| LV | 116/7 | 82 |
| PA | 29/16 mean 18 | 82 |
| PCWP | mean 12 | |
| RV | 110/12 | 96 |
| Aorta | 106/62 mean 83 | 93 |

**Calculations**

| | |
|---|---|
| Qp (L/min) | 5.63 |
| Qs (L/min) | 4.45 |
| Cardiac index (L/min/m$^2$) | 2.86 |
| Qp/Qs | 1.27 |
| PVR (Wood units) | 1.07 |
| SVR (Wood units) | 17.31 |

## FINDINGS
Hemodynamics are shown.

*Comments:* The LV was at systemic pressure levels, and there was no significant pressure gradient across the VSD.

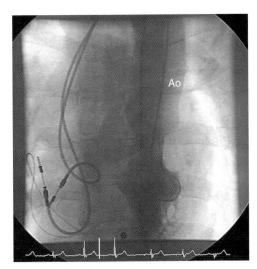

Figure 60-5 Systemic right ventriculogram.

## FINDINGS
The systemic RV had normal systolic function. There was little right-to-left shunt.

*Comments:* The pigtail catheter is situated in the anatomic right but systemic ventricle, giving rise to the aorta. The large, non-restrictive VSD is seen. Pacing wires are in the RA appendage (upturned wire), and one in the pulmonary ventricular apex (downward pointing wire), located to the right of the angiogram.

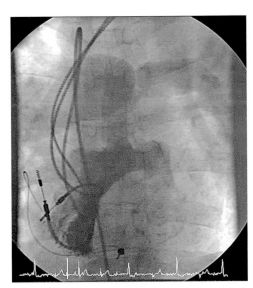

Figure 60-6 Pulmonary left ventriculogram.

## FINDINGS
Injection into the left (pulmonary) ventricle showed the valvar and subvalvar stenosis and confluent pulmonary arteries.

*Comments:* The right PA is dilated.

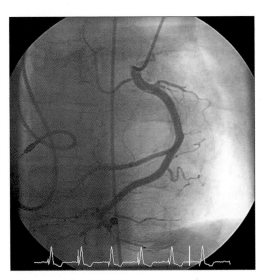

Figure 60-7 Right coronary angiogram.

## FINDINGS
There was no coronary artery stenosis.

The coronary artery on the left appears similar but a mirror image to a normal right coronary artery, and indeed supplies the morphologic RV. The vessel branches to supply a large ventricular acute marginal branch, then the posterior descending artery.

*Comments:* The patient did not have signs or symptoms suggestive of coronary artery disease, or risk factors for early atherosclerosis. Clinically, it was not important to assess the coronary arteries in this patient. However, coronary angiography is important prior to any surgical intervention for transposition, which was contemplated in this patient, not only because the surgeon may need to approach the patient differently depending on the course of the arteries, but because of the relatively frequent anomalous origin and course of coronary arteries.[8]

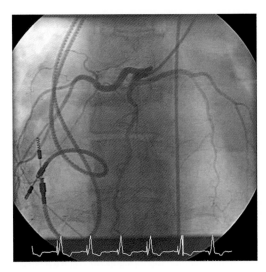

Figure 60-8 Left coronary angiogram.

# FINDINGS

Left coronary artery injection. No stenoses were present.

**Comments:** The occurrence of coronary anomalies in CCTGA is comparable to that seen in simple or D-TGA and TOF, even up to 45% of patients in one series.[8]

Proximally, the coronary artery pattern near the aortic sinus depends on the degree of aortopulmonary rotation. More peripherally, the coronary artery pattern is dictated by the relative location of the two ventricles with respect to each other, irrespective of atrial situs. The pattern tends to be similar to normal patients in that the circumflex artery will travel within the AV groove, and the left anterior descending artery (LAD) will course along the anterior septum.

## FOCUSED CLINICAL QUESTIONS AND DISCUSSION POINTS

1. What does the term *balanced* refer to in patients with complex ACHD?

*This term refers to the interaction between the large VSD and pulmonary stenosis and to the extent of pulmonary versus systemic blood flow, which in turn determines systemic saturations. The degree of pulmonary stenosis in our case was sufficient to prevent pulmonary arterial hypertension (much like a PA band placed in infancy), yet not severe enough to force a significant right-to-left shunt, even with the degree of exercise obtained. The patient was therefore "balanced" physiologically.*

*The coexistence of pulmonary stenosis with a VSD is not uncommon in patients with CCTGA,[6] but does not mean that all patients with this triad are similarly balanced.*

2. What interventional options could or should be considered for this patient?

*The first and most attractive option is to simply do nothing. The patient is asymptomatic, with excellent oxygen saturation, and it is impossible to improve on her current condition. The obvious advantages of this approach are that no intervention is necessary and the expectation would be that the patient continues to be asymptomatic. The disadvantage of this, however, is that she has a systemic RV, and long-term clinical outcome in patients with CCTGA is likely to include congestive heart failure by the fifth decade, often together with significant systemic AV valve regurgitation.[9,10] In addition, the presence of a large VSD leaves her potentially vulnerable to systemic thromboembolism, and to right-to-left shunting if her "balanced" state becomes less so over the long term. It is impossible to predict whether these would be likely occurrences over the course of her lifetime.*

*A second option is to close the VSD and relieve the pulmonary stenosis. This would leave the patient with a systemic RV with its inherent problems. If the patient was not already in heart block, the surgery could exaggerate the reported inherent risk (3% per year) and thus necessitate pacemaker implantation. This approach would not prevent future problems with systemic AV valve regurgitation and RV dysfunction,[11] and it may accelerate them. Following such a "physiologic" repair and the changed geometry (with lower left ventricular pressures and a new position of the interventricular septum) the systemic AV valve function may deteriorate, often leading to ventricular dilation and more tricuspid regurgitation from septal deviation. One potential treatment for systemic AV valve regurgitation in these patients is the creation of pulmonary stenosis, though with mixed success.[12,13] Furthermore, with this approach one assumes that the morphologic LV is capable of maintaining the pulmonary load independently of the RV (i.e., the systemic RV may be contributing to pulmonary blood flow through the stenosed outflow tract), so a detailed assessment of its function would be paramount.*

*Some degree of residual pulmonary stenosis following physiologic repair may therefore be desirable.*

*The third option would be of an "anatomic" repair. This would involve extensive surgery, namely a Rastelli tunnel from the VSD to the aorta, an RV-PA conduit (see Case 53), and atrial redirection (Mustard or Senning procedure).[14,15] The pacing wires would need to be reimplanted. Unless the VSD is located adjacent to the aortic valve intraventricular rerouting from the LV to the aortic orifice is not an easy task and may involve a fair volume of the native RV. In this particular patient, the VSD was of doubly committed and juxta-arterial type, which is rather unusual in the setting of discordant AV connections. Intra-atrial rerouting of blood (with a Senning or Mustard procedure) possesses its own difficulties and potential complications (see Case 49). In addition, the pacing leads would need to be routed through the venous pathways and mitral valve, creating potential problems of their own. Generally speaking, though theoretically feasible as a way to employ the morphologic LV as the systemic ventricle, an "anatomic" repair would be extensive and high-risk surgery, not often applicable to adult patients. It would be difficult to guarantee that this patient would be better off long-term from such an undertaking. When considered in early childhood for infants with major dysfunction of their systemic tricuspid valve and the RV, the potential risk/benefit ratio from this large undertaking may be more attractive.*

*A last alternative of cardiac transplantation is not relevant here because of the patient's excellent clinical condition. Importantly, though, the patient has normal pulmonary vascular resistance, and if the systemic ventricle fails in the future, she may be a suitable transplant candidate.*

3. What should the patient be counseled about the potential risks of any future pregnancy?

*There is no absolute contraindication to pregnancy in this patient; however, there is a risk of about 5% of maternal cardiac events.[16] Successful pregnancy (83%) can be achieved in most women with CCTGA. The rate of fetal loss and maternal cardiovascular morbidity is increased, and thus early planning is essential. One should also consider the risks of systemic thromboembolism from the transvenous pacing system when an intracardiac shunt is present,[17] which may potentially be higher during gestation.*

*The patient should be informed that the risk of recurrence of ACHD is approximately 5% compared to a background risk of 1%.*

*When considering the potential options explored previously, closure of the VSD will decrease her chances of either systemic thromboembolism or worsening cyanosis during pregnancy.*

4. What option is best for this patient?

*The various options were all explored at a multidisciplinary conference and in several discussions with the patient. It was openly acknowledged that for the most part no intervention was currently necessary given her optimally balanced physiology.*

*However, in considering her wishes for a low-risk successful pregnancy without risk of systemic thromboembolism, surgery was offered to maintain oxygen saturation, abolish the potential risk for paradoxical embolus, and obviate the need for anticoagulation. The anatomy was thought to be particularly suited for VSD closure and relief of LVOT obstruction, carrying a lower perioperative risk and not requiring concomitant pacing intervention.*

*This management decision may be rightly criticized, as the proposed operation would likely have only a small positive impact on future pregnancy. Furthermore, the patient would remain with a systemic RV after such a procedure and at even higher risk of requiring tricuspid valve replacement later on than she would have without surgery. As a rule, no intervention would usually be offered to a patient with such a well-balanced lesion.*

# FINAL DIAGNOSIS

Balanced CCTGA with nonrestrictive VSD and valvular pulmonary stenosis

# PLAN OF ACTION

"Physiologic" repair with relief of pulmonary stenosis and closure of VSD

# INTERVENTION

The patient's options were discussed thoroughly with her on several occasions, and surgery planned only after the clear consent and wish of both her and her fiancé.

Using a traditional surgical approach and cardiopulmonary bypass, closure of the doubly committed VSD was performed using a Gore-Tex patch. Then a porcine bioprosthetic valve/conduit (20-mm diameter) was placed between the pulmonary LV and main PA. The operation went smoothly, and there were no complications.

# OUTCOME

The patient made good recovery despite bilateral pleural effusions and a moderate pericardial effusion. Several days later she was walking without assistance. She was in paced rhythm, with good cardiac output and normal oxygen saturations in air.

Discharge echocardiography showed good biventricular function with no significant systemic tricuspid regurgitation and a normally functioning LV-PA conduit. However, she still had a small but restrictive VSD shunting from the systemic RV to the native PA (left to right) with a pressure gradient across the ventricular septum of 80 mm Hg. She was discharged home on a beta-blocker, diuretic, and aspirin.

Eighteen months after surgery, the patient had an uneventful pregnancy and gave birth to a healthy male infant under epidural anesthesia and with ventouse extraction.

Three years after repair, she remains well with mild tricuspid valve regurgitation and good biventricular function. She continues to take metoprolol and aspirin.

## Selected References

1. Von Rokitansky K: Pathologisch-anatomische Abhandlung. Vienna, W. Braumueller, 1875, pp 83–86.
2. Allwork SP, Bentall HH, Becker AE, et al: Congenitally corrected transposition of the great arteries: Morphological study of 32 cases. Am J Cardiol 38:910–923, 1975.
3. Anderson RC, Lillehei CW, Lester RG: Corrected transposition of the great vessels of the heart. Pediatrics 20:626–646, 1957.
4. Schiebler GL, Edwards JE, Burchell HB, et al: Congenitally corrected transposition of the great vessels: A study of 33 cases. Pediatrics 27(Suppl 2):851–888, 1961.
5. Masden RR, Franch RH: Isolated congenitally corrected transposition of the great arteries. In Hurst JW (ed): The Heart, 3rd ed. New York, McGraw-Hill, 1980, pp 59–83.
6. Beauchesne LM, Warnes CA, Connolly HM, et al: Outcome of unoperated adult who presents with congenitally corrected transposition of the great arteries. J Am Coll Cardiol 40:285–290, 2002.
7. Bitar FF, Shbaro R, Mroueh S, et al: Dextrocardia and corrected transposition of the great arteries (I,D,D) in a case of Kartagener's syndrome: A unique association. Clin Cardiol 21:298–299, 1998.
8. Ismat FA, Baldwin HS, Karl TR, et al: Coronary anatomy in congenitally corrected transposition of the great arteries. Int J Cardiol 86:207–216, 2002.
9. Graham TP, Bernard YD, Mellen BG, et al: Long-term outcome in congenitally corrected transposition of the great arteries. J Am Coll Cardiol 36:255–261, 2000.
10. Piran S, Veldtman G, Siu S, et al: Heart failure and ventricular dysfunction in patients with single or systemic right ventricles. Circulation 105:1189–1194, 2002.
11. Connelly MS, Liu PP, Williams WG, et al: Congenitally corrected transposition of the great arteries in the adult: Functional status and complications. J Am Coll Cardiol 27:1238–1243, 1996.
12. Koh M, Yagihara T, Uemura H, et al: Functional biventricular repair using left ventricle–pulmonary artery conduit in patients with discordant atrioventricular connections and pulmonary outflow tract obstruction: Does conduit obstruction maintain tricuspid valve function? Eur J Cardio-Thorac Surg 26:767–772, 2004.
13. Winlaw DS, McGuirk SP, Balmer C, et al: Intention-to-treat analysis of pulmonary artery banding in conditions with a morphological right ventricle in the systemic circulation with a view to anatomic biventricular repair. Circulation 111:405–411, 2005.
14. Langley SM, Winlaw DS, Stumper O, et al: Midterm results after restoration of the morphologically left ventricle to the systemic circulation in patients with congenitally corrected transposition of the great arteries. J Thor Cardiovasc Surg 125:1229–1241, 2003.
15. Davies B, Oppido G, Wilkinson JL, Brizard CP: Aortic translocation, Senning procedure and right ventricular outflow tract augmentation for congenitally corrected transposition, ventricular septal defect and pulmonary stenosis. Eur J Cardiothorac Surg 33:934–936, 2008.
16. Connolly HM, Grogan M, Warnes CA. Pregnancy among women with congenitally corrected transposition of great arteries. J Am Coll Cardiol 33:1692–1695, 1999.
17. Khairy P, Landzberg MJ, Gatzoulis MA, et al: Transvenous pacing leads and systemic thromboemboli in patients with congenital heart disease and intracardiac shunts: A multicenter study. Circulation 113:2391–2397, 2006.

# Intracardiac Thrombus in the Fontan Circulation

**Bengt Johansson and Elisabeth Bédard**

**Age: 24 years**
**Gender: Male**
**Occupation: Engineer**
**Working diagnosis: Tricuspid atresia with previous Fontan operation**

## HISTORY

The patient was born with tricuspid atresia and had a modified right BT shunt during the first year of life. A modified left BT shunt was created at the age of 2.

Four years later, an atriopulmonary Fontan operation was performed.

The patient remained well until he was 16, when he was started on warfarin after a possible pulmonary embolus, although no embolism could be confirmed on imaging.

One year later, at age 17, he was admitted with palpitations due to atrial flutter with 2:1 conduction and was successfully cardioverted to sinus rhythm.

In late adolescence, other episodes of paroxysmal "atrial flutter" occurred, each treated successfully with a combination of medication and cardioversion. Atrial fibrillation was noted at age 22. In response to his persisting arrhythmia, a catheterization and exercise study were performed at age 22. He began taking amiodarone and warfarin. A year later he was in sinus rhythm and stopped taking warfarin.

In general, the patient was well and completed his education. He was seen for routine follow-up.

**Comments:** BT and other systemic-to-pulmonary shunts are used to increase pulmonary blood flow in patients with cyanotic ACHD. They are used much less often now than in previous decades.

There are several modifications of the concept generally referred to as the Fontan operation.[1] In this patient, an atriopulmonary Fontan operation was performed, that is, the right atrium was connected to the pulmonary arteries. Contemporary approaches include variations of the total cavopulmonary connection with a "lateral tunnel" in the RA connecting the IVC with the pulmonary arteries and an extracardiac conduit leading the IVC venous return to the pulmonary arteries. In both these latter situations, SVC return is also to the pulmonary arteries via a bidirectional Glenn anastomosis.

"Silent" pulmonary emboli are relatively common in patients with a Fontan circulation[2] and may be easily overlooked.

Though this serves as an additional argument for anticoagulation in Fontan patients, there are presently no randomized trials to support the routine use of Coumadin in Fontan patients.

As with many other forms of ACHD, the occurrence of a clinical arrhythmia should instigate investigation for an underlying hemodynamic abnormality, such as new thrombus formation or other obstruction in the Fontan circuit.

Atrial flutter is extremely common in patients with a previous atriopulmonary Fontan operation. The prevalence increases as the patient ages.[3] Even in patients who seemingly tolerate the arrhythmia well, sinus rhythm should be restored promptly, as hemodynamic compromise may occur unexpectedly and rapidly. Often, TEE will be done to look for thrombus in the right atrium. Direct current (DC) cardioversion of a patient with a Fontan circulation is associated with increased risk, particularly of asystole or bradyarrhythmia immediately after conversion. Sedation and cardioversion should be done with caution and close attention.

## CURRENT SYMPTOMS

The patient was unlimited in his daily activities, including full-time office work. He felt he could climb stairs at his own pace. He experienced shortness of breath with heavy exercise but usually did not exert himself to that level. He had noted no new palpitations.

NYHA class: I

## CURRENT MEDICATIONS

Aspirin 75 mg daily

Amiodarone 200 mg daily

## PHYSICAL EXAMINATION

BP 118/72 mm Hg (right leg), HR 74 bpm, oxygen saturation 96%

Height 172 cm, weight 62 kg, BSA 1.72 m$^2$

Surgical scars: Pale bilateral thoracotomy scars and a pale midline sternotomy scar

Neck veins: Somewhat elevated above the sternal angle, without a persistent waveform

Lungs/chest: Chest was clear.

Heart: There was no RV lift. The apex was not palpable. The heart rhythm was irregular. The second heart sound was single. There were no murmurs.

Abdomen: The liver edge was not palpable and there was no ascites.

Extremities: There was no clubbing. The extremities were free of edema. Both radial pulses were absent, femoral pulses were normal bilaterally.

***Comments:*** The blood pressure may be difficult to measure in the ipsilateral arm of a patient with a previous BT shunt. In a case with a unilateral BT shunt it is important to be aware of this and measure the blood pressure in the contralateral arm to avoid false readings. In this case both arms had reduced pressure, and blood pressure had to be obtained in the leg.

This patient had a normal oxygen saturation. However, patients with a previous Fontan operation usually have a degree of arterial desaturation for several reasons, including open fenestrations (i.e., surgically created small ASDs), systemic venous collaterals, and pulmonary arteriovenous malformations (the latter mainly if there is or has been a classic Glenn shunt, i.e., an anastomosis between the SVC and the right pulmonary artery excluding the right lung from IVC venous return).

The JVP is typically difficult to see because of poor waveform and significant elevation in patients who have had a Fontan procedure.

The patient has an irregular heart rate, which is atrial fibrillation until proven otherwise. This should always be a cause for concern in a Fontan patient. The patient himself has noted no new palpitations. It is possible that his use of amiodarone has prevented a tachycardic response to new atrial arrhythmia, and thus the patient has not noted a change in heart rhythm. One might suspect the patient to have noted some change in exercise capacity, however.

The second heart sound is usually single in patients with a previous Fontan operation. There are typically no murmurs. Any easily audible or new murmurs should raise concern. For example, they may reflect progressive AV valve regurgitation and impairment of systemic ventricular function.

## LABORATORY DATA

| | |
|---|---|
| Hemoglobin | 13.5 g/dL (13–17) |
| Hematocrit/PCV | 43% (41–51) |
| MCV | 93 fL (83–99) |
| Platelet count | 293 × 10$^9$/L (150–400) |
| Sodium | 136 mmol/L (134–145) |
| Potassium | 4.6 mmol/L (3.5–5.2) |
| Creatinine | 0.9 mg/dL (0.6–1.2) |
| Blood urea nitrogen | 3.9 mmol/L (2.5–6.5) |

Liver and thyroid function tests were normal.

## ELECTROCARDIOGRAM

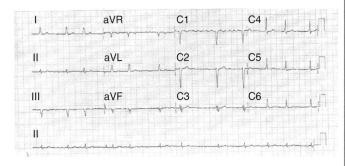

Figure 61-1 Electrocardiogram.

### FINDINGS
Heart rate: 72 bpm

Left axis deviation. Atrial fibrillation. Small R-waves and deep S-waves in V1 and V2. Dominant R-waves and no S waves in V5 and V6.

***Comments:*** Small R-waves and deep S-waves over right precordial leads and tall R-waves over left precordial leads, as well as left-axis deviation, are typical ECG features of tricuspid atresia with a dominant LV. Intra-atrial reentrant tachycardia or atypical atrial flutter is found in 57% of patients after Fontan procedure, and atrial fibrillation is not uncommon.

## CHEST X-RAY

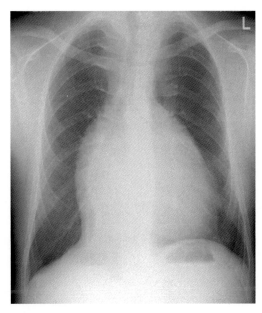

Figure 61-2 Posteroanterior projection.

### FINDINGS
Cardiothoracic ratio: 67%

Severe cardiomegaly with RA enlargement. Normal lung parenchyma.

***Comments:*** Severe RA enlargement is characteristic of Ebstein patients or aortopulmonary Fontan patients. Fontan patients with total cavopulmonary connection, in contrast, usually have a relatively small cardiac silhouette.

## EXERCISE TESTING

Exercise testing had been performed 2 years prior to presentation.

Exercise protocol: Modified Bruce
Duration (min:sec): 9:38
Reason for stopping: Fatigue
ECG changes: None (sinus tachycardia)

|  | Rest | Peak |
| --- | --- | --- |
| Heart rate (bpm): | 74 | 148 |
| Percent of age-predicted max HR: |  | 76 |
| $O_2$ saturation (%): | 96 | 98 |
| Blood pressure (mm Hg): | 118/72 | 142/78 |
| Double product: |  | 21,016 |
| Peak $V_{O_2}$ (mL/kg/min): |  | 23 |
| Percent predicted (%): |  | 54 |
| $Ve/Vco_2$: |  | 26 |
| Metabolic equivalents: |  | 6.5 |

***Comments:*** The peak $V_{O_2}$ is highly variable in subjects with a previous Fontan operation, but always well below expected for age. In 34 consecutive Fontan patients investigated, the mean peak $V_{O_2}$ was $19.8 \pm 5.8$ mL/kg/min.[4] This patient's performance is relatively reassuring.

In Fontan patients, there is virtually no increase in ejection fraction during exercise, in part because the Fontan ventricle is typically underfilled. Increased heart rate is the major adaptation that can increase cardiac output. Thus, these patients may be very sensitive to chronotropic incompetence.

When this study was performed, the patient was in sinus rhythm. The heart rate increase here is likely a major contributor to the patient's performance. Now that the patient is in atrial fibrillation, one doubts whether his exercise tolerance would be as good if objectively measured.

## ECHOCARDIOGRAM

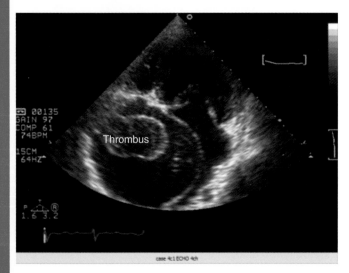

Figure 61-3 Apical four-chamber view.

## FINDINGS

There was severe enlargement of the RA with bulging of the atrial septum toward the LA. A large and rounded atrial thrombus was visualized inside the RA. Ventricular function was normal. There was no valvular regurgitation.

***Comments:*** Presence of RA or LA thrombus is usually best appreciated with TEE. In addition to evaluation of the RA size and assessment for atrial thrombus, echo images should include examination of the atriopulmonary connection, pulmonary artery size, AV valve, and main ventricular morphology. The thrombus here was unmistakable, and TEE was unnecessary.

## MAGNETIC RESONANCE IMAGING

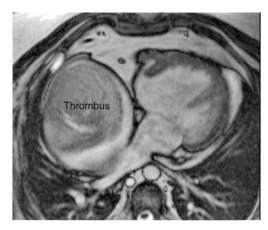

Figure 61-4 Oblique axial view.

## FINDINGS

Oblique axial image shows the large thrombus again in the severely enlarged RA. The single ventricle is also visible with mild mitral regurgitation.

***Comments:*** Here, the ventricle volumes were calculated as one ventricle, since the RV is hypoplastic. The "normal" volume values for a single ventricle are unknown. The ejection fraction here suggests mild dysfunction, which was consistent with the subjective appearance of the ventricle.

The signal characteristics within the thrombus vary, with various layers visible almost like rings of a tree. This suggests the thrombus is old and slowly growing with layer upon layer of thrombosis building over time.

### Ventricular Volume Quantification

|  | LV | (Normal range) |
| --- | --- | --- |
| EDV (mL) | 172 | (52–141) |
| ESV (mL) | 95 | (13–51) |
| SV (mL) | 77 | (33–97) |
| EF (%) | 45 | (57–75) |
| EDVi (mL/m²) | 100 | (62–96) |
| ESVi (mL/m²) | 55 | (17–36) |
| SVi (mL/m²) | 45 | (40–65) |

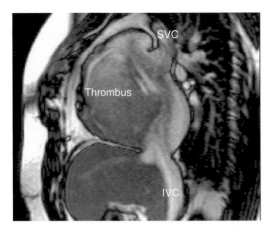

Figure 61-5 Oblique sagittal stady-state free precession cine.

## FINDINGS

Sagittal SSFP cine image through the enlarged RA showing the very large, rounded, laminated atrial thrombus (atrial size 9 × 7 × 7 cm). The flow from both caval veins passes unobstructed behind the thrombus to an unobstructed atriopulmonary connection.

**Comments:** This large thrombus developed in the setting of RA enlargement and slow volume flow. Thrombus formation is much more likely in such patients when they have atrial flutter or fibrillation, especially when they are not anticoagulated.

Flow through the RA must circumnavigate this large thrombus to reach the pulmonary arteries.

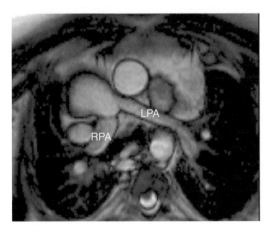

Figure 61-6 Oblique axial stady-state free precession cine.

## FINDINGS

The connection between RA and pulmonary arteries was intact and not obstructed, and flow was bidirectional. The left and right pulmonary arteries were relatively small.

**Comments:** One advantage of MRI is its ability to visualize the pulmonary artery branches. Small obstructions within the pulmonary arteries can be hemodynamically significant in a Fontan patient.

# CATHETERIZATION

## HEMODYNAMICS

Heart rate    70 bpm

|  | **Pressure** | **Saturation** (%) |
|---|---|---|
| SVC | mean 15 | 73 |
| IVC | mean 14 | 77 |
| RA | mean 14 |  |
| PA | mean 13 | 74 |
| PCWP | mean 9 |  |
| LA | mean 7 | 96 |
| LV | 124/8 |  |
| Aorta | 119/74 mean 87 | 96 |

### Calculations

| | |
|---|---|
| Qp (L/min) | 5.00 |
| Qs (L/min) | 5.46 |
| Cardiac index (L/min/m$^2$) | 3.17 |
| Qp/Qs | 0.92 |
| PVR (Wood units) | 1.20 |
| SVR (Wood units) | 13.38 |

## FINDINGS

Catheterization had been performed 2 years prior to presentation in an effort to address the more frequent atrial arrhythmia.

There was no evidence of an intracardiac shunt. The hemodynamics were excellent. The pulmonary vascular resistance was appropriately low for Fontan circulation.

**Comments:** Fenestrations were never performed as part of atriopulmonary Fontan connections. They were developed for use with lateral tunnel Fontans, and are also sometimes used with extracardiac Fontans.

There is no obstruction in the Fontan circuit that led to the atrial fibrillation. The arrhythmia seems to be the consequence simply of the huge RA usually seen in patients with this particular style of Fontan circulation.

This patient has a preserved cardiac index. Often patients with single ventricle palliation will have a relatively low cardiac index.

### FOCUSED CLINICAL QUESTIONS AND DISCUSSION POINTS

1. Should patients with a Fontan circulation routinely be offered anticoagulation with Coumadin?

   *Although there are no randomized data regarding anticoagulation in Fontan patients, in a consensus document on ACHD,[5] the Fontan circulation is generally considered a procoagulative state. Anticoagulation is recommended in patients with a fenestration in the Fontan circuit, "smoke" in the atria on echocardiography, or atrial arrhythmia. In this patient, there had also been a suspicion of previous pulmonary embolism. Further, he presented in atrial fibrillation, which should be treated with warfarin. Often, however, there are also patient preferences and institutional biases to consider as well as the accumulated risk of bleeding.[6]*

2. Is routine surveillance for thrombus in Fontan patients recommended?

   *Care of Fontan patients should include a search for atrial clots during the periodic outpatient follow-up. While transthoracic echocardiography is most often used, its sensitivity is clearly lower than is that of TEE and CMR. In the setting of new atrial flutter or fibrillation, TEE should usually be performed before cardioversion unless the patient is very unstable.*

3. **What is the treatment of choice for atrial thrombi in the setting of a Fontan circulation?**

*There is no good clinical trial evidence as to how atrial thrombi should be managed in Fontan patients. Small clots may be carefully observed and anticoagulation commenced if not already prescribed. Larger thrombi should probably be removed surgically. There is no specific clot size that is agreed on as an indication for surgery, but the mere presence of any thrombus should prompt discussions about proceeding with conversion of an atriopulmonary Fontan to a lateral tunnel or extracardiac Fontan. If the clot increases in size, if it obstructs blood flow, or if there is any evidence of embolism, aggressive management is warranted. Based on a retrospective review, thrombi that affect hemodynamics are generally dealt with surgically.[7] Mortality is substantially higher in these circumstances (75%, vs. 8% in hemodynamically stable patients). These are very difficult management issues that preferably should be handled in a tertiary adult congenital heart disease center. After much discussion in this case, given the thrombus and atrial arrhythmia, urgent planning of thrombectomy and Fontan conversion was recommended.*

## FINAL DIAGNOSIS

Tricuspid atresia

Prior atriopulmonary Fontan procedure

Atrial fibrillation

Large RA thrombus

## PLAN OF ACTION

Surgical removal of the RA clot and conversion to an extracardiac Fontan

## INTERVENTION

The patient stayed on anticoagulants until the time of surgery. A 22-mm Gore-Tex graft was placed between the IVC and the inferior aspect of the right pulmonary artery, forming a lateral tunnel. The clot was removed from the RA, and excess RA tissue was removed. The operation was difficult, and extreme surgical conditions did not allow for any attempt at arrhythmia ablation surgery.

## OUTCOME

In the immediate postoperative period, hemodynamic instability and inadequate hemostasis hampered attempts at sternal closure. After massive transfusions and skin-only closure, the patient was brought to the intensive care unit on maximal pressors.

The early postoperative phase was further complicated by a compartment syndrome in the left leg. Later recurrence of RA or lateral tunnel clot was diagnosed by TEE, but resolved with heparin treatment. With prolonged intubation, the patient developed acute respiratory distress syndrome and experienced several tension pneumothoraces, acute tubular necrosis requiring hemofiltration, and reoperation for sternal wound closure. After eventual tracheotomy, he was discharged home from the hospital 4 months after the operation.

One year after the operation he was doing reasonably well and had returned to work part time. He was able to climb three to four flights of stairs, which is remarkable in the context of the considerable postoperative muscle atrophy the patient experi-

enced. He remained anticoagulated with warfarin, as well as taking bisoprolol and digoxin for rate control of his persistent atrial fibrillation.

***Comments:*** Difficulties of Fontan conversion should never be underestimated. The fragile cardiovascular state in these patients can precipitate failure of multiple organ systems previously considered healthy. Bleeding from insufficient hepatic function, renal insufficiency, and acute respiratory distress syndrome are all manifestations of the brittle nature of these patients. Patients are particularly vulnerable when Fontan conversion is performed in emergent situations; thus surgery should be considered well in advance of trouble.

Atrial maze procedures for atrial arrhythmia are best planned well ahead of time jointly with electrophysiologists and surgeons. Though planned in this case, the surgeon did not feel able to offer a maze safely during the very difficult operation.

## POSTOPERATIVE MRI

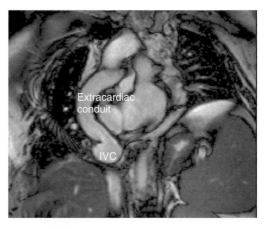

Figure 61-7 Coronal trueFISP image.

### FINDINGS

An extracardiac conduit was in place, bringing flow from the IVC up to the right pulmonary artery near the Glenn anastomosis.

***Comments:*** An early postoperative cardiac MRI again showed mildly impaired LV function. There is no evidence for new atrial clot formation.

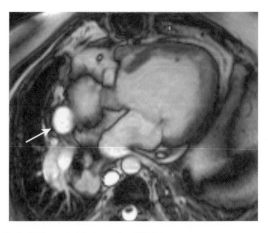

Figure 61-8 Oblique axial plane, trueFISP image.

**Comments:** The RA size has been dramatically reduced and the thrombus removed. Instead, the extracardiac tunnel can be seen coursing to the right of the RA (*arrow*).

## Selected References

1. Freedom R, Jia L, Shi-Joon Y: Late complications following the Fontan operation. In Gatzoulis MA, Webb GD, Daubeney PEF (eds): Diagnosis and Management of Adult Congenital Heart Disease. Philadelphia, Churchill Livingstone, 2003, pp 85–91.
2. Varma C, Warr MR, Hendler AL, et al: Prevalence of "silent" pulmonary emboli in adults after the Fontan operation. J Am Coll Cardiol 41:2252–2258, 2003.
3. Gelatt M, Hamilton RM, McCrindle BW, et al: Risk factors for atrial tachyarrhythmias after the Fontan operation. J Am Coll Cardiol 24:1735–1741, 1994.
4. Diller GP, Dimopoulos K, Okonko D, et al: Exercise intolerance in adult congenital heart disease: Comparative severity, correlates and prognostic implication. Circulation 112:828–835, 2005.
5. Therrien J, Warnes C, Daliento L, et al: Canadian Cardiovascular Society Consensus Conference 2001 update: Recommendations for the management of adults with congenital heart disease part III. Can J Cardiol 17:1135–1158, 2001.
6. Walker HA, Gatzoulis MA: Prophylactic anticoagulation following the Fontan operation. Heart 91:854–856, 2005.
7. Tsang W, Johansson B, Salehian O, et al: Intracardiac thrombus in adults with the Fontan circulation. Cardiol Young 17:646–651, 2007.

# Protein-Losing Enteropathy

**Marc Gewillig**

**Age: 16 years**
**Gender: Female**
**Occupation: Student**
**Working diagnosis: Univentricular heart, Fontan circulation**

## HISTORY

The patient had been diagnosed at birth with a functionally univentricular heart due to pulmonary valve atresia and severe tricuspid valve stenosis. At the age of 1 month a modified left BT shunt was created; at the age of 2 years an atriopulmonary Fontan connection was established.

She did clinically well with good exercise tolerance until the age of 15 years, when she began to feel noticeably more dyspneic than her peers during similar physical activities. Over the next few months her exercise tolerance reduced further. She sought medical attention at a tertiary care center.

She is a nonsmoker.

**Comments:** A newborn with this anatomical background will have limited pulmonary blood flow and severe cyanosis. The establishment of an aortopulmonary shunt, in this case subclavian artery to pulmonary artery, will enhance pulmonary blood flow, improve systemic oxygenation, and foster proper growth of the pulmonary arteries.

Most patients with a normally functioning Fontan circulation will be able to participate in normal daily activities. The biggest difference with peers is decreased exercise capacity, usually 50% to 70% of normal for young individuals.

## CURRENT SYMPTOMS

The patient's main complaint was shortness of breath with mild exertion. Four months prior to presentation she had developed intermittent facial edema with swollen eyelids. She also complained of a swollen abdomen. She did not complain of palpitations. Her bowel habits had not changed significantly.

NYHA class: III

**Comments:** Edema of nondependent areas, such as eyelid edema, suggests hypoalbuminemia and low osmotic pressure rather than heart failure.

Fontan patients have an increased incidence of coagulation factor deficiencies including protein C, protein S, and antithrombin III, as in any patient with hepatic congestion. Thrombosis is more likely to occur in patients with low cardiac output and more than usual atrial and systemic venous dilatation and blood stasis, as can be expected in any patient with an atriopulmonary connection. Some clinicians advocate anticoagulation for every patient with a Fontan circuit; however, there are clearly subgroups of patients with a very low risk.[1] Full anticoagulation should be prescribed in patients with previous thrombi, poor cardiac output (frequently associated with spontaneous contrast on echo), congestive heart failure, dilation of venous or atrial structures, and atrial flutter or fibrillation.

## CURRENT MEDICATIONS

Warfarin (target INR 2–3)

Yearly influenza vaccination

**Comments:** Immunization against influenza is recommended. Influenza is always associated with bronchitis, which increases pulmonary vascular resistance and is poorly tolerated by a Fontan patient (whose physiology requires low pulmonary vascular resistance).

## PHYSICAL EXAMINATION

BP 114/70 mm Hg, HR 85 bpm, oxygen saturation 93% on room air

Height 172 cm, weight 56 kg, BSA 1.64 m$^2$

Surgical scars: Left thoracotomy and median sternotomy scars

Neck veins: JVP was elevated to 7 cm above the sternal angle; there was no prominent A-wave.

Lungs/chest: Chest was clear.

Heart: There was no ventricular lift. There was a single first and second heart. No additional sounds or murmurs were present.

Abdomen: There was mild hepatomegaly but no ascites.

Extremities: There was moderate symmetric pitting edema of both ankles. There was peripheral cyanosis (reflecting sluggish tissue perfusion) but no clubbing.

**Comments:** Mild arterial desaturation is frequently seen in Fontan patients. However, in this patient the discrepancy between pulse oximetry and the peripheral cyanosis reflects poor cardiac output (with sluggish tissue perfusion and excessive oxygen extraction peripherally).

The RA in an atriopulmonary Fontan is usually dilated and overstretched; it does not generate a significant contraction.

Plastic bronchitis can be another expression of lymphatic leakage into the bronchi, chyle leaks into the bronchi forming casts that will impede adequate ventilation. This can be clinically very difficult to detect if the patient does not expectorate the casts. This diagnosis is then made, unfortunately, at autopsy.

Any Fontan patient with progressive respiratory insufficiency needs a bronchoscopy to exclude this possibility.

These auscultatory findings are typical of a Fontan patient: single S1 and S2, no murmurs.

## LABORATORY DATA

| | |
|---|---|
| Hemoglobin | 14.9 g/dL (11.5–15.0) |
| Hematocrit | 43% (36–46) |
| MCV | 93 fL (83–99) |
| MCH | 32.1 pg (27–32.5) |
| Sodium | 136 mmol/L (134–145) |
| Potassium | 3.9 mmol/L (3.5–5.2) |
| Creatinine | 0.8 mg/dL (0.6–1.2) |
| Total protein | **4.6 g/dL** (6.0–8.0) |
| Albumin | **2.7 g/dL** (3.5–5.2) |
| Alpha 1 antitrypsin | |
| Serum | 1.44 g/L (0.88–1.74) |
| Fecal | **4.2 g/L** (< 0.54 g/L) |
| Stool collection | Daily loss of **16%** (normal limit < 2%) after indium 111 transferrin administration |

***Comments:*** The hemoglobin is normal, as expected, as there is no resting central cyanosis.

Total protein and albumin are significantly decreased. These levels are invariably associated with edema.

In an adult, a normal liver can compensate loss of albumin up to 4 g per day. Losses beyond this will result in hypoalbuminemia.

The indium 111 or 51 Chr-albumin test indicates a large amount of undigested protein loss through the bowels. With this test protein (transferrin or albumin) labeled with indium 111 or 51 chromium is given intravenously; the patients are scanned at given intervals for several hours to localize the earliest site of protein loss; stools are collected for 5 days.[2] Normally less than 2% of the total dosage may appear in the stools.

The findings here confirm the diagnosis of PLE, a condition associated with chronically elevated central venous pressures and characterized by excessive protein loss in the stool.

## ELECTROCARDIOGRAM

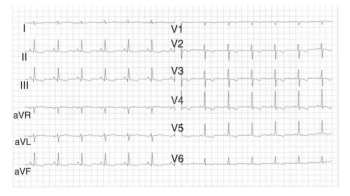

Figure 62-1 Electrocardiogram.

## FINDINGS

Heart rate: 76 bpm

PR interval: 144 msec

QRS axis: +84°

QRS duration: 82 msec

Normal sinus rhythm, probable RA enlargement. Nonspecific ST- and T-wave changes. (Note the lack of a 1-milliVolt. standardization.)

***Comments:*** Atrial enlargement would be expected in this patient.

## CHEST X-RAY

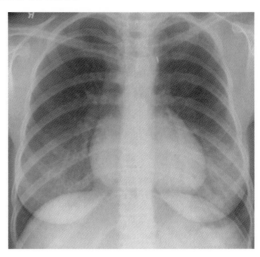

Figure 62-2 Posteroanterior projection.

## FINDINGS

Cardiothoracic ratio: 47%

The cardiac silhouette is at the upper limit of normal. The central pulmonary arteries are prominent but not dilated. The SVC is dilated. The prominent bulge at the right cardiac border indicates RA enlargement. Pulmonary vascular markings are at the lower limit of normal.

***Comments:*** Cardiac output in a Fontan circulation is diminished (50%–70% of normal for BSA).[3] A relatively small heart is therefore normal for a patient with Fontan physiology (see Case 63), unless clinical decompensation occurs or extreme RA enlargement occurs (see Case 61). A large cardiac silhouette reflects additional conditions other than "pure" Fontan physiology. These might include:

Abnormal loading conditions (volume overload) prior to the Fontan operation, resulting in overgrowth, overdilation, or reconfiguration of the ventricle(s) and atria

Ventricular dysfunction and dilation

Increased volume load due to residual shunts or valve regurgitation[4]

# ECHOCARDIOGRAM

## OVERALL FINDINGS

Relatively small LV with normal systolic function. No significant regurgitation of the left AV valve was present. The aortic valve was normal. The RA was enlarged, but no thrombus was present, and no obstruction visualized.

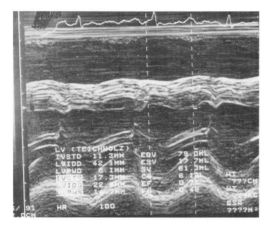

Figure 62-3 Parasteinal M-mode of the left ventricle (LV). The LV was not dilated and has good contractility and mild hypertrophy.

## FINDINGS

M-mode through the LV showed an end-diastolic dimension of 42 mm. The ventricle was underloaded, consistent with Fontan physiology. Ventricular contractility was still well preserved.

***Comments:*** Ventricular dysfunction, if present, may be due to (1) abnormal loading conditions prior to the Fontan operation, (2) an intrinsic abnormality of the abnormal ventricle itself, and/or (3) reduced transpulmonary blood flow and impaired LV filling. With the latter, Fontan physiology will chronically underload or deprive the ventricle, which may result in remodeling, reduced compliance, poor ventricular filling, and eventually continuously declining cardiac output. This mechanism/process is still poorly understood.

## CATHETERIZATION

|  | Pressure | Saturation (%) |
|---|---|---|
| SVC | mean 10 | 65 |
| RA | mean 10 | 66 |
| IVC | mean 10 | 68 |
| Right PA | mean 9 | 67 |
| Left PA | mean 9 | 67 |
| Left wedge | mean 7 |  |
| Right wedge | mean 7 |  |
| LV | 93/7 | 99 |
| Ao | 94/58 mean 75 | 99 |

**Calculations**

| | |
|---|---|
| Qp (L/min) | 3.20 |
| Qs (L/min) | 2.99 |
| Cardiac index (L/min/m²) | 1.83 |
| Qp/Qs | 1.07 |
| PVR (Wood units) | 0.62 |
| SVR (Wood units) | 21.77 |

## FINDINGS

Cardiac catheterization was performed to assess pulmonary arterial pressures and pulmonary vascular resistance, and to actively exclude an obstruction in the pulmonary blood flow, which might require intervention. The study demonstrated the systemic venous pressures to be mildly elevated, as expected with any Fontan circulation. Cardiac output was reduced, reflected by the decreased mixed venous saturation. Pulmonary vascular resistance was not elevated.

***Comments:*** Catheterization may reveal problems with the Fontan circuit (such as a gradient at one of the anastomotic sites or poor design), problems of the pulmonary vasculature (increased pulmonary vascular resistance, stenosis or hypoplasia, collateral flow through bronchial arteries), or cardiac problems (AV valve regurgitation, myocardial systolic or diastolic dysfunction, inappropriate afterload).

PLE is frequently reported despite "good hemodynamics."

Both preoperative and postoperative assessment can be misleading. Prior to operation, the pulmonary vascular resistance in low-flow conditions may not accurately reflect the hemodynamic conditions after the Fontan circulation is established. This is in part because pulmonary vascular impedance or capacitance is not measured, the lymphatic reserve is not assessed, previous long-standing increased pressure or flow through the pulmonary vasculature has led to altered resistance, or there has been diminished pulmonary vascular growth due to decreased flow.

Clinicians should recognize that in Fontan patients, low cardiac output causes significant underestimation of pulmonary vascular resistance; congestion cannot be assessed or quantified; and chronic diuretics blur most hemodynamic studies. Low-flow conditions make assessment using the Fick principle more difficult.

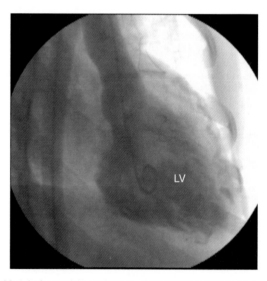

Figure 62-4 Left ventricle angiogram, right anterior oblique projection.

## FINDINGS

Good ventricular function was observed.

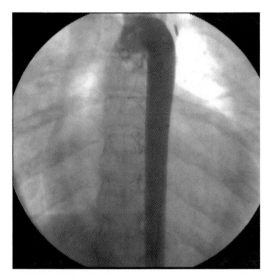

Figure 62-5 Anteroposterior aortogram.

## FINDINGS

No significant collateral arteries were seen.

**Comments:** Extensive collateral bronchial circulation needs to be excluded. Collaterals can be identified by the presence of a significant contrast flush in the lung parenchyma. Digital subtraction angiography and/or selective injections of thoracic vessels (subclavian artery, internal mammary arteries, intercostal arteries) may be required. If present, collaterals generally should be embolized.

Collaterals may grow in time; therefore this examination needs to be repeated during long-term follow-up.

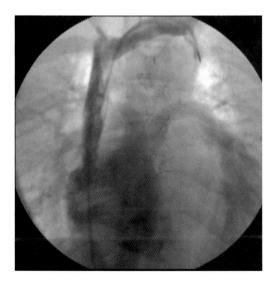

Figure 62-6 Injection in superior caval vein, anteroposterior projection.

## FINDINGS

The RA was severely dilated; there was significant energy loss from streamlined laminar flow in the SVC to the turbulent chaotic flow in the RA.

**Comments:** This pattern is consistent with a "functional" obstruction.[5]

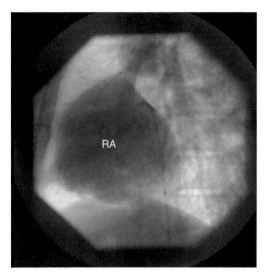

Figure 62-7 Right atrial angiogram profile.

## FINDINGS

The RA was severely dilated.

**Comments:** RA enlargement is expected in patients with an atriopulmonary-type Fontan circuit. Atrial enlargement promotes clot formation and arrhythmia. The dilated RA forms a "functional obstruction."

## SCINTIGRAPHY

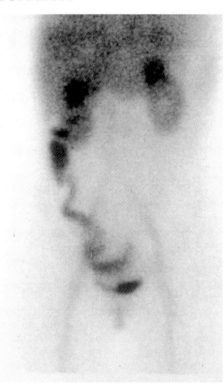

Figure 62-8 Scintigraphy of the abdominal cavity using 51 Chr-albumin.[2]

## FINDINGS

There was clear activity in liver, kidneys, and large veins (femoral, iliac, and caval); some collection in the bladder. There was abnormal leakage into the terminal ileum, with progression of counts into the ascending colon.

**Comments:** 51 Chr-albumin should remain in the intravascular space; therefore, scintigraphy will reflect the blood pool distribution.

The image suggests that chylous leakage in this patient is not diffuse, but concentrated in the terminal ileum. This finding opens the theoretical possibility of selective gut resection to "cure" PLE.

## FOCUSED CLINICAL QUESTIONS AND DISCUSSION POINTS

1. What is the basis for the patient's edema?

*This patient has leakage of lymph fluid into the terminal ileum. Lymphangiectasia is due to chronic systemic venous congestion and low flow in the Fontan circulation, and fosters this type of abnormality.*

2. What is the cause of chylous circulatory failure?

*The obstruction of lymphatic flow is mainly due to systemic venous congestion in a Fontan circuit. The differential diagnosis includes the following:*

1. *Left heart dysfunction: In this patient it has been excluded. Many Fontan patients have a large ventricle with adverse remodeling (due to either overuse or underfilling). However, even when ventricular dysfunction is present, circulatory failure may still be due to other causes.*
2. *Pulmonary vascular obstruction: In this patient the pulmonary circulation is free of hypoplasia, stenosis, or kinking (e.g., from a previous BT shunt); excessive collateral flow (bronchial arteries, or a palliative shunt); increased vascular resistance (though this may be undetected in low-flow states); or obstruction of one or more pulmonary veins.*
3. *Poor Fontan circulation: This is due primarily to anatomic obstruction or stenosis, or significant functional obstruction due to the dilated RA.*

*Hypoxemia induced pulmonary vasoconstriction can lead to PLE; a long stay at high altitude or even a long airplane flight can trigger PLE in some patients.[6] Most patients with a Fontan circuit will, however, tolerate such altitude conditions without a problem.*

3. What is the prognosis for this patient?

*The diagnosis of PLE usually carries a very poor prognosis. In an international multicenter study involving 35 centers and 3029 patients with Fontan repair (1975–1995) 114 patients were identified with PLE.[7] After diagnosis, the 5-year survival was 59%, with less than 20% surviving beyond 10 years. Slow onset and slow progression frequently mislead the clinician, resulting in a "soft" approach.*

4. What are the medical treatment options for PLE?

*A diet high in calories, high in protein and low in salt content, and high in medium-chain triglyceride fat supplements is usually recommended (without clinical proof of its efficacy). Diuretics can more or less control peripheral edema in most patients. Protein infusions (albumin, globulin) can be required on a weekly or monthly basis. In some patients specific anti-infection measures are necessary (chronic antibiotics, vaccines). All these measures are only palliative to treat symptoms; clinical resolution of PLE with only these measures is extremely rare, at less than 1%.[7]*

*Augmenting cardiac function or output with inotropic drugs or systemic vasodilators in this patient will not be helpful: the left heart is not usually the limiting factor in this type of Fontan circuit/situation.*

*Corticosteroids can significantly improve PLE,[8–10] although the mechanism remains unclear. Steroids act as a membrane sta-*

*bilizer, an inflammatory-immunologic mediator, which also improves cellular anabolism. The usual dose is prednisone 1 to 2 mg/kg/day with weaning after 2 weeks. This is successful in about 30% to 60% of the patients. Some patients are "cured" for several weeks, months, or years with a single course of treatment, while others will have an ongoing need for steroid therapy; some patients may also show no response at all. Side effects of chronic steroid therapy are substantial, and this should obviously be taken into account. Recently, budesonide (Entocort 3-mg capsule, slow release) has been introduced for treatment of inflammatory bowel disease.[11] Budesonide is 15 times more powerful than prednisolone with local effect in the ileum and ascending colon, but due to extensive biotransformation at first pass in the liver, it has hardly any systemic effect. Its efficacy on this type of PLE is currently under investigation; initial results are promising.*

*High molecular weight (unfractionated) heparin has been found to help some patients.[12] High molecular weight heparin is a proteoglycan sulfate membrane stabilizer; the minimal effective dose is unknown, but it is well below the anticoagulation dose. Most patients who respond will do so at the dosage of 3000 to 5000 units/day subcutaneously. Some patients will be cured after a single period of heparin, some patients will need ongoing treatment; at least one third of the patients will show no reaction. Side effects such as local hematoma and significant osteopenia are not uncommon.*

*Somatostatin (octreotide acetate) can in some patients improve PLE.[13] The dosage of 1 to 4 μg/kg/day subcutaneously or by depot intramuscular injection every 3 weeks can "cure" some patients (responders). For treatment of chylothorax much higher doses have been given, up to 40 μg/kg/day in three doses. Some patients will require ongoing administration on a daily, weekly, or monthly basis; but many patients will show no response whatsoever. Significant side effects such as sensitization have been described.*

5. What interventional and/or surgical treatment options could be considered for treatment of PLE?

*Several catheter techniques exist for PLE management:*

1. *Balloon dilation or stent implantation of a stenosed Fontan circuit or residual pulmonary vessel stenosis or hypoplasia.*
2. *Residual left-to-right shunts (native, surgical, arterial venous collaterals) can be embolized.*
3. *An appropriately sized fenestration with stent can safely be created through a percutaneous (or transhepatic) route.[14,15] The fenestration will decrease venous pressure and congestion, improve runoff, and increase cardiac output. However, this comes at the expense of arterial desaturation and cyanosis. As case reports demonstrate, PLE will nearly always improve following a proper fenestration,[16] but the range between "acceptable" PLE and "unacceptable" cyanosis may be narrow. This range frequently further narrows over months, probably because of secondary changes in the pulmonary vasculature. Many such patients will therefore require heart transplantation in the medium to longer term follow-up.*

*Cardiac pacing in patients with excessive bradycardia or AV dissociation can critically alter cardiac function and output and may have a beneficial effect on PLE.[17]*

*Resection of a limited part—the most affected part—of the intestine has been reported. However, experience is very limited, with few successful reports.[18] Even after a successful gut resection, the next weakest intestinal segment may start to leak again with time. However, if after optimization of hemodynamics PLE persists, and if chylous leakage is limited to a single gut segment, selected gut resection may be an option to consider.*

*Surgical conversion of atriopulmonary to cavopulmonary connection appears to be a valid option.[19] This procedure may carry a high mortality if there is significant AV valve regurgitation and ventricular dysfunction, but can improve venous flow through the* pulmonary vascular bed and reverse PLE.[5,19] Late Fontan take-down has been performed in some patients, but is associated with a high mortality.

Heart transplantation is the most reliable way to cure PLE but obviously comes with its own long-term problems.[20–22] Fontan patients are at increased risk of early mortality because of cachexia and immunologic deficiency. If successful, transplantation will improve the hemodynamic condition by increasing cardiac output and decreasing venous congestion. Chronic anti-rejection therapy may also favorably influence PLE. Thus, in most patients, PLE resolves after transplantation, and only rarely does the problem persist or relapse years later.

## FINAL DIAGNOSIS

PLE after Fontan with focal chylous leakage in the bowel

"Normal" left heart function

## PLAN OF ACTION

Conversion to total cavopulmonary circulation

## INTERVENTION

After careful consideration and planning, the patient underwent conversion to a total cavopulmonary connection. The top part of the SVC was anastomosed to the right pulmonary artery in an end-to-side fashion (bidirectional Glenn), and a 24-mm extracardiac conduit was placed between the IVC and the underside of the left pulmonary artery. A 5-mm fenestration into the RA was also created to limit congestion and enhance flow, at the expense of desaturation. Reduction of the RA with a right-sided maze procedure was also performed,[22] and an epicardial pacing system with backup spare wires was placed.

## OUTCOME

The operation was well tolerated, and the patient was extubated 6 hours after surgery. However, the patient had a slow recovery. Despite subcutaneous heparin she developed a thrombosis in the extracardiac conduit, thereby occluding the fenestration. She nevertheless made good progress and left the hospital 2 weeks after surgery.

The PLE resolved within 3 to 4 months from surgery, with a good clinical and functional result 3 years later.

The patient has been told that in time PLE may recur. If PLE develops without a clear predisposing factor, heart transplantation would have to be considered as the next surgical option.

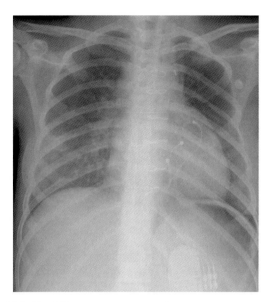

Figure 62-9 Chest X-ray.

### FINDINGS

Postoperative status; no cardiomegaly. One atrial and two ventricular epicardial pacing leads are well seen. The RA was prominent preoperatively, but is no longer visibly dilated.

**Comments:** If a pacing lead failure develops in the future, this cannot be resolved by a simple transvenous approach, but probably will require a resternotomy to find a good pacing position. Placement of spare epicardial leads at the time of elective surgery can therefore be very useful in patients with a Fontan circulation.

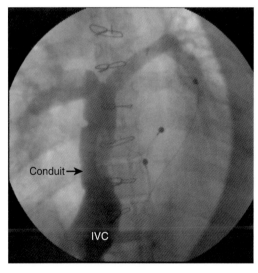

Figure 62-10 Inferior vena cava cavogram.

### FINDINGS

Angiogram in the extracardiac conduit 10 days after surgery. The IVC is connected with a 24-mm Gore-Tex conduit to the original pulmonary trunk. In the midportion a thrombus is observed, obstructing the fenestration. Note also the wash-in flow from the SVC in the proximal part of the right pulmonary artery.

**Comments:** During the catheterization the thrombus was never crossed with a catheter. The patient was maintained on heparin and Coumadin; the thrombus shrank without a functional or hemodynamic problem.

## Selected References

1. Monagle P, Karl TR: Thromboembolic problems after the Fontan operation. Semin Thorac Cardiovasc Surg Pediatr Card Surg Ann 5:36–47, 2002.
2. De Kaski MC, Peters AM, Bradley D, Hodgson HJ: Detection and quantification of protein-losing enteropathy with Indium-111 transferrin. Eur J Nucl Med 23:530–533, 1996.
3. Gewillig M, Kalis N: Pathophysiologic aspects after cavopulmonary anastomosis. Thorac Cardiovasc Surg 48:336–341, 2000.
4. Gewillig M: The Fontan circulation. Heart 91:839–846, 2005.
5. De Leval M, Kilner P, Gewillig M, Bull C: Total cavopulmonary connection: A logical alternative to atriopulmonary connection for complex Fontan operations. Experimental studies and early clinical experience. J Thorac Cardiovasc Surg 96:682–695, 1988.
6. McMahon CJ, Hicks JM, Dreyer WJ. High-altitude precipitation and exacerbation of protein-losing enteropathy after a Fontan operation. Cardiol Young 11:225–228, 2001.
7. Mertens L, Hagler D, Somerville J, et al: Protein losing enteropathy after the Fontan operation: An international multicenter evaluation. J Thorac Cardiovasc Surg 115:1063–1073, 1998.
8. Rothman A, Snyder J: Protein-losing enteropathy following the Fontan operation: Resolution with prednisone therapy. Am Heart J 121:618–619, 1991.
9. Rychik J, Piccoli DA, Barber G: Usefulness of corticosteroid therapy for protein-losing enteropathy after the Fontan procedure. Am J Cardiol 68:819–821, 1991.
10. Therrien J, Webb GD, Gatzoulis MA: Reversal of protein losing enteropathy with prednisone in adults with modified Fontan operations: Long term palliation or bridge to cardiac transplantation? Heart 82:241–243, 1999.
11. Siewert E, Lammert F, Koppitz P, et al: Eosinophilic gastroenteritis with severe protein-losing enteropathy: Successful treatment with budesonide. Dig Liver Dis 38:55–59, 2006.
12. Donnelly JP, Rosenthal A, Castle VP, Holmes RD: Reversal of protein-losing enteropathy with heparin therapy in three patients with univentricular hearts and Fontan palliation. J Pediatr 130:474–478, 1997.
13. Cheung Y, Leung M, Yip M: Octreotide for treatment of postoperative chylothorax. J Pediatr 139:157–159, 2001.
14. Mertens L, Dumoulin M, Gewillig M: Effect of percutaneous fenestration of the atrial septum on protein-losing enteropathy after the Fontan operation. Brit Heart J 72:591–592, 1994.
15. Stumper O, Gewillig M, Vettukattil J, et al: Modified technique of stent fenestration of the atrial septum. Heart 89:1227–1230, 2003.
16. Lemes V, Murphy AM, Osterman FA, et al: Fenestration of extracardiac Fontan and reversal of protein-losing enteropathy: Case report. Pediatr Cardiol 19:355–357, 1998.
17. Cohen MI, Rhodes LA, Wernovsky G, et al: Atrial pacing: An alternative treatment for protein-losing enteropathy after the Fontan operation. J Thorac Cardiovasc Surg 121:582–583, 2001.
18. Connor FL, Angelides S, Gibson M, et al: Successful resection of localized intestinal lymphangiectasia post-Fontan: Role of (99m) technetium-dextran scintigraphy. Pediatrics 112:242–247, 2003.
19. Conte S, Gewillig M, Eyskens B, et al: Management of late complications after classic Fontan procedure by conversion to total cavopulmonary connection. Cardiovasc Surg 7:651–655, 1999.
20. Mertens L, Hagler D, Canter C, et al: The outcome of heart transplantation for protein losing enteropathy after the Fontan operation. Circulation 100(Suppl 1):I–602, 1999.
21. Holmgren D, Berggren H, Wahlander H, et al: Reversal of protein-losing enteropathy in a child with Fontan circulation is correlated with central venous pressure after heart transplantation. Pediatr Transplant 5:135–137, 2001.
22. Mavroudis C, Deal BJ, Backer CL: The beneficial effects of total cavopulmonary conversion and arrhythmia surgery for the failed Fontan. Semin Thorac Cardiovasc Surg Pediatr Card Surg Ann 5:12–24, 2002.

# Fontan and Pregnancy

**Anselm Uebing**

**Age: 31 years**
**Gender: Female**
**Occupation: Supermarket clerk**
**Working diagnosis: Functionally univentricular heart after Fontan-type palliation, 16 weeks pregnant**

## HISTORY

The patient was cyanotic at birth and had her first palliative procedure (a classic left-sided BT anastomosis) in her native country at the age of 11 years. She felt well after this operation.

She immigrated to the United Kingdom at the age of 17 and by then had noticed dyspnea on exertion. She was investigated in a pediatric cardiology department and the diagnosis of functionally univentricular heart with pulmonary atresia was made. She underwent further surgery at the age of 20 years. A Fontan-type operation was performed with ligation of the BT anastomosis.

She felt much improved after this operation and her cyanosis resolved. She did not continue regular cardiological follow-up. She married at the age of 30. The couple did not practice any contraception. She became pregnant within a year and was referred at 16 weeks gestation from her local obstetrician.

**Comments:** The classic BT anastomosis was the first palliative procedure developed for "blue babies" and aims to increase pulmonary blood flow when pulmonary atresia or stenosis limits pulmonary blood supply.[1] It originally involved an end-to-side connection of the subclavian artery to the ipsilateral pulmonary artery. This procedure resulted in an absent arterial pulse in the arm. Later versions of the BT shunt used an interposition tube graft to connect the subclavian or a central systemic artery with a pulmonary artery. PAH—an uncommon complication of classic BT shunts—was addressed with this modification in which different sizes tubes were employed for different sizes of patients and for varying degrees of cyanosis. Arterial pulse in the ipsilateral arm was less affected.

Fontan-type operations were developed for patients with a univentricular heart to direct the systemic venous blood to the pulmonary arteries without the interposition of a subpulmonary ventricle, and to abolish right-to-left shunting. These operations therefore approached normalization of oxygen saturation at the cost of nonpulsatile pulmonary blood flow and elevated systemic venous pressure. The original Fontan operation consisted of the interposition of a valved conduit between the right atrium and the main pulmonary artery and has been modified many times since.[2]

It is common for patients with ACHD, complex or not, to leave proper follow-up, believing that their heart condition has been cured. Patients with ACHD need to know that lifelong follow-up is required for most of them and that further investigations and interventions might be needed. Women of reproductive age must be told of the impact of their heart condition on their childbearing potential. As cardiac disease, mostly congenital, is a leading cause of maternal death in developed countries, timely prepregnancy counseling must be offered to all women with congenital heart disease to prevent avoidable pregnancy-related risks and for crisis management.[3]

## CURRENT SYMPTOMS

The patient did not complain of any change in her well-being since becoming pregnant. She had not experienced shortness of breath nor had she noted a reduction in her exercise capacity.

She reported that she could walk without limitation on level ground and could climb three to four flights of stairs without any problems.

Furthermore, she has been free of palpitations, chest pain, and dizziness.

NYHA class: I

**Comments:** The risk for pregnant women with congenital heart disease of suffering an adverse cardiovascular event such as symptomatic arrhythmia, stroke, pulmonary edema, heart failure, or death increases with the anatomic complexity of the congenital heart lesion, the degree of cyanosis, myocardial dysfunction, poor functional class, and the severity of systemic outflow tract obstruction.[4,5]

The fact that this patient presented in good condition, feeling well, and unlimited in her exercise capacity was therefore indicative of a relatively good prognosis for the pregnancy, even though all pregnancies in Fontan patients should be considered relatively high risk.

## CURRENT MEDICATIONS

None

## PHYSICAL EXAMINATION

BP 110/70 mm Hg, HR 73 bpm, oxygen saturation 97%

Height 160 cm, weight 56 kg, BSA 1.58 m$^2$

Surgical scars: Scars from a left lateral thoracotomy and a median sternotomy

Neck veins: Jugular veins were difficult to assess but not grossly dilated. Normal waveforms not present.

Lungs/chest: Chest was clear.

Heart: The heart rate was regular. The cardiac impulse was not displaced. She had a normal first heart sound and a single and loud second heart sound with a grade 1/2 short systolic ejection murmur at the upper left sternal border and no diastolic or continuous murmurs.

Abdomen: No hepatomegaly

Extremities: No clubbing and no left arm pulses. The right radial artery and femoral artery pulses were normal.

***Comments:*** An oxygen saturation of 97% is optimal for a patient after a Fontan-type palliation and indicates that the vast majority of systemic venous blood enters the pulmonary arteries and that there are no major sources of right-to-left shunt within or outside the heart.

As central venous pressure is the driving force of blood flow through the lungs, it should be elevated in patients after a Fontan-type repair. An elevated JVP is therefore expected and not necessarily a matter of concern. The lack of pulsation of the jugular vein may indicate that the central venous pathways are disconnected from the atria, which is the case in newer modifications of the Fontan operation (e.g., total cavopulmonary connections).

A loud second heart sound in this patient may indicate the anterior position of the aorta and aortic valve. Pulmonary hypertension was certainly not present here and cannot be seen in a patient with a Fontan circulation where blood flows through the lungs passively driven by the venous pressure. A single second heart sound is common in Fontan patients, since antegrade flow from the heart to the pulmonary artery via the pulmonary valve is surgically interrupted as part of the Fontan procedure.

A low-grade systolic heart murmur at the upper sternal border indicates slight turbulent systolic blood flow within the heart or at the level of a heart valve. If there was blood flow across a severely stenotic pulmonary valve, the murmur would be much louder. Regurgitation of the mitral or tricuspid valve would be heard best at the lower sternal border. The patient's murmur is therefore most likely due to a mild stenosis of the aortic valve or some turbulence in the outflow tract. The lack of the left radial pulse and the left lateral thoracotomy are in keeping with a previous BT anastomosis.

## LABORATORY DATA

| | |
|---|---|
| Hemoglobin | 13.1 g/dL (11.5–15.0) |
| Hematocrit/PCV | 37% (36–46) |
| MCV | 87 fL (83–99) |
| Platelet count | $152 \times 10^9$/L (150–400) |
| Sodium | 140 mmol/L (134–145) |
| Potassium | 3.7 mmol/L (3.5–5.2) |
| Creatinine | 0.7 mg/dL (0.6–1.2) |
| Blood urea nitrogen | 4.4 mmol/L (2.5–6.5) |

### OTHER RELEVANT LAB RESULTS

| | |
|---|---|
| Total bilirubin | 19 μmol/L (3–24) |
| ALP | 70 U/L (67–372) |
| ALT | 21 IU/L (8–40) |
| AST | 28 IU/L (13–33) |
| Total protein | 63 g/L (62–82) |
| Albumin | 41 g/dL (37–53) |

***Comments:*** All laboratory tests were normal. There was no erythrocytosis and therefore no evidence of chronic cyanosis. At times Fontan patients have a relatively high hemoglobin to compensate for low-cardiac-output-introduced arterial oxygen saturation. This is not the case in this patient.

Hepatic dysfunction can be present in patients with a Fontan circulation as hepatic venous pressure is chronically elevated, although liver function tests are insensitive in assessing this.[6] A condition called PLE is another long-term complication related to the Fontan circulation. The patients lose protein into their intestine. Protein-losing enteropathy leads to low protein and

albumin levels and to peripheral edema (see Case 62). The exact pathophysiology of this condition is unclear, but the role of chronically elevated central venous blood pressures can be assumed.[7]

In summary, normal liver function tests and protein levels were additional indicators of a well-functioning Fontan circulation in this patient.

## ELECTROCARDIOGRAM

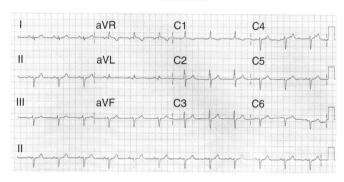

Figure 63-1 Electrocardiogram.

### FINDINGS

Heart rate: 73 bpm

QRS axis: +267°

QRS duration: 95 msec

PR interval: 154 msec

There was sinus rhythm with normal AV conduction.

There was a superior QRS axis. The tall R-wave in lead V1 and persistently negative S-waves in leads V4–6 suggest RV hypertrophy, although criteria for ventricular hypertrophy are very difficult to apply in the setting of a functionally single ventricle.

***Comments:*** Sinus rhythm and a normal pulmonary regurgitation interval are both favorable findings in a patient after Fontan-type surgery. Atrial scarring from surgery and RA enlargement from high systemic venous pressure commonly lead to atrial flutter/fibrillation or (less often) heart block.

## CHEST X-RAY

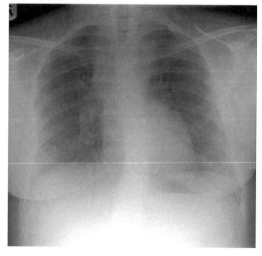

Figure 63-2 Posteroanterior projection, done 1 year before pregnancy.

## FINDINGS

Cardiothoracic ratio: 41%

There was situs solitus and levocardia (apex pointing to the left). There was a left-sided aortic arch and no cardiomegaly. The mediastinum appeared broadened. The usual pulmonary artery segment was absent. The right pulmonary artery was more prominent than the left. The peripheral pulmonary vascular markings were normal. Additionally, there were deformities of the left-sided ribs (ribs 2 to 3).

***Comments:*** This CXR showed some typical findings for a patient with a functionally univentricular heart after the Fontan-type operation. The absence of the pulmonary artery segment indicates hypoplasia or atresia of the main pulmonary artery. Broadening of the upper mediastinum can be explained by enlargement or displacement of the SVC as this vessel is connected to the pulmonary artery after a Fontan-type operation and operates at higher than normal pressures. A normal heart size on X-ray suggests good ventricular function without significant valvular lesions. Normal heart size on X-ray is very reassuring in any patient with ACHD especially when pregnancy is considered.

## EXERCISE TESTING

No exercise test performed

## ECHOCARDIOGRAM

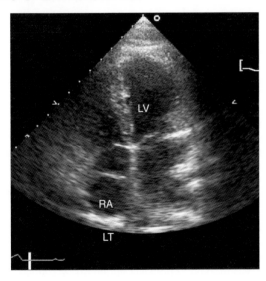

Figure 63-3 Apical four-chamber view.

## FINDINGS

Both ventricles showed normal function. There was no AV valve regurgitation. Both chambers were connected by a large and unrestricted VSD.

The aorta was arising anteriorly from the RV, and there was no aortic regurgitation. The pulmonary valve was atretic.

This showed both atria and ventricles connected normally and in their normal anatomic position. The RV was somewhat small. The RA contained the "lateral tunnel," connecting the IVC with the pulmonary artery system (cavopulmonary connection).

There was a fenestration in the tunnel wall with minimal continuous left-to-right shunting on color flow Doppler (not shown).

***Comments:*** This confirmed the diagnosis of a functionally univentricular heart after Fontan-type palliation with good function, and without hemodynamic or functional issues of concern.

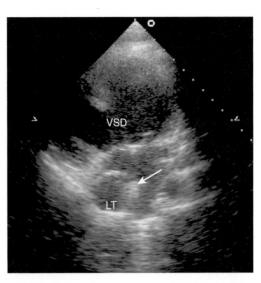

Figure 63-4 Apical four-chamber view with the transducer rotated anteriorly. LT, lateral tunnel.

## FINDINGS

This showed a large and unrestricted VSD.

The aorta arose anteriorly from the RV, and there was no aortic regurgitation. The pulmonary valve was atretic.

There was a fenestration in the tunnel (*arrow*) with minimal continuous left-to-right shunting on color flow Doppler.

***Comments:*** The echocardiogram confirmed the diagnosis of a functionally univentricular heart after Fontan-type palliation with good ventricular function, and without hemodynamic or functional issues of concern.

## MAGNETIC RESONANCE IMAGING

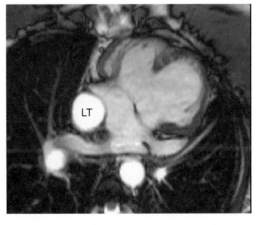

Figure 63-5 Oblique transaxial four-chamber view. LT, lateral tunnel.

## FINDINGS

This again showed normal size and systolic function of both ventricles, connected by a large VSD. The right ventricle was hypertrophied. Both AV valves were competent. The pulmonary veins drained normally into the left atrium.

The circular structure in the lateral RA again is the lateral tunnel directing the blood from the IVC to the pulmonary arteries.

### Ventricular Volume Quantification

|  | LV | (Normal range) | RV | (Normal range) |
|---|---|---|---|---|
| EDV (mL) | 70 | (52–141) | 61 | (58–154) |
| ESV (mL) | 28 | (13–51) | 19 | (12–68) |
| SV (mL) | 42 | (33–97) | 42 | (35–98) |
| EF (%) | 60 | (57–75) | 69 | (51–75) |
| EDVi (mL/m²) | **44** | (62–96) | **39** | (61–98) |
| ESVi (mL/m²) | 18 | (17–36) | **12** | (17–43) |
| SVi (mL/m²) | **27** | (40–65) | 27 | (38–62) |
| Mass index (g/m²) | — |  | — | (20–40) |

***Comments:*** A thorough estimate of ventricular function is crucial for pregnant women with ACHD, as the risk of serious cardiac events is increased if ventricular function is substantially impaired.[5]

Echocardiography and CMR are complementary if an estimate of cardiac function is needed in patients with complex congenital heart disease. MRI can be safely performed during pregnancy.

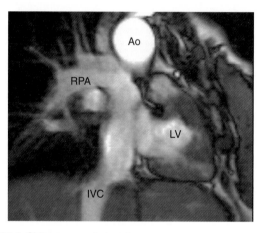

Figure 63-6 Oblique coronal plane image.

## FINDINGS

Oblique coronal plane aligned with the IVC, the lateral tunnel and the anastomosis with the right pulmonary artery.

This documented unrestricted blood flow from the IVC through the lateral tunnel into the large right pulmonary artery. The connection between the SVC and the pulmonary artery was also unobstructed. The ventricle was hypertrophied with good function.

***Comments:*** Documentation of unobstructed connections between the caval veins and the pulmonary arteries ("Fontan pathways") is very important for women with this cardiac physiology, since in pregnancy these pathways must accommodate a 30% to 50% increase in cardiac output.

This image depicts the typical anatomy of the so-called lateral tunnel Fontan, where the blood flow from the IVC is directed by an artificial Gore-Tex patch within the RA (or lateral tunnel) into the lower portion of SVC, which is then connected to the pulmonary artery. The "lateral tunnel Fontan" is considered to be advantageous in terms of blood flow dynamics as it allows relatively turbulence-free flow into the lungs resulting in minimal energy loss.[8]

A small ASD (or fenestration) connecting the lateral tunnel with the systemic atrium is a common practice in this type of Fontan palliation to allow the systemic ventricle to fill even if pulmonary perfusion is impaired. This is particularly beneficial

during the early postoperative course and may be closed by a transcatheter device later.[9]

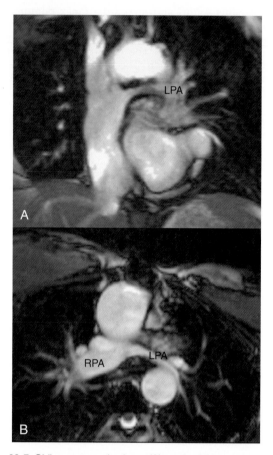

Figure 63-7 Oblique coronal plane (**A**) and oblique transverse (**B**) images.

## FINDINGS

This oblique coronal plane (*A*) again showed the lateral tunnel and the SVC unobstructed. The left pulmonary artery was hypoplastic, although there was no discrete stenosis.

The oblique transverse plane (*B*) shows the difference in diameter between the large right and hypoplastic left pulmonary artery.

***Comments:*** The patient's arterial oxygen saturation was 97% on room air indicating good pulmonary perfusion and absent right-to-left shunting.

There was marked hypoplasia but no discrete stenosis of the left pulmonary artery, suggesting a congenital origin rather stenosis secondary to the left BT shunt.

## CATHETERIZATION

Not performed

### FOCUSED CLINICAL QUESTIONS AND DISCUSSION POINTS

1. **What was this patient's initial cardiovascular status, and how has it been altered by surgery?**

*The patient has a functionally univentricular heart with normal atrial and ventricular arrangement (situs solitus and AV concordance) and a double outlet right ventricle with a small right* ventricle. The term **double-outlet RV** means that both great arteries arise predominantly (more than 50%) from the morphologic RV. A VSD is present that allows blood flow from the LV to reach the great arteries. The arrangement of the great arteries varies. In this patient the aorta was transposed anteriorly, and the pulmonary valve was atretic.

The patient had two palliative operations. The first (a classic BT anastomosis) improved pulmonary blood flow, and the second more definitive palliation (a lateral tunnel Fontan) eliminated her previous cyanosis and established a circulation with serial perfusion of the lungs and the body. Biventricular repair was not considered at the time because of the relatively small size of the RV. Other patients with a double-outlet RV can be repaired using a Rastelli operation (see Case 53).

2. What is the risk for pregnancy-related complications?

*Pregnancy carries significant risks for patients with a Fontan circulation.[10] The 30% to 50% increase in blood volume and cardiac output associated with pregnancy may worsen ventricular function and result in heart failure, ventricular enlargement, the development of AV valve regurgitation, and atrial arrhythmias.*

*Activation of the coagulation system during pregnancy increases the likelihood for thromboembolic complications fivefold (eightfold during the peripartum).[11] As blood volume increases during pregnancy, central venous pressure increases as well, potentially resulting in right-to-left shunting and/or heart failure.*

*This patient has been doing very well since her Fontan-type operation. She is clearly at the best functional spectrum of adult patients with Fontan physiology. Her favorable features are good ventricular function, no history of tachyarrhythmias or thromboembolic events, and good functional class.[4,5] Therefore, she could be considered at relatively low risk (approximately 1%–4%) for maternal adverse events during pregnancy.*

*The risk of fetal loss is higher in women with a Fontan circulation compared to the general population.[10] This probably reflects the relatively low cardiac output status of the Fontan circulation, the common coexistence of mild cyanosis, and other factors.*

*Maternal drugs (e.g., warfarin, amiodarone, or ACE inhibitors) may also affect the fetus. The fetal risk associated with the drugs must be weighed against the maternal risks of discontinuing them.*

3. What is the optimal management of the patient through gestation, labor, delivery, and the postpartum period?

*Close cardiovascular monitoring is mandatory throughout pregnancy, delivery, and the postpartum. Monitoring should focus on early signs of heart failure, arrhythmia, thromboembolic complications, and cyanosis. Clinical consensus suggests that low-dose aspirin should be given until the 35th week of pregnancy, then replaced by low molecular weight heparin for the remainder of pregnancy. Depending on the patient's clinical status, inpatient bed rest and oxygen supplementation (if needed) should be considered during the late weeks of pregnancy. If bed rest is necessary, anticoagulation with low molecular weight heparin should be administered instead of aspirin for thromboprophylaxis.*

*Women should lie in the lateral position to avoid supine hypotension from compression of the vena cava and the aorta, particularly during labor. Growth of the fetus should be monitored frequently.*

*Decisions about the mode of delivery should be made by obstetricians and anesthetists with expertise in ACHD and high-risk pregnancy management.[12] Vaginal delivery should be the aim, as it usually carries the lowest risk of complications such as hemorrhage, thromboembolism, and infection. To avoid pain and anxiety leading to an additional increase in cardiac output during delivery, epidural anesthesia should be introduced early, as it has*

*minimal effects on hemodynamic performance. Close and continuous monitoring of the mother and the fetus is crucial to avoid emergency situations.*

*After delivery the risk for thromboembolic complications persists, and anticoagulation should be continued until the patient is fully mobilized.*

## FINAL DIAGNOSIS

Situs solitus with usual atrial arrangement

Concordant AV connections

Double-outlet RV with D-transposition of the aorta and pulmonary atresia (small RV)

Large perimembranous outlet VSD

Prior right BT anastomosis

Total cavopulmonary connection as a lateral tunnel Fontan aged 20 years

Pregnancy (16 weeks)

## PLAN OF ACTION

Counseling of the patient regarding the maternal and fetal risk of pregnancy

Continuation of pregnancy with close cardiovascular monitoring and if necessary bed rest, anticoagulation, and oxygen supplementation late in pregnancy

Close monitoring of fetal growth

Fetal cardiac anomaly scan between the 16th and 20th weeks of gestation

## OUTCOME

The patient and her husband understood the risks involved and the need for close monitoring during pregnancy, accepted them, and opted to continue with the pregnancy. The patient remained well without any symptoms of sustained arrhythmia or heart failure. She continued to work full time until the 33rd week. Ventricular function was monitored by echocardiography after 24 weeks of pregnancy and remained unimpaired. The patient's oxygen saturation did not drop significantly nor did she develop systemic hypertension. Aspirin (75 mg) was commenced to prevent thromboembolic complications. Fetal growth was closely monitored with biweekly ultrasound. A fetal anomaly scan was normal without any evidence of heart disease in the fetus.

The patient was electively hospitalized from the 36th week of gestation until delivery to guarantee optimal and not delayed obstetric care, and to secure close monitoring of her clinical status at the end of pregnancy. Aspirin was stopped at the time of admission, and low molecular weight heparin was commenced (subcutaneous dalteparin 12,500 units daily).

After 39 weeks of gestation delivery was induced to guarantee optimal care on a weekday. Heparin was stopped on the day of induction and reinstated after delivery. The patient had epidural anesthesia by a team with experience in ACHD. Endocarditis prophylaxis was initiated (intravenous amoxicillin 1 g plus intravenous gentamicin 120 mg before delivery and amoxicillin 500 mg 6 hours after delivery). The delivery was uneventful. The patient gave birth to a healthy baby boy. Echocardiography of the newborn showed normal cardiac anatomy and function.

The patient recovered fully from delivery. She was supervised for 4 days on a regular ward thereafter. Aspirin was reinstated on the day of discharge when heparin was stopped.

At the day of discharge the oxygen saturation was 97% at rest on room air. The clinical status of the patient was unchanged from the day of presentation to our department until her post-delivery assessment 3 months after hospital discharge. She was in sinus rhythm, remaining asymptomatic with good biventricular function.

The couple wished to have a second child and they were advised that an interval of approximately 18 months prior to further pregnancy is recommended (primarily for obstetric and practical reasons; cardiovascular remodeling is usually complete within 6 to 12 months after delivery).

## Selected References

1. Blalock A, Taussig HB: Landmark article May 19, 1945: The surgical treatment of malformations of the heart in which there is pulmonary stenosis or pulmonary atresia. JAMA 251:2123–2138, 1984.
2. Fontan F, Baudet E: Surgical repair of tricuspid atresia. Thorax 26:240–248, 1971.
3. Steer, PJ: Pregnancy and contraception. In Gatzoulis MA, Swan L, Therrien J, Pantley GA (eds): Adult Congenital Heart Disease: A Practical Guide. Oxford, Blackwell, 2005, pp 16–35.
4. Siu SC, Sermer M, Harrison DA, et al: Risk and predictors for pregnancy-related complications in women with heart disease. Circulation 96:2789–2794, 1997.
5. Siu SC, Sermer M, Colman JM, et al: Prospective multicenter study of pregnancy outcomes in women with heart disease. Circulation 104:515–521, 2001.
6. Tomita H, Yamada O, Ohuchi H, et al: Coagulation profile, hepatic function, and hemodynamics following Fontan-type operations. Cardiol Young 11:62–66, 2001.
7. Mertens L, Hagler DJ, Sauer U, et al: Protein-losing enteropathy after the Fontan operation: An international multicenter study. PLE study group. J Thorac Cardiovasc Surg 115:1063–1073, 1998.
8. De Leval MR, Kilner P, Gewillig M, et al: Total cavopulmonary connection: A logical alternative to atriopulmonary connection for complex Fontan operations. Experimental studies and early clinical experience. J Thorac Cardiovasc Surg 96:682–695, 1988.
9. Bridges ND, Lock JE, Castaneda AR: Baffle fenestration with subsequent transcatheter closure. Modification of the Fontan operation for patients at increased risk. Circulation 82:1681–1689, 1990.
10. Canobbio MM, Mair DD, van der Velde M, et al: Pregnancy outcomes after the Fontan repair. J Am Coll Cardiol 28:763–767, 1996.
11. Heit JA, Kobbervig CE, James AH, et al: Trends in the incidence of venous thromboembolism during pregnancy or postpartum: A 30-year population-based study. Ann Intern Med 143:697–706, 2005.
12. Uebing A, Steer PJ, Yentis SM, Gatzoulis MA: Pregnancy and congenital heart disease. BMJ 332:401–406, 2006.

# Catheter Ablation for Atrial Arrhythmia

**Dominic J. Abrams, Mark J. Earley, and Richard J. Schilling**

**Age:** 32 years
**Gender:** Male
**Occupation:** Office worker
**Working diagnosis:** Double-inlet left ventricle with Fontan-type repair

## HISTORY

The patient was born with a double-inlet LV and an anterior, right-sided rudimentary RV. There was ventriculoarterial discordance, with the aorta located anteriorly. In the first year of life he underwent pulmonary artery banding and an atrial septectomy, followed at 9 years of age by an atriopulmonary Fontan procedure. The latter included a homograft placed between the RA appendage and the right pulmonary artery. The main pulmonary artery was divided at the site of previous banding and the ASD closed via the incision in the RA appendage.

He remained well until 4 years ago (28 years of age) when he was found incidentally to be in atrial tachycardia, although he reported no symptoms or palpitations. He underwent direct current cardioversion, which terminated his arrhythmia and revealed a slow junctional rhythm with occasional atrial capture and evidence of sick sinus syndrome.

Due to the sinus node disease an attempt was made to implant an atrial pacemaker transvenously. However, as both sensing and pacing parameters were inadequate, the procedure was abandoned. Consequently he was not started on antiarrhythmic agents.

The patient also suffered from PLE and marked body wasting (cardiac cachexia). Due to a constellation of complications of the Fontan circulation he had been referred for transplant assessment.

***Comments:*** Patients with double-inlet ventricle without pulmonary stenosis have an unprotected pulmonary vascular bed and therefore present with signs of heart failure in infancy when the pulmonary vascular resistance has fallen. Pulmonary artery banding is a palliative procedure to limit pulmonary blood flow and prevent pulmonary hypertension. Most patients with double-inlet LV also have ventriculoarterial discordance, meaning the aorta arises from the rudimentary RV. "Holmes heart" is a double inlet left ventricle with normal ventriculoarterial concordance.

The Fontan procedure performed here is a modification of Fontan's original technique[1] to separate the pulmonary and systemic circulations in the setting of "univentricular" physiology.

Atrial arrhythmias are a common complication following the modified Fontan, increasing with older age at surgery and longer follow-up.[2] They are an important cause of morbidity leading to heart failure, systemic AV valve regurgitation, atrial thrombus formation, and dilation of both the RA and LA.[3] As many as 50% of patients will have had an arrhythmia by the time they reach adulthood.[4]

Sinus node disease is not uncommon following the atriopulmonary Fontan. It may be caused by distortion of atrial structures induced by chronic stretch or by surgical injury to the sinoatrial node artery, which runs across the roof of the RA close to the site of atriopulmonary anastomosis. Sinus node disease has been associated with a higher incidence of atrial arrhythmias than in those with normal RA activation.[2] Atrial pacing is an effective way of maintaining an adequate atrial rate, which in itself may limit the development of further arrhythmias. However, the transvenous approach is often not recommended since it may predispose to venous obstruction and thrombus formation on the leads.[5] A transvenous approach was elected after consideration of risks and benefits. Careful planning was required before embarking on efforts to place a transvenous pacing wire. Securing adequate sensing and pacing thresholds in a highly scarred and hypertrophied chamber can be challenging, and asynchronous pacing due to loss of adequate sensing may be proarrhythmic.[6] Many centers would not attempt this, and instead would use epicardial pacing wires, though this method too has inherent drawbacks, especially long-term lead function. This approach was not felt to be suitable in this particular instance. However, some centers now report success with transvenous pacing.[7]

PLE is a difficult problem in the Fontan population (see Case 62). At times the best therapeutic option is cardiac transplantation.

## CURRENT SYMPTOMS

The patient described exercise limitation, although he was able to walk his dog slowly once a day. He was breathless at times while talking on the telephone. He was unaware of any palpitations or acceleration in his heart rate. Indeed, he had no symptoms during an episode of atrial tachycardia with 1:1 conduction and a ventricular rate of 190 bpm recorded on a 7-day ECG monitor.

***Comments:*** Young patients are often unaware of the presence of arrhythmia, but absence of symptoms at a heart rate of 190 bpm is unusual. Fontan patients can be particularly vulnerable to low cardiac output during tachyarrhythmias, which should therefore be taken seriously and treated promptly.

NYHA class: III

## CURRENT MEDICATIONS

Warfarin 6 mg daily

Ramipril 2 mg daily

Spironolactone 75 mg daily

Bumetanide 2 mg twice daily (loop diuretic)

Ferrous sulfate 200 mg daily

Folic acid 5 mg daily

Potassium chloride 16 mEq daily

## PHYSICAL EXAMINATION

BP 105/70 mm Hg, HR 84 bpm, oxygen saturation at rest 90%

Height 190 cm, weight 65 kg, BSA 1.85 m²

Surgical scars: Median sternotomy

Neck veins: JVP was visibly distended and compressible, but no waveform was seen even sitting upright.

Lungs/chest: Basal crepitations were audible in both lung fields.

Heart: Peripheral pulses were small in volume and character. Auscultation revealed a single second heart sound with no murmurs.

Abdomen: There was marked abdominal distension with evidence of ascites, and distended, tortuous superficial veins were evident on the thoracic and abdominal surfaces.

Extremities: There was wasting of the proximal muscle groups.

***Comments:*** The patient is mildly cyanosed, which is not uncommon in a Fontan patient. This may be due to a residual right-to-left shunt through an atrial communication or extracardiac venovenous collateral vessels and/or secondary-to-intrapulmonary shunting. At the time of Fontan surgery the patch across the left AV valve is commonly placed above the coronary sinus os to avoid the AV conducting system, which leaves coronary venous return draining into the systemic ventricle causing mild arterial desaturation (see Fig. 64-6).

The patient has an elevated JVP indicative of elevated RA pressure, a result of the Fontan circulation perhaps aggravated by his recent arrhythmia. Although the jugular vein is still in communication with the RA (unlike an extracardiac or lateral tunnel Fontan, see Case 63), no pulsations are seen because the RA is so severely dilated and hypertensive.

Abdominal distension secondary to ascites can be the result of both PLE and systemic venous hypertension.

## LABORATORY DATA

| | | |
|---|---|---|
| Hemoglobin | 16.3 g/dL | (13.0–17.0) |
| Hematocrit/PCV | **39%** | (41–51) |
| MCV | 90 fL | (83–99) |
| Platelet count | **128 × 10⁹/L** | (150–400) |
| White cell count | 4.7 × 10⁹/L | (3.6–9.2) |
| Lymphocyte count | **0.5 × 10⁹/L** | (1.0–4.5) |
| INR | 2.7 | |
| Sodium | 138 mmol/L | (134–145) |
| Potassium | 4.0 mmol/L | (3.5–5.2) |
| Creatinine | 1.1 mg/dL | (0.6–1.2) |
| Blood urea nitrogen | 6.0 mmol/L | (2.5–6.5) |
| ALT | 24 IU/L | (8–48) |
| ALP | 118 IU/L | (30–126) |
| Bilirubin (total) | 10 μmol/L | (3–24) |
| Total protein | **4.9 g/dL** | (6.2–8.2) |
| Albumin | **1.9 g/dL** | (3.7–5.3) |

Immunoglobulin A, G, M, E normal

***Comments:*** The mildly elevated hemoglobin represents secondary erythrocytosis, reflecting the residual right-to-left shunt.[8]

Albumin levels are severely reduced as a consequence of PLE. Lymphangiectasia of the intestinal bed causes loss of albumin, lymphocytes, and immunoglobulin into the gastrointestinal tract, reducing the plasma oncotic pressure and leading to generalized edema, effusions, and sometimes even pulmonary edema. While serum immunoglobulin levels were normal the lymphocyte count was low.

Abnormal hemodynamics and elevated central venous pressure as a result of the "failing" Fontan are felt to play an important role in the development of PLE.[8]

## ELECTROCARDIOGRAM

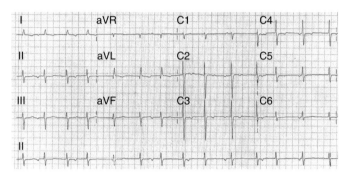

Figure 64-1 Electrocardiogram performed following DC cardioversion.

### FINDINGS

Heart rate: 84 bpm

QRS axis: –40°

QRS duration: 90 msec

Atrial pacemaker at 55 bpm and junctional rhythm with left-axis deviation. Nonspecific T-wave inversion.

***Comments:*** There is intermittent antegrade atrial capture.

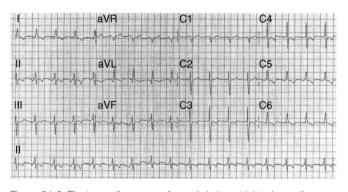

Figure 64-2 Electrocardiogram performed during atrial tachycardia.

### FINDINGS

Atrial rate: 200 bpm

Ventricular rate: 100 bpm

QRS axis: Left axis –36°

QRS duration: 88 msec

Atrial tachycardia (intra-atrial reentrant tachycardia) with 2:1 AV block.

***Comments:*** Inverted P-waves indicative of atrial activity can be clearly seen inferiorly (leads II, II, and aVF). Although this is suggestive of typical counterclockwise atrial flutter, subtle differences exist such as the longer isoelectric interval between P-waves, a feature common in ACHD. It is very difficult to differentiate between macroreentrant and focal atrial tachycardia from the P-wave morphology on the surface ECG.

## CHEST X-RAY

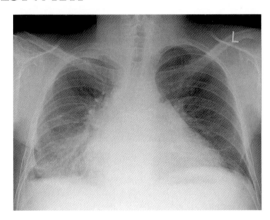

Figure 64-3 Posteroanterior projection.

### FINDINGS
Cardiothoracic ratio: 67%

Marked cardiomegaly with evidence of pulmonary edema. The right costophrenic angle was blunted suggesting a small pleural effusion.

***Comments:*** There is marked cardiomegaly, a significant proportion of which will be made up of the grossly dilated RA. Pulmonary edema can be clearly seen, a consequence of both hypoalbuminemia and possibly systolic and diastolic ventricular dysfunction. A small pleural effusion may be the result of reduced serum albumin. Lung volumes are also reduced, which may be caused by ascites, increasing intra-abdominal pressure and secondary splinting of the diaphragm.

## EXERCISE TESTING

| Exercise protocol: | Modified Bruce |
|---|---|
| Duration (min:sec): | 8:00 |
| Reason for stopping: | Dyspnea and arrhythmia |
| ECG changes: | Arrhythmia (1:1 AV conduction) |

| | Rest | Peak |
|---|---|---|
| Heart rate (bpm): | 84 | 210 |
| Percent of age-predicted max HR: | | 112 |
| O$_2$ saturation (%): | 90 | 88 |
| Blood pressure (mm Hg): | 105/70 | 140/90 |
| Peak Vo$_2$ (mL/kg/min): | | 13 |
| Percent predicted (%): | | 35 |
| Ve/Vco$_2$: | | 33 |
| Metabolic equivalents: | | 3.5 |

***Comments:*** Although low exercise tolerance is generally the norm in patients with a Fontan circulation, in this case exercise was likely limited by the emergence of the tachyarrhythmia with 1:1 conduction, which will need to be addressed before the patient's full cardiovascular exercise potential can be realized.

## ELECTROCARDIOGRAM

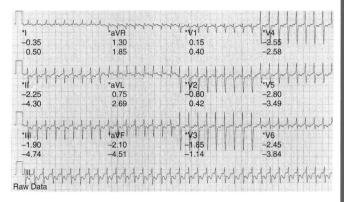

Figure 64-4 Electrocardiogram during exercise.

### FINDINGS
Heart rate: 200 bpm

QRS axis: Left axis −20°

QRS duration: 78 msec

Atrial tachycardia with 1:1 AV conduction.

***Comments:*** During exercise endogenous catecholamines may accelerate AV nodal conduction facilitating 1:1 conduction. P-waves are fused with the T-waves. Ventricular rates to this extent may produce profound hemodynamic compromise or syncope in patients with a single ventricular circulation and ventricular dysfunction.

Surprisingly, the patient remained asymptomatic during this episode and another episode of 1:1 conduction during a 7-day ECG recording. On cessation of exercise higher degrees of AV block resumed. An arrhythmia ablation procedure was planned.

## ECHOCARDIOGRAM

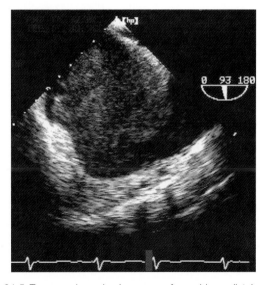

Figure 64-5 Transesophageal echo was performed immediately prior to an electrophysiology procedure.

### FINDINGS
The RA was grossly dilated with evidence of spontaneous contrast, but no thrombus was seen. The atriopulmonary anastomosis appeared to be widely patent. The LV function was

reduced with no mitral regurgitation; the VSD was nonrestrictive (i.e., there was no subaortic stenosis). There was no aortic regurgitation. The LA appendage was clear of thrombus.

***Comments:*** The need for transesophageal echo is dictated by the incessant tachycardia, which in the setting of an atriopulmonary Fontan is potentially thrombogenic, although the patient remains anticoagulated. Significant thrombus within the right atrium would preclude an ablation because of the risk of pulmonary embolism.

# MAGNETIC RESONANCE IMAGING

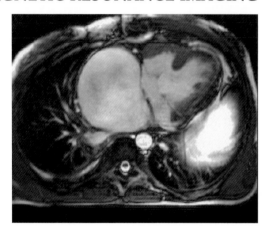

Figure 64-6 Oblique axial steady-state free precession cine (four-chamber view).

## FINDINGS

Double-inlet LV, hypoplastic RV, and a large VSD were seen. The ventricle was mildly to moderately dysfunctional. The RA was gigantic.

***Comments:*** The RA can be seen on the left-hand side of the image with the ventricular mass on the right-hand side. Efficiency of the ventricle is compromised in part by the large VSD. A small portion of the LA is visible immediately posterior to the RA. The diminutive RV is situated anterior to the unrestrictive VSD. A patch can be seen occluding the right AV valve, which has been placed superior to the os of the coronary sinus. In the moving image, movement of both the patch and valve with ventricular contraction can be clearly seen, with circular spontaneous contrast in the RA. Importantly, there seems to be external compression of the right-sided pulmonary veins "sandwiched" between the giant RA (anteriorly) and the spine (posteriorly).

### Ventricular Volume Quantification

|  | LV | (Normal range) | RV | (Normal range) |
|---|---|---|---|---|
| EDV (mL) | 110 | (77–195) | 26 | (88–227) |
| ESV (mL) | 64 | (19–72) | 18 | (23–103) |
| SV (mL) | 46 | (51–133) | 8 | (52–138) |
| EF (%) | 42 | (57–75) | 31 | (50–76) |
| EDVi (mL/m²) | 59 | (66–101) | 14 | (65–111) |
| ESVi (mL/m²) | 31 | (18–39) | 10 | (18–47) |
| SVi (mL/m²) | 28 | (43–67) | 4 | (39–71) |

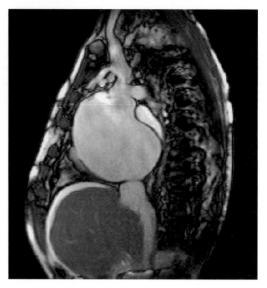

Figure 64-7 Sagittal oblique steady-state free precession cine of the right atrium.

## FINDINGS

The RA was extremely enlarged. No thrombus was present. Ascites was present.

***Comments:*** The MRI shows a grossly dilated RA supplied by the SVC and IVC (both dilated). The atrium measures 105 mm × 78 mm in this plane. The inferior atriocaval junction appears to be narrowed, although this is artifact from the plane selected. An infradiaphragmatic rim of ascitic fluid (white) can be seen on the superior surface of the liver. In the moving image, spontaneous contrast can clearly be seen as a result of the flow dynamics within the RA exacerbated by the arrhythmia.

The absence of thrombus is an important finding (see Case 61).

# CATHETERIZATION

## HEMODYNAMICS

Heart rate    88 bpm

|  | Pressure | Saturation (%) |
|---|---|---|
| SVC |  | 66 |
| IVC |  | 60 |
| RA | 30/19 mean 23 |  |
| PA | 26/16 mean 22 | 64 |
| PCWP | mean 18 |  |
| Aorta | 96/58 mean 67 | 90 |

### Calculations

| Qp (L/min) | 3.20 |
|---|---|
| Qs (L/min) | 4.26 |
| Cardiac index (L/min/m²) | 2.30 |
| Qp/Qs | 0.75 |
| PVR (Wood units) | 1.25 |
| SVR (Wood units) | 10.33 |

***Comments:*** A basic hemodynamic assessment was performed prior to the electrophysiology study.

RA hypertension is the result of the patient's hemodynamic and arrhythmic status. The LV end-diastolic pressure was presumably elevated but was not directly measured, as arterial access in a fully anticoagulated patient was felt to pose an unnecessary risk. The pulmonary capillary wedge pressure was elevated.

## FOCUSED CLINICAL QUESTIONS AND DISCUSSION POINTS

### 1. Why is arrhythmia so prevalent following the atriopulmonary Fontan procedure?

*Arrhythmia is a major cause of morbidity following the atriopulmonary Fontan procedure,[3] leading to ventricular dysfunction and heart failure, and increasing the risk of thrombus formation within the RA. All the complications of arrhythmia are in themselves "pro-arrhythmic." The prevalence of arrhythmia relates to a number of factors including a grossly dilated atrium with several natural and iatrogenic barriers to conduction, which may act as a central obstacle around which the reentrant wave front may propagate. Areas of scarring may occur in the absence of surgical intervention, which in some cases incorporate large areas of the atrial surface[9] and may coexist with natural barriers such as the orifice of the dilated inferior caval vein to create a central obstacle.[10] Narrow corridors of low-voltage myocardium between fixed conduction barriers slow wave front conduction sufficiently to allow the remainder of the circuit to repolarize and thereby maintain an "excitable gap" between the head and tail of the reentrant circuit. This is a fundamental principle of reentry. These corridors also make suitable sites for radiofrequency ablation. As the mechanism of arrhythmias in congenital heart disease is classically reentrant involving large areas of the atrial myocardium, these arrhythmias are commonly referred to as intra-atrial reentrant tachycardia or macroreentrant atrial tachycardia. These terms are better than atrial flutter, which to electrophysiologists infers a periannular counterclockwise circuit via the cavotricuspid isthmus, as seen most commonly in the structurally normal heart. While this does occur after the Fontan procedure (as in this case) it is a less frequent mechanism.*

### 2. Is radiofrequency ablation effective in patients following the modified Fontan procedure?

*Radiofrequency ablation of arrhythmias is possible, if challenging, after the modified Fontan. However arrhythmia recurrence has been a major problem,[4,11] often with a different electrocardiographic morphology seen at recurrence. This may in part relate to technical difficulties in the era before both three-dimensional mapping, when fluoroscopic visualization of an anatomically distorted chamber was taxing, and older nonirrigated catheters that may not have delivered sufficient power to create transmural lesions. Alternatively, the natural history of the RA may be a continually changing electrophysiological substrate allowing for the subsequent development of new arrhythmias. The continued advances in mapping and ablative technology, especially given the inadequacy and side effects of antiarrhythmic drugs, have led to unflagging interest in ablation in these patients, which in experienced centers is safe and well tolerated.[12]*

*More recent advances in mapping and ablative technology have led to both an increase in acute procedural success (arrhythmia termination) and an improvement in long-term outcome as defined by an improvement in a multiscale index of clinically relevant arrhythmia activity at more than 3 months following ablation.[13]*

*The CARTO electroanatomic mapping system (Biosense Webster, Diamond Bar, CA) allows the creation of a 3D map on which anatomical landmarks and areas of electrophysiologic interest such as scarring or double potentials may be annotated.*

*Electrogram timing relative to a fixed reference is superimposed on the chamber geometry to display activation. Both unipolar and bipolar electrogram amplitude may also be superimposed on the geometry to display voltage maps.*

*Irrigated radiofrequency ablation allows increased power delivery without a concomitant rise in temperature, thereby increasing lesion depth and size. This has been of benefit in areas of myocardial hypertrophy including the right atrium in congenital heart disease.[12]*

### 3. Is there a role for a pacemaker in preventing tachyarrhythmia?

*Given the high incidence of sinus node dysfunction in Fontan patients, pacing can be part of a strategy to maintain an appropriate sinus rate and try to limit the arrhythmia burden. Antitachycardia pacing is a useful adjunct to arrhythmia management. The device is capable of sensing atrial tachycardia and pacing at a faster rate to terminate the arrhythmia. While this technique was associated with initial complications of arrhythmia acceleration, the advent of second-generation devices such as the AT501 (Medtronic, Minneapolis, MN) has led to a renewed interest in this modality supported by a multicenter study.[14] Although the authors conclude that antitachycardia pacing is safe and efficacious, successfully terminating 54% of treatable rhythms, problems remain with appropriate detection of slower atrial tachycardias with 1:1 conduction and sinus tachycardia or ventricular tachycardia.*

*However, the relative merits of transvenous against epicardial pacing need to be considered in these complex patients. Transvenous pacing is not straightforward, and the risk of potential complications has been felt to be considerably high such that endocardial leads have been avoided.[6] The added potential for obstructing passive venous flow is also a consideration. However, epicardial leads are known to require ever increasing thresholds and eventually fail, making their use problematic as well. Several groups have now reported mid-term success with endocardial leads and no thromboembolic complications or venous pathway obstruction.[6,7] Longer-term follow-up for such complications versus freedom from arrhythmia will help guide these difficult decisions in the future.*

*When transvenous pacing is felt to be the preferred option, newer equipment aids deployment. The Medtronic SelectSecure lead has recently become available on the commercial market. It is an active fixation lead delivered via a steerable, peelaway sheath that allows for greater stability during implantation. While no scientific data are available on the use of the Select Secure in Fontan patients, many operators have found it to be of considerable benefit in ACHD.*

*In this particular case, the potential for sinus node dysfunction was felt high enough to warrant an attempt at pacemaker placement as part of the strategy of managing the patient's tachyarrhythmias. Despite the failed earlier attempt at adequate transvenous lead deployment and capture, this was still felt to be the preferred route in his clinical circumstances.*

### 4. Should surgical options be considered in this patient?

*The patient was declined for further congenital cardiac surgery because it was felt the intraoperative risk would be too high (PLE, systemic ventricular dysfunction); therefore, he was referred for transplantation. Conversion to a total cavopulmonary connection and arrhythmia surgery (modified maze procedure) is an effective strategy in carefully selected patients (see Case 65),[15] although in a proportion of patients the operative risk may outweigh the likelihood of potential benefits.*

*As with most aspects of the management of these patients, preprocedural planning and a carefully coordinated approach between electrophysiologist, cardiologist, and surgeon are fundamental to the best possible outcome.*

# FINAL DIAGNOSIS

Incessant atrial tachycardia late after the atriopulmonary Fontan procedure

# PLAN OF ACTION

Pacemaker placement

Electrophysiological intervention

# INTERVENTION

Due to concerns about an inadequate junctional response on termination of the atrial tachycardia in the face of sinus node disease, it was decided to insert a permanent atrial pacemaker and secure acceptable thresholds before attempting ablation. The device proposed was the Medtronic 501, which has antitachycardia pacing capabilities that may be useful in the event of arrhythmia recurrence. Due to difficulty with previous endocardial pacing, the Medtronic SelectSecure active fixation lead was used. The procedure went according to plan, and adequate capture was ensured.

The patient was thereafter referred for electrophysiology study and radiofrequency ablation of his incessant arrhythmia. Once femoral venous access had been secured the patient was given intravenous heparin to ensure continued anticoagulation during the ablative procedure.

Three-dimensional mapping was performed with the CARTO and ablation with an irrigated ablation NaviStar catheter.

An active fixation bipolar catheter was secured within the RA myocardium and used as the reference against which all other recorded electrograms were timed. A macroreentrant arrhythmia was identified. Radiofrequency ablation was performed across the more inferior portion of the mapped pathway (see Fig. 64-8), which successfully terminated the atrial tachycardia. Programmed atrial stimulation failed to re-induce the clinical or any other arrhythmias.

Following the procedure the patient returned to the ward. There were no complications.

# ELECTROPHYSIOLOGY

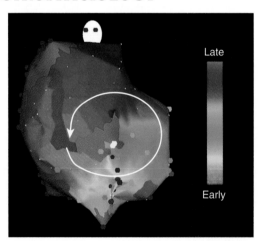

Figure 64-8 Electroanatomic activation map of the right atrium, depicted from the left anterior oblique view.

## Findings

Areas of scar and nonconductive tissue were present (depicted by gray).

Radiofrequency ablation (denoted by red dots) was performed across the cavotricuspid isthmus from the right AV valve patch to an area of scar approximating the IVC and successfully terminated the atrial tachycardia.

*Comments:* Activation is depicted by a color scheme, where earliest activation is red and latest purple. The wave front can be seen to rotate around a central barrier to conduction (the patch across the right AV valve) as depicted by the white arrow, reflecting an activation pattern consistent with typical counterclockwise atrial flutter traversing the cavotricuspid isthmus.

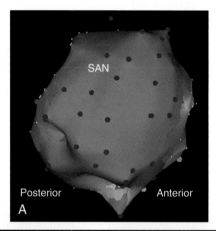

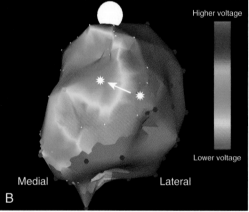

Figure 64-9 Electrophysiology study. SAN, sinoatrial node.

## Findings

Detailed electroanatomic mapping clearly demonstrated areas of viable myocardium as opposed to areas of low-voltage tissue and scar.

*Comments:* Here the RA is depicted from the right lateral view (*A*) and the posteroanterior view (*B*). Scar is depicted in gray. Bipolar voltage amplitude is depicted on a color scale with red denoting low-voltage and purple higher voltage tissue. The presumed position of the sinoatrial node (SAN) has been annotated to demonstrate the dense scarring in this area contributing to sinus node dysfunction. Note the distribution of low-voltage tissue approximating areas of scar. As the original pacing lead was likely placed close to the edge of scar tissue (asterisk on lateral side), a second lead was implanted to a more medial position with higher bipolar electrogram voltage (asterisk on medial side) in an attempt to minimize the loss of either sensing or pacing in the future.

Periannular tachycardias traversing the cavotricuspid isthmus similar to typical atrial flutter are less common following the Fontan than in patients who have undergone biventricular repair of ACHD,[9] although they may occur.

## OUTCOME

The patient has made marked clinical improvement since the restoration of sinus rhythm and the maintenance of ongoing AV synchrony by a permanent atrial pacing system. There has been no documented arrhythmia recurrence on 7-day Holter monitoring or on pacemaker telemetry. He has not been started on any antiarrhythmic medication.

A repeat cardiopulmonary exercise test demonstrated an increase in his maximal oxygen uptake ($MVo_2$) from 13 mL/kg/min preablation to 22 mL/kg/min, demonstrating a considerable improvement in his cardiopulmonary function. No tachyarrhythmia interfered with the test. He also reported a reduction in his ascites, an increase in his appetite, and a general sense of improvement in his quality of life.

While catheter ablation has been effective in arrhythmia control and, with it, functional improvement, legitimate concerns remain about the long-term detrimental effect of the marked RA dilatation. Because of his clinical improvement, discussions about appropriateness of surgery for conversion to a total cavopulmonary connection resurfaced. The patient was therefore scheduled for repeat hemodynamic assessment (measurement of pulmonary artery pressure and left ventricular end-diastolic pressure) as a prelude to renewed discussion for further surgery.

## Selected References

1. Fontan F, Baudet E: Surgical repair of tricuspid atresia. Thorax 26:240–248, 1971.
2. Fishberger LB, Wernovsky G, Gentles TL, et al: Factors that influence the development of atrial flutter after the Fontan operation. J Thorac Cardiovasc Surg 113:80–86, 1997.
3. Ghai A, Harris L, Harrison DA, et al: Outcomes of late atrial tachyarrhythmias in adults after the Fontan operation. J Am Coll Cardiol 37:585–592, 2001.
4. Walsh EP, Cecchin F: Arrhythmias in adult patients with congenital heart disease. Circulation 115:534–545, 2007.
5. Khairy P, Landzberg MJ, Gatzoulis MA, et al: Transvenous pacing leads and systemic thromboemboli in patients with intracardiac shunts: A multicenter study. Circulation 113:2391–2397, 2006.
6. Hansky B, Blanz U, Peuster M, et al: Endocardial pacing after Fontan-type procedures. Pacing Clin Electrophysiol 28:140–148, 2005.
7. Shah MJ, Nehgme R, Carboni M, Murphy JD: Endocardial atrial pacing lead implantation and midterm follow-up in young patients with sinus node dysfunction after the Fontan procedure. Pacing Clin Electrophysiol 27:949–954, 2004.
8. Mertens L, Hagler DJ, Sauer U, et al: Protein-losing enteropathy after the Fontan operation: An international multicenter study. PLE Study Group. J Thorac Cardiovasc Surg 115:1063–1073, 1998.
9. Nakagawa H, Shah N, Matsudaira K, et al: Characterization of reentrant circuits in macroreentrant right atrial tachycardia after surgical repair of congenital heart disease. Isolated channels between scars allow "focal" ablation. Circulation 103:699–709, 2001.
10. Mandapati R, Walsh EP, Triedman JK: Pericaval and periannular intra-atrial reentrant tachycardias in patients with congenital heart disease. J Cardiovasc Electrophysiol 14: 119–125, 2003.
11. Triedman JK, Bergau DM, Saul JP, et al: Efficacy of radiofrequency ablation for control of intraatrial reentrant tachycardia in patients with congenital heart disease. J Am Coll Cardiol 30:1032–1038, 1997.
12. Abrams JDJ, Earley MJ, Sporton SC, et al: Comparison of noncontact and electroanatomic mapping to identify scars and arrhythmia later after the Fontan procedure. Circulation 115: 1738–1746, 2007.
13. Triedman JK, Alexander ME, Love BA, et al: Influence of patient factors and ablative technologies on outcomes of radiofrequency ablation of intra-atrial re-entrant tachycardia in patients with congenital heart disease. J Am Coll Cardiol 39:1827–1835, 2002.
14. Stephenson EA, Casavant D, Tuzi J, et al: Efficacy of atrial anti-tachycardia pacing using the Medtronic AT500 pacemaker in patients with congenital heart disease. Am J Cardiol 92:871–876, 2003.
15. Deal BJ, Mavroudis C, Backer CL, et al: Comparison of anatomic isthmus block with the modified right atrial Maze procedure for late atrial tachycardia in Fontan patients. Circulation 106:575–579, 2002.

# Total Cavopulmonary Conversion: When and How

**Toru Ishizaka and Hideki Uemura**

**Age: 20 years**
**Gender: Female**
**Occupation: Office clerk**
**Working diagnosis: Tricuspid atresia and severe pulmonary stenosis, prior Fontan (atriopulmonary connection)**

## HISTORY

The patient was born at term but was cyanotic, and a diagnosis was made of tricuspid atresia with pulmonary stenosis. A right modified BT shunt was constructed at the age of 2 months, followed by the addition of a left-side modified BT shunt at 2 years. Subsequently, at the age of 5 years a Fontan circulation was established by means of an atriopulmonary anastomosis (direct anastomosis between the RA and the confluent pulmonary artery (PA) on the right posterior side of the ascending aorta). Her BT shunts were ligated. Her postoperative course was smooth and uneventful.

At the age of 6 years, a routine postoperative catheterization demonstrated no obstruction within the pulmonary circulation, a low cardiac index ($1.97 \, \text{L/min/m}^2$), and mild hypoxemia ($\text{Sao}_2$ 92%).

**Comments:** Tricuspid atresia is usually palliated by the creation of a Fontan circulation. The method originally reported by Fontan in 1971 involved the interposition of a homograft between the RA and the left PA on the right and posterior aspect of the ascending aorta. In that patient, the right PA had already been isolated from the left PA and the SVC had been anastomosed in a conventional Glenn fashion. Direct anastomosis of the RA to the confluent pulmonary arteries was described by Kreutzer in 1973.[1]

Generally our patient continued to do well through her primary and secondary education. She participated in physical training throughout and could climb three flights of stairs. During her follow-up visits, abnormal weight gain, edema, and hepatomegaly were occasionally noted when oral diuretics were not regularly taken or skipped.

At the age of 16 years, routine catheterization, 10 years after the Fontan procedure, demonstrated "normal" pressures through the venous pathways (SVC and IVC pressure of 13 mm Hg and PA pressure of 12 mm Hg), and again a low cardiac index ($1.5 \, \text{L/min/m}^2$). The arterial oxygen saturation was 96%. Contrast echocardiography showed a small right-to-left shunt at the atrial level, and cardiopulmonary exercise testing demonstrated a peak $\text{Vo}_2$ of $20.5 \, \text{mL/kg/min}$ with an anaerobic threshold of $13.65 \, \text{mL/kg/min}$.

She was seen again for routine clinical follow-up at age 20 years. She had started working full time.

## CURRENT SYMPTOMS

The patient could walk 2 km at a comfortable pace without stopping, but she could not run very far. She had not experienced palpitations or syncope.

NYHA class: II

## CURRENT MEDICATIONS

Furosemide 30 mg twice daily

Spironolactone 25 mg twice daily

Enalapril 5 mg daily

**Comments:** Diuretics and ACE inhibitors are commonly used in single ventricle patients (37% and 39%, respectively, from a large multicenter descriptive study),[2] although there is no clinical evidence supporting their use in this setting.[3]

## PHYSICAL EXAMINATION

BP 110/66 mm Hg, HR 70 bpm, oxygen saturation 94% on room air

Height 144 cm, weight 40 kg, BSA $1.26 \, \text{m}^2$

Surgical scars: Median sternotomy and bilateral posterolateral thoracotomy scars

Neck veins: No visible JVP

Lungs/chest: Normal vesicular breath sounds

Heart: The rhythm was regular. There was no murmur audible. The second heart sound was single.

Abdomen: The liver was palpable 2 cm below the ribs at the midclavicular line. There was no ascites.

Extremities: Mild cyanosis was noted. There was no edema.

**Comments:** Because the jugular veins are no longer in direct communication with an atrium that fills and empties in the typical manner, the usual rise and fall of the venous pulse (including x and y descent) are not seen in the Fontan patient. Various patterns of jugular venous distension may reflect respiratory changes in flow, but clinical interpretation of the neck veins is difficult, and the usual rules are not easily applied.

## LABORATORY DATA

| | | |
|---|---|---|
| Hemoglobin | **15.5 g/dL** (11.5–15.0) | |
| Hematocrit/PCV | **46.8%** (36–46) | |
| MCV | 90.3 fL (83–99) | |
| Platelet count | **144 × 10⁹/L** (150–400) | |
| Sodium | 139 mmol/L (134–145) | |
| Potassium | 4.2 mmol/L (3.5–5.2) | |
| Creatinine | 0.61 mg/dL (0.5–1.0) | |
| Blood urea nitrogen | 14 mg/dL (6–24) | |
| Total bilirubin | 1.0 mg/dL (0.2–1.2) | |
| AST | 22 U/L (0–40) | |
| ALT | 17 U/L (0–35) | |
| Total cholesterol | **105 mg/dL** (130–220) | |

### OTHER RELEVANT LAB RESULTS
| | |
|---|---|
| BNP | **267.1 pg/mL** (<20.0) |
| Renin activity | **11.2 ng/mL/hr** (0.5–2.5) |
| Aldosterone | **24.0 ng/dL** (3–16) |

***Comments:*** Activation of the renin-angiotensin-aldosterone system in ACHD is increasingly recognized.[5] The pattern of neurohormonal activation perhaps justifies empiric use of pharmacotherapy to counteract such activation, though no clinical trials exist to support or refute this.

There was minimal erythrocytosis, which is associated with mild cyanosis.

It is known that the total cholesterol level is often lower in patients with cyanotic ACHD.[4]

## ELECTROCARDIOGRAM

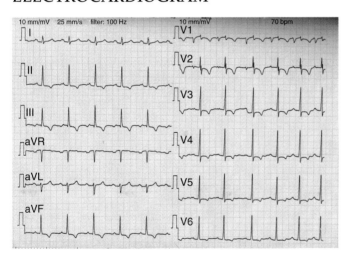

Figure 65-1 Electrocardiogram.

### FINDINGS
Heart rate: 68 bpm

QRS axis: +85°

QRS duration: 100 msec

***Comments:*** The P-wave is wide and biphasic in the limb leads. In V1, the P-wave illustrates high negative voltage with a sharp deflection, probably related to a dilated or hypertro-

phied morphologic RA. The P-wave is broad and notched in leads I and II, suggesting LA overload as well.

In addition, there are widespread and nonspecific T-wave inversions.

## CHEST X-RAY

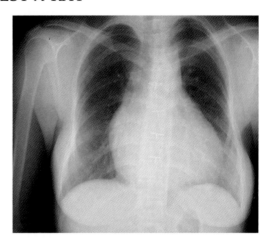

Figure 65-2 Posteroanterior projection.

### FINDINGS
Cardiothoracic ratio: 64%

Cardiomegaly. The RA shadow was enlarged, with the rightward border of the SVC and the IVC shadow more obviously seen than normal. The pulmonary vasculature was normal or reduced. No sign of pulmonary venous congestion was seen. Left aortic arch with situs solitus was noted. There was evidence of previous sternotomy.

***Comments:*** The aortic knob appeared less prominent, indicating a prolonged low cardiac output. The enlarged cardiac silhouette is mainly due to RA enlargement.

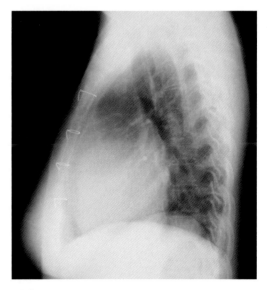

Figure 65-3 Lateral view.

### FINDINGS
Enlargement of the RA. Retrosternal filling of uncertain origin.

# EXERCISE TESTING

| Exercise protocol: | Modified Bruce |
| Duration (min:sec): | 6:00 |
| Reason for stopping: | Dyspnea |
| ECG changes: | Wandering P-wave morphology. No ST change. Nonsustained atrial tachycardia (HR 180–200 bpm) during latter portion of the test. |

| | Rest | Peak |
| --- | --- | --- |
| Heart rate (bpm): | 80 | 138 |
| Percent of age-predicted max HR: | | 69 |
| O$_2$ saturation (%): | 94 | 94 |
| Blood pressure (mm Hg): | 110/66 | 134/76 |
| Peak Vo$_2$ (mL/kg/min): | | 15.9 |
| Percent predicted (%): | | 48 |
| Ve/Vco$_2$: | | 30 |
| Metabolic equivalents: | | 4.3 |

***Comments:*** The amplitude and dispersion of the P-wave may be abnormal long after an atriopulmonary Fontan palliation.[6]

An arrhythmia had not been seen during exercise in the last examination at 16 years of age.

Her exercise capacity is low, and even lower compared with her previous values.

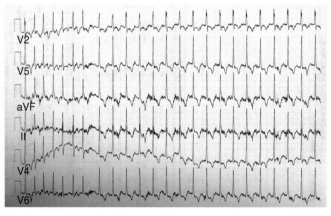

Figure 65-4 Holter electrocardiogram.

## FINDINGS

Atrial tachycardia seen during exercise.

***Comments:*** Maximum HR is 131 bpm, minimum HR is 61 bpm. Maximum R-R is 1.0 sec.

Three types of P-waves are seen; two types with a rate of 60 bpm and another with a rate of 90 bpm, appearing alternately.

# ECHOCARDIOGRAM

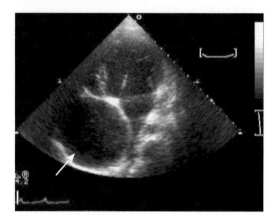

Figure 65-5 Apical four-chamber view.

## FINDINGS

The RA was severely enlarged, measuring 70 mm × 60 mm (*arrow*). No thrombus was present in the RA. There was mild-to-moderate aortic regurgitation through the center of the valve orifice. The SVC was normal in size (11 mm, flow velocity was normal at 0.29 m/sec), but the IVC was dilated (18 mm × 22 mm). Flow velocity in the hepatic vein was normal at 0.28 m/sec. There was tiny bidirectional flow between the hypoplastic RV cavity and RA. The left PA had a slight narrowing at its origin from the pulmonary trunk. The LV was within normal limits (LVEDd 49 mm), with mildly reduced systolic function (LV ejection fraction 47%). There was only trace mitral regurgitation.

***Comments:*** Until this echo investigation found a small communication between the RA and the small RV, the diagnosis had been tricuspid atresia. The finding changes the anatomic diagnosis to critical tricuspid stenosis, which is a small but noteworthy distinction. With critical tricuspid stenosis, mild desaturation after the Fontan procedure can be partly explained. A small right-to-left shunt at the atrial level shown on contrast echocardiography (see "History") probably reflected the flow across the very severe tricuspid stenosis. Because of tricuspid stenosis, there must be a VSD between the main LV and the rudimentary RV.

While not perfect, the findings suggest satisfactory Fontan physiology. The enlarged RA has the potential to be both arrhythmogenic and thrombogenic.

# CT ANGIOGRAPHY

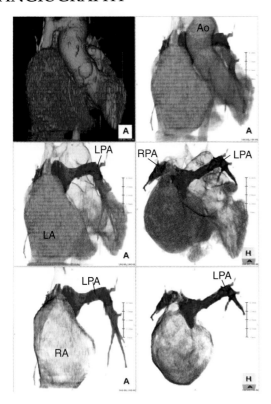

Figure 65-6 Computed tomography angiogram.

## FINDINGS

The connection between the RA and PA was widely patent. The RA cavity, IVC, and the coronary sinus were markedly dilated.

Contrast injected via an upper arm vein was stagnant and flowed slowly into the RA. A small amount of contrast from the RA entered the LA around the origin of the right pulmonary veins. The ostia of the right pulmonary veins into the LA were flattened and compressed by the remarkably dilated RA, but there did not seem to be significant pulmonary vein stenosis.

No thrombus was present within the RA. The right and the left PAs were confluent and generally slender, about 8 mm bilaterally.

**Comments:** There was a deformity of the hilar PA, particularly the left, which appeared pulled superiorly (*center right*). This was presumably related to the previous BT shunts, which can distort the branch PAs. At the time of the Fontan procedure, these tubes were ligated, but not divided.

Not all of the myocardium had uniform enhancement, suggesting the presence of perfusion abnormalities or myocardial scar. This finding, however, may merely reflect the abnormal flow patterns from Fontan physiology and should not be interpreted in the same way as in a patient with a normal circulation.

# CATHETERIZATION

## HEMODYNAMICS

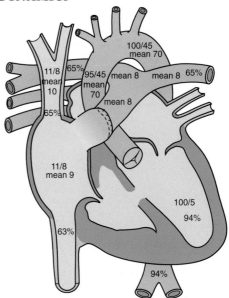

Figure 65-7 Preoperative catheterization.

**Calculations**

| | |
|---|---|
| Qp (L/min) | 2.13 |
| Qs (L/min) | 2.39 |
| Cardiac index (L/min/m²) | 1.89 |
| Qp/Qs | 0.89 |
| PVR (Wood units) | 1.41 |
| SVR (Wood units) | 25.57 |

## FINDINGS

There was moderate aortic insufficiency and trace mitral regurgitation.

The LVEDV was 120.3 mL (103% of normal) ESV 57.8 mL, EF 52%.

Right PA diameter was 11 mm (57% of normal), left PA diameter was 12 mm (72% of normal). The PA index (Nakata index) was 165.

**Comments:** All the pressures are ideal. The flows are quite low as on previous studies. Chronic diuretic therapy has probably lowered systemic venous pressures too much, and cardiac output would probably be better off without diuretics.

In the past, it was considered that a certain degree of hypoplasia of the pulmonary arteries should be regarded as a risk factor for repair of TOF. Several methods for standardization of the pulmonary arterial size were proposed. They included the McGoon ratio, the Nakata index, the pulmonary arterial area index, and so on. These methods of standardization were based on the hypothesis that an angiographic diameter of the PA at the hilum represents the degree of development of intrapulmonary vascular bed on that side. This, of course, is not always the case, particularly when there is a localized stenosis of the RVOT, or when an arborization abnormality is present as seen in the setting of major aortopulmonary collateral arteries. These standardized values were eventually applied beyond biventricular physiology, since pulmonary arterial size was considered an important factor for a successful Fontan procedure.

The pulmonary arterial index proposed by Nakata et al[7] is calculated by the following formula:

$$[(RPA\ diameter/2)^2 + (LPA\ diameter/2)^2 \times \pi]/BSA$$

In this particular patient:

$$[(11/2)^2 + (12/2)^2 \times 3.14]/1.26 = 165$$

The normally anticipated value will be between 250 and 350, depending on the BSA.[7]

# ANGIOGRAM

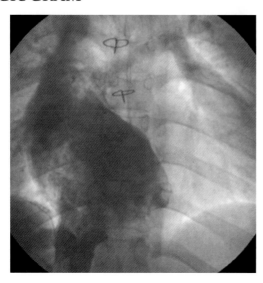

Figure 65-8 Anteroposterior projection.

## FINDINGS

The RA and coronary sinus were markedly dilated, and there was stagnant flow in the systemic venous pathway.

*Comments:* The findings here are typical of a Fontan patient with a dilated atrium.

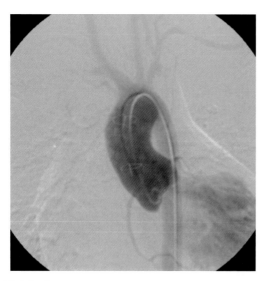

Figure 65-9 Angiogram.

## FINDINGS

Moderate aortic regurgitation.

*Comments:* A jet is coming through the center and the superior half of the aortic orifice. Dilation of the aortic root and the ascending aorta is not obvious. The catheter position is very close to the aortic valve.

# FOCUSED CLINICAL QUESTIONS AND DISCUSSION POINTS

1. **What are disadvantages of the traditional Fontan circulation?**

*There are a number of hemodynamic, morphologic, electrophysiologic, and functional aspects of the original Fontan circulation that make it suboptimal. While the hemodynamic effects of the Fontan procedure occur immediately, morphologic changes gradually occur that reflect the unfavorable hemodynamics.*

*In many respects the creation of the Fontan circulation by an atriopulmonary connection means the end of a cyanotic circulation but the beginning of RA disease. Gross dilatation of the RA is an inevitable byproduct of chronically raised systemic venous pressure. The dilated RA induces stagnant flow within the chamber, often leading to local thrombosis.[8] Thromboembolism, even microscopic, can in turn impair pulmonary circulation. The overdistended RA can also reduce the right lung capacity. The right pulmonary veins commonly appear compressed by the dilated RA.*

*Furthermore, RA dilation increases the risk of atrial arrhythmia, and reentry circuits are apt to be present around the surgical scar. The sinus node usually suffers from chronotropic incompetence because of the chronically increased RA pressure. The free wall of the RA can also have histopathologic changes after some duration of raised atrial pressure[9] and contribute to arrhythmia.*

2. **What are the advantages of total cavopulmonary connection (TCPC) over the traditional Fontan circulation?**

*Conversion to TCPC involves routing the IVC flow through a conduit directly to the PA, and routing the SVC flow also directly to the PA (bidirectional Glenn shunt). The IVC channel can be constructed entirely outside of the heart (extracardiac) or may pass through the atrial cavity (usually called a lateral tunnel). Therefore, an extracardiac Fontan is a form of TCPC. To exclude all the atrial walls from the IVC channel, interposition of a prosthetic tube as a conduit is one established option. If a lateral tunnel technique is used for the IVC channel, some part of the atrial musculature and the site of the sinus node remain in the wall where higher venous pressure is persistently posed.*

*Commonly, depending on the surgeon, a small windowlike communication, or fenestration, is created between the conduit and the atrium, which helps avoid excessive pressure elevation in the TCPC pathway at the cost of mild cyanosis.*

*Converting to TCPC theoretically makes fluid kinetic energy loss smaller, since venous blood flows through a conduit of normal caliber rather than through a giant RA. Also, venous blood through the coronary sinus can drain to the functionally LA chamber, decreasing the pressure of the cardiac veins and increasing preload to the dominant ventricle just as a fenestration. The downside of this is persistent minor desaturation (usually an oxygen saturation of 95% would be expected).*

*At the time of surgery, the free wall of the atrium as well as the atrial septum can be resected, and the overall atrial size can be reduced.[10,11] This helps avoid some of the thrombotic and arrhythmogenic properties of the large RA.*

*However, subsequent to conversion to TCPC, access to the atrium with a percutaneous venous catheter becomes impossible unless a fenestration is constructed, and is difficult even if one is present. Therefore issues involving pacing or arrhythmia ablation become very difficult to address afterward, and should be dealt with as completely as possible prior to TCPC conversion. If antiarrhythmic therapy is accomplished preoperatively by transcatheter technique, the surgeon can reduce to some extent the bypass time in these already high-risk procedures.*

### 3. Is TCPC likely to reduce the risk of atrial arrhythmia?

*Even after TCPC conversion together with antiarrhythmic surgery, persistent or recurrent arrhythmia is still frequent in patients who had already experienced sustained atrial fibrillation or flutter.[10] In other words, it may be too late to convert to TCPC without arrhythmic morbidity.*

*Most studies of the maze procedure cite success in very different types of patients.[12] For example, in a patient with mitral valve disease an atrial size of over 40 mm and/or history of atrial arrhythmia longer than 10 years are conditions favoring a successful maze procedure. Yet, there is a fundamental difference between this situation and a TCPC conversion; one is for the LA, and the other for the RA. The atria are morphologically different. In mitral disease, LA pressure is often severely elevated, while it is usually relatively lower in the Fontan circulation. Therefore, an arrhythmogenic focus around the pulmonary venous orifice is much less likely in the atriopulmonary Fontan compared with mitral valve disease. In tricuspid atresia, for example, the architecture of the RA muscle is not normal. Because of the absence of the tricuspid valve orifice, a floor of muscles covers the wall separating the rudimentary RV, where a hollow space for the tricuspid valve is present in the normal heart. When antiarrhythmic surgery is to be employed for the abnormal RA, an additional blocking line through this area is required.[11] In addition to these structural differences, the RA becomes much larger than that seen in typical mitral valve disease, and hence the size criteria are not applicable. Furthermore, sinus node dysfunction may be related to chronically raised venous pressure in the Fontan circulation.*

*In these respects, 10 years after the atriopulmonary connection might be already theoretically too late for successful antiarrhythmic surgery.*

### 4. What is the optimal timing for an elective TCPC conversion?

*At our institution, we began to employ TCPC as an initial Fontan completion in 1988. Our procedural intention was, from the beginning, to place the sinus node as well as the coronary sinus within the low-pressure atrial cavity rather than the high-pressure systemic venous circuit.[13] In these patients, we have not encountered progressive arrhythmia problems in long-term follow-up, with the exception of patients with visceral heterotaxy.*

*We started conversion from atriopulmonary Fontan to TCPC concomitantly with the maze procedure in August 1995.[11] When this particular patient was discussed, the institution's growing clinical experience with TCPC and antiarrhythmic surgery included 10 patients all over 15 years old, with no surgical deaths. Hemodynamic improvement was seen after the procedure in all patients. Therefore, there was some enthusiasm at that time that a more efficient circulation with TCPC would foster fewer arrhythmic problems. Further, the data suggested that perhaps earlier conversion to TCPC rather than waiting for significant complications to occur was advantageous. To justify earlier conversion in terms of atrial arrhythmia, we subsequently investigated consecutive changes in P-wave morphology in patients who previously underwent atriopulmonary connection type of Fontan procedure.[6]*

*Nonetheless, the long-term results after such a combination of procedures had yet to be determined. The patients are fragile, with various degrees of hepatic dysfunction due to chronic venous stasis, and show evidence of a chronically low cardiac output. The surgery is long and complex and stressful on the cardiovascular system. At many institutions, even those with expertise in congenital heart disease, mortality from TCPC conversion is rather high. Thus, even now, substantial controversy exists regarding whether to offer a patient an elective TCPC conversion, and what the ideal clinical indications ought to be.*

*Other morphologic problems that can progress or recur in the Fontan setting may trigger reoperation, and conversion to TCPC could be concomitantly carried out. These include AV or aortic valve regurgitation or subaortic stenosis as a result of the potential abnormalities seen in hearts with univentricular physiology.*

### 5. Should this patient undergo a TCPC conversion?

*This patient underwent initially a Fontan-type procedure by means of atriopulmonary connection. It was a modification of the procedure described by Kreutzer et al,[1] in which an atriopulmonary anastomosis was created in front of the aortic root. Though routine postoperative catheter investigation demonstrated a slightly elevated systemic venous pressure and low cardiac index, her clinical condition was stable with a reasonable quality of life.*

*Now 14 years after her initial procedure, repeat investigation showed mild cyanosis due to a small shunt from RA to LA or to the ventricle, a markedly dilated RA, and mild-to-moderate aortic regurgitation. In addition, findings of decreasing exercise tolerance and self-limited atrial rhythm disturbances attracted the clinicians' attention.*

*Furthermore, the BNP level was over 250, which is unequivocally high even for the atriopulmonary Fontan circulation.*

*In this particular patient, she had not experienced palpitations, and no atrial fibrillation or flutter had been documented. Exercise testing recorded a short run of atrial tachyarrhythmia. Together with marked P-wave abnormalities, it seemed reasonable to predict that clinical atrial arrhythmia would develop sooner or later.*

*After extensive discussion at multidisciplinary meetings, the group strongly felt that TCPC conversion and antiarrhythmic surgery should not be postponed.*

### 6. What additional surgical procedures ought to be considered?

*In this patient, aortic regurgitation could be treated concomitantly with conversion to TCPC, though it is not an indication for surgery itself. Nonetheless, since aortic regurgitation can contribute to improper hemodynamics in these fragile patients, it is reasonable to address this if surgery is planned for other procedures. While there are studies that address the coexistence of AV valve regurgitation in the pre- and the post-Fontan circulation, aortic regurgitation has not been mentioned as a major issue. Clinical experience with this problem will likely grow as the number of patients increase. In particular, aortic valve dysfunction may be more prominent in Fontan patients with a previous Damus-Kaye-Stansel anastomosis or the Norwood procedure.*

*It is important that the left-sided valves function normally in TCPC circulation. In this patient, the aortic root is not markedly dilated. Probably, aortic regurgitation is more likely related to abnormalities of the valve leaflets. If repair of the valve turns out to be challenging, replacement is also an option. Mitral regurgitation is mild. This lesion can be ignored if total cardiac arrest time is prolonged for other reasons.*

*Permanent pacemaker implantation remains controversial. After TCPC conversion, placement of a transvenous approach becomes virtually impossible. Thus, atrial and ventricular epicardial pacing leads ought to be placed. If atrial flutter occurs after TCPC conversion, the cardiologist may use a beta-blocker. To maintain and to control the ventricular rate, ventricular leads should be considered. The optimal location for placement of ventricular pacing leads remains controversial. To allow an intelligent antitachyarrhythmic pacing generator to work, which was not available when this patient was discussed, bipolar leads are required for both the atrium and the ventricle.*

## FINAL DIAGNOSIS

Severe tricuspid stenosis with pulmonary stenosis

Prior atriopulmonary Fontan procedure

Hugely dilated RA

Mild-to-moderate aortic regurgitation, mild mitral regurgitation

Atrial tachyarrhythmia on exercise with P-wave abnormalities

## PLAN OF ACTION

TCPC conversion

Cryo-maze procedure

Aortic valvuloplasty or replacement, mitral valve plasty

## INTERVENTION

On sternotomy and during dissection of the heart, atrial tachycardia and wandering atrial pacemaker were noted. The SVC was transected and anastomosed to the superior aspect of the right PA in a bidirectional fashion. The IVC was isolated, and an extracardiac conduit of 24 mm Gore-Tex tube graft was interposed between the IVC and the inferior aspect of the central PA. The RA free wall was grossly resected, leaving the sinus node intact. The atrial septum was resected extensively. The maze procedure was carried out using cryoablation for the LA side, for the atrial septum, and for the floor around the severely hypoplastic right AV junction. The tiny orifice leading to the RV was left intact, as the orifice would no longer provide a communication between the systemic venous channel and the ventricular chamber subsequent to TCPC conversion using an extracardiac conduit.

The aortic valve had an obvious fusion between the right coronary and the noncoronary cusps, forming a bicuspid-like valve. These leaflets had been thickened. A gap between these leaflets was fixed, and commissures were plicated at the sinotubular junction to make the apposition of the leaflets deeper. The mitral valve annulus was also plicated by the so-called Kay method at both the medial and the lateral commissures. The cardiopulmonary bypass time was 280 minutes, with an aortic cross-clamp time of 139 minutes.

Permanent epicardial pacemaker leads were implanted on the remaining RA wall (bipolar) and on the RV (monopolar or unipolar).

## OUTCOME

In the early postoperative period there was an episode of spontaneous intra-abdominal bleeding. An emergency laparotomy showed bilateral ovarian cysts, and the left ovarian gland was bleeding. The cysts were resected by a gynecologist. A right pleural effusion noted postoperatively resolved on diuretics.

Histopathology revealed that the resected portion of the RA free wall contained patchy and severe fibrosis, as well as considerable myocyte degeneration. The atrial septum also had degeneration of myocytes and severe fibrosis, with the intimal layer containing fibrous thickening.

Postoperatively, the following three drugs were restarted:

Furosemide 20 mg once daily

Spironolactone 25 mg once daily

Enalapril 5 mg daily

A year later the patient's serum BNP level was 28 pg/mL (normal < 20). Echocardiography showed improved fractional shortening and ejection fraction (LVDD/SD 45/33 mm, LVEF 61%). There was trivial mitral and no aortic regurgitation. Flow in the SVC and IVC was normal.

## EXERCISE TESTING

Exercise protocol: Modified Bruce
Duration (min:sec): 5:30
Reason for stopping: Dyspnea
ECG changes: Rare ectopic beats

| | Rest | Peak |
|---|---|---|
| Heart rate (bpm): | 80 | 104 |
| Percent of age-predicted max HR: | | 52 |
| O$_2$ saturation (%): | 94 | 94 |
| Blood pressure (mm Hg): | 110/60 | 130/70 |
| Peak Vo$_2$ (mL/kg/min): | | 18.2 |
| Percent predicted (%): | | 61 |
| Metabolic equivalents: | | 4.9 |

Eleven months after TCPC conversion, the measured exercise tolerance is not remarkably improved. This was not uncommon in our series of patients undergoing TCPC conversion. Improvement may take longer. It may also be that long-standing low cardiac output has already spoiled normal growth of the pulmonary vascular bed. Indeed, this patient had relatively small pulmonary arteries. Research suggests that the pulmonary arterial size does not increase at a normal rate after the Fontan procedure.[14] One positive finding from the exercise test was that there was no further atrial arrhythmia.

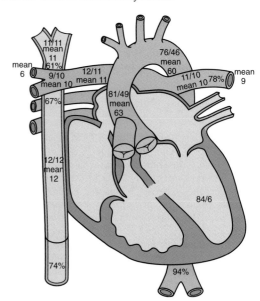

Figure 65-10 Eleven months after conversion.

## REST

**Calculations**

| | |
|---|---|
| BSA | 1.25 m$^2$ |
| Qp | 3.63 L/min (2.91 L/min/m$^2$) |
| Qs | 3.63 L/min (2.91 L/min/m$^2$) |
| Rp | .96 units (1.20 units × m$^2$) |
| Rs | 13.21 units (16.52 units × m$^2$) |
| Qp/Qs | 1.00:1 PD    Rp/Rs = .073 |
| Heart rate | 91 bpm |
| O$_2$ consum. | 120 mL/min/m$^2$ |
| Hemoglobin | 13.8 g/dL |
| F$_{IO_2}$ | 21% |
| pH | 7.45 |
| Pco$_2$ | 38.0 mm Hg |
| Po$_2$ | 62.7 mm Hg |
| Hco$_3$ | 25.7 |

**ThermoCO**

| o$_2$ (%) | | Syst | Diast | Mean |
|---|---|---|---|---|
| 61 | SVC | 11 | 11 | 11 |
| | RA | 12 | 12 | 12 |
| | PA | 12 | 11 | 11 |
| 67 | RPA | 9 | 10 | 10 |
| 78 | LPA | 11 | 10 | 10 |

| **Right** | | **Left** | | |
|---|---|---|---|---|
| 6 | Wedge | 9 | | |

| o$_2$ (%) | | Syst | Diast | Mean |
|---|---|---|---|---|
| | LV | 84 | 6 | |
| | aAo | 81 | 49 | 63 |
| 94 | dAO | 76 | 76 | 60 |

LVEDV 94.9 mL (83%), LVESV 45.4 mL, LVEF 52%

RPA 10.2 mm (53% of normal), LPA 9.0 mm (54% of normal)

PA index (Nakata index) 116

The data are all those of a normally functioning Fontan circulation. The cardiac output and index (3.6 L/min and 2.9 L/min/m$^2$, respectively) are higher than prior to the revision, supporting the notion of improved hemodynamics with an extracardiac Fontan circuit.

## VENOGRAM

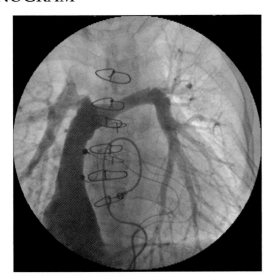

Figure 65-11 Venogram from the inferior vena cava.

### FINDINGS

The TCPC connection is visible.

**Comments:** The IVC channel is smoothly connected to the pulmonary arteries. The hepatic effluent can enter into both lungs. In the moving image, flow to the lungs appeared less turbulent than before.

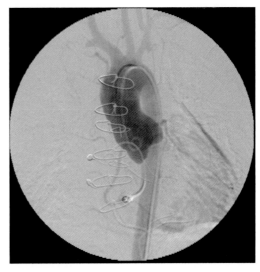

Figure 65-12 Aortic regurgitation was no longer present.

## Selected References

1. Kreutzer G, Galindez E, Bono H, et al: An operation for the correction of tricuspid atresia. J Thorac Cardiovasc Surg 66:613–621, 1973.
2. Engelfriet P, Boersma E, Oechslin E, et al: The spectrum of adult congenital heart disease in Europe: Morbidity and mortality in a 5 year follow-up period. The Euro Heart Survey on adult congenital heart disease. Eur Heart J 26:2325–2333, 2005.
3. Vonder Muhll I, Liu P, Webb G: Applying standard therapies to new targets: The use of ACE inhibitors and B-blockers for heart failure in adults with congenital heart disease. Int J Cardiol 97(Suppl 1):25–33, 2004.
4. Fyfe A, Perloff JK, Niwa K, et al: Cyanotic congenital heart disease and coronary artery atherogenesis. Am J Cardio 96:283–290, 2005.
5. Bolger A, Sharma R, Li W, et al: Neurohormonal activation and the chronic heart failure syndrome in adults with congenital heart disease. Circulation 106:92–99, 2002.
6. Koh M, Yagihara T, Uemura H, et al: Optimal timing of the Fontan conversion change in the P-wave characteristics precedes the onset of atrial tachyarrhythmias in patients with atriopulmonary connection. J Thorac Cardiovasc Surg 133:1295–1302, 2007.
7. Nakata S, Imai Y, Takanashi Y, et al: A new method for the quantitative standardization of cross-sectional areas of the pulmonary arteries in congenital heart diseases with decreased pulmonary blood flow. J Thorac Cardiovasc Surg 88:610–619, 1984.
8. Kao JM, Alegos JC, Gran PW, et al: Conversion of atriopulmonary to cavopulmonary anastomosis in management of late arrhythmias and atrial thrombosis. Ann Thorac Surg 58:1510–1514, 1994.
9. Yoshikawa Y, Ishibashi-Ueda H, Uemura H, et al: Pathologic findings in atrial musculature seven years after the intraatrial tunnel Fontan. Ann Thorac Surg 73:663–664, 2002.
10. Mavroudis C, Backer CL, Deal BJ, Johnsrude CL: Fontan conversion to cavopulmonary connection and arrhythmia circuit cryoablation. J Thorac Cardiovasc Surg 115:547–556, 1998.
11. Kawahira Y, Uemura H, Yagihara T, et al: Renewal of the Fontan circulation with concomitant surgical intervention for atrial arrhythmia. Ann Thorac Surg 71:919–921, 2001.
12. Kobayashi J, Kosakai Y, Nakano K, et al: Improved success rate of the Maze procedure in mitral valve disease by new criteria for patients' selection. Eur J Cardio-Thorac Surg 13:247–252, 1998.
13. Uemura H, Yagihara T, Kawashima Y, et al: What factors affect ventricular performance after a Fontan-type operation? J Thorac Cardiovasc Surg 110:405–415, 1995.
14. Addachi I, Yagihara T, Kagisaki K, et al: Preoperative small pulmonary artery did not affect the midterm results of Fontan operation. Eur J Cardio-Thorac Surg 32:156–162, 2007.

# Arrhythmia Intervention at the Time of Total Cavopulmonary Conversion

**Barbara J. Deal and Constantine Mavroudis**

**Age: 31 years**
**Gender: Female**
**Occupation: Schoolteacher**
**Working diagnosis: Tricuspid atresia, Fontan repair**

## HISTORY

This patient with tricuspid atresia underwent a classic right BT shunt at 5 months of age. At 12 years of age, she underwent a modified Fontan procedure and division of her right BT shunt with an uncomplicated postoperative course. Her atriopulmonary Fontan operation consisted of anastomosis of the dome of the RA to the underside of the RA.

At 24 years of age, she developed atrial arrhythmias with ventricular rates reaching 200 to 220 bpm. Medical treatment for tachycardia included digoxin and beta-blockers. She had multiple episodes of tachycardia requiring direct current cardioversion.

The following year she had a left-sided cerebrovascular accident, with transient left hemiparesis. Cardiac catheterization showed a mean RA pressure of 14 mm Hg (A-wave 20, V-wave 16), pulmonary artery mean pressure of 14, and an LV pressure of 110/5 bpm; a wedge pressure could not be obtained. The RA was markedly dilated with sluggish flow, with a right-to-left shunt noted at the atrial level. Ventricular function was described as "good," with mild atrioventricular valve regurgitation. Procainamide was initiated. She had exercise intolerance and depression at this time.

At 28 years of age she underwent the first of three catheter ablation procedures. At her first electrophysiology study, RA macroreentrant tachycardia of two different morphologies was easily inducible. Lengthy lines of ablation were delivered in the RA inferior isthmus region, between the SVC and the atriopulmonary anastomosis, and between the SVC and the ASD patch. Tachycardia recurred promptly after a rather long ablation procedure. Propafenone was initiated.

Her second ablation was attempted the following year, at 29 years of age, using a CARTO 3D mapping system. She was again noted to have intra-atrial reentry tachycardia with a cycle length of 315 msec. Ablation was performed at the lateral right atrial wall between the area of the crista terminalis and the previous surgical atriotomy scar, and within the coronary sinus. The procedure was considered acutely successful. Her antiarrhythmic medications other than digoxin were discontinued. Following the second ablation, she experienced daily frequent short bursts of tachycardia, at slower rates of 120 to 140 bpm, with dizziness after termination of episodes. She was noted to have marked sinus bradycardia with 3 to 4 second pauses after termination of tachycardia.

She had a second cerebrovascular accident with transient hemiparesis at 30 years of age. Exercise intolerance was pro-gressive. She experienced abdominal fullness and swelling of her lower extremities, as well as brawny induration of both lower legs. She had frequent loose stools.

Her third catheter ablation was attempted, at 31 years of age. At this time, she had sustained intra-atrial tachycardia that was easily induced, with 1:1 AV conduction and an atrial cycle length of 350 msec. A high-energy radiofrequency generator was used and lesions were placed in regions near the tricuspid valve, without affecting the tachycardia. Three additional tachycardia circuits were identified, and after termination of sinoventricular tachycardia a >6-second asystolic pause occurred. Of note, despite multiple attempts, the coronary sinus could not be entered during this procedure. The patient was discharged on antiarrhythmic therapy and referred for arrhythmia surgery.

***Comments:*** In older Fontan-type patients, tricuspid atresia is the most common underlying congenital heart defect. This surgical approach was later extended to patients with more complex lesions, including heterotaxy syndromes, and hypoplastic left heart syndrome.

The technique of doing a BT shunt has changed over time. The classic BT shunt involves an end-to-side anastomosis between a severed subclavian artery and the ipsilateral pulmonary artery. The current technique does not interrupt the subclavian artery. A Gore-Tex graft is placed between the subclavian and pulmonary arteries with end-to-side connections of each anastomosis. The pulse and blood pressure are absent or reduced in the classic BT shunt, and normal or reduced with the modern technique.

Initial palliation consisting of systemic pulmonary shunt at several months of age suggests the presence of pulmonary stenosis; patients with pulmonary atresia would undergo initial palliation during the first week of life. Patients with excessive pulmonary flow would have undergone pulmonary artery banding as the initial procedure.

Typically, sinoventricular tachycardia develops about 8 years after Fontan repair. Although the patient became symptomatic at age 24 years, continuous 24-hour electrocardiographic monitoring likely would have shown the development of sinus bradycardia, atrial ectopy, and nonsustained atrial tachycardia prior to the development of sustained tachycardia.

The development of a cerebrovascular accident suggests right atrial thrombus due to sluggish atrial flow, in addition to right-to-left atrial-level shunting.

Fontan patients typically do not complain of exercise intolerance until fatigue has progressed significantly; they usually have maintained a sedentary lifestyle. They may be able to walk on a flat surface for lengthy periods, but they are usually unable to run, or to go up a flight of stairs quickly, due to their inability to augment cardiac output abruptly.

The most common mechanism of sinoventricular tachycardia in Fontan patients is a macroreentrant atrial tachycardia in the RA. Atrial dilatation and prior surgical incisions/patches create the environment for conduction slowing and reentry. Focal atrial tachycardia, which may represent microreentrant circuits, may occur in up to 10% of patients.

In patients with lateral-tunnel-type Fontan repairs, or patients with double-inlet LVs with prior partitioning of the atria, the tachycardia circuit may be localized on the pulmonary venous side of the atrial partition, and thus not be easily accessible to an ablation catheter.

The acute success rates of ablation in patients with congenital heart disease are improved by the use of 3D mapping techniques, as well as noncontact mapping systems allowing mapping of single beats of atrial tachycardia. However, the short-term recurrence of tachycardia during the first 6 months is greater than 60%.

## CURRENT SYMPTOMS

Daily palpitations, associated with faintness; weight loss (10 pounds over the last year); increasing exertional fatigue. Hypothyroidism had developed 8 years previously, and the patient was on replacement.

Our patient stopped working as a schoolteacher due to progressive fatigue. She took daily naps and had abdominal swelling and lower extremity edema if she had a busy day in the house.

She reported feeling depressed much of the time.

NYHA class: III–IV

***Comments:*** Weight loss is common in patients with right heart failure due to a sensation of abdominal fullness and nausea after eating small amounts of food.

Change in work status/habits may be indicative of exercise intolerance. Daily naps are frequent; again, patients rarely volunteer the information about napping.

Depression is very common among adult Fontan patients with arrhythmias and exercise intolerance; at least half of patients report the use of antidepressant medications.

## CURRENT MEDICATIONS

Digoxin 0.125 mg daily

Lasix 20 mg daily

Potassium chloride 80 mEq daily

Lisinopril 15 mg daily

Warfarin 4 mg daily

Aspirin 81 mg daily

Synthroid 150 µg daily

***Comments:*** Anticoagulation is essential in Fontan patients with dilated atria and/or atrial arrhythmias, due to the increased risk of thrombus formation and strokes (see Case 61).

There is an increased incidence of thyroid disorders in Fontan patients, in addition to amiodarone-induced thyroid disease.

## PHYSICAL EXAMINATION

Overall well-appearing adult female in no distress with thin arms

BP 110/70 mm Hg, HR 65 bpm, oxygen saturation 93%

Height 163 cm, weight 61 kg, BSA 1.66 m$^2$

Surgical scars: Midline sternotomy scars and right lateral thoracotomy scar

Neck veins: Jugular veins could not be seen.

Lungs/chest: Mild rhonchi over the right lower lobe

Heart: The LV impulse was increased, and a regular rhythm present with a single S1 and S2, with no gallop, and a grade 1/6 systolic murmur was audible at the apex.

Abdomen: The abdomen was protuberant, with the liver 3 cm below the right costal margin. No venous distension over the abdomen.

Extremities: There was digital erythema with mild clubbing. Mild dark brownish discoloration of lower extremities was seen. There was trace edema.

### PERTINENT NEGATIVES
There was no goiter, ascites, or scoliosis.

***Comments:*** Muscle wasting in the upper extremities is common in Fontan patients with advanced congestive failure.

Mild desaturation at rest is common in Fontan patients due to right-to-left shunting at the atrial level and/or intrapulmonary shunting.

Cardiomegaly may result in decreased aeration of the right lower lobe.

Single first and second heart sounds reflect AV valve atresia and single ventricular outflow (since pulmonary outflow is obliterated when a Fontan procedure is performed).

Mitral regurgitation is progressive with ventricular dilatation, and frequently abnormal mitral valve morphology is present. Hepatomegaly is often difficult to appreciate due to the degree of hepatic enlargement and general abdominal fullness.

Chronic desaturation results in clubbing; dependent edema and sluggish venous return produce plethora of the extremities. In patients with a "failed Fontan," chronic venous stasis changes of the lower extremities are more common than edema.

Ascites is an advanced finding, often associated with PLE.

Scoliosis is common in patients with repeated thoracotomies and contributes to restrictive lung disease.

## LABORATORY DATA

| | |
|---|---|
| Hemoglobin | **15.8 g/dL** (11.5–15.0) |
| Hematocrit/PCV | **46.5%** (36–46) |
| MCV | 89.7 fL (83–99) |
| Platelet count | $170 \times 10^9$/L (150–400) |
| Sodium | 139 mmol/L (134–145) |
| Potassium | 3.9 mmol/L (3.5–5.2) |
| Creatinine | 0.6 mg/dL (0.6–1.2) |
| Blood urea nitrogen | **10 mmol/L** (2.5–6.5) |

## OTHER RELEVANT LAB RESULTS

| | | |
|---|---|---|
| Magnesium | **1.6 mg/dL** | (1.8–2.4) |
| Phosphorus | 3.3 mg/dL | (3.0–4.5) |
| Calcium | 9.8 mg/dL | (8.8–10.8) |
| Free T4 | 1.6 ng/dL | (0.89–1.76) |
| TSH | 1.76 mU/L | (0.35–5.10) |
| Total protein | **8.1 g/dL** | (6.0–8.0) |
| Albumin | 4.5 g/dL | (3.1–4.6) |
| AST | 31 IU/L | (16–52) |
| ALT | 28 IU/L | (2–30) |
| Alk Phos | 142 IU/L | (55–274) |
| Total bilirubin | **2.2 mg/dL** | (0.2–1.0) |
| Direct bilirubin | **0.4 mg/dL** | (<0.3) |

***Comments:*** Mild erythrocytosis is not uncommon in Fontan patients. Erythropoiesis is stimulated by the low cardiac output and typical mild desaturation.

## ELECTROCARDIOGRAM

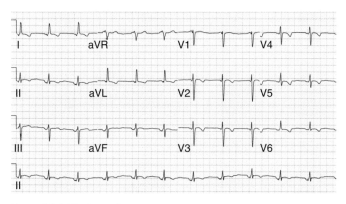

Figure 66-1 Electrocardiogram.

### FINDINGS

Heart rate: 67 bpm

QRS axis: –5°

QRS duration: 112 msec

Low atrial rhythm, left-axis deviation. Atrial abnormality, non-specific repolarization abnormality.

***Comments:*** Left-axis deviation is usually present in tricuspid atresia type 1b.

LV hypertrophy with repolarization abnormalities is commonly present in tricuspid atresia, single ventricle.

## CHEST X-RAY

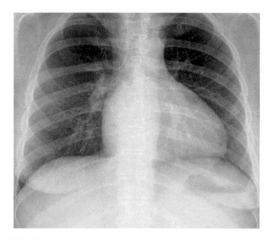

Figure 66-2 Posteroanterior projection.

### FINDINGS

Cardiothoracic ratio: 60%

Moderate cardiomegaly, with a prominent RA shadow and left ventricular contour, was seen. There were normal pulmonary vascular markings.

***Comments:*** Marked cardiomegaly is not common in Fontan patients and, when present, usually reflects massive RA enlargement (see Case 61).

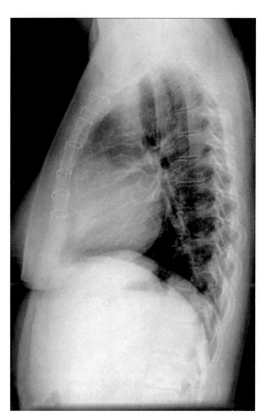

Figure 66-3 Lateral view.

## FINDINGS

The retrosternal space was filled in. The pulmonary artery branches were small. There were sternal wires.

**Comments:** Mild elevation of diaphragms is suggested, and may be due to hepatomegaly and/or ascites.

## EXERCISE TESTING

| Exercise protocol: | Modified Bruce |
| Duration (min:sec): | 5:40 |
| Reason for stopping: | Dyspnea, pallor, nausea, cool extremities |
| ECG changes: | Sinus with atrial ectopy |

| | Rest | Peak |
| --- | --- | --- |
| Heart rate (bpm): | 65 | 130 |
| Percent of age-predicted max HR: | | 69 |
| $O_2$ saturation (%): | 93 | 81 |
| Blood pressure (mm Hg): | 110/70 | 140/90 |
| Peak $Vo_2$ (mL/kg/min): | | 15.2 |
| Percent predicted (%): | | 50 |
| Metabolic equivalents: | | 5.4 |

**Comments:** Exercise capacity is almost always substantially reduced in Fontan patients. Peak $Vo_2$ in healthy Fontan patients is reduced to approximately 65% of predicted for age. In the series by Diller and colleagues,[1] peak $Vo_2$ averaged 19.8 mL/kg/min in single ventricle adults. The peak $Vo_2$ of 15.2 mL/kg/min therefore is markedly reduced, even for older Fontan patients.

Exertional pallor and clamminess are unusual for Fontan patients and more suggestive of a coronary perfusion abnormality.

## ECHOCARDIOGRAM

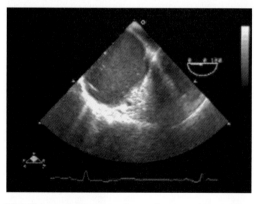

Figure 66-4 Transesophageal echocardiogram, transverse view, 0 degrees; view of right atrium.

## FINDINGS

Giant RA with an absent right AV connection.

**Comments:** Note marked RA dilatation with spontaneous microcavitations giving a "smoky" appearance due to stasis of blood flow.

## MAGNETIC RESONANCE IMAGING

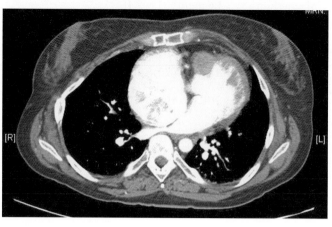

Figure 66-5 Axial view.

## FINDINGS

Marked RA dilatation. The right pulmonary veins are compressed between the huge RA and the spine.

**Comments:** Compression of the right pulmonary venous return by the huge RA is best visualized by either CT or MR, and may be difficult to appreciate by echocardiogram or catheterization.

## CATHETERIZATION

### HEMODYNAMICS

Heart rate    62 bpm

| | Pressure | Saturation (%) |
| --- | --- | --- |
| SVC | 10 | 64 |
| IVC | 10 | 68 |
| RA | 9 | 65 |
| PA | mean 8 | 65 |
| LV | 100/7 | 93 |
| Aorta | 104/68 mean 78 | 93 |

| Calculations | |
| --- | --- |
| Qp (L/min) | 2.44 |
| Qs (L/min) | 2.88 |
| Cardiac index (L/min/m²) | 1.73 |
| Qp/Qs | 0.85 |
| PVR (Wood units) | 0.41 |
| SVR (Wood units) | 23.29 |

### FINDINGS

Normal mean RA pressure for a Fortan was found, with only 1 mm Hg pressure drop to the pulmonary arteries, which is not striking; however, a 2-mm gradient is a significant degree of obstruction in these patients.

There was normal pulmonary capillary wedge pressure and normal left ventricular end-diastolic pressure.

**Comments:** Patients with markedly dilated RA occasionally do not show significant elevation of RA pressure.

In the presence of low cardiac output and a boggy RA, a measurable gradient to the pulmonary arteries may be underestimated. Visualization of anatomic narrowing becomes important in these situations.

Obstruction may occur at several points: the atriopulmonary anastomosis, the branch pulmonary arteries, the pulmonary venous return to the LA, the mitral inflow, and, in patients with transposition, in the subaortic outflow region.

The dilated RA may compress venous return, particularly from the right lung. Assessment of pulmonary capillary wedge pressure versus end-diastolic pressure is important to assess pulmonary venous obstruction.

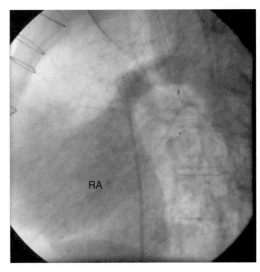

Figure 66-7  Lateral view, atriopulmonary Fontan.

## FINDINGS

A hugely dilated RA is seen, with a relatively small outlet to the pulmonary arteries.

**Comments:** Atrial dilatation is typically better appreciated in the lateral view, as seen here.

### FOCUSED CLINICAL QUESTIONS AND DISCUSSION POINTS

1. **What is the best way to assess the clinical status in older Fontan patients?**

   *Due to their long period of adaptation to their hemodynamic status, it is unusual for Fontan patients to complain of symptoms of fatigue or exercise intolerance until they reach an advanced state of decompensation, or until symptoms related to tachycardia intervene. Hence, in addition to a clinical history of exercise intolerance, it is important to obtain objective information on which to gauge functional status. Assessment should include watching for increased cardiomegaly on chest radiographs, evidence of peripheral edema including chronic venous stasis changes of the lower extremities, and periodic exercise testing with measurement of peak Vo₂.*

2. **What is the preferred imaging modality for detecting problems with the Fontan flow?**

   *The onset of atrial tachycardia often correlates with the presence of marked atrial dilatation with or without obstruction of the Fontan circuit. Echocardiograms typically cannot adequately assess distortion of the atriopulmonary connection or pulmonary venous obstruction. Catheterization pressure measurements with angiograms of the RA, or CMR, are more sensitive for detecting hemodynamically important abnormalities.*

3. **What types of Fontan patients with sinoventricular tachycardia are optimal candidates for catheter ablation treatment?**

   *Repeated catheter ablations or chronic amiodarone use may control symptoms enough to allow the progression of ventricular dysfunction or the development of atrial fibrillation or stroke.*

   *Ablation is best suited to patients with a lateral-tunnel–type repair without significant atrial dilatation or elevation of atrial pressures.*

4. **Should this patient be offered a total cavopulmonary connection (TCPC)?**

   *Conversion of a classical atriopulmonary Fontan connection to a TCPC, that is, establishing a route for venous blood to flow*

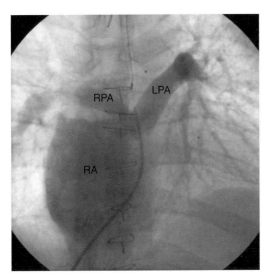

Figure 66-6  Anteroposterior view, right atrium in atriopulmonary Fontan.

## FINDINGS

There was marked RA dilatation. Narrowing of the takeoff of the right pulmonary artery was noted.

**Comments:** Despite measuring essentially normal RA pressure, visualization of the degree of atrial dilatation and relative flows to each lung is important. In this case, there is acute angulation of takeoff of the right pulmonary artery, with more prominent flow to the left pulmonary artery.

In this patient, obstruction of the os of the coronary sinus was demonstrated with coronary angiography, correlating with the earlier finding at the last ablation, in which the coronary sinus could not be cannulated. The coronary sinus and coronary veins were markedly dilated.

Coronary angiography should be performed in adult patients undergoing reoperation to assess variations in anatomy as well as the possibility of coronary artery disease.

Aortic dilatation is common among single ventricle patients; rarely the ascending aorta becomes aneurysmal in size.

*directly to the pulmonary arteries, bypassing the RA, is a high-risk operation, and best performed at experienced centers with high volume. The procedure can be done in conjunction with surgical maze and RA resection to prevent further arrhythmia and thrombus formation (see Case 61), but mortality is not trivial. From the published experience of 111 cases with roughly 5 years of follow-up, there were seven deaths, plus six eventually requiring transplantation (two of whom died).[2] Furthermore, despite aggressive arrhythmia management at the time of surgery, there was still a 25% arrhythmia recurrence rate. Criteria for offering conversion are not well established, as has been discussed (see Case 65).*

*Patients most likely to benefit from arrhythmia surgery with Fontan conversion to a TCPC have evidence of obstruction of pulmonary flow or marked RA dilatation. Fontan revision or conversion to TCPC without arrhythmia surgery has been shown to result in prompt recurrence of tachycardia, albeit with improved hemodynamics.*

*Left-sided arrhythmia surgery is performed for atrial fibrillation, or for reentrant tachycardias located in the LA. In patients with double-inlet LV, the tricuspid valve and coronary sinus are usually partitioned to the pulmonary venous atrium, and at least one tachycardia circuit is usually LA.*

*Patients more likely to be considered for transplant have evidence of PLE, severe AV valve regurgitation, and/or severe ventricular dysfunction thought not to be secondary to a reversible cause. Moderately depressed ventricular function caused by frequent atrial tachycardia, persistent atrial fibrillation, bradycardia, chronic antiarrhythmic therapy, obstruction of pulmonary flow, or massive atrial dilatation may improve following Fontan conversion.*

## FINAL DIAGNOSIS

Tricuspid atresia type 1b with Fontan palliation

Recurrent atrial reentry tachycardia

Obstruction of coronary sinus

## PLAN OF ACTION

Fontan conversion to TCPC with arrhythmia surgery

## INTERVENTION

### Arrhythmia Surgery: Epicardial Electrophysiology Study

After cannulation for bypass, atrial reference electrograms were positioned medial to the atriopulmonary anastomosis, and two decapolar catheters were positioned over the epicardial atrial surface, extending posteriorly. Atrial tachycardia was reproducible, initiated with atrial pacing, and the atrial epicardium was mapped. Four distinct tachycardia circuits were present, including typical atrial flutter, two morphologies mapped to the LA, and atrial fibrillation.

A modified RA maze procedure was performed, with resection of the anterior RA wall measuring 11.5 × 4.5 cm, 6 to 9 mm thick, and removal of the RA appendage, measuring 3.5 × 3 cm. Cryoablation lesions were delivered at −150°C, with lesions from the coronary sinus os to the IVC, from the inferior rim of the ASD patch to the superior os of the coronary sinus, from the base of the resected RA appendage to the superior rim of the atrial defect, and from the posterior atrial defect to the cut edge of the lateral RA, across the crista terminalis.

A modified Cox-maze III procedure was performed in the LA, with lesions as follows: encircling lesion around the pulmo-nary veins, resection of the LA appendage (measuring 3 × 1.6 cm), and lesions between the pulmonary veins to the base of the resected appendage, and to the posterior mitral annulus. A circular lesion was delivered to the epicardial surface of the huge coronary sinus, aligned with the endocardial mitral lesion.

### HEMODYNAMIC SURGERY

Inspection of her RA showed a web of fibrous tissue occluding the os of the coronary sinus; this web was resected. The atrio-pulmonary anastomosis was taken down, with an extracardiac total cavopulmonary anastomosis created using a 24-mm Gore-Tex graft. The large Dacron ASD patch was removed, as was the Dacron patch over the dome of the LA. A bidirectional Glenn procedure was performed.

**Comments:** The coronary sinus os was completely occluded by fibrous tissue, thought to be caused by ablation in the region of the os. This obstruction caused elevated coronary venous pressure and may have caused her symptoms of chest pain and pallor.

### PACEMAKER IMPLANTATION

An epicardial dual-chamber antitachycardia pacemaker was implanted (Medtronic AT 501). The atrial lead was positioned on the remaining RA tissue, anterior to the suture line, and near the AV groove. The ventricular lead was positioned on the apical surface of the anterior LV.

**Comments:** Chronic atrial pacing is usually maintained at rates higher than 70 bpm, to minimize bradycardia and atrial ectopy, and to optimize cardiac output.

Due to the possibility of development of late recurrent sino-ventricular tachycardia and/or late AV block, dual-chamber leads are usually implanted, as well as an antitachycardia pacing generator.

## OUTCOME

The patient received amiodarone intravenously, and atrial pacing at 110 bpm initially, decreased over the following days. She was extubated on postoperative day 1 and was discharged on day 11. At follow-up visit, her pacemaker was programmed AAIR, that is, with a lower rate of 80 bpm and an upper tracking rate of 150 bpm. Discharge medications included Coumadin and amiodarone 200 mg (to be tapered over 3 months). After approximately 1 year of follow-up, she is off antiarrhythmic medications, with no recurrence of tachycardia. She has returned to work full time as a schoolteacher.

**Comments:** Early postoperative atrial fibrillation may occur in as many as one third of patients undergoing LA maze surgery. Intravenous amiodarone markedly reduces this potential. Amiodarone is typically discontinued 3 months postoperatively.

Anticoagulation is maintained for at least 1 year postoperatively with a target INR of 2.0. The optimal duration of anticoagulation therapy is not known.

## Selected References

1. Diller GP, Dimopoulos K, Okonko D, et al: Exercise intolerance in adult congenital heart disease: Comparative severity, correlates, and prognostic implication. Circulation 112:828–835, 2005.
2. Mavroudis C: J. Maxwell Chamberlain Memorial Paper for congenital heart surgery. 111 Fontan conversions with arrhythmia surgery: surgical lessons and outcomes. Ann Thorac Surg 84:1457–1465, 2007.

# Bibliography

Cox JL, Boineau JP, Schuessler RB, et al: Modification of the maze procedure for atrial flutter and atrial fibrillation: I. Rationale and surgical results. J Thorac Cardiovasc Surg 110:473–484, 1995.

Deal BJ, Mavroudis C, Backer CL, et al: Impact of arrhythmia circuit cryoablation during Fontan conversion for refractory atrial tachycardia. Am J Cardiol 83:563–568, 1999.

De Leval MR, Kilner P, Gewillig M, Bull C: Total cavopulmonary connection: A logical alternative to atriopulmonary connection for Fontan operations. Experimental studies and early clinical experience. J Thorac Cardiovasc Surg 96:682–695, 1988.

Marcelletti CF, Hanley FL, Mavroudis C, et al: Revision of previous Fontan connections to total extracardiac cavopulmonary anastomosis: A multicenter experience. J Thorac Cardiovasc Surg 119:340–346, 2000.

Mavroudis C, Backer CL, Deal BJ, Johnsrude CL: Fontan conversion to cavopulmonary connection and arrhythmia circuit cryoablation. J Thorac Cardiovasc Surg 115:547–556, 1998.

Peters NS, Somerville J: Arrhythmias after the Fontan procedure. Br Heart J 68:199–204, 1992.

Theodoro DA, Danielson GK, Porter CJ, Warnes CA: Right-sided maze procedure for right atrial arrhythmias in congenital heart disease. Ann Thorac Surg 65:149–153, 1998.

# Timing and Merits of Transplantation in a Fontan Patient

**Anji T. Yetman and Shelley D. Miyamoto**

**Age: 25 years**
**Gender: Female**
**Occupation: Student**
**Working diagnosis: Tricuspid atresia with transposition**

## HISTORY

The patient was diagnosed with tricuspid atresia, transposed great vessels, and moderate subvalvar pulmonary stenosis shortly after birth. The bulboventricular foramen (VSD) was moderate in size, and the patient was felt to have balanced circulation with adequate systemic and pulmonary blood flow. The patient underwent balloon atrial septostomy and was discharged home with oxygen saturations of 80% to 85%. The patient remained well during early childhood. At the age of 5 years, the patient underwent a classic RA-PA Fontan procedure.

Over the next 10 years the patient developed a slow but steady decline in exercise tolerance. In addition, she complained of symptoms of periorbital and pedal edema. She underwent serial evaluation for PLE but was noted to have a normal albumin and only mildly elevated stool alpha-1-antitrypsin.

During this time period the patient developed frequent palpitations and syncope. She was documented to have sinus bradycardia with intermittent atrial flutter with 2:1 conduction (Fig. 67-1) as well as nonsustained ventricular tachycardia.

Echocardiography demonstrated marked right atrial and coronary sinus enlargement, mildly reduced systemic ventricular function, and a 20 mm Hg gradient across the subaortic VSD.

Cardiopulmonary stress testing demonstrated moderate impairment in exercise capacity and an increase in gradient across the VSD. The patient underwent cardiac catheterization confirming elevated Fontan pressures in the setting of an increased left ventricular end-diastolic pressure and a restrictive VSD.

**Comments:** Twenty-three percent of patients born with tricuspid atresia will have D-transposition of the great vessels. While the majority of patients with tricuspid atresia and normally related great vessels will require surgical intervention in the first few months of life for augmentation of pulmonary blood flow, those with transposition commonly have a clinical course marked by heart failure.[1] Heart failure in this *latter* situation may occur secondary to unrestricted pulmonary arterial blood flow with or without inadequate systemic blood flow, as the aorta may arise from a diminutive outflow chamber with a potentially restrictive VSD. Any restriction at the site of the bulboventricular foramen (subaortic VSD) will further increase pulmonary blood flow at the expense of systemic blood flow (see Fig. 67-5). Surgical options include pulmonary artery banding to restrict pulmonary blood flow,[1] a Damus-Kaye-Stansel procedure plus Blalock-Taussig shunt to bypass aortic outflow tract obstruction and control pulmonary blood flow,[2] or a palliative arterial switch procedure[3] wherein ventriculoarterial continuity is restored by connecting the aorta to the larger LV and connecting the pulmonary artery to the smaller RV. Such a procedure entails coronary artery translocation to the neoaorta. The latter option not only ensures unobstructed aortic blood flow but also restores the morphologic LV to its position as the systemic ventricle. Pulmonary artery banding has been associated with restriction of the bulboventricular foramen, or VSD,[4] and late adverse outcome following the Fontan procedure.[5]

PLE is a serious late complication occurring in 4% to 13% of Fontan patients.[3] Clinical features include hypoalbuminemia, ascites, pleural effusions, diarrhea, malaise, and lymphocytopenia.[4] Fecal alpha-1-antitrypsin levels increase prior to the development of hypoalbuminemia and clinical symptoms.[5] The mortality rate is 40% to 56% within 5 years.[3] Medical therapies effective in some, but not all, include high-dose spironolactone,[6] heparin,[7] and corticosteroids.[8] The mechanism of PLE remains poorly understood and does not necessarily relate to poor Fontan hemodynamics.[6] Fontan revision[9] and orthotopic heart transplantation[3] have sometimes been successful in refractory cases.

Other long-term complications following the atriopulmonary Fontan include thromboembolism in 10% to 25%, sinus node dysfunction and atrial arrhythmias in 20% to 56%,[9] Fontan pathway obstruction, coronary sinus hypertension, decreased ventricular function, and increasing cyanosis secondary to collateral circulation and right-to-left shunting of various types.

The natural history of the VSD in tricuspid atresia is a relative decrease in size with an associated increase in LV-to-RV obstruction (with a form of subaortic stenosis in patients with transposed great arteries). This is often precipitated by volume unloading, as occurs with the Fontan or Glenn procedure.[10]

# ELECTROCARDIOGRAM

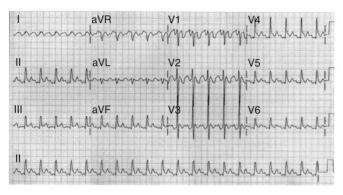

Figure 67-1 Electrocardiogram.

## FINDINGS

Heart rate: 120 bpm

QRS axis: +69°

QRS duration: 148 msec

The patient has atrial flutter with 2:1 AV conduction.

**Comments:** Intra-atrial tachycardia is not uncommon in patients following a classic RA-PA Fontan connection. Restoration of normal sinus rhythm is thought to improve hemodynamics in these patients. Rate control in isolation is not advisable. In the face of a grossly dilated RA, medical therapies may not be effective. Consideration should be given to a Fontan conversion with a maze procedure, or in some cases to ablative therapy alone.

# CHEST X-RAY

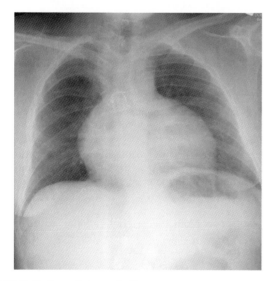

Figure 67-2 Posteroanterior projection.

## FINDINGS

Cardiomegaly with RA prominence. Normal pulmonary vascular markings. There is a bioprosthetic valve in the atriopulmonary connection (unusual).

**Comments:** The patient had marked cardiomegaly with severe RA enlargement, which is to be expected following her classic Fontan procedure. The mediastinum is narrow second-

ary to the absence of the main pulmonary artery shadow, which typically comprises the upper left heart border. The main pulmonary artery lies posterior to the aorta in this patient with transposed great vessels. It has been tied off as part of the Fontan procedure to avoid competitive blood flow with subsequent elevation of the pulmonary artery pressures. There is no evidence of pulmonary venous congestion.

# EXERCISE TESTING

| Exercise protocol: | 15 W ramp protocol on cycle ergometer |
| Duration (min:sec): | 6:00 |
| Reason for stopping: | Presyncope |
| ECG changes: | Normal sinus rhythm with intact AV conduction |

| | Rest | Peak |
| --- | --- | --- |
| Heart rate (bpm): | 106 | 145 |
| Percent of age-predicted max HR: | | 74 |
| O$_2$ saturation (%): | 96 | 92 |
| Blood pressure (mm Hg): | 100/72 | 130/110 |
| Peak Vo$_2$ (mL/kg/min): | | 16 |
| Percent predicted (%): | | 43 |
| Ve/Vco$_2$: | | 40 |
| Metabolic equivalents: | | 4.4 |

## OTHER FINDINGS

The patient had a blunted heart rate slope.

The Vo$_2$ work slope was reduced at 6 (60% predicted).

The peak oxygen pulse was reduced at 10 mL/beat (65% predicted).

A previous test 2 years prior demonstrated a peak Vo$_2$ of 27.9 mL/kg/min (75% predicted).

**Comments:** The exercise test employed an incremental ramp protocol with increments of $\frac{1}{4}$ Watt per kg of body weight per minute. The protocol is designed to achieve an exercise duration of between 8 and 12 minutes. This duration is designed to achieve a maximal cardiac and pulmonary effort.

Oxygen saturation at rest was 96% and at peak exercise was 92%, which was within normal limits for the test altitude (5200 feet).

There has been a significant reduction in her exercise capacity from a study 2 years previously. A reduction in ventilatory efficiency is common in patients following a Fontan procedure. This may be secondary to elevated pulmonary artery pressures, elevated left heart filling pressures, chest wall deformities secondary to previous thoracotomy or VQ mismatch. Chronotropic incompetence is also common following Fontan palliation and will adversely affect exercise capacity.

Exercise testing with collection of metabolic data is a useful diagnostic tool for determining the timing of listing for heart transplantation.[11] Such testing has been documented to be safe with a low risk of adverse events in outpatients with congestive heart failure in the setting of palliated congenital heart defects.[12] A peak oxygen consumption of less than 14 mL/kg/min is used as a criterion for listing in an adult population without congenital heart disease.[11] This value is not applicable to the child or young adult with congenital heart disease who will often have a higher peak Vo$_2$ at the time of heart transplantation.[12] A more applicable cutoff value may be a peak oxygen consumption less than 50% predicted.[12] Similarly, a peak oxygen pulse of less than 10 mL/beat, which has been used as an indication for heart transplantation in the adult without congenital heart disease, may not be applicable in this instance.[12]

# ECHOCARDIOGRAM

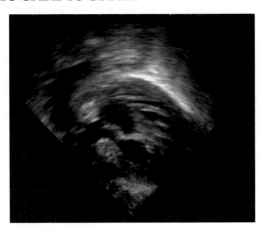

Figure 67-3 Subcostal 2D echo.

## FINDINGS

Subcostal imaging demonstrates a single great vessel (the aorta) arising from the small RV outlet chamber. The LV communicates with the aorta via the bulboventricular foramen, which appears small and approximately the same size as the aortic valve.

**Comments:** TTE images are limited in this patient. The fixed orifice of the bulboventricular foramen may also have a further component of dynamic narrowing that will further compromise cardiac output during exercise.

## CATHETERIZATION

### HEMODYNAMICS

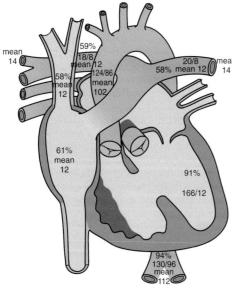

Figure 67-4 Hemodynamic data.

## FINDINGS

Cardiac catheterization prior to Fontan revision demonstrated mild elevation of Fontan pressures with no gradient within the Fontan circuit suggestive of stenosis. Low mixed venous saturations were indicative of low cardiac output. TEE performed at the time of the study demonstrated no clot within the Fontan circuit. The patient was fully saturated for this altitude (5200 feet). LV end-diastolic pressure was mildly elevated. There was a significant gradient between the systemic LV through the bulboventricular foramen to the aorta (44 mm Hg at rest).

**Comments:** Prior to consideration of Fontan revision it is important to determine (1) the cause of previous Fontan "failure" and (2) the suitability of the patient for a successful Fontan revision. Attention needs to be paid to pulmonary artery pressures and the transpulmonary gradient, pulmonary artery size, the presence of aortopulmonary and veno-venous collaterals, systemic ventricular function, systemic AV valve insufficiency, and the presence or absence of outflow tract obstruction.

# ANGIOGRAM

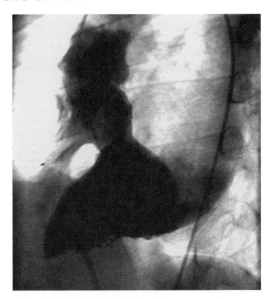

Figure 67-5 Left anterior oblique projection.

## FINDINGS

The aorta was seen arising primarily from the rudimentary RV. The diameter of the bulboventricular foramen was smaller than the aortic valve diameter in keeping with LVOT obstruction.

**Comments:** Note the arterial catheter approach retrograde in the aorta, across the aortic valve, through the bulboventricular foramen, and into the LV.

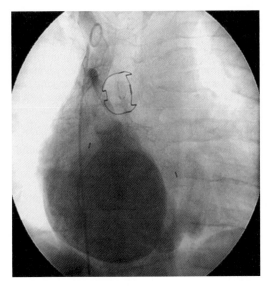

Figure 67-6 Anteroposterior projection.

## FINDINGS

Classic RA-PA Fontan connection. This patient has had a modification of this procedure with placement of a valved conduit between the RA and pulmonary artery. There was marked dilation of the RA and coronary sinus (*bottom right*), with stasis of flow as demonstrated by the very slow clearing of dye.

*Comments:* The classic RA-PA connection is no longer performed, having been replaced by other versions of the Fontan procedure associated with better hemodynamics. These include the extracardiac conduit wherein a Gore-Tex conduit is connected to the IVC inferiorly and the pulmonary artery superiorly. This approach excludes the RA from the Fontan circuit. This may lead to a reduced incidence of atrial dysrhythmias in the long term. The conduit may be fenestrated with a small connection to the RA in high-risk patients. The lateral tunnel Fontan involves an intracardiac tunnel within the atria. It too is thought to lead to improved hemodynamics and a lower incidence of long-term arrhythmias, although the suture lines within the atrial wall can be arrhythmogenic.

## HISTORY

The patient subsequently underwent Fontan revision with placement of a 24-mm fenestrated extracardiac conduit, right atrial plication, RA maze procedure, enlargement of the VSD, and placement of an epicardial dual-chamber pacing system.

Following surgery the patient had marked cyanosis, which slowly improved to a resting oxygen saturation of 88%. The patient had further desaturation with exercise. One year after surgery the patient underwent device occlusion of the fenestration. The procedure was well tolerated. The patient had significant symptomatic improvement and experienced normal exercise tolerance lasting 10 years.

The patient then developed NYHA class III symptoms. She was no longer able to attend college classes. Exercise testing demonstrated a significant reduction in oxygen consumption.

Repeat cardiac catheterization with angiography was performed showing no obstruction of the Fontan circuit, mild elevation of pulmonary pressures, and a reduced cardiac index. Symptoms persisted despite maximal medical management. She was evaluated for orthotopic heart transplantation. During the process of heart transplant evaluation the patient had clini-

cal deterioration that necessitated the placement of an indwelling catheter for home milrinone therapy.

*Comments:* Conversion to an extracardiac Fontan with concomitant arrhythmia surgery has been shown to improve arrhythmias and NYHA class in atriopulmonary Fontan patients.[9]

Indications for Fontan fenestration closure include an oxygen saturation of less than 90% and ability to tolerate test occlusion. Closure has been associated with improved oxygenation, reduced use of anticongestive therapy, and improved somatic growth in children.[13]

Serial cardiopulmonary exercise testing provides objective assessment of aerobic capacity and may be used to determine whether the limitation in exercise tolerance is secondary to low cardiac output, pulmonary pathology, or peripheral muscle disease.

Many patients require supportive care while awaiting transplantation. Continuous IV home milrinone therapy has been shown to be safe and effective.[14]

## CURRENT SYMPTOMS

The patient's symptoms were fatigue, anorexia, dyspnea, and exercise intolerance.

NYHA class: III

## CURRENT MEDICATIONS

Milrinone infusion 0.5 µg/kg/min

Enalapril 10 mg twice daily

Lasix 40 mg twice daily

Spironolactone 25 mg daily

Coumadin 5 mg daily (to maintain INR of 2.0–3.0)

*Comments:* Some cardiologists recommend routine anticoagulation following the Fontan procedure in childhood. At present, there are no large, randomized controlled trials to support this practice.

Intracardiac thrombus may become a serious problem following the Fontan procedure, especially in patients with additional risk factors. Thrombus within the Fontan circuit may result in obstruction to the pathway, chronic pulmonary embolic disease with ventilation/perfusion mismatch, or elevation of pulmonary vascular resistance.[15] All will adversely affect Fontan hemodynamics. In Fontan patients reaching adulthood an average of 15 years following surgery, documented thromboembolic events are present in 25%. The associated mortality rate is high at more than 30%.[16]

Patients felt to be at high risk for thromboses, including those with systemic ventricular dysfunction, atrial arrhythmias, and a classic RA-PA Fontan connection, may benefit from anticoagulation.

## PHYSICAL EXAMINATION

The patient was in good spirits and in no acute distress.

BP 98/72 mm Hg, HR 106 bpm atrially paced, oxygen saturation 96%, afebrile

Height 159.5 cm, weight 50 kg, BSA 1.49 m$^2$

Surgical scars: Well-healed median sternotomy scar without keloid formation

Neck veins: No facial suffusion. No prominence of superficial vessels. Elevated JVP to the angle of the jaw at 30 degrees.

Lungs/chest: Good air entry bilaterally with no adventitious sounds

Heart: A regular heart rhythm was present, with a precordium normal to palpation. There was a normal first heart sound, a single second heart sound, and an S3 gallop. There were no murmurs.

Abdomen: The abdomen was soft, nontender, and mildly protuberant. The liver was palpable 3 cm below the costal margin and was firm but nontender. No splenomegaly or masses were present. There was positive shifting dullness and a fluid thrill to suggest ascites.

Extremities: The extremities were warm and well perfused with no clubbing or cyanosis, and 2+ pulses were present and equal throughout. There was 1+ pedal edema.

**Comments:** The patient has had device closure of her fenestration and thus is now fully saturated.

The patient has findings consistent with right heart failure. In the face of elevated LV filling pressures or even a slight increase in pulmonary vascular resistance, which may be secondary to "clinically silent" pulmonary embolism,[17] Fontan pressures will be elevated leading to impaired flow through the Fontan circuit.

## LABORATORY DATA

| | |
|---|---|
| Hemoglobin | 12 g/dL (11.5–15.0) |
| Hematocrit/PCV | 38% (36–46) |
| MCV | 85 fL (83–99) |
| Platelet count | $160 \times 10^9$/L (150–400) |
| Sodium | **132 mmol/L** (134–145) |
| Potassium | 4.2 mmol/L (3.5–5.2) |
| Creatinine | 1.1 mg/dL (0.6–1.2) |
| Blood urea nitrogen | **20 mg/dL** (5–17) |
| Protein | 5.5 g/dL (5.5–8.0) |
| Albumin | 3.5 g/dL (3.5–5.5) |

### OTHER RELEVANT LAB RESULTS

Blood typing: O-positive blood

Cytomegalovirus (CMV) negative

Markedly elevated plasma renin activity (PRA): human leukocyte antigen (HLA) class I titer 5% and class II titer of 94% with broad reactivity

**Comments:** Increased PRA (>10%) represents immunologic sensitization to foreign HLA antigens, which occur as a result of exposure to blood transfusions, homograft tissue, and even assist devices. Elevation in PRA tends to be more common in patients with congenital heart defects undergoing heart transplantation.[18] The presence of anti-HLA antibodies has been associated with hyperacute, acute, and chronic rejection.[18] There is evidence that these antibodies may play a role in the development of transplant cardiac allograft vasculopathy. Therapies to lower the PRA include plasmapheresis followed by IVIG administration, azathioprine, and cyclophosphamide.

### FOCUSED CLINICAL QUESTIONS AND DISCUSSION POINTS

1. What are the causes of congestive heart failure in the Fontan patient?

*Symptoms of right or left heart failure may develop in the Fontan patient. Symptoms may occur secondary to "Fontan" and "pump" failure. The patient must be evaluated to identify and potentially relieve any obstruction to flow through the Fontan circuit. Sources of obstruction include anastomotic strictures, pulmonary artery stenoses, thrombus within the circuit, pulmonary emboli, and elevated pulmonary artery pressures secondary to competitive flow from collaterals. CMR provides excellent noninvasive imaging of the Fontan pathway. Pump failure with associated elevation of LV filling pressures will also impede Fontan flow. Myocardial dysfunction may occur secondary to multiple cardiac surgeries, outflow tract obstruction, or a variety of other reasons.*

2. Is heart transplantation indicated in this patient?

*Indications for heart transplantation in patients following Fontan palliation include congestive heart failure, intractable arrhythmias, recurrent thrombosis refractory to medical therapy, PLE, and plastic bronchitis.*

*While a peak oxygen consumption of less than 14 mL/kg/min and a peak oxygen pulse of less than 10 are used as cutoff points for consideration for heart transplantation in adults with acquired heart disease, they are, as mentioned earlier, not applicable to the patient with congenital heart disease.*

3. Should this patient have had primary heart transplantation rather than a Fontan?

*In high-risk Fontan candidates, primary cardiac transplantation may provide a better chance of survival. Previous surgery, immunodeficiency, and malnutrition associated with PLE, lymphocytotoxic antibodies, longer wait list times, higher pulmonary vascular resistance, emergency status, and perioperative bleeding all contribute to mortality.[19] These factors must be weighed into the decision regarding early or later listing for transplantation.*

## FINAL DIAGNOSIS

Congestive heart failure secondary to progressive myocardial dysfunction in a patient with a total cavopulmonary connection

## PLAN OF ACTION

List for heart transplantation

## INTERVENTION

The decision was made to list the patient for heart transplantation with a status of 1B. Efforts were made to lower the PRA including IVIG 1 g/kg weekly for 2 weeks and then monthly for 3 months and then every other month. Azathioprine was started at 2 mg/kg/day. The PRA was checked monthly but remained elevated. Because of the elevated PRA, the patient required a cross-match with potential donors. Multiple donors were refused secondary to positive cross-match results. Efforts to lower the PRA were intensified through the use of plasmapheresis (five-times volume exchange) followed by IVIG.

The patient was ultimately transplanted with a CMV-positive donor organ 25 months after initial listing and after a 4-month hospital stay on intensified inotropic support.

The patient received plasmapheresis at the time of bypass in a final effort to lower her PRA. The patient could not separate from bypass secondary to acute biventricular failure of the donor organ. A biventricular Bio-Medicus assist device was placed. Ventricular function improved over 48 hours, and the assist device was removed. Other than transient renal insufficiency, the postoperative course was uncomplicated. Postoperatively the patient developed transient acute tubular necrosis with a peak BUN of 190 and creatinine of 1.4.

**Comments:** Cardiac transplantation in patients with single ventricle physiology involves several unique surgical challenges resulting in longer bypass and ischemic times.[20] Reconstructive surgery to restore normal systemic venous return and to address pulmonary artery distortion is commonly required.[20] Ideally, a congenital heart surgeon should be involved in planning and/or carrying out the procedure(s). Despite these challenges, outcomes are comparable to those for patients transplanted for other etiologies.[20]

The primary causes of death early after heart transplantation in children and young adults are rejection with early graft failure and RV failure secondary to pulmonary hypertension. Optimal therapy of pulmonary hypertension with oxygen, nitric oxide, and/or sildenafil[21] and aggressive use of assist devices may assist in getting through this critical period.

## OUTCOME

Following induction immunosuppression and eventual transition to maintenance therapy with cyclosporine and mycophenolate mofetil, the patient was discharged to home. Secondary to mismatched CMV status (recipient negative and donor positive), the patient was treated with oral gancyclovir for 1 month posttransplant. Ongoing medical problems included renal insufficiency with renal tubular acidosis requiring treatment with bicarbonate and potassium replacement for 2 months.

Late complications included systemic CMV requiring hospitalization for IV fluids and gancyclovir at 3 months posttransplant. In the first year posttransplantation the patient had two episodes of rejection with the first episode (ISHLT 3A) triggered by the CMV infection. She had two subsequent biopsy-confirmed episodes of rejection with the last documented episode occurring at 3 years posttransplant. The patient was hemodynamically stable during all episodes and was treated with steroids and antibody therapy and subsequent alteration of maintenance immunosuppressive therapy (cyclosporine was discontinued and tacrolimus added). Following the CMV illness at 3 months, the patient had no further infectious illnesses requiring hospitalization.

Other late medical problems included osteopenia but no osteoporosis or fractures. The patient remained normotensive posttransplant with a normal lipid profile and normal fasting glucose. She was highly compliant with her medical regime and was a nonsmoker.

At 1 year posttransplantation the patient was active running local 5K charity races and attending the gym 3 days per week. She reported a sense of well-being and a good quality of life.

The patient underwent cardiopulmonary stress testing using a bicycle ergometer. After 10 minutes she achieved a peak workload of 150 Watts, peak heart rate of 160 bpm (82% of predicted), and peak BP of 170/60. Oxygen saturation at peak exercise was 92%, which was within normal limits for this altitude. The patient stopped secondary to presyncope. Her peak $Vo_2$ was 25 mL/kg/min (65% of predicted), anaerobic threshold 19 mL/kg/min (65% of predicted), with a $Ve/Vco_2$ slope of 40. At peak exercise the patient developed symptomatic 2:1 AV block, which persisted after testing (see Fig. 67-7). A 24-hour ECG was recorded. The patient had two brief syncopal spells during the 24-hour period, both of which were associated with an episode of 2:1 AV block.

A routine coronary angiogram was performed. The patient had mild transplant cardiac allograft vasculopathy (CAV) (mild CAV is defined as less than 50% lesion in any branch segment). The vasculopathy was medically managed as per our institution's protocol with pravastatin and anti-T-cell antibody therapy while being monitored in hospital on telemetry. The decision was made to place a pacemaker if the second-degree AV block persisted following additional rejection therapy.

The patient had resolution of heart block with documentation of normal AV conduction after 24 hours of medical treatment. There were no further episodes of heart block on initial 48-hour Holter monitoring and serial Holter monitoring out to 2 years. In addition, the patient had no further syncopal spells. There was no further progression of transplant CAV on repeat coronary evaluations as of 2 years posttreatment.

**Comments:** CMV infection in transplant patients has been associated with rejection in the transplanted heart. Use of prophylactic gancyclovir in the CMV seronegative recipient of a CMV-positive donor has been shown to effectively prevent CMV infection in this high-risk population. However, CMV mismatching represents a risk factor for 1-year mortality.[22]

Late CMV infection has been associated with the development of transplant CAV. The mechanism of this association is unclear, but the viral infection may initiate a destructive immune response that can lead to rejection and/or CAV.[23] Two or more episodes of rejection in the first year after transplant have also been shown to correlate with CAV.[24-26]

A wide range of medical problems can occur after heart transplant secondary to the use of calcineurin inhibitors including hypertension, hyperlipidemia, diabetes, chronic renal insufficiency, and gout. The chronic use of glucocorticoids will exacerbate many of these problems and is the primary cause of posttransplant osteoporosis.[27]

In adult heart transplant recipients, exercise capacity remains reduced at 50% to 70% of predicted[28] despite marked symptomatic improvement. Factors responsible for exercise impairment include a reduced heart rate reserve, impaired lung diffusion capacity, LV diastolic dysfunction, and peripheral vasoconstriction.[28] Cardiac rehabilitation has been shown to be effective in improving exercise tolerance.[29]

Transplant patients have been documented to have a reduction in ventilatory efficiency that appears to relate to abnormal lung diffusion capacity.[28] This impairment may relate to long-standing congestive heart failure prior to transplantation or may be due to impaired cardiac output in these patients. Chronotropic incompetence is common in transplant patients and will adversely affect exercise capacity.

Assessment for CAV is an important aspect of rejection surveillance in heart transplant patients. Evaluation of coronary flow reserve and intimal thickening on coronary intravascular ultrasound often precede changes seen on coronary angiography. Coronary angiography is required to assess the severity of vasculopathy.

Rejection and/or CAV were the most likely cause of the new-onset high-grade AV block. New-onset Wenckebach heart block has been associated with rejection and CAV[30] and is not considered benign in this population. High-grade second-degree AV block has also been correlated with CAV.[31] Rhythm disturbances may predate noticeable changes on coronary angiography.[31] Routine use of pravastatin has been demonstrated to reduce the risk of developing CAV following transplantation in adults.[32]

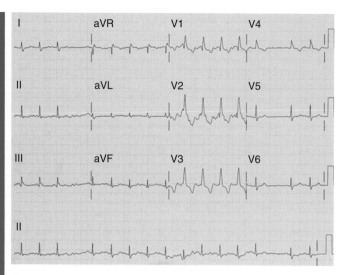

Figure 67-7 Electrocardiogram.

# FINDINGS

Heart rate: 100 bpm

QRS axis: +119°

QRS duration: 135 msec

Normal sinus rhythm with intermittent 2:1 AV block. Right bundle branch block.

***Comments:*** The baseline elevated heart rate is unchanged from previous findings and is common in patients after heart transplantation.

As a result of the ECG abnormality, a 24-hour Holter monitor was placed and demonstrated a minimum HR of 110 bpm, an average HR of 113 bpm, and a maximal HR of 126 bpm. The reduction in HR variability is normal following heart transplantation.

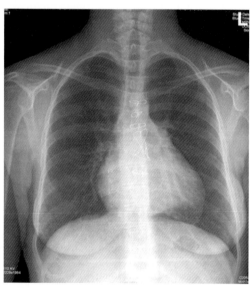

Figure 67-8 Posteroanterior projection.

# FINDINGS

Cardiothoracic ratio: 55%

A mildly enlarged cardiac silhouette was seen, in contrast to marked cardiomegaly prior to transplantation. Normal pulmonary vascular markings. Prior median sternotomy.

***Comments:*** The patient has evidence of previous sternotomy with sternotomy wires in place. There is no evidence of wire fracture. There is mild cardiomegaly. Cardiomegaly following heart transplantation may occur secondary to ventricular dysfunction caused by rejection, or CAV. Other causes of cardiomegaly may include RA dilation secondary to tricuspid insufficiency, or right heart dilation in the setting of persistent pulmonary arterial hypertension. Pulmonary vascular markings are normal.

The patient had mild transplant CAV by angiography using the cardiac transplant research database criteria,[33] which defines mild CAD as less than 50% lesion in any branch segment; moderate CAD as greater than 50% lesion in one primary vessel, or greater than 50% in branches of two vessels; and severe disease as a greater than 50% lesion in two primary vessels, or greater than 50% in branches of all three systems, or 50% left main lesion.

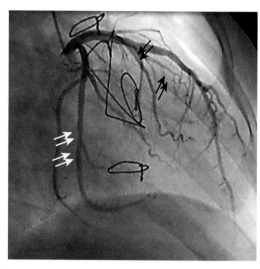

Figure 67-9 Left coronary artery angiogram in the right anterior oblique projection. Areas of mild irregularity in branches of the left anterior descending artery (*black arrows*) and the left circumflex artery (*white arrows*).

***Comments:*** Assessment for coronary vasculopathy is an important aspect of rejection surveillance in heart transplant patients. Evaluation of coronary flow reserve and intimal thickening on coronary intravascular ultrasound often precedes changes seen on coronary angiography. Coronary angiography is required to assess the severity of vasculopathy.

## Selected References

1. Adams FH, Emmanouilides GC, Riemenschneider TA: Moss Heart Disease in Infants, Children, and Adolescents, 4th ed. Philadelphia, Lippincott Williams & Wilkins, 1989.
2. Lacour-Gayet F, Serraf A, Fermont L, et al: Early palliation of univentricular hearts with subaortic stenosis and ventriculoarterial discordance: The arterial switch option. J Thorac Cardiovasc Surg 104:1238–1245, 1992.
3. Brancaccio G, Carotti A, D'Argenio P, et al: Protein-losing enteropathy after Fontan surgery: Resolution after cardiac transplantation. J Heart Lung Transplant 22:484–486, 2003.
4. Powell AJ, Gauvreau K, Jenkins KJ, et al: Perioperative risk factors for development of protein-losing enteropathy following a Fontan procedure. Am J Cardiol 88:1206–1209, 2001.
5. Fujii T, Shimizu T, Takahashi K, et al: Fecal alpha1-antitrypsin concentrations as a measure of enteric protein loss after modified Fontan operations. J Pediatr Gastroenterol Nutr 37:577–580, 2003.

6. Ringel RE, Peddy SB: Effect of high-dose spironolactone on protein-losing enteropathy in patients with Fontan palliation of complex congenital heart disease. Am J Cardiol 91:1031–1032, A9, 2003.

7. Donnelly JP, Rosenthal A, Castle VP, Holmes RD: Reversal of protein-losing enteropathy with heparin therapy in three patients with univentricular hearts and Fontan palliation. J Pediatr 130:474–478, 1997.

8. Zellers TM, Brown K: Protein-losing enteropathy after the modified Fontan operation: Oral prednisone treatment with biopsy and laboratory proved improvement. Pediatr Cardiol 17:115–117, 1996.

9. Kim WH, Lim HG, Lee JR, et al: Fontan conversion with arrhythmia surgery. Eur J Cardiothorac Surg 27:250–257, 2005.

10. Hiramatsu T, Imai Y, Kurosawa H, et al: Midterm results of surgical treatment of systemic ventricular outflow obstruction in Fontan patients. Ann Thorac Surg 73:855–860; discussion, 860–861, 2002.

11. Mancini DM, Eisen H, Kussmaul W, et al: Value of peak exercise oxygen consumption for optimal timing of cardiac transplantation in ambulatory patients with heart failure. Circulation 83:778–786, 1991.

12. Das BB, Taylor AL, Boucek MM, et al: Exercise capacity in pediatric heart transplant candidates: Is there any role for the 14 ml/kg/min guideline? Pediatr Cardiol 27:226–229, 2006.

13. Goff DA, Blume ED, Gauvreau K, et al: Clinical outcome of fenestrated Fontan patients after closure: The first 10 years. Circulation 102:2094-2099, 2000.

14. Brozena SC, Twomey C, Goldberg LR, et al: A prospective study of continuous intravenous milrinone therapy for status IB patients awaiting heart transplant at home. J Heart Lung Transplant 23:1082–1086, 2004.

15. Walker HA, Gatzoulis MA: Prophylactic anticoagulation following the Fontan operation. Heart 91:854–856, 2005.

16. Van den Bosch AE, Roos-Hesselink JW, van Domberg R, et al: Long-term outcome and quality of life in adult patients after the Fontan operation. Am J Cardiol 93:1141–1145, 2004.

17. Varma C, Warr MR, Hendler AL, et al: Prevalence of "silent" pulmonary emboli in adults after the Fontan operation. J Am Coll Cardiol 41:2252–2258, 2003.

18. Balfour IC, Fiore A, Graff RJ, Knutsen AP: Use of rituximab to decrease panel-reactive antibodies. J Heart Lung Transplant 24:628–630, 2005.

19. Carey JA, Hamilton JR, Hilton CJ, et al: Orthotopic cardiac transplantation for the failing Fontan circulation. Eur J Cardiothorac Surg 14:7–13; discussion 13–14, 1998.

20. Jayakumar KA, Addonizio LJ, Kichuk-Chrisant MR, et al: Cardiac transplantation after the Fontan or Glenn procedure. J Am Coll Cardiol 44:2065–2072, 2004.

21. Kulkarni A, Singh TP, Sarnaik A, et al: Sildenafil for pulmonary hypertension after heart transplantation. J Heart Lung Transplant 23:1441–1444, 2004.

22. Taylor DO, Edwards LB, Boucek MM, et al: The Registry of the International Society for Heart and Lung Transplantation: Twenty-first official adult heart transplant report—2004. J Heart Lung Transplant 23:796–803, 2004.

23. Pietra B, Boucek M: Coronary artery vasculopathy in pediatric cardiac transplant patients: The therapeutic potential of immuno-modulators. Paediatr Drugs 5:513–524, 2003.

24. Boucek MM, Edwards LB, Keck BM, et al: Registry for the International Society for Heart and Lung Transplantation: Seventh official pediatric report—2004. J Heart Lung Transplant 23:933–947, 2004.

25. Pahl E, Naftel DC, Kuhn MA, et al: The impact and outcome of transplant coronary artery disease in a pediatric population: A 9-year multi-institutional study. J Heart Lung Transplant 24:645–651, 2005.

26. Uretsky BF, Murali S, Reddy PS, et al: Development of coronary artery disease in cardiac transplant patients receiving immunosuppressive therapy with cyclosporine and prednisone. Circulation 76:827–834, 1987.

27. Lindenfeld J, Page RL, II, Zolty R, et al: Drug therapy in the heart transplant recipient. Part III: Common medical problems. Circulation 111:113–117, 2005.

28. Al-Rawas OA, Carter R, Stevenson RD, et al: Exercise intolerance following heart transplantation: The role of pulmonary diffusing capacity impairment. Chest 118:1661–1670, 2000.

29. Haykowsky M, Riess K, Figgures L, et al: Exercise training improves aerobic endurance and musculoskeletal fitness in female cardiac transplant recipients. Curr Control Trials Cardiovasc Med 6:10, 2005.

30. Kertesz NJ, Towbin JA, Clunie S, et al: Long-term follow-up of arrhythmias in pediatric orthotopic heart transplant recipients: Incidence and correlation with rejection. J Heart Lung Transplant 22:889–893, 2003.

31. Cannon BC, Denfield SW, Friedman RA, et al: Late pacemaker requirement after pediatric orthotopic heart transplantation may predict the presence of transplant coronary artery disease. J Heart Lung Transplant 23:67–71, 2004.

32. Mahle WT, Vincent RN, Berg AM, Kanter KR: Pravastatin therapy is associated with reduction in coronary allograft vasculopathy in pediatric heart transplantation. J Heart Lung Transplant 24:63–66, 2005.

33. Costanzo MR, Naftel DC, Pritzker MR, et al: Heart transplant coronary artery disease detected by coronary angiography: A multiinstitutional study of preoperative donor and recipient risk factors. Cardiac Transplant Research Database. J Heart Lung Transplant 17:744–753, 1998.

# Early Appraisal of Adults with Norwood Correction

**Eapen Thomas and Sara Thorne**

**Age: 14 years**
**Gender: Female**
**Occupation: Student**
**Working diagnosis: Hypoplastic left heart syndrome**

## HISTORY

The patient was born at term gestation by normal delivery. She had normal Apgar scores and her birth weight was 3.2 kg. Her mother did not have an antenatal fetal echocardiogram.

She developed tachypnea and cyanosis 30 hours after birth. Clinical examination at that time revealed a saturation of 68% on 70% oxygen, a gallop rhythm, a grade 2/6 systolic murmur at the left upper sternal edge, and a clear chest. Arterial blood gases showed severe hypoxia with a $Po_2$ of 35 mm Hg. CXR demonstrated borderline cardiomegaly.

The baby was started on a prostaglandin E1 infusion and then transferred to a tertiary children's hospital for further management. Her oxygen saturation improved to 90% on the prostaglandin E1 infusion. An echocardiogram on arrival revealed situs solitus with normal systemic and pulmonary venous connections. The LV was markedly hypoplastic with a patent mitral valve and intact interventricular septum. There was subaortic atresia. A restrictive secundum ASD was noted with a single right SVC. The ascending aorta and arch were of reasonable size measuring 50 mm at the sinuses and 35 mm at the transverse arch. There was no aortic coarctation. A PDA with right-to-left shunting was noted.

She underwent a successful first-stage Norwood procedure on day 7 under hypothermic circulatory arrest. She had an uneventful postoperative period and was discharged home on digoxin, furosemide, and amiloride.

She remained well at home with normal development and satisfactory weight gain. Her resting $O_2$ saturation gradually dropped and was 68% at the age of 3 months. Cardiac catheterization revealed a good caliber neoaorta with no coarctation. There was some stenosis of the left pulmonary artery. The RV angiogram revealed good systolic function.

The patient underwent elective stage II palliation (bidirectional cavopulmonary shunt, see Fig. 68-7) at 3.5 months of age, along with further enlargement of the ASD and bovine pericardial patch repair of the left pulmonary artery. At the time of discharge her resting oxygen saturation was 80% on room air and her ventricular function was good by echocardiography.

She remained under close clinical follow-up. By the age of 3 years, her parents expressed concern that her exercise tolerance and oxygen saturations had decreased. Cardiac catheter assessments were done at 1.5 and 3 years of age. These revealed good cavopulmonary connection with good-sized branch pulmonary arteries and a transpulmonary gradient of 8 mm Hg.

At the age of 3.5 years, she had her third staged palliative procedure: elective Fontan surgery (total cavopulmonary connection, see Fig. 68-8). In this procedure the RA-PA connection was completed with a pulmonary homograft patch. A lateral tunnel, constructed using Gore-Tex with a 3.5 mm fenestration, directed the IVC flow into the pulmonary artery.

She was extubated on the day of operation and was transferred to the ward on the following day. She remained hemodynamically stable with a resting oxygen saturation of 90% on room air. She had a significant pleural effusion requiring drainage. A transthoracic echocardiogram performed at the time of discharge showed good ventricular function, trivial tricuspid regurgitation, a patent fenestration, and no pericardial or pleural effusions. Prior to discharge she was fully anticoagulated.

Repeat cardiac catheterization at age 5 showed the oxygen saturation in the RV and aorta to be 92% with an RA mean pressure of 17 mm Hg and a left atrial mean pressure of 13 mm Hg. This did not change significantly with balloon occlusion of the lateral tunnel fenestration. There were no venovenous collaterals. The treating cardiologist opted not to close the fenestration.

Several years later, further cardiac catheterization revealed satisfactory Fontan circulation hemodynamics with mean pressures in the IVC, Fontan tract, SVC, and branch pulmonary arteries all reading 15 mm Hg. The fenestration in the Fontan pathway remained patent.

At age 14, she returned for routine clinical follow-up.

***Comments:*** Infants with hypoplastic left heart syndrome (HLHS) are usually normal in appearance at birth. Symptoms are commonly noted after 24 to 48 hours but may appear in an hour or two in response to ductus arteriosus constriction, as the circulation is duct-dependent.

Clinical features in the early neonatal period are influenced by the severity of obstruction at the foramen ovale. Babies with severe obstruction of the foramen ovale usually have severe early symptoms with severe cyanosis and metabolic acidosis. Usually there is no initial significant respiratory distress, but tachypnea and dyspnea may develop. With severe hypoxemia and metabolic acidosis, hypoglycemia and hypocalcaemia can occur.

In HLHS, constriction of the arterial duct leads to reduced tissue perfusion with anaerobic metabolism and oliguria. In the presence of moderate restriction of the foramen ovale, pulmonary edema develops progressively as pulmonary vascular resistance falls. Constriction of the ductus arteriosus in this setting will dramatically decrease systemic perfusion and increase pulmonary blood flow further aggravating pulmonary edema. If there is evidence of constriction of the arterial duct, prostaglandin E1 is indicated to maintain duct patency and to increase systemic blood flow and perfusion.

Norwood and his colleagues achieved the initial surgical palliation of HLHS.[1] This first operation is usually performed within the first week of life. The procedure involves transection of the pulmonary trunk proximal to its bifurcation and its anastomosis to the hypoplastic ascending aorta, incorporating a patch of homograft material to augment the ascending aorta, arch, and distal aorta. An atrial septectomy is performed, and a Blalock-Taussig shunt constructed (see Fig. 68-6).

Recent data from Toronto demonstrated consistent improvement in the mortality rate for first-stage surgery from 1990 through 2000. For the period 1998–2000, the mortality rate was 19%, lower than the 59% mortality for the period 1990–1993.[2]

Risk factors for poor outcome from a Norwood procedure include low birth weight, diminutive ascending aorta, atresia of both aortic and mitral valves, severe extracardiac anomalies, poor preoperative clinical status, Turner syndrome, RV dysfunction, and older age at the time of first palliation.[3] Factors contributing to perioperative morbidity and mortality are recurrent obstruction of the aortic arch (11%–37% incidence), acute shunt thrombosis, and tricuspid valve regurgitation.[4,5]

During the stage II bidirectional cavopulmonary anastomosis the SVC is divided and its cranial end is anastomosed to an incision in the superior aspect of right pulmonary artery. The cardiac end of the SVC is oversewn. This operation is usually performed at the age of 3 to 6 months. It facilitates ventricular volume unloading as well as promoting regression of the ventricular mass and reducing any atrioventricular valve regurgitation.[6]

Risk factors identified with early mortality in patients having the stage II bidirectional cavopulmonary shunt include younger age at the time of surgery (<2 months), mean pulmonary artery pressure more than 18 mm Hg, abnormal pulmonary venous connection, heterotaxy, and severe atrioventricular valve regurgitation.

There is no unanimous agreement as to the optimum age for stage III Fontan surgery but it is usually performed between 4 and 6 years in HLHS. This surgery may carry more risk in the adult and in the infant, although it can be carried out in children as young as 2 years and in adults with potentially excellent results.[7-9] In patients younger than 10 years there is a favorable decrease in ventricular dimensions, volumes, and wall stress after Fontan-type surgery as compared to those undergoing the surgery after age 10 years.[10]

Fenestration in the Fontan tract results in lower superior and IVC and RA pressures and an improved cardiac output, at the expense of usually mild desaturation. It may also reduce the severity and duration of postoperative pleural effusions.[11]

Thromboembolic events have been well documented both acutely and late after Fontan surgery. Varma and colleagues demonstrated clinically silent pulmonary emboli in 17% of an adult population with Fontan surgery.[12] Rosenthal and colleagues documented an overall rate of 3.9 per 100 patient years of thromboembolic events with a time from Fontan operation to the thrombotic event of 6.1 ± 5 years.[13]

## CURRENT SYMPTOMS

The patient denies any symptoms. She participates in all her desired daily activities without restriction, and denies chest pains or palpitations.

NYHA class: I

## CURRENT MEDICATIONS

Warfarin 5 mg daily

Lisinopril 5 mg daily

***Comments:*** ACE inhibitors such as lisinopril are not established therapy in patients with Fontan procedures. There are no clinical trial data to suggest they are effective in protecting ventricular function or preserving favorable ventricular shape, but they are often used on clinical grounds.

## PHYSICAL EXAMINATION

BP 98/68 mm Hg, HR 75 bpm, oxygen saturation 92%, falling to 82% on exertion

Height 144 cm, weight 43 kg, BSA 1.31 m$^2$

Surgical scars: Midline sternotomy scar

Neck veins: Hard to evaluate and a waveform not seen

Lungs/chest: Clear to auscultation

Heart: Rhythm was regular, there was a normal S1, a single S2, and no murmur.

Abdomen: Liver edge palpable

Extremities: Normal without edema, skin was warm

***Comments:*** This physical exam is favorable for a Fontan patient. A saturation of 90% to 95% on room air is typical, dropping on exercise. The absence of edema argues against both heart failure and PLE. The absence of a murmur is as expected, and argues against substantial AV valve regurgitation.

## LABORATORY DATA

| | | |
|---|---|---|
| Hemoglobin | **15.4 g/dL** | (11.5–15.0) |
| Hematocrit/PCV | 45% | (36–46) |
| MCV | 86 fL | (83–99) |
| Platelet count | $203 \times 10^9$/L | (150–400) |
| Sodium | 140 mmol/L | (134–145) |
| Potassium | 4 mmol/L | (3.5–5.2) |
| Creatinine | 0.8 mg/dL | (0.6–1.2) |
| Blood urea nitrogen | 4 mmol/L | (2.5–6.5) |

***Comments:*** Mild degree of erythrocytosis may relate to the mild desaturation at rest (due to the fenestration) that is exacerbated with exercise.

## ELECTROCARDIOGRAM

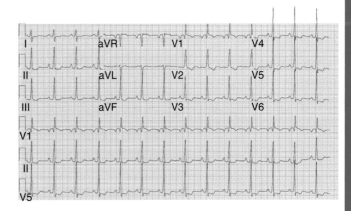

Figure 68-1 Electrocardiogram.

## FINDINGS

Heart rate: 83 bpm

QRS axis: +91°

QRS duration: 102 msec

Normal sinus rhythm. Incomplete RBBB, RV hypertrophy, non-specific ST-T wave abnormalities.

***Comments:*** RV hypertrophy is present. The prominent R-waves in the left precordial leads are hard to explain since the LV is hypoplastic. It should be remembered that the RV occupies a dominant portion of the left hemithorax; hence much of the depolarization represented by these leads is still right ventricular.

## CHEST X-RAY

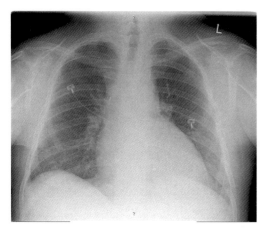

Figure 68-2 Anteroposterior projection.

## FINDINGS

Cardiothoracic ratio: 56%

The cardiac silhouette is enlarged, with pulmonary vasculature appearance within normal limits. A clip reflects takedown of the BT shunt. Sternotomy wires are present.

***Comments:*** CXR following the classical Fontan procedure usually demonstrates a normal or mildly enlarged cardiac silhouette. The presence of significant cardiomegaly may reflect severe enlargement of the RA after an atriopulmonary Fontan procedure, significant AV valve regurgitation, or ventricular dysfunction (see Cases 61 and 62).

## EXERCISE TESTING

Not indicated

## ECHOCARDIOGRAM

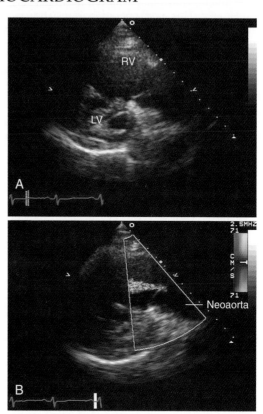

Figure 68-3 Parasternal long-axis view.

## FINDINGS

There was a hypoplastic LV located posteriorly. The RV was enlarged (*A*). There was mild regurgitation of the neoaortic valve (*B*).

***Comments:*** The hypoplastic LV is clearly visible. Function of the systemic RV can be difficult to gauge in this view.

The term neoaortic valve refers to the native pulmonary valve now functioning as the aortic valve after the Norwood palliation. Mild dysfunction of this valve is common.

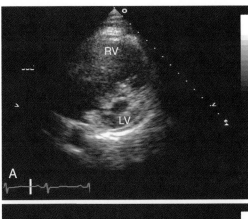

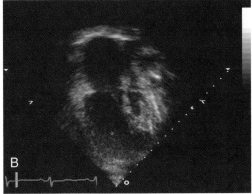

Figure 68-4 Short-axis view (**A**), apical four-chamber view (**B**).

## FINDINGS

The RV was severely enlarged, with a small, hypoplastic LV.

***Comments:*** There is still visible function of the hypoplastic LV. This can be seen when there is residual filling and emptying from the mitral and native aortic valves or a VSD. In contrast, the RV is significantly enlarged.

## CATHETERIZATION

### HEMODYNAMICS

Heart rate    78 bpm

|  | Pressure | Saturation (%) |
|---|---|---|
| SVC | mean 15 | 72 |
| IVC |  | 75 |
| RA | mean 15 | 72 |
| PA | mean 15 | 72 |
| PCWP | mean 12 |  |
| LA | mean 12 | 94 |
| RV (systemic) | 98/12 | 92 |
| Aorta | 95/69 mean 75 | 92 |

**Calculations**

| | |
|---|---|
| Qp (L/min) | 2.93 |
| Qs (L/min) | 3.95 |
| Cardiac index (L/min/m$^2$) | 3.01 |
| Qp/Qs | 0.74 |
| PVR (Wood units) | 1.03 |
| SVR (Wood units) | 15.18 |

This was undertaken to assess the hemodynamics and to consider the need for fenestration closure, because although her resting arterial oxygen saturation was 92%, she desaturated on exercise and had marginally elevated hemoglobin, reflecting hypoxia.

## FINDINGS

The pressures within her Fontan circuit show a mean of 15 mm Hg with no evidence of obstruction. The transpulmonary gradient is 3 mm Hg.

***Comments:*** Her LV end-diastolic pressure and LA pressures are higher than ideal, but acceptable. These are good Fontan hemodynamics, with a small right-to-left shunt.

The fenestration may not be the only source of cyanosis, and the angiogram should exclude the presence of venovenous collaterals or fistulae.

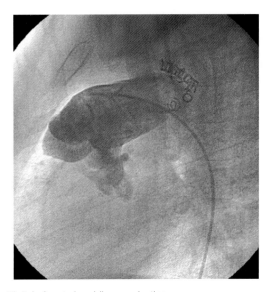

Figure 68-5 Left anterior oblique projection.

## FINDINGS

The aortic arch was mildly dilated. The native aortic valve was visible below the neoaortic valve. There was mild regurgitation of the neoaortic valve. There was no arch obstruction.

***Comments:*** Mild enlargement of the neoaorta is not uncommon in Norwood patients.

The native aortic valve, arising from the hypoplastic LV, can be seen opening and closing on cine imaging because there is still mild residual flow from the hypoplastic LV.

Coils are visible. This image was taken after coiling of aortopulmonary collaterals. These constitute a left-to-right shunt and impose a disadvantageous volume load on the systemic RV. Therefore, they are often coil occluded.

### FOCUSED CLINICAL QUESTIONS AND DISCUSSION POINTS

1. **What is the morphologic spectrum of HLHS?**

   *The concept of "hypoplastic aortic tract complex" was first introduced by Dr. Maurice Lev in 1952. This described a group of congenital cardiac lesions with severe aortic stenosis or aortic atresia, severe stenosis or atresia of the mitral valve, and hypoplastic ascending aorta associated with a small LV.*

   *Noonan and Nadas recognized these patients' clinical presentation with severe cardiac failure and inadequate systemic perfu-*

sion akin to infants with aortic isthmus atresia or interruption and suggested the term hypoplastic left heart syndrome.[14] Others subsequently unified the following features: (1) aortic stenosis or atresia, (2) mitral stenosis or atresia, (3) varying degrees of left ventricular hypoplasia, (4) patent foramen ovale or less commonly intact atrial septum, (5) patent ductus arteriosus, and (6) LV endocardial sclerosis.

## 2. What are the stages of the Norwood palliation procedure?

### Stage I Palliation
*An atrial septectomy is performed to allow pulmonary venous blood to reach the RV. The pulmonary arterial trunk is disconnected from the pulmonary arteries and the arterial duct is ligated. The diminutive ascending aorta is opened and anastomosed to the main pulmonary artery (Damus-Kaye-Stansel procedure) and enlarged with a homograft patch. Thus the RV, which now receives pulmonary and systemic venous blood, ejects via the pulmonary valve into the newly formed aorta. The sole source of pulmonary blood supply is via a Blalock-Taussig shunt.*

*The Sano modification of the stage I procedure, in which a right ventricle to pulmonary artery conduit is placed instead of the BT shunt, may result in improved hemodynamics.*

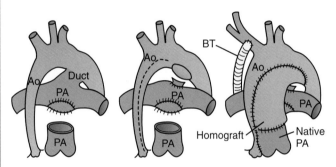

Figure 68-6 Stage I palliation. Ao, ascending aorta; PA, pulmonary artery.

### Stage II Palliation
*As the child grows she will outgrow the BT shunt and become increasingly cyanosed. At this age, usually around 4 to 5 months, the pulmonary vascular resistance should have fallen sufficiently to allow a venous shunt. The BT is ligated, and a bidirectional Glenn (cavopulmonary shunt) is performed.*

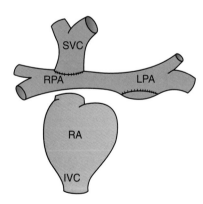

Figure 68-7 Stage II palliation.

### Stage III Palliation
*Completion of the Fontan operation is usually performed at 4 to 6 years of age.*

*A total cavopulmonary connection is performed, either as an extracardiac total cavopulmonary connection or a lateral tunnel procedure, bringing IVC flow directly to the pulmonary arteries.*

*The left pulmonary artery may need reconstruction because of trapping between the left main bronchus and the neoaorta.*

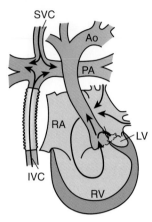

Figure 68-8 Stage III palliation. Total cavopulmonary circulation is achieved by connecting the inferior vena cava with the pulmonary artery via either a lateral tunnel or an extracardiac conduit (shown here). Ao, neoaorta.

## 3. What specific clinical issues should clinicians expect to encounter during the follow-up of young adults with Fontan-type palliation of HLHS?

*These patients face the well-known long-term complications of Fontan circulation. These include atrial enlargement, atrial arrhythmias, thromboembolic events, hepatic dysfunction, PLE, worsening cyanosis, myocardial dysfunction and failure, systemic outflow tract obstruction, obstruction to pulmonary veins, plastic bronchitis, and adverse neurodevelopmental outcome.*

*There are additional potential complications related specifically to the Norwood palliation. These are illustrated in Figure 68-8 and are as follows: (1) recoarctation of the aorta, (2) left pulmonary artery stenosis, (3) restriction of interatrial communication, (4) possible ischemia from diminutive coronary arteries, (5) systemic RV dysfunction, and (6) tricuspid valve regurgitation.*

### Potential Complications in the Norwood Procedure

| | |
|---|---|
| Coarctation and arch repair site: | recoarctation |
| Left pulmonary artery: | stenosis |
| Atrial septal defect: | restrictive |
| Coronary arteries arising from hypoplastic ascending aorta: | ischemia |
| Systemic RV: | function |
| Tricuspid valve: | regurgitation |

## 4. What routine investigations should be performed in the follow-up of young adults who are palliated for HLHS?

*Survivors of the Norwood palliation strategy are just now reaching adulthood, and little is known about their long-term clinical risks and how these patients should best be followed. A rational clinical follow-up should include the following:*
1. *ECG to document any arrhythmia, ischemia, or other abnormalities including pre-excitation.*
2. *CXR to document cardiothoracic ratio, look for any evidence of aortic coarctation, pulmonary venous congestion, pulmonary embolism or infarction, pleural effusion, and scoliosis.*
3. *TTE to assess ventricular function including segmental wall motion, the degree of RV hypertrophy, AV valve regurgitation and its degree; atrial size, pulmonary venous obstruction; restriction of the interatrial communication; ventricular outflow obstruction; neoaortic valve function; IVC and SVC*

flow, thrombus in the systemic venous circuit; patency of and gradient across the fenestration; and aortic arch coarctation.

4. *MRI:* This is a very useful modality in experienced hands to obtain complementary information on ventricular function as well as the other issues listed above. MRI is also particularly helpful in demonstrating anatomic details of those structures, some of which cannot be reliably assessed by standard echocardiography, such as aortic arch repair and left pulmonary artery stenosis.

5. *Functional assessment:* There is a paucity of data as to whether these patients are likely to suffer from coronary ischemia, even subclinically. Considering that the coronary arteries originate from a diminutive ascending aorta, stress testing may be warranted, and coronary angiography should be performed if there is any evidence of myocardial ischemia.

5. **What should the patient be advised regarding exercise, contraception, and future pregnancy?**

*Moderate cardiovascular exercise is reasonable and should be encouraged not only for improved cardiovascular fitness but for overall well-being.*

*There is very little experience about contraception and pregnancy in Norwood patients, although the general understanding about Fontan patients should apply. Such strategies have been discussed elsewhere. Generally, estrogen is thrombogenic and may be contraindicated even when patients are on warfarin (consensus view, not evidence-based), whereas certain progestogen-only pills (such as Cerazette, available in the UK, but not in the United States) are safe. The Mirena coil is effective, but care must be taken at insertion to avoid vasovagal syncope and cardiovascular collapse. Amenorrhea may be an added benefit, particularly when menorrhagia is worsened by anticoagulation. Implanon is a single-rod, nonbiodegradable implantable contraceptive that contains the progestin etonogestrel and is highly effective.*

*Pregnancy outcome in HLHS patients with Fontan-type circulation is not known. The risk from pregnancy is likely to be dependent on how good the prepregnancy hemodynamics are (i.e., good RV function with no significant tricuspid regurgitation and no ischemia, aortic, or Fontan circuit obstruction or arrhythmias). One may anticipate morbidity from deteriorating ventricular function and atrial arrhythmias in some patients.*

*Cannobio and colleagues reported on 33 pregnancies after the Fontan operation. There were 15 (45%) live births, 13 spontaneous abortions, and 5 elective terminations. Mean gestational age of the infants was 36.5 weeks and median weight 2344 g. Thus, there was an increased risk of miscarriage and low birth weight babies. There were no cardiac complications except one patient who had supraventricular tachycardia that reverted to sinus rhythm.*[15]

## FINAL DIAGNOSIS

HLHS with Norwood palliation and a fenestrated lateral tunnel Fontan

## PLAN OF ACTION

Routine clinical follow-up

## INTERVENTION

None

## OUTCOME

The patient was educated again about her anatomy, her current clinical state, the importance of routine clinical care, and good oral hygiene. Early discussions about contraception and the impact of future pregnancy decisions were begun. She was encouraged to maintain an active lifestyle. She returned 1 year later after an uneventful year.

## Selected References

1. Norwood WI, Lang P, Castenada AR: Experience with operations for hypoplastic left heart syndrome. J Thorac Cardiovasc Surg 82:511–519, 1981.
2. Azakie A, Merklinger SL, McCrindle BW: Evolving strategies and improving outcomes of the modified Norwood procedure: A 10-year single institution experience. Ann Thorac Surg 72:1349–1353, 2001.
3. Gaynor JW, Mahle WT, Cohen MI: Risk factors for mortality after the Norwood procedure. Eur J Cardio-Thorac Surg 22:82–89, 2002.
4. Lang P, Norwood WI: Haemodynamic assessment after palliative surgery for hypoplastic left heart syndrome. Circulation 68:104–108, 1983.
5. Zellers T: Balloon angioplasty for recurrent coarctation of the aorta in patients following staged palliation for hypoplastic left heart syndrome. Am J Cardiol 84:231–233, 1999.
6. Forbes TJ, Gajarski R, Johnson GL: Influence of age on the left ventricular volume, mass and ejection fraction. J Am Coll Cardiol 28:1301–1307, 1996.
7. Freedom RM: The Fontan operation: Indications, outcome, and survival data. In Braunwald E (series ed), Freedom RM (vol ed): Atlas of Heart Diseases. Congenital Heart Diseases. Philadelphia, Mosby, 1997, pp 17-1–17-10.
8. Gentles TL, Mayer JE, Jr, Gauvreau K: Fontan operation in five hundred consecutive patients: Factors influencing early and late outcome. J Thorac Cardiovasc Surg 114:376–391, 2002.
9. Veldtman GR, Nishimoto A, Siu S: The Fontan procedure in adults. Heart 86:330–335, 2001.
10. Sluysmans T, Sanders SP, van der Velde M: Natural history and patterns of recovery of contractile function in single left ventricle after Fontan operation. Circulation 86:1753–1756, 1992.
11. Senaki H, Masutani S, Kobayashi J: Ventricular afterload and ventricular work in Fontan circulation: Comparison with normal two-ventricle circulation and single-ventricle circulation with Blalock-Taussig shunts. Circulation 105:2885–2892, 2002.
12. Varma C, Warr MR, Hendler AI: Prevalence of "silent" pulmonary emboli in adults after the Fontan operation. J Am Coll Cardiol 41:2252–2258, 2003.
13. Rosenthal DN, Friedman AH, Kleinman CS: Thromboembolic complications after Fontan operations. Circulation 92(Suppl 9):II287–II293, 1995.
14. Noonen JA, Nadas AS: The hypoplastic left heart syndrome: An analysis of 101 cases. Pediatr Clin North Am 5:1029–1056, 1958.
15. Canobbio MM, Mair DD, van der Velde M, Koos BJ: Pregnancy outcomes after the Fontan repair. J Am Coll Cardiol 28:763–767, 1996.

Case 69

# Complications of Ventricular Septation in a Patient with a Single Ventricle

**Masahiro Koh, Toshikatsu Yagihara, and Hideki Uemura**

**Age: 17 years**
**Gender: Male**
**Occupation: High school student**
**Working diagnosis: Double-inlet left ventricle**

## HISTORY

Soon after birth, the patient developed heart failure and was diagnosed with double-inlet LV with ventriculoarterial discordance (transposition). Heart failure was due to volume overload from increased pulmonary flow. He was treated medically until he underwent banding of the pulmonary trunk at the age of 1 year. When he was 10 years old, he was referred for further surgical treatment. His mean pulmonary arterial pressure was 37 mm Hg with a Qp/Qs value of 1.58, so Fontan repair was not an option. Eventually, ventricular septation was chosen as a definitive repair and was performed uneventfully.

While he did reasonably well for some time on diuretics with supplemental albumin infusions and afterload reduction therapy, his physical abilities gradually became more limited. He developed dependent edema. At age 17, he developed severe edema. Echocardiography showed progressive and severe regurgitation across the right-sided AV valve.

In addition to having edema and ascites, the patient had mild diarrhea. Hypoalbuminemia was detected, and an intestinal scintigram revealed the evidence of gastrointestinal protein loss. He was diagnosed as having PLE. Several treatment options were employed with little alleviation of his symptoms.

He had repeated hospitalizations for treatment of congestive failure, and had quite severe exercise intolerance. He was reinvestigated in anticipation of further discussion about potential interventions.

**Comments:** In hearts with double-inlet LV, both the left-sided and the right-sided AV valves insert to the morphologically left and dominant ventricle. The morphologic RV is usually small and incomplete, lacking its inlet portion.

There are two types of double-inlet LV. The more common type, with the aorta arising anteriorly from the hypoplastic RV and the pulmonary trunk arising from the dominant LV (ventriculoarterial discordance), was present in this patient. This is often designated as [S, L, L] type according to Van Praagh's classification. Without pulmonary stenosis (or banding), pulmonary vascular resistance will become too high to allow for Fontan correction. The alternative arrangement, in which the aorta arises from the dominant LV and the pulmonary trunk arises from the hypoplastic RV (ventriculoarterial concordance), is known as Holmes heart.

Ventricular septation, an uncommon procedure, involves the creation of a ventricular septum using a patch. Heart block is common because the course of the conduction bundles is very close to the intended suture line for attaching the patch. To minimize this probability, the surgeon may omit placing a deep stitch at the likely crossing point of the conduction axis, though this may result in a small residual baffle leak and left-to-right shunt. Such was the case in this patient, as seen later at catheterization.

The dominant LV was dilated (240% of a normal LV). The inlet valves had separate orifices with no tendinous cords shared. If the ventricular volume was smaller than 200% of normal, or if the inlet valves had some of the tension apparatus shared or had a common orifice, ventricular septation would not have been elected.

PLE is known to occur when right heart function is severely impaired and when systemic venous pressure remains chronically high.[1] The lymphatic drainage system of the intestine is congested. This problem is encountered most frequently in Fontan patients (see Case 62).[2,3] For quantitative evaluation of PLE, alpha-1-antitrypsin measurement in the stool is the test of choice.

In double-inlet LV, the AV valves are often structurally abnormal. In some hearts, both of the inlet valves have two leaflets, and, in others, they are bilaterally trifoliate. Either valve can be regurgitant.

## CURRENT SYMPTOMS

The patient was severely restricted by dyspnea in performing his usual activities. He became breathless walking up one flight of steps and often had to stop half way. Frequent hospitalizations were interrupting his school work. He did not have palpitations, dizziness, lightheadedness, or chest pain.

NYHA class: III

# CURRENT MEDICATIONS

Enalapril 2.5 mg daily

Furosemide 80 mg daily

Spironolactone 150 mg daily

Potassium L-aspartate 1800 mg daily

Digoxin 0.2 mg daily

Chlorthiazide 2 mg daily

Denopamine 20 mg daily

Coenzyme Q10, 30 mg daily

**Comments:** Denopamine is a partial beta-1 agonist developed and tried in Japan. Its sympathomimetic action has been used for the treatment of coronary vasospasm and heart failure.[4]

# PHYSICAL EXAMINATION

BP 100/70 mm Hg, HR 85 bpm, regular rhythm, oxygen saturation 97%

Height 155 cm, weight 45 kg, BSA 1.39 m$^2$

Neck veins: Jugular veins could not be assessed.

Lungs/chest: Sounds were clear with no rales.

Heart: There was a 3/6 pan-systolic murmur at the fourth left intercostal space.

Abdomen: Abdomen was soft and flat, mild hepatomegaly.

Extremities: Lower extremities were edematous to the shins.

**Comments:** We expected the JVP to be elevated, but could not confirm this. Absence of a large V-wave may not necessarily exclude right AV valve regurgitation if the atrium is large and extremely compliant. The murmur was likely due to right or perhaps left AV valve regurgitation, or could represent residual left-to-right shunt through a leak in the VSD patch.

# LABORATORY DATA

| | |
|---|---|
| WBC | 5.34 μ10$^3$/μL (4.0–9.0) |
| Hemoglobin | 14.9 g/dL (13.0–17.0) |
| Hematocrit/PCV | 44.0% (41–51) |
| Platelet count | 246 x 10$^9$/L (150–350) |
| Sodium | **135 mmol/L** (138–145) |
| Potassium | 3.6 mmol/L (3.4–4.9) |
| Creatinine | **0.4 mg/dL** (0.7–1.3) |
| Blood urea nitrogen | 11 mg/dL (6–24) |
| Total protein | **4.4 g/dL** (6.5–8.2) |
| Albumin | **2.7 g/dL** (3.6–5.5) |
| Globulin | **1.7 g/dL** (2.0–3.0) |
| A/G | 1.6 (1.3–2.5) |
| Total bilirubin | 0.5 mg/dL (0.2–1.2) |
| Direct bilirubin | 0.2 mg/dL (0–0.4) |
| Indirect bilirubin | 0.3 mg/dL (0.2–0.8) |
| AST | 21 U/L (0–40) |
| ALT | 23 U/L (0–35) |
| ALP | 83 U/L (32–97) |
| GTP | **101 U/L** (13–68) |
| LDH | 160 U/L (100–225) |
| Triglycerides | **208 mg/dL** (30–130) |
| HDL-cholesterol | **24 mg/dL** (40–55) |
| Uric acid | 6.1 mg/dL (3.8–8.0) |
| Ca | **8.1 mg/dL** (8.8–10.5) |
| BNP | **75.6 pg/mL** (<20.0) |

**Comments:** Many of the abnormalities present are consistent with PLE, including hypoproteinemia and hypoalbuminemia. The elevated BNP level indicates cardiac failure.

# ELECTROCARDIOGRAM

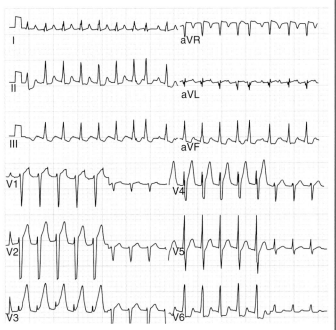

Figure 69-1 Electrocardiogram.

### FINDINGS

Heart rate: 112 bpm

QRS axis: +74°

QRS duration: 108 msec

Atrial tachycardia. Diffuse ST changes.

Holter ECG: Sinus rhythm with occasional atrial and ventricular ectopics.

**Comments:** The patient had a past history of transient atrial tachycardia recorded when he was 15 years old. Because such nonsustained arrhythmias can be recurrent and clinically silent, ambulatory ECG monitoring is often prudent. Persistent tachycardia can depress ventricular function.

# CHEST X-RAY

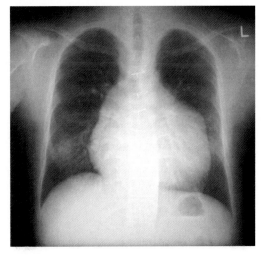

Figure 69-2 Posteroanterior projection.

## FINDINGS

Cardiothoracic ratio: 65%

Enlarged cardiac silhouette with RA enlargement, prior sternotomy, increased breast shadows bilaterally (unusual for a male).

**Comments:** Enlargement of the RA chamber is striking and fits with suspected severe right AV valve regurgitation. The left border of the cardiac silhouette is unusual; it is probably related to the abnormally located RV chamber giving rise to the anterior aorta.

Gynecomastia is suspected, which is commonly seen with long-term administration of high-dose spironolactone.

## ECHOCARDIOGRAM

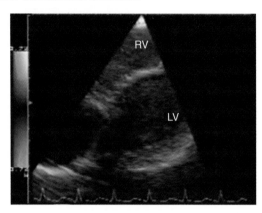

Figure 69-3  Apical four-chamber view.

## FINDINGS

The functional "left ventricular" chamber was moderately to severely dilated (67 mm) with a low fractional shortening (10%) and paradoxical movement of the prosthetic ventricular septum. The functional "right ventricular" chamber was also dilated. There was a residual VSD through the partition. Severe regurgitation of the right AV valve was seen, and the RA was extremely dilated. The IVC was engorged and did not collapse with inspiration (indicating high RA pressure).

**Comments:** Subsequent to ventricular septation for double-inlet LV, both the systemic and the pulmonary ventricular chambers are composed of morphologically LV mass, because the very small morphologically RV does not have functional value in this patient. Therefore, the terms LV and RV do not accord with their true morphologic meanings after ventricular septation.

The ventricular septum (visible here) is made of noncontractile prosthetic material. During systole, the artificial ventricular septum, which is noncontractile, bulges toward the pulmonary ventricular chamber as LV pressure rises, and appears to move paradoxically by echocardiography, thus contributing to the low fractional shortening of the systemic ventricle. In contrast, shortening of the pulmonary ventricular chamber is exaggerated because of the motion of the artificial septum. Considering this peculiar motion of the artificial septum, the surgeon will typically place the partition such that the systemic ventricular chamber is larger than the pulmonary chamber, and hence the

echocardiographic measurements are not necessarily indicative of pathology.

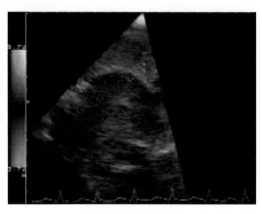

Figure 69-4  Parasternal short-axis view.

## FINDINGS

A large regurgitant jet appeared through a gap between the anterior leaflet and the septal leaflet of the right-sided AV valve.

**Comments:** In this view, the septum has a slightly different configuration but again is thin and echogenic because it is composed of synthetic material. The right AV valve jet can be seen at the left of the image.

## CATHETERIZATION

### HEMODYNAMICS

Heart rate    85 bpm

|  | **Pressure** | **Saturation** (%) |
|---|---|---|
| SVC | mean 8 | 70 |
| IVC |  | 70 |
| RA | mean 8 | 71 |
| RV | 29/6 |  |
| PA | 20/8 mean 13 | 78 |
| PCWP | 5 |  |
| LV | 89/4 | 98 |
| Aorta | 90/69 mean 60 | 94 |

| **Calculations** | |
|---|---|
| Qp (L/min) | 4.73 |
| Qs (L/min) | 3.94 |
| Cardiac index (L/min/m$^2$) | 2.83 |
| Qp/Qs | 1.20 |
| PVR (Wood units) | 1.69 |
| SVR (Wood units) | 13.20 |

**Comments:** Relatively low pressures in the RA and the SVC might be considered inconsistent with the diagnosis of PLE. However, note that the patient was on strict fluid restriction and diuretics, so heart failure control has been optimized.

Curiously, pulmonary arterial pressure was within the normal range, and calculated pulmonary vascular resistance was relatively low, which may make the patient a candidate for Fontan palliation. There is evidence of a small left-to-right shunt, presumed to be at the site of prior VSD patch closure.

## Ventricular Volume Quantification*

| | LV | (Normal range) | RV | (Normal range) |
|---|---|---|---|---|
| EDV (mL) | 187 | (77–195) | **87** | (88–227) |
| ESV (mL) | **113** | (19–72) | 30 | (23–103) |
| SV (mL) | 74 | (51–133) | 57 | (52–138) |
| EF (%) | **40** | (57–74) | 65 | (48–74) |
| EDVi (mL/m²) | **134** | (68–103) | **62** | (68–114) |
| ESVi (mL/m²) | **81** | (19–41) | 22 | (21–50) |
| SVi (mL/m²) | 53 | (44–68) | 41 | (40–72) |

***Comments:*** End-diastolic volumes and ejection fractions of the systemic and the pulmonary ventricular chambers calculated from angiography reflect the presence of the artificial septum, which showed noncontracting passive and paradoxical motion. The normal ranges in the table are from MRI data and are for comparison only. It is impossible to know what the normally expected volume ought to be for a septated ventricle.

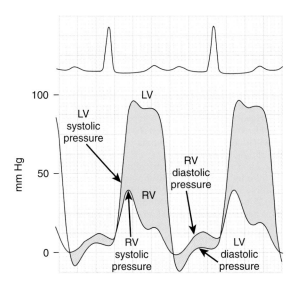

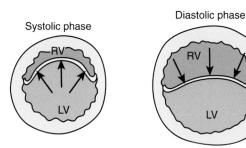

Figure 69-5 Schematic representation of pressure findings in septation.

***Comments:*** Because the septum is nonfunctional and thin, its motion is entirely dependent on the relative pressure difference between the RV and LV throughout the cardiac cycle. Thus, as the pressure rises in the LV during systole, the septum will deviate toward the RV. In diastole, if RV pressure is higher than LV pressure, as in this case, the septum will deviate toward the LV.

## FOCUSED CLINICAL QUESTIONS AND DISCUSSION POINTS

1. **What is the etiology of the patient's symptoms?**

   *The principal problem in this particular patient is PLE, which began just 18 months after ventricular septation and has been insidiously progressive over the following 7 years. PLE is believed to be related to chronic hepatic engorgement from elevated central venous pressure as occurs in Fontan patients, and is unusual in a patient with two ventricles. The pathogenesis of PLE is complex (see Case 62), and the mechanism in this patient is not clear.*

   *Progressive regurgitation across the right-sided AV valve is the most likely cause of symptomatic right heart failure in this patient. It is recognized as one of the most common sequelae of ventricular septation. Although the right-sided valve is under lower pressure than the left, it is much more frequently affected. One potential rationale is the abnormal architecture of the inlet valves, but a more practical explanation relates to the artificial septal patch. The leaflet adjacent to the patch is liable to adhere to the patch. If the leaflet becomes adherent to the patch, a considerable gap is created in the valvar orifice. This process may be noted within a year after surgery.*

2. **Should the patient undergo repair or replacement of the right AV valve?**

   *Because the pulmonary arterial pressure is not elevated, one could expect clinical improvement by correcting the hemodynamic problems, namely the AV valve regurgitation.*

   *Because of this structural distortion of the valvar leaflet, repair of the valve is probably not possible. Replacement using a mechanical valve is the most likely choice. Arguments regarding the type of valve to use in a young person are well known. Bioprostheses in young patients usually degenerate and become dysfunctional sooner than they do in older patients, though in theory their potential longevity ought to be better in the subpulmonary ventricle as compared to the systemic ventricle.*

   *Replacement of the inlet valve may produce complete AV block. Surgical complete AV block should be avoided whenever possible, as a paced rhythm, even in a DDD mode, may compromise cardiovascular function. Further, pacing leads would need to be placed through the newly inserted valve or epicardially.*

3. **Should the ventricular patch defect be closed?**

   *An additional procedure that could help somewhat is closure of the residual intraventricular shunt. If an actual hole is recognizable during surgery, closure is prudent. Nonetheless, the surgeon should again consider the risk of iatrogenic complete AV block. In double-inlet LV the conduction system typically runs a long course anterosuperiorly to the VSD. Thus, naturally progressing AV block may also occur regardless of the surgeon's intervention, and efforts to spare the conduction system may not be worthwhile.*

   *PLE in Fontan patients may be improved by the addition of a fenestration, or intracardiac communication. The residual VSD is probably not contributing importantly to the PLE. Because of our patient's 6-year history of the PLE that gradually progressed, there is a concern that the PLE could persist even after successful surgery.*

4. **Is ventricular septation favorable to Fontan circulation?**

   *Theoretically, biventricular repair is considered advantageous compared to the Fontan procedure in terms of hemodynamic features and exercise tolerance because of the presence of a pumping chamber to the pulmonary circulation. Some reports compared postoperative conditions after ventricular septation and the Fontan procedure in patients with double-inlet LV, and described that ventricular septation provided lower systemic venous pressure, larger cardiac output, and better exercise capacity.[5-8]*

*However, in the setting of severe right AV valve regurgitation, overall cardiovascular function may compare unfavorably with the Fontan circulation. In patients in whom ventricular septation is achievable, the Fontan procedure may still be the option of choice. Improvement in surgical strategy for functionally univentricular hearts together with better minimally invasive techniques has led to better outcome in the early and intermediate follow-up after the Fontan procedure. Because of this, when biventricular repair would mean extensive, high-risk surgery, some argue that the Fontan strategy is preferable.[9]*

*Another possible option is creation of a bidirectional cavopulmonary anastomosis, with the SVC anastomosed to the pulmonary arteries, or the so-called one-and-a-half ventricular physiology. Since only flow from the IVC is ejected through the right heart, the ventricle is off-loaded. This procedure would be an option in this patient because of his low pulmonary vascular resistance. However, this option remains controversial.*

*Whenever possible, most clinicians would favor a biventricular repair. Thus, in this patient, with reasonable RV function, we decided to first restore competency of the right-sided AV valve and reevaluate.*

## FINAL DIAGNOSIS

Right heart failure after ventricular septation for double-inlet LV associated with tricuspid regurgitation and residual interventricular shunt

Protein-losing enteropathy

## PLAN OF ACTION

Replacement of the right-sided AV valve

Closure of the residual VSD

## INTERVENTION

Tricuspid valve replacement using a St. Jude 31-mm valve, closure of residual interventricular communication, and plication of the dilated RA

## OUTCOME

The patient tolerated the surgical procedure well, and his postoperative course was uneventful. He remained in regular sinus rhythm in follow-up. The prosthesis implanted was functioning well on stable anticoagulation with warfarin. No residual interventricular shunt was detected on follow-up echocardiography. AV conduction was intact.

Hypoalbuminemia improved considerably. He was eventually weaned off strict restriction of water intake and resumed his daily activity. Serum total protein level was 7.0 mg/dL 2 years after the surgery.

## Selected References

1. Davidson JD, Waldmann TA, Goodman DS, Gordon RS: Protein-losing enteropathy in congestive heart failure. Lancet 1:899, 1961.
2. Mertens L, Hagler DJ, Sauer U, et al: Protein-losing enteropathy after the Fontan operation: An international multicenter study. J Thorac Cardiovasc Surg 115:1063–1073, 1998.
3. Thorne SA, Hooper J, Kemp M, Somerville J: Gastro-intestinal protein loss in late survivors of Fontan surgery and other congenital heart disease. Eur Heart J 19:814–820, 1998.
4. Nishio R, Matsumori A, Shioi T, et al: Denopamine, a beta 1-adrenergic agonist, prolongs survival in a murine model of congestive heart failure induced by viral myocarditis: Suppression of tumor necrosis factor-alpha production in the heart. J Am Coll Cardiol 32:808–815, 1998.
5. Kurosawa H, Imai Y, Fukuchi S, et al: Septation and Fontan repair of univentricular atrioventricular connection. J Thorac Cardiovasc Surg 99:314–319, 1990.
6. Ohuchi H, Arakaki Y, Yagihara T, Kamiya T: Cardiopulmonary responses to exercise after repair of univentricular heart. Int J Cardiol 58:17–30, 1997.
7. Uemura H, Yagihara T: Ventricular septation in patients with double inlet left ventricle. In Redington AN, Brawn WJ, Deanfield JE, Anderson RH (eds): The Right Heart in Congenital Heart Disease. London, Greenwich Medical Media, 1998, pp 163–167.
8. Koh M, Yagihara T, Uemura H, et al: Biventricular repair for right atrial isomerism. Ann Thorac Surg 11:1806–1816, 2006.
9. Delius RE, Rademecker MA, de Leval MR, et al: Is a high-risk biventricular repair always preferable to conversion to a single ventricle repair? J Thorac Cardiovasc Surg 112:1561–1569, 1996.

# Fever in a Patient with a Single Ventricle

**Ed Nicol**

**Age: 45 years**
**Gender: Male**
**Occupation: Sound engineer**
**Working diagnosis: Univentricular heart with pulmonary stenosis**

## HISTORY

The patient presented to his local hospital at the age of 9 years with mild cyanosis and dyspnea and an inability to keep up with his peers. The initial diagnosis was that of a large VSD, but subsequent cardiac catheterization at age 22 ultimately showed dextrocardia, functionally univentricular LV with a large VSD and a rudimentary RV, ventriculoarterial discordance, and subvalvar and valvar pulmonary stenosis.

He underwent a classic right BT shunt soon after his cardiac catheterization to enhance his pulmonary blood flow. Following surgery he was initially hemodynamically stable and less cyanosed with an improved exercise capacity. Two years after the BT shunt, at age 24, he developed paroxysmal atrial tachycardias, predominantly atrial fibrillation, but also atrial flutter (intra-atrial reentry tachycardia). Cardiac catheterization at the time showed mild pulmonary arterial hypertension with a mean pulmonary pressure of 25 mm Hg and high pulmonary blood flow. His ECG showed left atrial overload reflecting his increased pulmonary blood flow. He was treated with verapamil and digoxin, which controlled his symptomatic tachycardia until the age of 41.

The patient eventually developed persistent atrial fibrillation, and despite increased antiarrhythmic therapy and anticoagulation he was admitted in gross cardiac failure secondary to uncontrolled atrial fibrillation. A transthoracic echocardiogram showed a large RA thrombus and moderate pulmonary hypertension with impaired systemic ventricular function. Due to his ongoing hemodynamic instability he was direct current (DC) cardioverted despite the thrombus in his atrium. He experienced a systemic thromboembolic event (a transient ischemic episode, presenting with pins and needles in the left limbs and left side of his face). He was subsequently switched from verapamil to amiodarone (due to concern over his LV function) and had his dose of warfarin increased prior to being discharged. However, unfortunately, within a month he was readmitted with a gastrointestinal bleed secondary to a gastric ulcer after some alcoholic birthday celebrations.

**Comments:** The classic BT shunt was the first palliative procedure developed for blue babies and aimed to increase pulmonary blood flow if pulmonary atresia or stenosis was present.[1] It involved the end-to-side anastomosis of the subclavian artery to the ipsilateral pulmonary artery.

Fontan-type operations were developed for patients with a functional "univentricular" heart to direct the systemic venous blood to the pulmonary arteries without the interposition of a subpulmonary ventricle. These operations therefore led to normalization in oxygen saturation at the cost of nonpulsatile pulmonary blood flow and elevated central venous pressure. The original Fontan operation consisted of the interposition of a valved conduit between the RA and the main pulmonary artery[2] and has been modified many times since. Pulmonary arterial hypertension, even mild, is an absolute contraindication to any Fontan procedure, as blood must be able to flow through the pulmonary vasculature driven only by the systemic venous pressure.

Due to the presence of pulmonary arterial hypertension the patient was not considered suitable for a Fontan procedure. Although he remained well on follow-up, a routine CMR scan showed aneurysms at both ends of the BT shunt, that is, just above the right pulmonary artery and at the origin of the right subclavian artery anastomosis. Hypotensive therapy was therefore commenced to reduce the risk of further aneurysmal dilatation. Subsequent MRI scans over the following few years showed no further dilatation of the conduit aneurysm, and the atrial tachycardias remained quiescent. The patient complained of occasional intermittent palpitations but had no limitation of his exercise capacity or impact on his work, which involved long hours and much heavy lifting.

## CURRENT SYMPTOMS

Dry cough, night sweats, and rigors were his predominant symptoms. Intermittent muscular chest pain was noted. He experienced diarrhea intermittently for several weeks. He felt himself slowing down at work and was increasingly tired on minimal exertion.

NYHA class: II

**Comments:** The history of this combination of symptoms, though somewhat vague and nonspecific in some respects, should alert the clinician to the possibility of a significant systemic illness such as infective endocarditis. Given the aneurysmal nature of the anastomotic graft sites and the likelihood of altered and turbulent flow this would represent a natural nidus for infection, as would the original stenotic native pulmonary valve.

# CURRENT MEDICATIONS

Furosemide 80 mg daily

Digoxin 250 µg daily

Amiodarone 200 mg daily

Perindopril 2 mg daily

Thyroxine 100 µg daily

Omeprazole 20 mg daily

Warfarin (target INR of 2–3)

# PHYSICAL EXAMINATION

BP 110/60 mm Hg, HR 58 bpm, temp 37.5° C, oxygen saturation 80% on room air

Height 165 cm, weight 64 kg, BSA 1.71 m$^2$

Surgical scars: Right thoracotomy scar

Neck veins: JVP was 4 cm above the sternal angle with normal venous waveform.

Lungs/chest: Vesicular breath sounds, no wheeze or crepitations

Heart: Regular rhythm. There was a prominent ventricular lift over the right precordium with a nondisplaced right-sided apex, grade 4 ejection systolic murmur at the upper left sternal border, and single second heart sound. In addition, a grade 3 continuous murmur could be heard over the right chest.

Abdomen: No organomegaly; soft, nontender abdomen

Extremities: Moderate clubbing and cyanosis, normal left radial and bilateral femoral pulses, but absence of a right radial pulse. There were no Janeway lesions or Roth spots identified.

***Comments:*** The lack of fever does not exclude subacute endocarditis.

The right thoracotomy scar and the lack of a right radial pulse are suggestive of a previous right BT shunt, when, in the past, the subclavian artery was transected and anastomosed end to side to the pulmonary artery. Since about 1980, a tube graft, often Gore-Tex has been used to make such a side-by-side connection between the subclavian and the ipsilateral pulmonary artery without the complete interruption of the subclavian artery. This type of shunt provided better control of the degree of additional pulmonary blood flow through the shunt and abolished the risk of pulmonary arterial hypertension (compared to the old, classic BT shunt).

The single second heart sound is indicative of the stenotic pulmonary valve. The loud ejection systolic heart murmur is consistent with turbulent flow across a severe valvar obstruction. In addition there is a loud and long heart murmur due to the turbulent flow in the aneurysmal BT shunt. Usually, such murmurs can be heard continuously in the back. The large unrestrictive VSD would not cause a murmur due to the lack of gradient from the left-to-right cardiac chambers.

# LABORATORY DATA

| | |
|---|---|
| Hemoglobin | 13.4 g/dL (13.0–17.0) |
| Hematocrit/PCV | 38% (41–51) |
| MCV | **79 fL (83–99)** |
| Platelet count | 170 × 10$^9$/L (150–400) |
| WCC | 9.0 × 10$^9$/L (3.6–9.2) |
| Neutrophils | **7.5 × 10$^9$/L (1.7–6.1)** |
| Lymphocytes | 1.1 × 10$^9$/L (1.0–3.2) |
| Sodium | **133 mmol/L (134–145)** |
| Potassium | 4.2 mmol/L (3.5–5.2) |
| Creatinine | 0.7 mg/dL (0.6–1.2) |
| Blood urea nitrogen | 3.7 mmol/L (2.5–6.5) |
| Iron | **6.7 µmol/L (12.6–26.0)** |
| Ferritin | 50 µg/L (32–284) |
| Transferrin saturation | **14% (20–45)** |

***Comments:*** The indolent nature of endocarditis is often reflected in only subtle changes in the hematologic and biochemical markers.

It is not unusual for the total white cell count to remain normal in endocarditis, as in this case. Neutrophilia and raised C-reactive protein (see below) indicate a likely bacterial infection.

The normal hemoglobin is also worrying in this case, as the patient has resting saturations of 80%. A compensatory erythrocytosis (rather than polycythemia, see Case 17) would be expected with hemoglobin levels between 18 and 20 g/dL.[3] His relative anemia is likely due to iron deficiency, although subacute endocarditis may have also been contributory; the former (iron deficiency) should be treated with oral iron supplementation or intravenous iron if the oral form is not tolerated.

## OTHER RELEVANT LAB RESULTS

| | |
|---|---|
| Bilirubin | 16 µmol/L (3–24) |
| ALP | **55 U/L (67–372)** |
| ALT | 21 IU/L (8–40) |
| Total protein | 62 g/L (62–82) |
| Albumin | **23 g/dL (37–53)** |
| CRP | **95 mg/L (0–10)** |

Blood cultures: Positive growth
Gram stain showed gram positive cocci in chains.

**Urinalysis**

| | |
|---|---|
| WBC | <10/mm$^3$ |
| RBC | >100/mm$^3$ |

***Comments:*** The low albumin level may also relate to the systemic infection, although other causes such as nephrotic syndrome and/or PLE should be excluded (the latter is exceedingly rare in patients with non–Fontan type of palliation for univentricular heart circulation).

The growth of the gram-positive cocci in blood culture samples confirms the diagnosis of endocarditis, unless an alternative source of bacteremia is unequivocally identified. Treatment with a minimum of 4 weeks of intravenous antibiotics would be prudent given the underlying anatomy. In the absence of positive blood cultures the diagnosis of endocarditis remains a clinical one and somewhat speculative, although it should be seriously considered in a patient such as ours with an underlying shunt and a severely stenotic valve with complex ACHD.

# ELECTROCARDIOGRAM

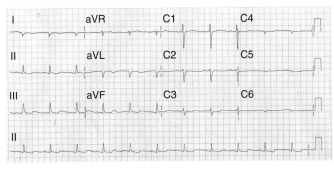

Figure 70-1 Left-sided electrocardiogram.

## FINDINGS

Heart rate: 67 bpm

PR interval: 213 msec

QRS axis: +115°

QRS duration: 100 msec

Sinus rhythm with borderline first-degree heart block. There is a dominant R-wave in lead V1. Nonspecific ST depression in the inferior leads compatible with digoxin administration. There is a right-axis deviation. Subtle bifid P-waves in the inferior leads suggest LA enlargement.

***Comments:*** The dominant R-wave in V1 is a result of this left-sided ECG being taken on a patient with dextrocardia. Note the progressively smaller electrical complexes laterally, as there is greater distance from the myocardial mass in the right thoracic cavity.

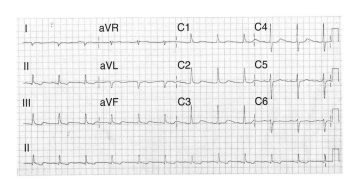

Figure 70-2 Right-sided electrocardiogram.

## FINDINGS

Heart rate: 69 bpm

PR interval: 230 msec

QRS axis: +111°

QRS duration: 104 msec

Sinus rhythm with first-degree heart block. There is a reversal of the usual R-wave progression in the anterior leads compared to the left-sided ECG. Downsloping ST depression in the inferior leads consistent with digoxin effect.

***Comments:*** With a right-sided ECG, the precordial leads are placed in mirror image positions leading to the right axillary line. The limb leads are unchanged. Hence, there will still be abnormal P-waves and right-axis deviation. Now, however, the R-wave progression can be interpreted more similarly to a patient with levocardia. Note the early (V1–3) prominent R-wave and late (V5–6) S-wave in these leads, consistent with RV hypertrophy. V1 and V2 should be reversed but are otherwise the same, which is not seen in this comparison.

# CHEST X-RAY

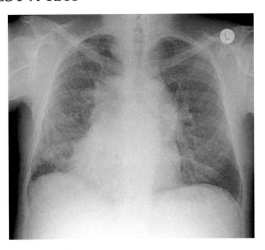

Figure 70-3 Posteroanterior projection.

## FINDINGS

Cardiothoracic ratio: 50%

Situs solitus, dextrocardia, left aortic arch. Cardiothoracic ratio at the upper limit of normal. The right superior mediastinal border has a markedly abnormal contour (possibly related to the shunt aneurysm) with dilated central pulmonary arteries. Pulmonary vascular markings within normal range (at the upper limit of normal on the right).

***Comments:*** There is no radiographic evidence of a right thoracotomy. The right BT shunt, however, was done late—at the age of 22—hence no disruption of symmetry of the ribs on the right side can be seen.

# EXERCISE TESTING

Not performed

# ECHOCARDIOGRAM

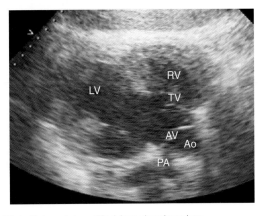

Figure 70-4. Subcostal modified four-chamber view.

## FINDINGS

Double-inlet LV, ventriculoarterial discordance (pulmonary artery arising from the LV with an anterior aorta) with a large

VSD. The aorta overrides the VSD by approximately 50%. The pulmonary valve was dysplastic and stenotic with a peak gradient of 98 mm Hg. RV and LV systolic function was normal with a large LV cavity (69 mm in diastole). No vegetations were identified on any of the four valves. There was mild left AV valve regurgitation.

***Comments:*** This off-plane subcostal view demonstrated double-inlet LV with a small rudimentary RV. Because the aortic valve overrides the VSD toward the left side, this could be classified as double-outlet LV as well, a rare combination. In contrast, double-outlet RV is more commonplace, and usually exists as a variant of transposition of the great arteries, such that there is fibrous discontinuity between the mitral valve and aortic valve, with a subpulmonary VSD.

# MAGNETIC RESONANCE IMAGING

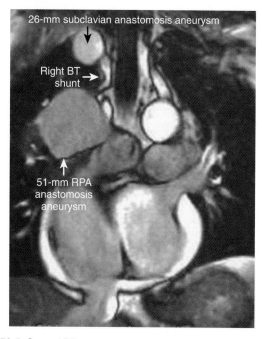

Figure 70-5 Coronal BT shunt; coronal plane steady-state free precession cine.

## FINDINGS

There was a normal functioning morphologic LV. The right BT shunt showed significant aneurysms both proximally and at the right pulmonary artery anastomosis. There was a small, native main pulmonary artery. A moderate pericardial effusion was present.

***Comments:*** Although MRI is not the test of choice for endocarditis, it can be incredibly helpful in clarifying anatomical relationships, quantifying ventricular function, and demonstrating the presence and structure of the pulmonary arteries. The aneurysms within the BT shunt seen here may be potential sites for bacterial infection. The pericardial effusion does not appear to have any hemodynamic effect, but is a notable finding in the context of infection.

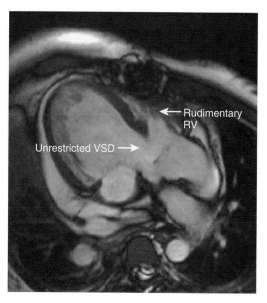

Figure 70-6 Univentricular heart; oblique axial steady-state free precession cine (four-chamber view).

## FINDINGS

The apex of the heart was toward the right. The more anterior RV was rudimentary. The LV was dilated but had normal function. Large, unrestricted VSD. Moderate pericardial effusion, especially posterior.

***Comments:*** In general, there are several features that distinguish a morphologic RV from LV. First, the RV is almost always anteriorly located (i.e., closer to the sternum), as is the case here. The RV is more heavily trabeculated, often has a large moderator band, and the tricuspid insertion is usually 10 mm or so closer to the apex than is the mitral. Though the latter three characteristics do not necessarily apply in this rudimentary ventricle with a large VSD, one can feel somewhat confident calling this the RV based on its anterior position.

Note that the tricuspid valve overrides the ventricular septum (more than 50%), thus the classification of double-inlet LV.

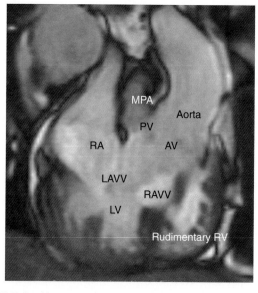

Figure 70-7 Double-outlet left ventricle; oblique coronal steady-state free precession cine.

# FINDINGS

The aorta arises anteriorly and to the left of the more posterior pulmonary artery. The peak velocity through the small pulmonary valve was 3.9 m/sec (60 mm Hg).

**Comments:** This image illustrates further the relationship of the great arteries to each other and to the two ventricles. Thus, it highlights the double-outlet LV with the anterior aorta and smaller, more posterior main pulmonary artery.

# CATHETERIZATION

Not performed

## FOCUSED CLINICAL QUESTIONS AND DISCUSSION POINTS

### 1. What is the diagnosis?

*Anatomically, the patient has a functionally univentricular heart with normal atrial arrangement, double-inlet LV, and transposed great arteries. The aorta arises anteriorly with a small main pulmonary artery arising posteriorly. There is by definition a VSD as well, since there would be no communication with an RV otherwise.*

*Placement of a BT shunt was performed in adult life to enhance pulmonary blood supply and, in turn, to improve systemic oxygenation. Subsequent cardiac catheterization showed mild PAH, making the patient unsuitable for a Fontan-type of operation. Some may argue that the catheterization should have been performed prior to the construction of the BT shunt, and, if applicable, the patient should have been considered for a staged Fontan operation on a native lesion. However, the patient was dealt with in a different era, and Fontan operation itself is no more than a palliation, associated with mid- and long-term complications, which are also more problematic in the older patient. No other reparative procedure was possible in this patient apart from transplantation.*

*Clinically, the patient has endocarditis. Though the exact site of infection is not certain, bacteremia with likely streptococcus in the setting of these symptoms should be treated for 4 to 6 weeks of antibiotics regardless of whether vegetations are found. Presumably the infection involves either the pulmonary valve or the aneurysmal BT shunt.*

### 2. What is the risk of endocarditis in congenital heart disease?

*Congenital heart disease is the substrate for infective endocarditis in 10% to 20% of cases in adults under 50 years of age.[4] PDA, VSD, and bicuspid aortic valves are all common predisposing factors.[5]*

*Generally, patients with congenital heart disease remain at risk throughout life. Furthermore, subsequent intervention is high risk. The incidence of endocarditis increases with age from 4.2 out of 100,000 patient-years (under 30) to 15 to 30 out of 100,000 patient-years (from the sixth to eighth decade). In the adult population some 55% to 75% have an underlying predisposition to endocarditis such as ACHD, rheumatic heart disease, degenerative valve disease, or intravenous drug abuse.[6] Previous cardiovascular operation, the use of foreign material, dental or other surgical procedures without recommended antibiotic prophylaxis, and cardiac catheterization all contribute to the increased incidence of endocarditis in this population.[7]*

*In adults, viridans streptococci are responsible for 45% to 65% of all cases of endocarditis but are usually of low virulence and cause a subacute clinical picture. Staphylococcus aureus is the second most prevalent bacteria, yet is often associated with a more aggressive form of acute endocarditis with rapid tissue and valve destruction.*

*Patients should be well educated about their specific risk of endocarditis, that is, they should be able to identify the possible signs and symptoms of it and know the recommended antibiotic prophylaxis, which has recently changed.[8] Even with the new guidelines, cyanotic patients are still advised to use prophylaxis. Regular dental inspection and fastidious attention to oral hygiene should be emphasized in all patients.*

### 3. What are the indications for surgical intervention in infective endocarditis?

*It has been demonstrated that a combination of appropriate antibiotic therapy and timely surgical intervention reduces mortality when compared to antibiotics alone.[9,10] Surgery is indicated to remove vegetative material, particularly with embolic potential on the "systemic" side, drain abscesses if present, remove infected synthetic material (mechanical valves or conduits), and restore compromised hemodynamics (such as valvular dysfunction or dehiscence). Large vegetations on the anterior mitral valve (particularly if > 10 mm) or increasing vegetation size despite antimicrobial therapy increases the risk of systemic embolization.[11]*

*Timing of surgery should be determined on a case-by-case basis, but the evidence suggests earlier intervention offers the greatest benefit when the embolization risk is at its greatest and other predictors of a complicated course are present.[12]*

*The prospect of surgery in this patient, with "univentricular" heart, cyanosis, and some PAH, was clearly not appealing. Though the anatomical substrate for endocarditis was present, and indeed the diagnosis was confirmed on positive blood cultures, there was no demonstrable vegetation, abscess, or hemodynamic embarrassment. Furthermore, there was no prosthetic material used during his only previous shunt operation. Without a clearly defined rationale, therefore, surgery was neither indicated nor pursued.*

### 4. What is the importance of aneurysmal dilatation of a BT shunt?

*The bulges seen in the BT shunt could be true aneurysms or potentially pseudoaneurysms, though the latter seems less likely. Such aneurysms have been very occasionally seen in the setting of a classic BT shunt, but not so in modified BT shunts. Though a risk of rupture is undoubtedly present, given the location of these aneurysms and the fragile nature of our patient, one would not pursue surgical repair of the aneurysm electively.*

# FINAL DIAGNOSIS

Dextrocardia with situs solitus

Double-inlet LV, transposition of great arteries

Severe valvar and subvalvar pulmonary stenosis

Aneurysmal BT shunt (proximally and at the right pulmonary artery anastomosis)

Acute bacterial endocarditis

Iron deficiency anemia

# PLAN OF ACTION

Hospitalization for 6 weeks of intravenous antibiotic therapy

Treatment of iron deficiency anemia

# INTERVENTION

None at present

# OUTCOME

The patient was admitted from the outpatient clinic and antibiotic treatment initiated only after multiple specimens were obtained, including several blood cultures. The isolation of *Streptococcus mitis* was subsequently made, and appropriate parenteral antibiotic therapy was given including penicillin and gentamycin. Initially, the patient felt better, and his inflammatory markers decreased.

Approximately 2 weeks into his course, his temperature climbed and his C-reactive protein doubled. TEE showed two small vegetations on the anterior pulmonary valve leaflet. Additionally, the patient was found to have moderate restrictive lung disease probably related to amiodarone therapy, but a rheumatoid factor assay of 1/5120 also raised the possibility of rheumatoid lung disease.

Despite 3 weeks of intensive parenteral antibiotic therapy the patient continued to deteriorate clinically. At a multidisciplinary meeting it was felt that surgery to replace the infected pulmonary valve was indicated. There was intense discussion relating to the need to take down the right BT shunt. Arguments for removing the BT shunt at the time of pulmonary valve surgery were that infection might have been present there also and that any expansion of the aneurysm into the right upper lobe might have made his restrictive lung disease worse. Eventually, a decision was made to proceed with removal of both the pulmonary valve and the BT shunt.

The operation was done after careful planning. At the time of surgery, there were two small nodules on the valve but no destructive endocarditis. The infected pulmonary valve was replaced with a 15-mm pulmonary homograft. A small pulmonary valve prosthesis was chosen to provide a somewhat restricted flow into the main pulmonary artery to prevent any reactive endothelial change and subsequent development of PAH.

The pulmonary anastomosis aneurysm measured 100 mm in diameter and was very thin walled. There was no macroscopic evidence of infection within the shunt. The aneurysm was dissected away with primary repair to the right pulmonary artery.

Given the increased pulmonary blood flow through the pulmonary valve prosthesis, it was felt that there was no need to create an additional source of pulmonary blood supply in the form of an arterial or venous shunt. Indeed, postoperatively the patient's oxygen saturations remained stable in the lower 80s on room air. Postoperative recovery was uneventful, and following a short stay in intensive care the patient was transferred back to the telemetry ward. Subsequent CMR images showed a patent main pulmonary artery with a small pseudoaneurysm and thrombus overlying the site of the previous BT shunt insertion.

Microbiological study of the explanted tissue showed both the native pulmonary valve and BT shunt to be infected with *S. mitis*. The hospital stay was prolonged due to episodes of paroxysmal atrial fibrillation requiring cardioversion, as well as further fevers. A prolonged course of parenteral and then oral antibiotic therapy was, nevertheless, given, and the patient was discharged home 2 months following his initial admission.

The patient has since remained well, and 1 year after his surgery he reports improved exercise tolerance with no recurrence of fevers. His resting oxygen saturations are 85% on room air, he has a long ejection systolic heart murmur of grade 4/6 intensity radiating to the back, and he is no longer iron deficient as he is on daily oral iron supplementation.[13]

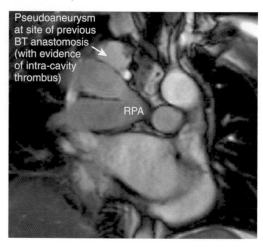

Figure 70-8 Postoperative magnetic resonance image of right pulmonary artery; oblique coronal plane steady-state free precession cine.

***Comments:*** The right BT shunt has been partially removed. There was evidence of a small pseudoaneurysm at the site of the previous BT–right pulmonary artery anastomosis and immediately above the repaired right upper lobe pulmonary artery. This remained stable in size on subsequent scans.

The pulmonary homograft was competent with no regurgitation but a peak forward velocity of 3.5 m/sec.

## Selected References

1. Blalock A, Taussig HB: Landmark article May 19, 1945: The surgical treatment of malformations of the heart in which there is pulmonary stenosis or pulmonary atresia. JAMA 251:2123–2138, 1984.
2. Fontan F, Baudet E: Surgical repair of tricuspid atresia. Thorax 26:240–248, 1971.
3. Broberg C, Jayaweera AR, Diller G, et al: The optimal relationship between resting oxygen saturation and hemoglobin in adult patients with cyanotic congenital heart disease can be determined and correlates with exercise capacity. American Heart Association Scientific Sessions, Atlanta, GA, November 2006. Circulation 114:II503, 2006.
4. Hogevik H, Olaison L, Andersson R, et al: Epidemiological aspects of infective endocarditis in an urban population: A 5-year prospective study. Medicine 74:324–339, 1995.
5. Morris CD, Reller MD, Menashe VD: Thirty-year incidence of endocarditis after surgery for congenital heart defect. JAMA 279:599–603, 1998.
6. Sandre RM, Shafran SD: Infective endocarditis: A review of 135 cases over 9 years. Clin Infect Dis 22:276–286, 1996.
7. Knirsch W, Haas NA, Uhlemann F, et al: Clinical course and complications of infective endocarditis in patients growing up with congenital heart disease. Int J Cardiol 101:285–291, 2005.
8. Wilson W, Taubert KA, Gewitz M, et al: Prevention of infective endocarditis: Guidelines from the American Heart Association. American Heart Association Rheumatic Fever, Endocarditis, and Kawasaki Disease Committee, Councils on Cardiovascular Disease in the Young, Clinical Cardiology, and Cardiovascular Surgery and Anesthesia, and the Quality of Care and Outcomes Research Interdisciplinary Working Group. Circulation 116:1736–1754, 2007. Epub 2007 Apr 19.
9. Al Jubair K, Al Fagih M, Ashmeg A, et al: Cardiac operations during active endocarditis. J Thorac Cardiovasc Surg 104:487, 1992.
10. Sexton DJ, Spelman D: Current best practices and guidelines: Assessment and management of complications in infective endocarditis. Cardiol Clin 21:273–282, 2003.

11. Baddour LM, Wilson WR, Bayer AS, et al: Diagnosis, antimicrobial therapy, and management of complications: A statement for healthcare professionals from the Committee on Rheumatic Fever, Endocarditis, and Kawasaki Disease, Council on Cardiovascular Disease in the Young, and the Councils on Clinical Cardiology, Stroke, and Cardiovascular Surgery and Anesthesia, American Heart Association. Endorsed by the Infectious Diseases Society of America. Circulation 111:e394–e434, 2005.

12. Erbel R, Rohmann S, Drexler M, et al: Improved diagnostic value of echocardiography in patients with infective endocarditis by transesophageal approach: A prospective study. Eur Heart J 9: 43–53, 1988.

13. Spence MS, Balaratnam MS, Gatzoulis MA: Clinical update: Cyanotic adult congenital heart disease. Lancet 370:1530–1532, 2007.

# Eisenmenger Syndrome

# Long-Term Survival in Eisenmenger Syndrome

**Emmeline F. Hou, George Pantely, and Victor Menashe**

**Age: 70 years**
**Gender: Female**
**Occupation: Retired bookkeeper**
**Working diagnosis: Unrepaired ventricular septal defect with Eisenmenger physiology**

## HISTORY

The patient was discovered to have a murmur in her early adult years as part of a premarriage physical, and a VSD was suspected. This led eventually to a cardiac catheterization at age 25, in 1958. The study demonstrated systemic RV pressure with a bidirectional shunt through a VSD. No repair could be offered.

After her marriage, the patient conceived at age 26. The child was delivered 2 months prematurely and significantly underweight. Growing up, this child was developmentally delayed and had many special needs. The patient had one other pregnancy resulting in a spontaneous abortion. A third pregnancy was ectopic, resulting in tubal ligation.

In addition to a tubal ligation, she has had a right pyeloplasty done for ureteropelvic obstruction secondary to trauma from a motor vehicle accident, and has undergone cataract surgery.

The patient was regularly followed over the next several decades, during which time she worked as a bookkeeper and housewife. Generally, she felt well and capable of meeting life's various demands.

She traveled whenever occasion permitted and never had difficulty with long distance air travel.

In recent years, she had intermittent palpitations, sometimes with associated dizziness. Continuous ECG monitoring documented infrequent episodes of nonsustained ventricular tachycardia. She never had a sustained arrhythmia requiring treatment. She did not experience hemoptysis or cerebrovascular events.

She noted intermittent mild hyperviscosity symptoms of headache and paresthesia of the fingers and toes. She developed flares of gout, which were treated with allopurinol. She was not treated with phlebotomy. She used supplemental oxygen of 2 L by nasal cannula chronically.

She presented for her biannual clinical review.

**Comments:** Although Victor Eisenmenger described the first case history and postmortem details of a patient with a large VSD and the pathological features of pulmonary hyper-

tension in 1897,[1] it was in the 1958 Croonian lectures by Paul Wood that Eisenmenger syndrome was finally understood and described in full as a pathophysiological concept. The term *Eisenmenger complex* came into use to describe "pulmonary hypertension at systemic level due to high pulmonary vascular resistance with reversed or bi-directional shunt," with Wood stating, "It matters very little where the shunt happens to be. The distinguishing feature is not anatomy, but the physiological behaviour of the pulmonary circulation."[2]

This patient was first evaluated just as Paul Wood's concept was being publicized, including his warning that repair of defects at this stage should not be performed. The advent of cardiopulmonary bypass around this time allowed some centers to offer correction. However, its use was not widespread.

Pregnancy in Eisenmenger syndrome is associated with substantial risk to mother and fetus. The maternal mortality rate is thought to be 30% to 50% with death usually occurring during delivery or within 1 week postpartum.[3,4] Spontaneous abortion occurs in 20% to 40% of pregnancies, premature delivery in 50%, and perinatal mortality is as high as 28%.[4,5] Most infants have intrauterine growth retardation in keeping with low maternal cardiac output and oxygen delivery during pregnancy.[4] A review of 125 pregnancies in patients with pulmonary vascular disease, of which 73 pregnancies occurred in the setting of Eisenmenger syndrome, observed a maternal mortality rate of 36% in Eisenmenger syndrome and a neonatal mortality of 13%.[6] Although pregnancy should be discouraged in women with Eisenmenger syndrome and elective abortion is advised, successful delivery has been possible under the guidance of a multidisciplinary team including cardiologists, obstetricians, anesthesiologists, and neonatologists.

In Eisenmenger patients who survive beyond the fifth decade, there is an increased likelihood for needing noncardiac surgery such as cholecystectomy. These patients have had a reported perioperative mortality rate as high as 30% with noncardiac surgery.[7] However, with modern surgical techniques, anesthesia, and monitoring, the risk of death should be substantially improved.

It is important that anesthesia for noncardiac surgery be administered by a cardiac anesthesiologist with experience in patients with Eisenmenger syndrome. A minor fall in systemic pressure can increase right-to-left shunting and potentiate cardiovascular collapse. Surgery should be performed under local anesthesia when feasible and appropriate; otherwise, anesthesia that is least likely to decrease the systemic blood pressure and vascular resistance is recommended. Although epidural anesthesia has been used successfully in minor surgeries, general anesthesia is preferred.[8,9] Prolonged fasting and volume depletion should be avoided prior to surgery, and maintenance intravenous fluids should be used appropriately. All intravenous lines should be equipped with air filters, and antibiotic prophylaxis against endocarditis should be provided, in harmony with recent guidelines.[10] Systemic arterial hypotension should be treated aggressively, and blood loss should be minimized and treated promptly with blood products. A "normal" hematocrit will not provide adequate arterial oxygenation, and a higher hematocrit must be maintained. Routine use of a pulmonary artery catheter is not necessary, but a central venous pressure catheter and an arterial line are recommended in monitoring patients.[8]

Most patients with Eisenmenger syndrome are symptomatic with complaints of exertional dyspnea or fatigue, palpitations, edema, and syncope. However, by adjusting their lifestyle accordingly, the majority are able to maintain an acceptable quality of life despite a decreasing exercise tolerance and increasing cyanosis during follow-up.

Although many providers may still recommend that these patients should not fly, Eisenmenger syndrome is not a contraindication to commercial air travel. A survey of 50 Eisenmenger syndrome patients showed no significant events compared to acyanotic patients,[11] and experimental studies have shown that these patients have built-in coping mechanisms such that the effects of low oxygen tension are not as pronounced as in normal individuals.[12] Advice to take precautions against thrombus formation during flight is worthwhile, as emboli may cross to the systemic circulation and cause a stroke or transient ischemic attack. Patients traveling from sea level to high-altitude destinations may notice more significant dyspnea on exertion, not surprisingly, and should be told of this likelihood and to restrict their physical activities.

Many patients with cyanotic heart disease die suddenly, although it is uncertain whether this is arrhythmic in origin. Unlike patients in other categories such as repaired TOF or patients with systemic RVs, unoperated patients with Eisenmenger syndrome present less commonly with symptomatic, sustained arrhythmia. Indeed, the development of atrial flutter or fibrillation in Eisenmenger syndrome can be a preterminal event.

Hyperviscosity symptoms include fatigue, headache, muscle aches, joint aches, gum bleeding, and easy bruising. Phlebotomy is sometimes prescribed to alleviate these symptoms. Most centers rightly discourage phlebotomy, however, as it can induce or enhance preexisting iron deficiency. Very occasionally phlebotomy may be tried for the alleviation of hyperviscosity symptoms (that can mimic the symptoms of iron deficiency) and then usually in conjunction with iron supplementation to avoid iron deficiency.[13]

## CURRENT SYMPTOMS

The patient was able to walk half a mile in 60 minutes and performed the household cooking. However, she was unable to do much of the housecleaning.

NYHA class: III

***Comments:*** Although most Eisenmenger patients complain of exertional dyspnea and/or fatigue, a retrospective analysis of 188 Eisenmenger patients demonstrated that their perception of life was good and more than 70% maintained a satisfactory functional Ability index of 1 or 2 for more than 10 years.[5] The Ability index stresses positive aspects of function rather than negative aspects.

Ability index 1: A normal life and full-time work or school

Ability index 2: Able to work with intermittent symptoms, but there is some interference with daily life

Ability index 3: Unable to work and limited in all activities

Ability index 4: Extreme limitation, dependent, almost housebound

## CURRENT MEDICATIONS

Furosemide 40 mg daily

Digitalis 125 µg daily

Potassium 20 mEq daily

Allopurinol 200 mg daily

***Comments:*** Eisenmenger patients should be kept well hydrated, and diuretics should be used judiciously. Allopurinol should be used to prevent gout rather than to treat asymptomatic hyperuricemia.

## PHYSICAL EXAMINATION

BP 110/70 mm Hg, HR 72 bpm, oxygen saturation 82% on room air

Height 144 cm, weight 47 kg, BSA 1.51 m$^2$

Oropharynx: Prominent central cyanosis

Neck veins: JVP was 8 cm above the sternal angle, and with a prominent V-wave.

Lungs/chest: Auscultation of the chest was normal.

Heart: There was a parasternal impulse with an easily palpable pulmonary closure sound. The rhythm was regular. The pulmonary component of S2 was prominent. A grade 2 systolic ejection murmur and a grade 2 high-pitched diastolic murmur were heard over the pulmonary area. A grade 3 holosystolic murmur was heard over the tricuspid area. There were no gallops.

Abdomen: Soft and nontender; hepatomegaly not present

Extremities: Extremities were warm, and there was trace pedal edema. The nail beds had significant clubbing and cyanosis.

Neurologic: No focal deficits

***Comments:*** The JVP may be normal or elevated, with a prominent V-wave if moderate or severe tricuspid regurgitation is present.

Signs of pulmonary hypertension include a right parasternal heave, palpable pulmonary valve closure, and a loud pulmonary heart sound. In the setting of a VSD, the second heart sound may be single. A high-pitched, diastolic pulmonary regurgitation murmur and a holosystolic murmur of tricuspid regurgitation may also be heard. In many patients a pulmonary ejection click and soft systolic ejection murmur are audible and are attributed to dilation of the main pulmonary artery.

Peripheral edema is absent unless RV failure occurs.

In a 1996 retrospective study of 162 patients with cyanotic congenital heart disease, 14% of patients had cerebrovascular events. This risk was increased in the setting of hypertension, atrial fibrillation, history of phlebotomy, and microcytosis (mean corpuscular volume < 82 fL). Microcytosis had the strongest risk association and was still associated with increased events after hypertension atrial fibrillation was excluded.[14]

## LABORATORY DATA

| | |
|---|---|
| Hemoglobin | **18.5 g/dL** (11.5–15.0) |
| Hematocrit | **55.8%** (36–46) |
| MCV | 95.3 fL (83–99) |
| Platelet count | **$125 \times 10^3$ cells/μL** (150–400) |
| Creatinine | 0.9 mg/dL (0.6–1.1) |
| Blood urea nitrogen | 19 mg/dL (6–20) |
| Serum iron | 102 μg/dL (40–150) |
| Iron binding capacity | 297 μg/dL (225–410) |
| Serum ferritin | 218 ng/mL (10–291) |
| Transferrin saturation | 34% (20–50) |
| Uric acid | 5.7 mg/dL (2.5–6.2) |

**Comments:** The degree of secondary erythrocytosis is closely associated with the severity of chronic hypoxemia. Compensated secondary erythrocytosis refers to a stable hemoglobin and hematocrit in an iron-replete state. Hyperviscosity symptoms are typically absent or mild even at hematocrit levels higher than 70%. Decompensated secondary erythrocytosis has been used to describe patients with iron deficiency and a constant cycle of phlebotomy for seemingly excessive erythrocytosis. Hyperviscosity symptoms can be severe and limiting, yet symptoms of iron deficiency can be very similar, and thus the correct etiology can be difficult to determine.[13] The two indications for phlebotomy are moderate-to-severe hyperviscosity symptoms and preoperative phlebotomy to improve hemostasis.[15]

Patients with cyanotic heart disease are at increased risk for both bleeding and thrombosis due to abnormalities in platelet and coagulation pathways. Bleeding is typically mild and self-limited, although severe hemoptysis is the most common and serious complication. Despite these hemostatic abnormalities, patients are not protected against thrombotic complications. Thrombosis is associated with low velocity blood flow in dilated pulmonary arteries, and with ventricular dysfunction.[16] The incidence of large pulmonary arterial thrombosis is 20% to 30%.[16–18] Although anticoagulation has been shown to reduce morbidity and mortality in patients with idiopathic PAH, there are no data to support the use of anticoagulation in adults with Eisenmenger syndrome. Strong indications for anticoagulation in Eisenmenger syndrome may include atrial flutter or fibrillation, recurrent thromboembolic events in the absence or iron deficiency or dehydration, mechanical heart valves, and other high-risk anatomy.

Serum uric acid is often increased in cyanotic ACHD. A retrospective study of 94 Eisenmenger patients in 2000 showed that serum uric acid was raised in these patients compared to age- and sex-matched control patients, and that the level of uric acid increased in proportion to the severity of the NYHA functional class.[19] In a multivariate analysis including clinical, echocardiographic, and laboratory variables, the serum uric acid level was identified as an independent predictor of mortality.

## ELECTROCARDIOGRAM

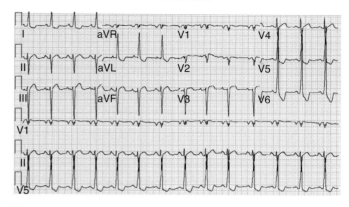

Figure 71-1 Electrocardiogram.

### FINDINGS
Heart rate: 82 bpm

QRS axis: −54°

QRS duration: 112 msec

The rhythm is sinus. There is biatrial enlargement and LV hypertrophy with repolarization abnormality.

**Comments:** This ECG does not have any alarming high-risk markers such as supraventricular or ventricular arrhythmias.

Supraventricular tachycardia is common with 36% of Eisenmenger patients having this rhythm on 24-hour Holter monitoring. A history of supraventricular tachycardia requiring treatment is an independent predictor for mortality, with a hazard ratio of 3.44.[20] It often heralds clinical deterioration with heart failure, peripheral embolism, or cardiovascular collapse.[5,17] An increased precordial voltage as an index for RV hypertrophy has also been identified as an independent predictor of death with a hazard ratio of 1.61 per 1 mV increase.[20] Though many Eisenmenger patients have ECG findings consistent with RV hypertrophy, they were not present here.

## CHEST X-RAY

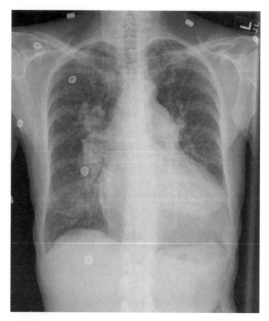

Figure 71-2 Posteroanterior projection.

## FINDINGS

Cardiothoracic ratio: 63%

There was severe cardiomegaly. The main and central pulmonary arteries were enlarged consistent with pulmonary hypertension.

***Comments:*** Chest radiography usually reveals dilated central pulmonary arteries and decreased number and size of peripheral vessels, sometimes described as "pruning." Patients with Eisenmenger syndrome and a VSD usually have a normal or minimally increased cardiothoracic ratio. The degree of cardiomegaly in this patient with a VSD is unusual and may reflect pulmonary and tricuspid regurgitation or LV disease.

## ECHOCARDIOGRAM

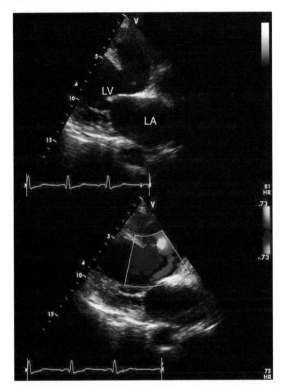

Figure 71-3 Parasternal long-axis view with and without 2D Doppler.

## FINDINGS

The LV cavity size is severely increased with an LV diastolic internal dimension at 72 mm. The LA is also severely dilated, measuring 56 mm.

A large, nonrestrictive VSD is seen. Bidirectional shunting is noted on color Doppler.

There is mild mitral regurgitation.

***Comments:*** Because the pulmonary arterial pressure is at systemic level, the pressure gradient and flow across the intracardiac defect may be small and therefore difficult to visualize by color flow Doppler imaging.

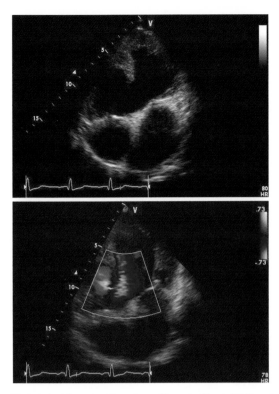

Figure 71-4 Apical four-chamber view with and without 2D Doppler.

## FINDINGS

Using biplane Simpson's method, the LV ejection fraction is low at 46%. There is mild global dysfunction.

The RV is severely enlarged and hypertrophied. There is severe global RV dysfunction.

Both atria are severely dilated.

The large VSD with bidirectional shunting across the defect on color Doppler is again appreciated.

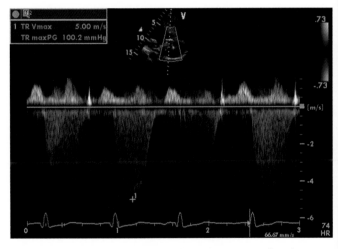

Figure 71-5 Tricuspid flow velocity with continuous-wave Doppler.

## FINDINGS

On color Doppler, there is mild-to-moderate tricuspid regurgitation. The tricuspid regurgitant velocity is 5 m/sec.

The IVC is dilated with inspiratory collapse less than 50%. Assuming an RA pressure of 20 mm Hg, the RV systolic pressure is severely elevated at 120 mm Hg.

**Comments:** This echocardiogram demonstrates the hallmark of Eisenmenger complex: severe pulmonary hypertension at systemic level with reversed or bidirectional shunt.

When assessing the severity of pulmonary hypertension, the systemic blood pressure should be recorded.

# MAGNETIC RESONANCE IMAGING

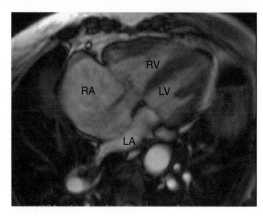

Figure 71-6 Steady-state free precession cine, oblique axial plane (four-chamber view).

## FINDINGS

RV hypertrophy with mildly reduced systolic function. There was mild tricuspid regurgitation. The LV also had mildly reduced systolic function but was normal in size. There was severe RA enlargement.

### Ventricular Volume Quantification

|  | LV | (Normal range) | RV | (Normal range) |
|---|---|---|---|---|
| EDV (mL) | 82 | (52–141) | 78 | (58–154) |
| ESV (mL) | 42 | (13–51) | 44 | (12–68) |
| SV (mL) | 40 | (33–97) | **34** | (35–98) |
| EF (%) | **49** | (60–78) | **44** | (59–83) |
| EDVi (mL/m²) | 60 | (50–84) | 57 | (45–82) |
| ESVi (mL/m²) | **31** | (12–30) | 32 | (6–32) |
| SVi (mL/m²) | **29** | (34–59) | **25** | (33–57) |
| Mass index (g/m²) | 65 | (49–78) | **63** | (14–35) |

**Comments:** In patients with Eisenmenger syndrome, ventricular dysfunction tends to occur in both ventricles concurrently, rather than the RV failing first.[16] Although the VSD cannot be seen in this view, its effects on the RV are readily apparent. RA enlargement is the result of chronically elevated RV end-diastolic pressure and tricuspid regurgitation. The RA is compressing the relatively normal-sized LA.

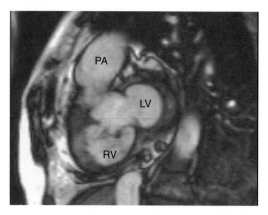

Figure 71-7 Steady-state free precession cine, oblique sagittal plane (basal short-axis view).

## FINDINGS

A large perimembranous VSD was seen, with bidirectional shunting.

**Comments:** The image illustrates the typical finding in Eisenmenger syndrome of RV hypertrophy. The lack of ECG evidence of RV hypertrophy is surprising. It may be due in part to biventricular dysfunction.

# EXERCISE TESTING

| Exercise protocol: | Modified Bruce |
|---|---|
| Duration (min:sec): | 2:15 |
| Reason for stopping: | Dyspnea, headache |
| ECG changes: | None |

|  | Rest | Peak |
|---|---|---|
| Heart rate (bpm): | 72 | 137 |
| Percent of age-predicted max HR: |  | 91 |
| $O_2$ saturation (%): | 82 | 64 |
| Blood pressure (mm Hg): | 110/70 | 138/70 |
| Peak $\dot{V}O_2$ (mL/kg/min): |  | 11 |
| Percent predicted (%): |  | 25 |
| Ve/Vco₂: |  | 184 |
| Metabolic equivalents: |  | 4.1 |

| Pre-exercise: | $O_2$ saturation 82% on room air |
|---|---|
| 6-minute walk test: | 228 m |
| Postexercise: | Heart rate 118 bpm |
|  | $O_2$ saturation 68% on room air |

**Comments:** Objective measurement of exercise capacity can be a routine part of management of Eisenmenger patients to objectively measure their capacity, and can be done safely with appropriate supervision and caution. A 2005 prospective study of 149 adolescents and adults with congenital heart disease compared self-reported quality of life with measured cardiopulmonary exercise capacity on an upright bicycle. Despite an overall good correlation of objective exercise capacity as measured by cardiopulmonary exercise testing with self-reported exercise capacity and self-reported general health, a substantial number of patients overestimated their physical capabilities on the quality of life self-assessment.[21]

Cardiopulmonary exercise testing, however, can be risky and time consuming and requires special expertise. Furthermore, patients may not be able to reach their anaerobic threshold or may be unable to perform a bicycle or treadmill exercise test due to physical disability or delayed mental development. In contrast, a 6-minute walk test can easily be performed, is cost effective, and the distance covered in 6 minutes has been demonstrated to correlate well with peak oxygen uptake on cardiopulmonary exercise testing in adults with complex congenital cardiac disease.[22]

In this patient's case, both tests confirm her extreme exertional limitation. Despite this, she was still doing more activity than might be expected from these test results, which again highlights the perseverance of many congenital heart patients.

## FOCUSED CLINICAL QUESTIONS AND DISCUSSION POINTS

1. **What is the long-term prognosis and survival of patients with Eisenmenger syndrome?**

*The longevity of patients with Eisenmenger syndrome has perhaps been underestimated for many years, and overall is better than that of patients with other forms of PAH. One retrospective study looking at the survival of adults with severe primary pulmonary hypertension and adults with Eisenmenger syndrome found a survival rate of 35% at 3 years for those with primary pulmonary hypertension and 77% at 3 years for those with Eisenmenger syndrome.[23]*

*Many surviving patients with Eisenmenger syndrome do well into their third decade of life but become more symptomatic as they age. There are no prospective data available regarding survival rates and long-term prognosis. In one retrospective study with a population of 201 Eisenmenger patients, there was an 80% survival rate at 10 years, a 77% survival rate at 15 years, and a 42% survival rate at 25 years after initial presentation.[24] Another retrospective study of a pediatric and adult population of Eisenmenger patients found a survival rate of 75% at the age of 30 years, 70% at the age of 40 years, and 55% at the age of 50 years.[5]*

*Longevity in adults with Eisenmenger syndrome is influenced by the underlying cardiac abnormality. Eisenmenger patients with simple ACHD had a later clinical deterioration than those with complex ACHD, 26.7 years versus 18.6 years, and a significantly better actuarial survival rate.[5] In one series the 5-year actuarial survival rate after initial visit was best in patients with truncus arteriosus (91%) and in patients with a VSD (67%). It was worst in patients with univentricular heart (34%).[17]*

2. **What are the risk factors for mortality in Eisenmenger syndrome?**

*Although no large prospective study has analyzed risk factors for death, retrospective studies have demonstrated a number of strong predictors for death. These include age at presentation or symptoms, deterioration in Ability index or poor functional class, complex ACHD, syncope, supraventricular tachycardia, elevated mean RA pressure (>7 mm Hg), low oxygen saturation (So$_2$ < 85%), RV dysfunction, increased precordial ECG voltage as an index for RV hypertrophy, and elevated serum uric acid concentration.[5,19,20]*

*Premature death occasionally relates to potentially avoidable complications due to noncardiac surgery, infection, or excess phlebotomy. About 8% of patients will die from hemoptysis, but a history of hemoptysis has not been demonstrated to worsen one's prognosis.[20]*

3. **Vasodilator therapy has been used in the management of primary pulmonary hypertension. Is this applicable to patients with Eisenmenger syndrome?**

*The defining pathophysiology in Eisenmenger syndrome is the presence of a nonrestrictive communication between pulmonary and systemic circulations with consequent increased pulmonary blood flow and transmission of near systemic pressure to the pulmonary arteries. This is the driving force for the development of severe pulmonary vascular disease.*

*There have been many attempts to assess the reactivity of the pulmonary vasculature and to reduce pulmonary vascular resistance in patients with PAH. The use of vasodilator therapy has been the mainstay of treatment of idiopathic PAH. Four vasodilator agents have been approved for the treatment of pulmonary arterial hypertension in the United States and Europe: intravenous epoprostenol, inhaled prostacyclin analogue iloprost, subcutaneous and intravenous prostacyclin analogue treprostinil, and oral endothelin–receptor antagonist bosentan (see Case 81). These agents have many adverse effects in terms of safety, tolerability, and drug delivery.*

*More recently, there has been a randomized double-blind placebo control study (BREATHE-5) showing safety and efficiency of bosentan, a dual-receptor endothelin antagonist, in improving functional class, the 6MWT, and pulmonary hemodynamics in patients with Eisenmenger syndrome.[25]*

*The oral phosphodiesterase inhibitor sildenafil has also been approved for the treatment of PAH. A double-blind, placebo-controlled study of 278 patients with symptomatic PAH (either idiopathic or with connective tissue disease, or repaired congenital systemic to pulmonary shunts) was randomized so that patients received placebo or sildenafil (20, 40, or 80 mg) orally three times daily for 12 weeks. The primary end point was the change from baseline to week 12 in the distance walked in 6 minutes. The distance walked in 6 minutes significantly increased from baseline in all treatment groups compared to placebo therapy. Among the 222 patients who completed a year of sildenafil, the improvement in distance walked in 6 minutes was 51 meters.[26] The study also assessed change in mean pulmonary artery pressure and World Health Organization functional class. The mean pulmonary artery pressures in the sildenafil groups were significantly decreased, and there was a significant improvement in World Health Organization class. There did not appear to be a dose–response relationship associated with exercise capacity or tolerability. The most frequent side effects were flushing, dyspepsia, and diarrhea.*

*Although this study included patients with repaired congenital systemic to pulmonary shunts, it did not include Eisenmenger patients with uncorrected congenital shunts.*

## FINAL DIAGNOSIS

Unoperated VSD with Eisenmenger physiology and severe exercise intolerance

## PLAN OF ACTION

Pulmonary vasodilator treatment

## INTERVENTION

None

## OUTCOME

The patient and caregivers believed she had already done much better clinically than anyone would have thought. However, in an effort to make the patient feel better, and given the reported safety of sildenafil therapy, this was explored with the patient and she agreed to try the medication.

The patient was initially placed on sildenafil at 80 mg three times a day and had marked improvement in her exercise tolerance. Within 3 months of starting the medication, she was able to go shopping, which she previously had not been able to do. She was able to walk a half mile in 40 minutes. Her sildenafil dose was eventually reduced to 20 mg three times a day, and she continued to maintain the same level of improvement she had initially.

Several months later she presented with an episode of brief hemoptysis, approximately a half cup of bright red blood. She was observed in the hospital but had no further hemoptysis.

One month later she presented with rapid atrial flutter to a local emergency department. She felt generally weak and unwell but reverted to sinus rhythm while under observation and was discharged home on amiodarone. A follow-up 24-hour ECG showed several runs of nonsustained ventricular tachycardia. Given her advanced state, it was felt that an implantable cardioverter-defibrillator was not indicated.

Over the ensuing weeks her condition continued to deteriorate. She was seen in clinic several times, each time showing slightly worse oxygen saturation. She appeared feeble and needed more assistance from her husband getting around in the clinic.

Several weeks later her husband called to say she had passed away quietly in her bed at home. She was 72 years old.

***Comments:*** The sildenafil improved her quality of life for several months, after which she experienced her first episode of hemoptysis, then her first episode of atrial flutter, often a pre-terminal rhythm when it occurs in Eisenmenger patients. We do not know why these events occurred when they did, but her survival to age 72 was exceptional.

Pulmonary vasodilators are being used increasingly in patients with PAH related to congenital heart disease, though data on their mid- and long-term use and refining selection criteria for such advanced therapies are obviously needed.

## Selected References

1. Eisenmenger V: Die angeborenen Defecte der kammerscheidewand des Herzens. Z Klin Med 32(Suppl):1–28, 1897.
2. Wood P: The Eisenmenger syndrome or pulmonary hypertension with reversed central shunt. BMJ 2:701–709, 755–762, 1958.
3. Avila WS, Grinberg M, Snitcowsky R, et al: Maternal and fetal outcome in pregnant women with Eisenmenger syndrome. Eur Heart J 16:460–464, 1995.
4. Gleicher N, Midwall J, Hocheberger D, Jaffin H: Eisenmenger syndrome and pregnancy. Obstet Gynecol Surv 24:721–741, 1979.
5. Daliento L, Somerville J, Presbitero P, et al: Eisenmenger syndrome: Factors relating to deterioration and death. Eur Heart J 19:1845–1855, 1998.
6. Weiss B, Zemp L, Seifert B, et al: Outcome of pulmonary vascular disease in pregnancy: A systematic overview from 1978 through 1996. J Am Coll Cardiol 31:1650–1657, 1998.
7. Liberthson RR: Eisenmenger's physiology, pulmonary vascular obstruction. In Liberthson RR (ed): Congenital Heart Disease: Diagnosis and Management in Children and Adults. Boston, Little, Brown, 1989, pp 87–93.
8. Ammash NM, Connolly HM, Abel MD, Warnes CA: Noncardiac surgery in Eisenmenger syndrome. J Am Coll Cardiol 33:222–227, 1999.
9. Foster J, Jones RM: The anesthetic management of the Eisenmenger syndrome. Ann R Coll Surg Engl 66:353–355, 1984.
10. Wilson W, Taubert KA, Gewitz M, et al: Prevention of infective endocarditis: Guidelines from the American Heart Association. American Heart Association Rheumatic Fever, Endocarditis, and Kawasaki Disease Committee, Councils on Cardiovascular Disease in the Young, Clinical Cardiology, and Cardiovascular Surgery and Anesthesia, and the Quality of Care and Outcomes Research Interdisciplinary Working Group. Circulation 116(15): 1736–1754, 2007.
11. Broberg CS, Uebing A, Cuomo L, et al: Adult patients with Eisenmenger syndrome report flying safely on commercial airlines. Heart 93:1599–1603, 2007.
12. Harnick E, Hutter PA, Hoorntje TM, et al: Air travel and adults with cyanotic congenital heart disease. Circulation 93:272–276, 1996.
13. Broberg CS, Bax BE, Dalington OO, et al: Blood viscosity and its relationship to iron deficiency, symptoms, and exercise capacity in adults with cyanotic congenital heart disease. J Am Coll Cardiol 48:356–365, 2006.
14. Ammash N, Warnes CA: Cerebrovascular events in adult patients with cyanotic congenital heart disease. J Am Coll Cardiol 28: 768–772, 1996.
15. Vongpatanasin W, Brickner ME, Hillis LD, et al: The Eisenmenger syndrome in adults. Ann Intern Med 128:745–755, 1998.
16. Broberg CS, Ujita M, Prasad S, et al: Pulmonary arterial thrombosis in Eisenmenger syndrome is associated with biventricular dysfunction and decreased pulmonary flow velocity. J Am Coll Cardiol 50:634–642, 2007.
17. Niwa K, Perloff JK, Kaplan S, et al: Eisenmenger syndrome in adults: Ventricular septal defect, truncus arteriosus, univentricular heart. J Am Coll Cardiol 34:223–232, 1999.
18. Silversides CK, Granton JT, Konen E, et al: Pulmonary thrombosis in adults with Eisenmenger syndrome. J Am Coll Cardiol 42: 1982–1987, 2003.
19. Oya H, Nagaya N, Satoh T, et al: Haemodynamic correlates and prognostic significance of serum uric acid in adult patients with Eisenmenger syndrome. Heart 84:53–58, 2000.
20. Cantor WJ, Harrison DA, Moussadju JS, et al: Determinants of survival and length of survival in adults with Eisenmenger syndrome. Am J Cardiol 84:677–681, 1999.
21. Hager A, Hess J: Comparison of health-related quality of life with cardiopulmonary exercise testing in adolescents and adults with congenital heart disease. Heart 891:517–520, 2005.
22. Niedeggen A, Skobel E, Haager P, et al: Comparison of the 6-minute walk test with established parameters for assessment of cardiopulmonary capacity in adults with complex congenital cardiac disease. Cardiol Young 15:385–390, 2005.
23. Hopkins WE, Ochoa LL, Richardson GW, et al: Comparison of the hemodynamics and survival of adults with severe primary pulmonary hypertension or Eisenmenger syndrome. J Heart Lung Transplant 15:100–105, 1996.
24. Saha A, Balakrishnan KG, Jaiswal PK, et al: Prognosis for patients with Eisenmenger syndrome of various aetiology. Int J Cardiol 45:199–207, 1994.
25. Galiè N, Beghetti M, Gatzoulis MA, et al: Bosentan therapy in patients with Eisenmenger syndrome: A multicenter, double-blind, randomized, placebo-controlled study. Circulation 114: 48–54, 2006.
26. Galiè N, Ghofrani HA, et al: Sildenafil citrate therapy for pulmonary arterial hypertension. Sildenafil Use in Pulmonary Arterial Hypertension (SUPER) Study Group. N Engl J Med 353:2148–2157, 2005.

# Iron Deficiency in Cyanotic Heart Disease

**Craig S. Broberg and Per Lunde**

**Age: 40 years**
**Gender: Female**
**Occupation: Lawyer**
**Working diagnosis: Eisenmenger syndrome**

## HISTORY

At birth the patient had a large VSD with congestive heart failure. A pulmonary artery band was placed at 1 year of age. Catheterization at age 3 confirmed the anatomical diagnosis, but her pulmonary vascular resistance was elevated. Her parents were told an operation to correct the defect could not be offered.

She had an otherwise uneventful childhood and upbringing, but gradually became cyanotic and clubbed. She completed her education and began a busy full-time career. She had been told she should not have children, and never married.

Gradually her exercise tolerance deteriorated. At the age of 30, she had her first of several episodes of significant hemoptysis. Her hemoglobin fell as low as 12 g/dL. Each episode resolved spontaneously. She was placed on a waiting list for a heart-lung transplant, but 3 years later her condition was no worse and she was told she was too well for transplant. Since then, she has had smaller episodes of hemoptysis each year. She continued to work but did so mainly from her own home and at a slower pace.

Within the last year she felt her physical capacity dwindle further, and she sought additional medical attention.

The patient had heavy menstrual flow every month. She had never had a therapeutic phlebotomy. There was no evidence of gastrointestinal bleeding. She was not a vegetarian.

***Comments:*** Pulmonary artery (PA) banding to prevent pulmonary vascular disease does not always succeed. If the band is not tight enough to produce significant stenosis, pulmonary vascular disease will develop in a relatively short period of time. Indeed, in some patients, pulmonary vascular resistance never falls after birth (pulmonary hypertension of the newborn).

Hemoptysis is common in Eisenmenger syndrome (see Cases 73 and 74) but has no known bearing on prognosis.[1] It can be a cause of relative anemia, and transfusions or iron supplementation may be necessary to restore the hemoglobin to an appropriately increased level (see Case 73).

Heart-lung transplantation is often considered as an option in Eisenmenger patients with severe disability. However, the long-term survival from heart-lung transplantation is usually worse than from Eisenmenger syndrome itself.

Factors related to blood loss and iron deficiency are worth exploring in any patient with cyanotic heart disease.

## CURRENT SYMPTOMS

The patient is unable to climb a flight of steps without stopping and has to rest when pushing a shopping cart through the supermarket. She is able to continue working, however, and spends most of her day at her desk in her home office.

NYHA class: III

***Comments:*** In the care of adults with congenital heart disease, it is remarkable how many patients with disabling lesions are able to continue full-time gainful employment for long periods despite their medical problems. Chronic disability can be very well tolerated by a determined patient.

## CURRENT MEDICATIONS

None

## PHYSICAL EXAMINATION

BP 120/80 mm Hg, HR 90 bpm, oxygen saturation 73% (finger), 80% (earlobe), and 71% (toe)

Height 165 cm, weight 59 kg, BSA 1.64 m$^2$

Surgical scars: Left thoracotomy scar

Neck veins: The venous pulsations were seen 5 cm above the sternal angle, with pronounced x and y descents.

Lungs/chest: No rales or wheezes were heard in the chest.

Heart: The rhythm was regular, with a normal first heart sound, loud pulmonary component of the second heart sound, and soft systolic ejection murmur. There was an RV lift.

Abdomen: Thin, no ascites or organomegaly

Extremities: Symmetrical clubbing of fingers and toes, but no edema

***Comments:*** Not all vascular beds, or oximeters, are created equal. Even when there is no differential cyanosis, oxygen saturation measured transcutaneously will vary between body sites. In cyanotic heart disease, this variation can be considerable. Even when the fingernail bed is clean and without fingernail polish (a common source of error), earlobe saturations will usually be 6% points higher. The earlobe is rich in arterial flow and will respond faster to changes in oxygen saturation[2] than the finger, for example, and there is less oxygen uptake to affect the photometric reading. Usually this difference is inconsequential, but ought to be appreciated so that a consistent oximetry method is maintained.

Eisenmenger patients will usually have normal central venous pressure in the absence of tricuspid valve regurgitation or RV dysfunction. The pattern seen here was not expected.

The loud pulmonary component of the second heart sound is the hallmark of pulmonary hypertension.

It is surprising that the PA banding did not create a louder ejection systolic murmur. The band must have been very loose.

## LABORATORY DATA

| | |
|---|---|
| Hemoglobin | **17.4 g/dL** (11.5–15.0) |
| Hematocrit/PCV | **55%** (36–46) |
| MCV | **77 fL** (83–99) |
| Platelet count | $208 \times 10^9$/L (150–400) |
| Sodium | 135 mmol/L (134–145) |
| Potassium | 4.2 mmol/L (3.5–5.2) |
| Creatinine | 0.65 mg/dL (0.6–1.2) |
| Blood urea nitrogen | 5.2 mmol/L (2.5–6.5) |
| Iron | **9.9 μmol/L** (12.6–26.0) |
| Ferritin | **14 μg/L** (30–233) |
| TIBC | 80 μmol/L (50–80) |
| Transferrin | 3.2 g/L (2.0–3.2) |
| Transferrin saturation | **12%** (20–45) |
| TSH | 0.81 IU/L (0.32–5.0) |
| Urate | 345 μmol/L (210–440) |
| Erythropoietin | **110.8 IU** (5.0–25.0) |
| $P_{50}$ of the oxygen-hemoglobin dissociation curve | **31 mm Hg** (27) |

**Comments:** The hemoglobin is a bit too low for her level of desaturation (see "Focused Clinical Questions and Discussion Points"). She is iron deficient, and it is reasonable to expect this is the reason for her relatively low hemoglobin/hematocrit.

The MCV is low here, consistent with her iron deficiency. However, microcytosis is often not seen despite low iron stores, and thus MCV is usually not an adequate screening test for iron deficiency in cyanotic heart disease.[3]

Plasma urate level, often elevated because of the relatively high turnover of red blood cells in cyanotic patients, has been shown to have prognostic implications.[4] If a gout flare has occurred, daily allopurinol should be offered.

The $P_{50}$ of the oxygen-hemoglobin dissociation curve is right-shifted, meaning oxygen will be released at a lower oxygen tension at the tissue level.[5] Elevated erythropoietin occurs in response to low oxygen delivery.[6] Though these tests are not standard clinical laboratory tests, in this case they both indicate that her hemoglobin is insufficient for her systemic oxygen delivery needs.

## ELECTROCARDIOGRAM

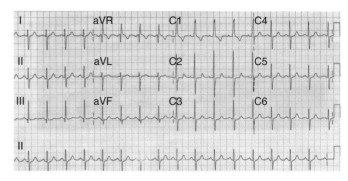

Figure 72-1 Electrocardiogram.

### FINDINGS

Heart rate: 101 bpm

QRS axis: +148°

QRS duration: 86 msec

Sinus rhythm, prominent R-wave in V1 with deep persistent S-waves to V6 and right-axis deviation, consistent with RV hypertrophy

**Comments:** These are typical findings of a patient with chronic pulmonary hypertension. There is evidence of RV hypertrophy, even though RA overload is not seen. There is no AV or intraventricular conduction delay.

## CHEST X-RAY

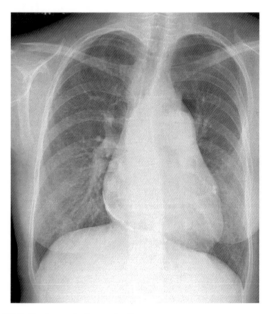

Figure 72-2 Posteroanterior projection.

## FINDINGS

Cardiothoracic ratio: 59%

Mildly enlarged cardiac silhouette. There was a prominent central and left pulmonary artery, with normal lung parenchyma. Abnormal calcification within the pericardium along the RA and RV border was also seen. Mild scoliosis and evidence of previous left thoracotomy were also present.

**Comments:** The CXR is compatible with Eisenmenger syndrome. There is a dilated central and left pulmonary artery without any pulmonary plethora, compatible with pulmonary hypertension. It is not clear why the right PA branch is not more prominent.

The abnormal pericardial calcification seen here is a surprise, and could indicate possible constrictive pericarditis. The frequency of calcific pericardial disease varies depending on the population studied and when the CXR was done. When tuberculous disease is excluded, available literature suggests that pericardial calcification is found in less than 40% of patients with constrictive pericarditis. It is most often found in patients with idiopathic constrictive pericarditis (82%) and suggests that calcification is a nonspecific response to a chronic inflammatory process. It rarely follows cardiac surgery (12%).[7,8]

## EXERCISE TESTING

| Exercise protocol: | Modified Bruce |
| --- | --- |
| Duration (min:sec): | 4:14 |
| Reason for stopping: | Dyspnea and headache |
| ECG changes: | Downsloping ST depression in II, III, aVF |

| | Rest | Peak |
| --- | --- | --- |
| Heart rate (bpm): | 90 | 146 |
| Percent of age-predicted max HR: | | 81 |
| O$_2$ saturation (%): | 73 | 47 |
| Blood pressure (mm Hg): | 120/80 | 135/75 |
| Peak Vo$_2$ (mL/kg/min): | | 9.25 |
| Percent predicted (%): | | 34 |
| Ve/Vco$_2$: | | 139 |
| Metabolic equivalents: | | 3.0 |

**Comments:** As a group, patients with Eisenmenger syndrome have the lowest exercise capacity of any group of congenital heart patients,[9] and there are likely several reasons for this. This particular patient was able to exercise for only 4 minutes, which is low even for the Eisenmenger group, in our experience. The drop in oxygen saturation is expected in a cyanotic patient.

The significance of ST depression in these patients is not yet certain, but probably relates to low oxygen delivery rather than epicardial coronary disease.

All patients with cyanotic heart disease have a higher Ve/Vco$_2$ slope than acyanotic patients. Yet here the Ve/Vco$_2$ slope is very high, even higher than average for a cyanotic patient, in whom the mean for Eisenmenger patients was 70 ± 10.[10] Still, the significance of this is not certain, and the value of this slope does not correlate with outcome.[10]

## ECHOCARDIOGRAM

### OVERALL FINDINGS

The RV was mildly dysfunctional. There was mildly reduced LV function. The RA was enlarged. The mitral and tricuspid valves functioned normally.

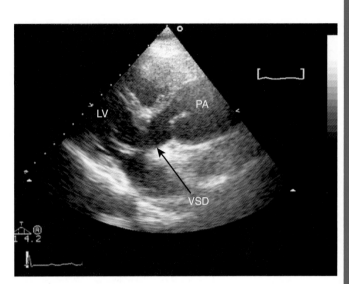

Figure 72-3 Parasternal long-axis view.

### FINDINGS

A subpulmonary VSD was present, with fibrous discontinuity between the aortic annulus and the mitral annulus.

**Comments:** At first glance it would appear in this view that the LV empties through a long, angled outflow tract to the aorta, and that a VSD is not visible. The aortic valve annulus, normally contiguous with the mitral annulus, is separated from the mitral annulus and displaced anteriorly. What appears to be a continuation of the septum at a right angle continuing to the aorta is actually a large muscular band of the hypertrophied RV, and the semilunar valve visible in this view is actually the pulmonic valve. The aorta is more anterior and out of plane and arises purely from the RV.

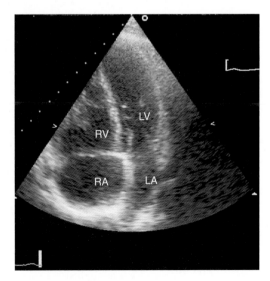

Figure 72-4 Apical four-chamber view.

## FINDINGS

The RV was dilated and hypertrophied with mild dysfunction. There was restricted filling of both ventricles based on E/A wave patterns, and septal motion towards the LV during early diastole. The RA was enlarged. The mitral and tricuspid valves functioned normally.

***Comments:*** Abnormal motion of the interventricular septum and posterior wall in constrictive pericarditis has long been recognized. The characteristic findings on M-mode echocardiography are an early diastolic notching due to variations in interventricular relaxation dynamics and flattening of the posterior wall.[11] More recently, Doppler tissue imaging has been used to classify patterns of ventricular filling on a spectrum and has improved the interpretation of abnormal septal motion in patients with constrictive pericarditis.[12]

However, in the presence of RV hypertrophy and a VSD, the septal dynamics are already very different from normal, and thus interpretation of the usual findings to support constriction may not apply. The abnormal septal motion, for example, is unusual since the large VSD means generally that the RV and LV have equal pressure throughout the cardiac cycle. Eisenmenger patients do not normally have a restrictive filling pattern on Doppler echocardiography, and hence the findings here are not expected. Overall, the combination of an elevated central venous pressure and restrictive filling here suggests that the abnormal pericardium may be of hemodynamic significance.

## MAGNETIC RESONANCE IMAGING

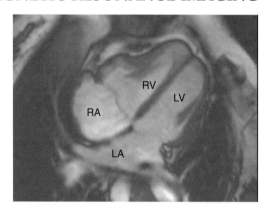

Figure 72-5 Oblique transaxial plane, four-chamber view.

### Ventricular Volume Quantification

|  | LV | (Normal range) | RV | (Normal range) |
|---|---|---|---|---|
| EDV (mL) | 89 | (52–141) | 107 | (58–154) |
| ESV (mL) | 43 | (13–51) | 55 | (12–68) |
| SV (mL) | 46 | (33–97) | 52 | (35–98) |
| EF (%) | **52** | (58–76) | **49** | (53–77) |
| EDVi (mL/m²) | **54** | (59–93) | 65 | (57–94) |
| ESVi (mL/m²) | 26 | (16–34) | 33 | (14–40) |
| SVi (mL/m²) | **28** | (39–63) | 32 | (19–39) |
| Mass index (g/m²) | 48 | (48–77) | 46 | |

## FINDINGS

The LV had mildly reduced function and was not enlarged; the RV was severely hypertrophied and had mildly reduced function. The mass of the RV and LV was similar.

There were regions of dark signal representing thickened pericardium between the bright layers of epicardial and pericardial fat anterior to the RV. The AV valves were both competent.

***Comments:*** The volume measurements confirmed the echocardiographic assessment of mild biventricular dysfunction. Eisenmenger patients with a VSD tend to have similar morphologic features for both the RV and LV, as is generally seen here. Mass, for example, is nearly equal, as is ejection fraction.[13]

Despite the anatomical defect, the four-chamber view appears fairly normal, apart from the hypertrophied RV (anteriorly). The VSD is not seen. The thickened pericardium and pattern of restricted filling are noted, and unusual.

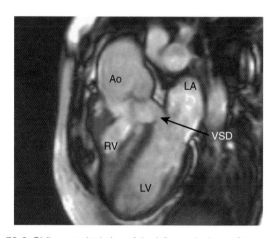

Figure 72-6 Oblique sagittal cine of the left ventricular outflow tract.

## FINDINGS

Double-outlet RV with a large subpulmonary VSD. The aorta arose from the RV. A VSD was present without obstruction. There was no significant PA stenosis.

***Comments:*** In the presence of a VSD, the RV stroke volume should be equal to the volume passing through the aorta and returning to the RA. Similarly, the LV stroke volume should be equal to the volume of blood passing through the pulmonary artery and returning to the LA. Hence the Qp/Qs ratio should equal the LV/RV stroke volume ratio, in the absence of significant AV valve regurgitation. This is the opposite for a normal person, or in the presence of an ASD or PDA, in which the pulmonary artery/aortic flow ratio equals the RV/LV stroke volume ratio. The absence of pulmonary stenosis is consistent with incomplete banding at birth.

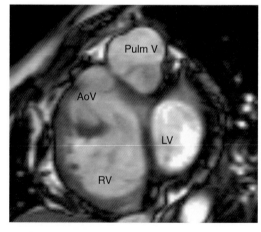

Figure 72-7 Short-axis view, basal level.

## FINDINGS

The aorta was displaced anteriorly, and there was no fibrous continuity between the aortic valve (seen at left, just opening) and the mitral valve (orifice seen at right).

***Comments:*** Between the mitral and aortic valves lies the pulmonic valve (seen in cross section), which is the reason for classifying the VSD as "subpulmonary," since it lies more below the pulmonary valve.

The finding of fibrous discontinuity between the mitral and aortic valves as present here implies the loss of normal relationship of the great vessels, which themselves are parallel to each other and not criss-crossing. This morphologic feature is the hallmark of the classic description of double-outlet RV (see "Focused Clinical Questions and Discussion Points").

# COMPUTED TOMOGRAPHY

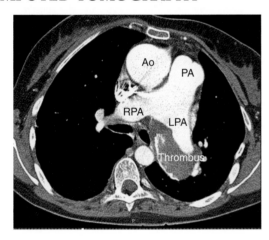

Figure 72-8 Computed tomography pulmonary angiography.

## FINDINGS

CT pulmonary angiography was performed to search for thrombus within the pulmonary arteries.

There was obvious dilatation of the left pulmonary artery, which was more than half filled with a mural thrombus. The aorta was located anteriorly.

***Comments:*** Pulmonary artery thrombosis is a common finding in Eisenmenger patients, with a prevalence of approximately 20%.[14,15] CT pulmonary angiography is the gold standard for detection of intrapulmonary thrombus, since other modalities, which look for lumen obstruction, may not demonstrate the mural quality of the thrombus. Large thrombi such as these can also be seen by MRI.[15,16] The pulmonary arteries are dilated and there is calcification in the wall of the left pulmonary artery, a sign of chronic PAH.

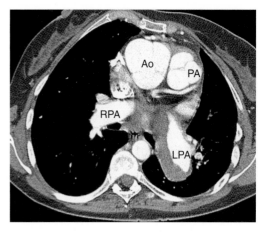

Figure 72-9 Computed tomography pulmonary angiogram.

## FINDINGS

Thrombus was seen in the more distal left pulmonary artery. A large left circumflex coronary artery was also seen.

***Comments:*** The CT gives several other interesting findings including confirmation of the anatomical diagnosis. The aortic and pulmonary valve planes are seen at the same level, and the aorta is displaced from its usual position posterior and to the right of the pulmonary valve, to a position more anterior to the pulmonary valve. These suggest D-TGA; however, this is not the case here, since both great vessels originate from the RV.

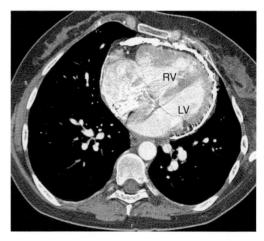

Figure 72-10 Computed tomography pulmonary angiogram.

## FINDINGS

Heavily calcified and thickened pericardium was present.

***Comments:*** The pericardium of this patient is definitely thickened, as suggested by MRI, and is densely calcified. The combination of this with the echocardiographic findings of constriction confirms the diagnosis of constrictive pericarditis.

# CATHETERIZATION

Not performed

## Focused Clinical Questions and Discussion Points

### 1. What is the anatomic diagnosis?

*This patient has a double-outlet RV with a large VSD. Review of her early chart notes revealed that this was known at her first diagnostic catheterization. She has obvious changes of chronic pulmonary vascular disease and is cyanotic, and so has Eisenmenger syndrome.*

*Double-outlet RV simply means that both great arteries predominantly (>50%) originate from the RV. This could be part of the spectrum of TOF if the aorta overrides the septum by more than 50%, and in such a case the VSD can be termed* subaortic. *More classically, however, the term* double-outlet right ventricle *applies to the diagnosis seen here and is part of the spectrum of TGA. The aorta is abnormally located and separated from the mitral valve—that is, there is fibrous discontinuity between the aortic and mitral valve annuli—and the VSD can be termed* subpulmonic. *Some morphologists argue that this latter form is the only true definition of double-outlet RV.*

### 2. What is the cause of her recent deterioration?

*The workup has identified two important problems, namely iron deficiency and constrictive pericarditis. Iron deficiency is common in cyanotic ACHD, and is likely multifactorial,[17] though often related to menorrhagia, therapeutic phlebotomy, or frequent hemoptysis. This patient had experienced two of these events. Because of this, her hemoglobin is too low for her level of desaturation, and iron deficiency should be treated. Low hemoglobin reduces systemic oxygen transport[18] and may contribute to poorer exercise function.[17]*

*Because of iron deficiency, this patient's hemoglobin level is far lower than is considered appropriate for her degree of cyanosis.[19]*

*In cyanotic adults, a target optimal hemoglobin level can be found by using this formula: optimal hemoglobin = 60 − ½ (% oxygen saturation).[20]*

*Hence, in this case, using a baseline saturation of 73%, her predicted optimal hemoglobin would be 25 g/dL, far higher than it currently is. Most likely the above formula becomes less accurate at saturations this low, but it still may be a helpful guideline to assess for functional anemia.*

*Her other problem, constrictive pericarditis, is clearly chronic. It is more difficult to know how much this is contributing to her symptoms. She gives no history suggesting acute inflammatory pericarditis or tuberculous pericarditis. Constrictive pericarditis as a complication of prior surgery is less likely, as pulmonary banding was the only procedure performed. In addition, pericardial calcification is rarely seen following cardiac surgery, even if constrictive physiology occurs. Constrictive pericarditis in her case is most likely idiopathic, the most frequent cause of constrictive pericarditis and most commonly associated with pericardial calcification.[7]*

### 3. How should this patient be treated?

*Treatment of iron deficiency in Eisenmenger syndrome is controversial. Some authors emphasize concern about inducing severe secondary erythropoiesis and hyperviscosity symptoms,[21] and recommend treating with iron supplementation only until the first detectable rise in hematocrit.[22,23] However, practice styles vary, and others have not reported adverse consequences of more complete iron supplementation.[17,24] A reasonable compromise may be to replace iron until the transferrin saturation is within the normal range (>20%). A rise in hemoglobin usually follows within weeks.*

*Should the patient be on warfarin? The rationale for treating the pulmonary artery thrombus with warfarin is not straightforward, particularly given her repeated episodes of hemoptysis (see Case 74). Deaths from warfarin in Eisenmenger patients have been reported. Though anticoagulation has been recommended for decades,[25] there has been no clinical trial showing any benefit of anticoagulation in this setting.[16] This patient was offered warfarin, but her own research into its potential risks and benefits in patients like her made her decline. She is taking aspirin, the benefits of which are similarly unknown in this setting.*

*Treatment of constrictive pericarditis is more problematic. Ideally, the patient would undergo pericardial stripping. But this procedure carries a significant morbidity and mortality even if isolated, and patients with calcific constrictive pericarditis have a higher perioperative mortality compared to patients with constrictive pericarditis without calcification.[8] In a patient with the comorbidities of severe cyanosis and pulmonary vascular disease, these risks are, of course, even greater. In addition, she has not suffered dependent edema or ascites from the constriction, and surgery was not pursued.*

# FINAL DIAGNOSIS

Double-outlet RV

Nonrestrictive VSD

Eisenmenger physiology

Iron deficiency

Constrictive pericarditis

Intramural pulmonary artery thrombosis

# PLAN OF ACTION

Treatment with iron supplementation

Medical management of constriction (as required)

# OUTCOME

The patient began taking ferrous sulfate 200 mg (65 mg of elemental iron) orally twice a day. She developed severe constipation and could not tolerate the drug. Therefore, she was given weekly intravenous iron dextran infusions together with measurement of hemoglobin and transferrin saturation, with a goal to continue until her transferrin saturation rose to above 20% (normal levels). After 6 weeks of injections, she felt much better and did not wish to continue. She took a transcontinental vacation and did well. Though her exercise capacity was still limited, she felt able to resume her usual daily activities.

|  | Base | Wk 2 | Wk 4 | Wk 6 | 5 mo |
|---|---|---|---|---|---|
| Hgb (g/dL) | 17.4 | 17.2 | 18.5 | 19.9 | **20.5** |
| Hct (%) | 55 | 56 | 57 | 62 | **64** |
| MCV (fL) | 77 | 84 | 85 | 85 | 85 |
| Iron (µmol/L) | 9.9 | 5.0 | 7.7 | 11.1 | 11.4 |
| Ferritin (µg/L) | 14 | 18 | 38 | 61 | 22 |
| Transferrin (sat) % | 12 | 6 | 13 | 16 | 14 |

After 5 months, her iron levels had dropped further, but her hemoglobin had climbed. Often repletion of iron initially allows for adequate erythropoiesis, but does not fully replenish normal levels of iron storage, and thus levels may continue to fall after treatment subsides.

With a higher hemoglobin, formal exercise testing was repeated. She exercised for 5 minutes and 39 seconds (4:14 at baseline), reached a heart rate of 162, had a peak $Vo_2$ of 10.3 mL/kg/min (38% of predicted), which represents a small increase from prior testing using an identical protocol. No doubt a significant portion of her continued exercise limitation is due to pulmonary hypertension and/or abnormal filling related to her constrictive pericarditis.

The patient has also since started oral advanced therapy for PAH (see Case 81) with a good clinical response and further objective improvement of her exercise tolerance.

## Selected References

1. Daliento L, Somerville J, Presbitero P, et al: Eisenmenger syndrome: Factors relating to deterioration and death. Eur Heart J 19:1845–1855, 1998.
2. De Kock JP, Reynolds KJ, Tarassenko L, Moyle JT: The effect of varying LED intensity on pulse oximeter accuracy. J Med Eng Technol 15:111–115, 1991.
3. Kaemmerer H, Fratz S, Braun SL, et al: Erythrocyte indexes, iron metabolism, and hyperhomocysteinemia in adults with cyanotic congenital cardiac disease. Am J Cardiol 94:825–828, 2004.
4. Oya H, Nagaya N, Satoh T, et al: Haemodynamic correlates and prognostic significance of serum uric acid in adult patients with Eisenmenger syndrome. Heart 84:53–58, 2000.
5. Gidding SS, Stockman JA 3rd: Effect of iron deficiency on tissue oxygen delivery in cyanotic congenital heart disease. Am J Cardiol 61:605–607, 1988.
6. Gidding SS, Stockman JA 3rd: Erythropoietin in cyanotic heart disease. Am Heart J 116:128–132, 1988.
7. Bertog SE, Thambidorai SK, Parak K, et al: Constrictive pericarditis: Etiology and cause-specific survival after pericardiectomy. J Am Coll Cardiol 43:1445–1452, 2004.
8. Ling LH, Oh JK, Breen JF, et al: Calcific constrictive pericarditis: Is it still with us? Ann Intern Med 132:444–450, 2000.
9. Diller GP, Dimopoulos K, Okonko D, et al: Exercise intolerance in adult congenital heart disease: Comparative severity, correlates, and prognostic implication. Circulation 112:828–835, 2005.
10. Dimopoulos K, Okonko DO, Diller GP, et al: Abnormal ventilatory response to exercise in adults with congenital heart disease relates to cyanosis and predicts survival. Circulation 113:2796–2802, 2006.
11. Engel PJ, Fowler NO, Tei CW, et al: M-mode echocardiography in constrictive pericarditis. J Am Coll Cardiol 6:471–474, 1985.
12. Sengupta PP, Mohan JC, Mehta V, et al: Doppler tissue imaging improves assessment of abnormal interventricular septal and posterior wall motion in constrictive pericarditis. J Am Soc Echocardiogr 18:226–230, 2005.
13. Broberg C, Prasad SK, Gatzoulis MA: The interventricular relationship with Eisenmenger syndrome: Findings with cardiac magnetic resonance and late gadolinium enhancement. J Am Coll Cardiol 49:263A, 2007.
14. Broberg CS, Ujita M, Prasad S, et al: Pulmonary arterial thrombosis in Eisenmenger syndrome is associated with biventricular dysfunction and decreased pulmonary flow velocity. J Am Coll Cardiol 50:634–642, 2007.
15. Silversides CK, Granton JT, Konen E, et al: Pulmonary thrombosis in adults with Eisenmenger syndrome. J Am Coll Cardiol 42:1982–1987, 2003.
16. Broberg C, Ujita M, Babu-Narayan S, et al: Massive pulmonary artery thrombosis with haemoptysis in adults with Eisenmenger's syndrome: A clinical dilemma. Heart 90:e63, 2004.
17. Broberg CS, Bax BE, Okonko DO, et al: Blood viscosity and its relation to iron deficiency, symptoms, and exercise capacity in adults with cyanotic congenital heart disease. J Am Coll Cardiol 48:356–365, 2006.
18. Berman W Jr, Wood SC, Yabek SM, et al: Systemic oxygen transport in patients with congenital heart disease. Circulation 75:360–368, 1987.
19. Diller G-P, Dimopoulos K, Broberg CS, et al: Presentation, survival prospects and predictors of death in Eisenmenger syndrome: A combined retrospective and case control study. Eur Heart J 27:1737–1742, 2006.
20. Broberg C, Jayaweera AR, Diller G, et al: The optimal relationship between resting oxygen saturation and hemoglobin in adult patients with cyanotic congenital heart disease can be determined and correlates with exercise capacity. American Heart Association Scientific Sessions, Atlanta, Ga, November 2006. Circulation 114:II-503, 2006.
21. Rosove MH, Perloff JK, Hocking WG, et al: Chronic hypoxaemia and decompensated erythrocytosis in cyanotic congenital heart disease. Lancet 2:313–315, 1986.
22. Territo MC, Rosove MH: Cyanotic congenital heart disease hematologic management. J Am Coll Cardiol 18:320–322, 1991.
23. Thorne SA: Management of polycythaemia in adults with cyanotic congenital heart disease. Heart 79:315–316, 1998.
24. Gaiha M, Sethi HP, Sudha R, et al: A clinico-hematological study of iron deficiency anemia and its correlation with hyperviscosity symptoms in cyanotic congenital heart disease. Indian Heart J 45:53–55, 1993.
25. Wood P: The Eisenmenger syndrome or pulmonary hypertension with reversed central shunt. BMJ 2:701–709, 1958.

# Management of Acute Hemoptysis

**Erwin Oechslin**

**Age: 36 years**
**Gender: Female**
**Occupation and lifestyle information: Clerk and frequent traveler**
**Working diagnosis: Patent ductus arteriosus and Eisenmenger syndrome**

## HISTORY

The patient was diagnosed with a PDA after she experienced cardiac and pulmonary problems during infancy. At age 5 years, the continuous murmur disappeared and the clinical findings were consistent with PAH. Further investigations were recommended but not performed. There were no follow-up visits.

At age 13, the patient had symptomatic thoracolumbar scoliosis and was considered for surgery. She complained of dyspnea on exertion. Preoperative clinical assessment and heart catheterization confirmed PAH. Pulmonary vascular resistance was at systemic level with no response to vasodilators. Angiograms showed a dilated left pulmonary artery and a hypoplastic right pulmonary artery. In addition, the right lower lobe was fed by an aortopulmonary collateral arising from the abdominal aorta. There was no pulmonary sequestration. With these findings understood, orthopedic surgery was performed. The vertebral column was stabilized with two Harrington rods extending from the distal thoracic into the lumbar region. The perioperative course was uneventful.

At age 32 the patient was diagnosed with restrictive pulmonary disease (forced vital capacity [FVC] 2.0 L, 60% predicted; inspiratory vital capacity 2.0 L, 60% predicted; total lung capacity 3.2 L, 68% predicted; RV 1.2 L, 86% predicted) and moderately reduced CO diffusing capacity (DLCO 4.7 mmol/kPa/min, 54% predicted). Obstructive lung disease was mild (FEV1/FVC 71% predicted).

A 6-minute walk test (6MWT) was performed 2 years later. She walked 450 m. Her oxygen saturation (right fingers) was 90% at rest but fell to 63% after the test. She remained active without noticeable limitation.

Recently, after completing an uneventful 12-hour-long intercontinental flight, the patient felt a "crackling" in her right chest and experienced rapidly progressive, severe dyspnea associated with cough and minor hemoptysis. Intravenous heparin (bolus injection of 5000 units, followed by a continuous infusion of 25,000 units per 24 hours) was administered in a regional hospital. D-dimers were negative. She was treated with 10 L/min supplemental oxygen and 10 mg intravenous furosemide before referral to a tertiary care center for further investigation and therapy.

There was no history of bleeding events, thromboembolic complications, hyperviscosity symptoms, or gouty arthritis. The patient was not a smoker.

***Comments:*** The medical history is characteristic for a patient with an isolated large PDA. Nonrestrictive PDAs are rare in adults living in the developed countries because most nonrestrictive PDAs are diagnosed and closed during childhood. PDAs are more common in females.[1,2] As neonatal pulmonary vascular resistance falls after birth, the left-to-right shunt increases. The affected child may present with left heart failure before the age of 3 months.[3] Congestive heart failure and recurrent pulmonary infections may occur during infancy. In the setting of a nonrestrictive PDA, endothelial injury triggers a cascade of events initiating progressive pulmonary vascular disease. As pulmonary vascular disease progresses and pulmonary vascular resistance increases after the first year of life, the systemic-to-pulmonary shunt decreases. The continuous murmur disappears when pulmonary arterial hypertension is established. The disappearance of this murmur can be misinterpreted as spontaneous PDA closure.

Thoracic deformities (mainly scoliosis and kyphoscoliosis) often cause restrictive pulmonary disease in congenital heart patients. A ventilation–perfusion mismatch may further reduce oxygenation and contribute to symptoms and reduced exercise capacity in these patients.

Patients with Eisenmenger PDA are less symptomatic and have a better long-term outcome than other Eisenmenger patients, especially those with severe pulmonary hypertension and complex disease (truncus arteriosus, atrioventricular septal defect, univentricular connection, transposition complexes, etc.). After left heart failure resolves during infancy, right heart failure may develop during adulthood because of severe PAH. Our patient did not present with right heart failure symptoms or infective endocarditis.

Pulmonary emboli and/or intrapulmonary hemorrhage are the major diagnostic considerations in this setting. On the basis of the medical history, heart failure or pulmonary infection causing dyspnea and hemoptysis is less likely.

## CURRENT SYMPTOMS

The patient's main symptom acutely was severe dyspnea with ongoing hemoptysis.

NYHA class: III

## CURRENT MEDICATIONS

Minulet (oral contraceptive containing 0.075 mg gestoden and 0.03 mg ethinylestradiol)

Heparin 25,000 U intravenously every 24 hours

**Comments:** A reliable method of contraception is essential in a female with Eisenmenger syndrome.[4,5] The benefits of oral contraceptives must be balanced against the risks including systemic hypertension, venous thrombosis, and fluid retention. The patient has been taking this oral contraceptive for many years without any complication. Some ACHD experts would not have supported the use of oral contraceptives in a patient like this. There were case reports of oral contraceptive use being associated with accelerated pulmonary hypertension in the 1960s,[6] but the lower dose preparations used today may not be contraindicated.

Anticoagulation is the therapy of choice in the setting of confirmed pulmonary emboli but is contraindicated in the presence of intrapulmonary hemorrhage.

## IMMUNIZATION STATUS

The patient is immunized against influenza and pneumococcal pneumonia.

**Comments:** Pneumonia is the cause of death in 7% of patients with PAH. Immunization against pneumococcal infections and influenza is recommended.[7]

## PHYSICAL EXAMINATION

BP 130/95 mm Hg, HR 106 bpm, RR 22/min, oxygen saturation at rest 86% (right hand), on room air 80% (feet), increasing to 94% on 10 L/min supplemental oxygen

Height 158 cm, weight 55 kg, BSA 1.55 m$^2$

Surgical scars: Surgical scar on the back

Neck veins: JVP was not elevated (2 cm above sternal angle), with normal A- and V-waves. The hepatojugular reflex was negative.

Lungs/chest: There was moderate kyphoscoliosis and hypoplasia of the right chest. Crackles were present in the right lung. The left lung was clear.

Heart: The heart rhythm was regular (106 bpm). The apex was located in the right sixth intercostal space and was laterally displaced. There was a right ventricular lift. No thrill was present. The first heart sound was normal. The second heart sound was narrowly split with a loud pulmonary component; there was no clear variation with respiration. There was neither a diastolic murmur nor a continuous murmur. Peripheral pulses were normal.

Abdomen: No hepatomegaly

Extremities: Differential cyanosis was present. Toe clubbing was present. There was no edema.

**Comments:** The demonstration of differential cyanosis is diagnostic of an Eisenmenger PDA (see Fig. 73-8).

There is no evidence of right heart failure.

Location of the apex in the right chest suggests dextrocardia.

The second heart sound is typically single in patients with Eisenmenger VSD, because both ventricles act as single ventricle due to the large interventricular communication. The second heart sound is narrowly split with a loud pulmonary component in patients with Eisenmenger PDA.

In general, the second heart sound becomes widely split when RV function is depressed and ejection time prolonged; this phenomenon results from delayed closure of the pulmonary valve.[8]

The loud pulmonary second heart sound and the RV lift are both due to PAH.

## PERTINENT NEGATIVES
There were no findings of infectious disease.

## LABORATORY DATA

|  | Day 1* | Day 2* |
|---|---|---|
| Hemoglobin | **20.7 g/dL** | **17.6 g/dL** (11.5–15.0) |
| Hematocrit/PCV | **62%** | **53%** (36–46) |
| MCV | 97 fL | 96 fL (83–99) |
| Platelet count | $163 \times 10^9$/L | $169 \times 10^9$/L (150–400) |
| Sodium | 141 mmol/L (136–145) | |
| Potassium | 3.7 mmol/L (3.6–4.5) | |
| Creatinine | 0.70 mg/dL (0.6–1.2) | |
| Blood urea nitrogen | 3.6 mmol/L (1.7–8.3) | |
| Ferritin | 29 µg/L (10–150) | |

*Day 1: Day of admission

**Comments:** Secondary erythrocytosis is a physiologic response to chronic hypoxemia and refers to the isolated increase in red blood cells, hemoglobin, and hematocrit as is appropriate in the setting of cyanotic ACHD (this is in contrast to polycythemia rubra vera, which is a proliferative disorder including all three cell lines). There is a close relationship between the degree of secondary erythrocytosis and the severity of hypoxemia.

A hemoglobin of 20.7 g/dL is appropriate for a patient with Eisenmenger PDA and an oxygen saturation of less than 85% in the lower extremities. There was a significant fall in hemoglobin/hematocrit from day 1 to day 2 caused by a major intrapulmonary hemorrhage even though hemoptysis was a minor feature of her presentation. A hemoglobin of 17.6 g/dL is mildly suboptimal in the setting of cyanotic ACHD.[11] There is no evidence of iron depletion since the ferritin is still in the range of normal, although ferritin is an acute phase reactant and thus not entirely accurate during an acute illness. Transferrin saturations would be a better marker under these circumstances.

## OTHER RELEVANT LAB RESULTS

| | |
|---|---|
| CRP | 3 mg/L (<5) |
| ProBNP | **651 ng/L** (<153) |
| CK | 52 U/L (<167) |
| Troponin | <0.01 µg/L (<0.10) |
| INR* | **1.4** (<1.2) |

*The amount of sodium citrate was appropriately adjusted to hematocrit.

**Comments:** The mildly elevated INR (1.4) is the result of reduced vitamin-K-dependent clotting factors (II, VII, IX, X) in patients with cyanotic ACHD. A low platelet count is frequently observed in this population.

Laboratory precautions are required for accurate measurement of the coagulation parameters in cyanotic patients because secondary erythrocytosis increases hematocrit and decreases plasma volume. Adjustment of the amount of liquid anticoagulants is essential for accurate measurement of the coagulation parameters.[12–14]

ACHD is a chronic heart failure syndrome, which is reflected by the mildly elevated proBNP.[15] However, this proBNP level is far too low to support the diagnosis of dyspnea due to heart failure in this patient. The mildly elevated proBNP is caused by the severely increased RV systolic pressure.

## ELECTROCARDIOGRAM

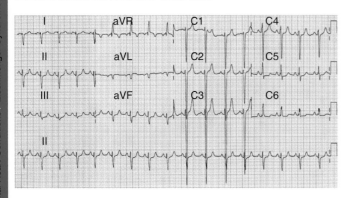

Figure 73-1 Electrocardiogram.

### FINDINGS

Heart rate: 100 bpm

QRS axis: +210°

PR interval: 148 msec

QRS duration: 92 msec

Sinus rhythm with a tall P-wave (2.5 mm in lead II); peaked P-waves are evident in lead C4–6. There is precordial voltage evidence of LV hypertrophy, not supported elsewhere.

***Comments:*** It is crucial to confirm the position of both the limb and precordial leads before interpretation of the ECG. In the setting of situs solitus with dextrocardia, the limb leads are left unchanged and the precordial leads are recorded from the right anterior chest.[16] This lead position is appropriate because the atrial situs is normal (i.e., the sinus node is located at the junction of the right SVC and the morphologic RA on the right) and the base-to-apex axis points to the right. In situs solitus with dextrocardia, the atrium is depolarized from a normally positioned sinus node.

In all patients with dextrocardia, ECG interpretation depends on knowledge of the lead positions used regardless of what they were.

The biphasic P-wave in lead I may be caused by the abnormal position of the heart because of kyphoscoliosis. Accuracy of the ECG interpretation is limited in the presence of severe thoracic deformity.

## CHEST X-RAY

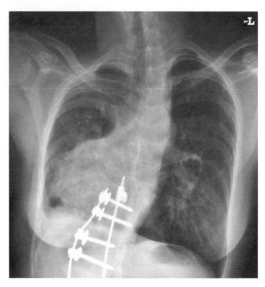

Figure 73-2 Posteroanterior projection.

### FINDINGS

Cardiothoracic ratio: 54%

There is abdominal situs solitus (left-sided stomach bubble). The cardiac shadow is predominantly located in the right chest and is to the right of the midline (dextroposition), and the apex seems to point to the right (dextrocardia). The aortic arch is left-sided. Hypoplasia of the right chest is present. The cardiac silhouette is poorly delineated from the diaphragm consistent with retrocardial acinar consolidation. The right heart silhouette is not clear. A right pleural effusion may be present. The left lung is clear.

The left pulmonary artery is enlarged, and the pulmonary vessels narrow toward the periphery of the lungs ("pruning"). Kyphoscoliosis is evident, and two Harrington rods extending from the distal thoracic to the lumbar region are in place. There is a malformation of the ribs (right- and left-sided ribs 6 and 7 are bifurcated).

***Comments:*** Bronchial and abdominal situs are a good guide to identify atrial morphology, because there is concordance between atrial and bronchial/abdominal morphology. There is abdominal situs solitus: the liver is on the right, the stomach on the left. Bronchial bifurcation is also normal, reflecting situs solitus of the lungs. Thus, there is cardiac situs solitus.[16] This is also supported by the same (left-sided) location of the descending aorta (left-sided aortic arch), LA, and stomach bubble.

Cardiac position describes the location of the heart within the chest with respect to its location (levo-, dextro-, and mesoposition) *and* the orientation of the apex: levocardia (base-apex axis to the left; left hemidiaphragm lower than the right), dextrocardia (base-apex axis to the right; right hemidiaphragm lower than the left), and mesocardia (base-apex axis in the midline). There is dextroposition and there seems to be dextrocardia; however, the right hemidiaphragm is higher than the left hemidiaphragm indicating the apex is not on the right. This interpretation is limited by the thoracic deformity. The base-to-apex axis is best described by echocardiography or MRI using the apical and subcostal four-chamber views.

The cardiothoracic ratio must be interpreted cautiously because of the thoracic deformity. Meticulous evaluation for potential thoracic deformities is important in patients with congenital heart disease.

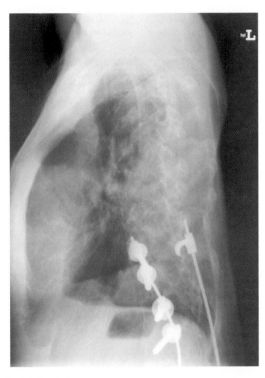

Figure 73-3 Lateral view.

## FINDINGS

The thoracic deformity is evident. Two Harrington rods are in place. There is no clear calcification in the area of the PDA. There is retrosternal filling in keeping with RV dilatation and hypertrophy.

**Comments:** The lateral projection adds limited information on this occasion.

## EXERCISE TESTING

Not performed

# ECHOCARDIOGRAM

## OVERALL FINDINGS

There was cardiac situs solitus (the morphologic RA is on the right to the morphologic LA). This subcostal view provides a perfect apical four-chamber view suggesting mesocardia (base-apex axis is in the midline).

The atrioventricular connection and ventriculoarterial connection (not shown) were concordant. There was concentric hypertrophy and normal systolic function of the RV.

The right ventricular systolic pressure was 108 mm Hg over right atrial pressure, and the RA pressure was estimated to be 5 mm Hg; RV systolic pressure is calculated at 113 mm Hg (systolic blood pressure was 124 mm Hg on the right arm at that time); tricuspid regurgitation was trace. There was no obstruction of the RVOT. LV size and systolic function were normal.

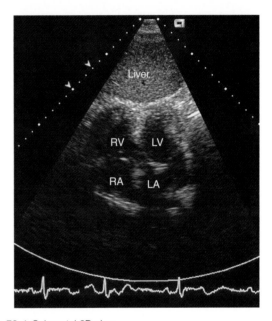

Figure 73-4 Subcostal 2D view.

**Comments:** A perfect apical four-chamber view obtained from the subcostal window indicates mesocardia. However, severe thoracic deformity limits any information regarding cardiac orientation (base-apex axis). All other image modalities indicate dextrocardia.

Atypical additional views are required to obtain adequate images to interpret the anatomy/morphology in patients with congenital heart disease and thoracic deformity. A patient with dextrocardia should be examined in the right lateral position.

RVOT obstruction has to be excluded in the presence of an elevated RV pressure. If pulmonary hypertension is present, systemic systolic pressure must be measured at the same time to calculate the ratio between the pulmonary and systemic systolic pressures.

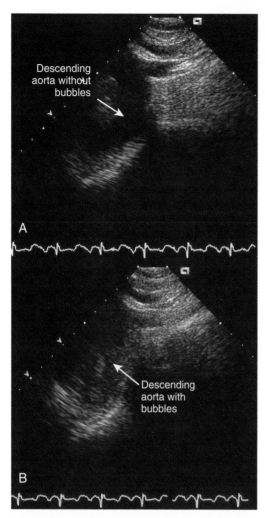

Figure 73-5 Suprasternal view. Two-dimensional echo before and after injection of agitated saline.

## FINDINGS

Descending aorta before injection of agitated saline (*A*); descending aorta after injection of agitated saline (*B*).

Agitated saline was injected in the right brachial vein (bubble study). The bubbles appeared in the RA, RV, and pulmonary artery, but no bubbles appeared in the LA, LV, ascending aorta, and aortic arch. However, bubbles appeared in the descending aorta early after injection.

***Comments:*** Bubbles appearing in the descending aorta indicate a right-to-left shunt at the arterial level between the pulmonary artery and proximal descending aorta (PDA).

Image quality of the parasternal and apical views is poor due to severe chest deformity and two Harrington rods extending from the distal thoracic to the lumbar region.

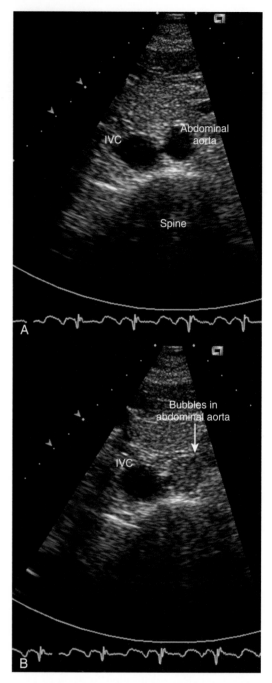

Figure 73-6 Subcostal view with probe perpendicular to spine. Two-dimensional echo before and after injection of agitated saline.

## FINDINGS

Abdominal aorta before injection of agitated saline (*A*); abdominal aorta after injection of agitated saline (*B*).

Agitated saline was injected in the right brachial vein (bubble study). There were no bubbles in the LA, LV, and ascending aorta/aortic arch. However, bubbles appeared in the descending aorta and abdominal aorta.

The relative position of the great vessels just below the diaphragm helps to identify cardiac situs. The IVC is located to the right of the abdominal aorta (situs solitus). The location of the IVC and abdominal aorta is atypical because of severe thoracic deformity.

***Comments:*** Bubbles appearing in the abdominal aorta indicate a right-to-left shunt at the arterial level (PDA).

# COMPUTED TOMOGRAPHY

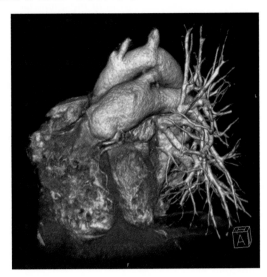

Figure 73-7 Three-dimensional reconstruction of the computed tomography scan of the heart and great arteries.

## FINDINGS

The large PDA (14 mm) entered the aorta distal to the origin of the left subclavian artery. The branching of the left pulmonary artery and left pulmonary veins was nicely visualized. The arteries arising from the left-sided aortic arch were normal.

***Comments:*** This 3D reconstruction visualizes very clearly the anatomic and hemodynamic background of differential cyanosis in patients with Eisenmenger PDA and reversed (right-to-left) shunt (see also Fig. 73-8). The thoracic aorta distal to the origin of the left subclavian artery receives desaturated blood from the pulmonary artery, which is delivered to the lower extremities. Differential cyanosis is missed when the cyanotic feet are not examined.

The subclavian and carotid arteries are fed by oxygenated blood. The presence of leg fatigue and the relative lack of dyspnea in patients with Eisenmenger PDA are typical and are caused by the exercise-induced increase in right-to-left shunt and cyanosis in the lower limbs; in contrast, hypoxia-induced stimulation of the respiratory system and carotid body is precluded in Eisenmenger PDA, but not in other causes of Eisenmenger syndrome.[12]

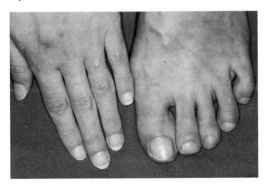

Figure 73-8 Differential cyanosis. (From Oechslin E: Zyanose. In Siegenthaler W [ed]: Differenzialdiagnose, 19th ed. Auflage, Georg Thieme Verlag, 2005, Fig. 21.20B, p 710.)

## FINDINGS

This picture was taken 1 year before the current problem and shows the differential cyanosis: The fingers are pink, the toes are cyanotic. Clubbing of the toes is minimal.

***Comments:*** Differential cyanosis is diagnostic of a reversed (right-to-left) shunt due to pulmonary hypertension in patients with an Eisenmenger PDA.

The anatomic substrate to explain the mechanism of differential cyanosis is presented in Figure 73-7.

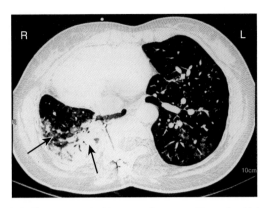

Figure 73-9 Chest computed tomography scan with contrast injection.

## FINDINGS

Pulmonary emboli and thrombus formation were excluded.

There was extensive acinar consolidation consistent with intrapulmonary hemorrhage in the right lower lobe (*black arrows*). There were also minor opacifications in the other lobes of both lungs (aspiration).

The main pulmonary artery (not seen in this view) measured 31 mm in diameter. The left pulmonary artery was dominant (21 mm in diameter), the right pulmonary artery was hypoplastic (12 mm in diameter). There was no pulmonary artery aneurysm.

Dextrocardia was present.

***Comments:*** The first important question is to exclude pulmonary emboli in a patient with rapidly progressive dyspnea after a long-distance flight (and thus at risk for deep vein thrombosis). Secondly, adults with Eisenmenger syndrome are at risk for thrombus formation in the enlarged or aneurysmal proximal pulmonary arteries.[10,17-19]

The extensive intrapulmonary hemorrhage in the right lower lobe is the cause for the rapidly progressive dyspnea and the minor hemoptysis. Opacifications in the other lobes are probably caused by blood aspiration.

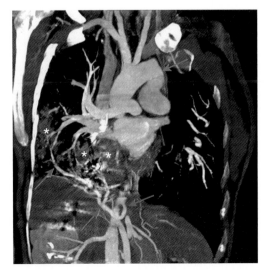

Figure 73-10 Chest computed tomography scan with contrast injection.

## FINDINGS

The MAPCA (*red arrows*) arising from the abdominal aorta (just proximal to the celiac trunk) and passing through the liver (segment VII/VIII) was the main finding. It branched immediately before passing through the diaphragm and fed the right lower lobe. Acinar consolidation (asterisks) was visualized in the right lower lobe. The aortic arch with its normal branching pattern was left sided. Active bleeding could not be visualized.

The nonrestrictive connection between the left pulmonary artery and the proximal descending aorta was visualized (*green arrow*).

**Comments:** MAPCAs arising from the abdominal aorta are rare in the setting of isolated PDA.[20,21] The importance of these MAPCAs in isolated PDA is not clear; they may contribute to LV volume overload and heart failure during infancy. MAPCAs occur in the setting of impaired pulmonary blood flow, which may have been the case in our patient with hypoplasia of the right pulmonary artery. MAPCAs are frequently seen in patients with pulmonary atresia and VSD.

The histologic structure of the MAPCAs is different from that of normal arteries. MAPCAs are fragile and may rupture. These MAPCAs in the right lower lobe are the likely source of the intrapulmonary hemorrhage and minor hemoptysis.

## CATHETERIZATION

Not performed

## FOCUSED CLINICAL QUESTIONS AND DISCUSSION POINTS

1. What was the cause of intrapulmonary hemorrhage in this patient?

*Pulmonary hemorrhage may be caused by pulmonary infection or pulmonary infarction secondary to pulmonary emboli originating from the proximal pulmonary arteries.[10,17–19] Pulmonary emboli and infarction may also be caused by thromboembolism from deep vein thrombosis. However, there was no clinical evidence of deep vein thrombosis or of pulmonary emboli by CT scan.*

*The rupture of pulmonary artery aneurysms is usually fatal. MAPCAs are fragile and can rupture and cause pulmonary hemorrhage. This is the likely cause of intrapulmonary bleeding in our patient. The role of the long-distance flight is not known.*

*Hemoptysis is the external manifestation of a respiratory hemorrhage and does not reflect the extent of the intrapulmonary hemorrhage at all. The patient had only minor hemoptysis, which one might erroneously assume indicated a minor hemorrhage. However, the severity of dyspnea and the significant fall of hemoglobin drew attention to a more serious problem. There is frequently a discrepancy between the amount of external and internal bleeding as in our patient.*

2. Is hemoptysis life-threatening?

*Every hemoptysis must be regarded as potentially life-threatening (approximately 8% of Eisenmenger patients will eventually die of hemoptysis[17]; although most episodes are minor and self-limiting. These events require meticulous evaluation.[11,12,22–27]*

3. What is the first diagnostic step to evaluate an Eisenmenger patient with hemoptysis?

*The CXR is the first diagnostic step. If there is no acinar consolidation or infiltration, further imaging modalities do not add any information to the management and are not required. However,*

*a CT scan is required in the presence of an acinar consolidation or infiltration to assess the severity of intrapulmonary hemorrhage or to visualize thrombus formation in situ in the proximal pulmonary arteries.[10,17–19] Bronchoscopy does not have any diagnostic or therapeutic role in this setting. The procedure may harm the patient (worsen hemorrhage due to increase in intrapulmonary pressure or increase shunt and cyanosis from sedation) without providing useful information, and should be avoided.*

4. What are the general therapeutic measures in treating acute hemoptysis in a patient with Eisenmenger syndrome?

*The patient should optimally be admitted to a tertiary care referral center whenever a consolidation or infiltration is present on the chest radiograph.[23,25] If there is no infiltration and the external bleeding (hemoptysis) is only minor, the patient may be treated as an outpatient, although the threshold for hospital admission should be low.*

*Physical activity must be reduced (typically bed rest) and the patient kept calm in a quiet room. Any cough must be suppressed with medication. The patient should be positioned on the ipsilateral side of the bleeding to avoid blood aspiration into the contralateral lung.*

*Aspirin, nonsteroidal anti-inflammatory drugs, and oral anticoagulants must be discontinued. Because cyanotic patients are known to have hemostatic abnormalities[12–14] any deficiency that might impair hemostasis must be corrected. Specifically, this may include administration of platelets, especially if platelet count is less than 100,000/μL, or administration of fresh frozen plasma, factor VIII, vitamin K, desmopressin, and so on.*

*Although the hematocrit and hemoglobin may remain supranormal, one must consider that the value may be inappropriately low depending on the degree of cyanosis. In this patient, a drop in hemoglobin was noted even with only mild hemoptysis. Transfusion may be warranted to restore oxygen-carrying capacity to appropriate levels.*

*Pulmonary infectious disease may cause hemoptysis and must be treated appropriately. Sputum culture should be taken in the presence of suspected infection.*

5. Is there a role for transcutaneous intervention?

*The majority of hemorrhagic episodes will eventually self-terminate. If the hemorrhage continues, angiography to identify the culprit vessel may be an option. Selective embolization of the vessel supplying the source of blood loss (often bronchial artery collaterals), if identified, may be considered in the setting of severe and/or incessant bleeding (see Case 74). This is a procedure that should be performed by an interventionalist with expertise in congenital heart disease at a high-volume referral center. Though successful case reports exist, data on the mid- to long-term benefits of this approach are not available.*

6. Is there any role for oral anticoagulants in this cyanotic patient with secondary erythrocytosis to prevent thromboembolic complications long term?

*Secondary erythrocytosis is a physiologic response to chronic hypoxemia and is not a risk factor per se for thromboembolic events.[14,28,29] The patient never experienced thromboembolic complications or sustained supraventricular arrhythmias, which may be an indication for oral anticoagulation. Laboratory precautions have to be considered in cyanotic patients with secondary erythrocytosis.[12–14] Although debates about the use of anticoagulants in Eisenmenger syndrome are ongoing,[17] there are no data to support their routine use.*

## FINAL DIAGNOSIS

Situs solitus with dextrocardia and dextroposition

PDA with Eisenmenger syndrome

MAPCA arising from the proximal abdominal artery and supplying the right lower lobe

Intrapulmonary hemorrhage in the right lower lobe presumably from a ruptured MAPCA

## PLAN OF ACTION

Hospital admission, bed rest, monitoring of vital signs, suppression of nonproductive cough

## INTERVENTION

None

## OUTCOME

The clinical condition and course of the patient remained stable after hospital admission without any additional intervention. She was discharged home 5 days later.

Iron supplements were not prescribed because the major bleeding was internal and there was no external loss of iron.

Physiotherapy as an outpatient was organized.

Paracetamol/acetaminophen was prescribed, as nonsteroidal anti-inflammatory drugs were contraindicated.

The patient was reassessed 6 weeks after discharge. There were no further episodes of hemoptysis. Her clinical condition and exercise tolerance improved dramatically (NYHA class II). Her oxygen saturation was 93% on room air measured in the right hand and 85% in the toes. Her hemoglobin/hematocrit had increased to an appropriate level. There was no hematological evidence of iron deficiency.

### LABORATORY DATA

| | |
|---|---|
| Hemoglobin | **19.8 g/dL** (11.5–15.0) |
| Hematocrit/PCV | **60%** (36–46) |
| MCV | 96 fL (83–99) |
| Platelet count | $245 \times 10^9$/L (150–400) |
| ProBNP | **443 ng/L** (<153) |

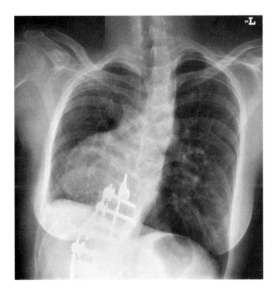

Figure 73-11 Posteroanterior projection.

### FINDINGS

Cardiothoracic ratio: 53%

In contrast to the CXR on admission, the right cardiac silhouette was clearly delineated. There was a clear delineation between the diaphragm and the cardiac silhouette as well. Otherwise, the findings were unchanged.

**Comments:** The acinar consolidations on the conventional CXR have resolved.

## ACKNOWLEDGMENTS

The author acknowledges Dr. R. Jenni, Echocardiography Laboratory, and Dr. B. Marincek, Institute of Diagnostic Radiology, University Hospital, Zurich, Switzerland. This chapter was written when Dr. Oechslin was Section Head of the Adult Congenital Heart Disease Program at this institution.

## Selected References

1. Campbell M: Natural history of patent ductus arteriosus. Br Heart J 30:4–13, 1968.
2. Perloff JK: Patent ductus arteriosus. In Perloff JK (ed): Clinical Recognition of Congenital Heart Disease, 5th ed. Philadelphia, WB Saunders, 2003, pp 403–429.
3. Peirone AR, Benson LN: The patent arterial duct. In Freedom RM, Yoo SJ, Mikaillan H, Williams WG (eds): The Natural and Modified History of Congenital Heart Disease. New York, Blackwell, 2004, pp 72–90.
4. Connolly HM, Warnes CA: Pregnancy and contraception. In Gatzoulis MA, Webb GD, Daubeney PEF (eds): Diagnosis and Management of Adult Congenital Heart Disease. London, Churchill Livingstone, 2003, pp 135–144.
5. Warnes CA: Pregnancy and pulmonary hypertension. Int J Cardiol 97:11–13, 2004.
6. Oakley C, Somerville J: Oral contraceptives and progressive pulmonary vascular disease. Lancet 1:890–893, 1968.
7. Galie N, Torbicki A, Barst R, et al: Guidelines on diagnosis and treatment of pulmonary arterial hypertension of the European Society of Cardiology. Eur Heart J 25:2243–2278, 2004.
8. Constant J: Essentials of Bedside Cardiology, 2nd ed. Totowa, NY, Humana Press, 2003, p 150.
9. Perloff JK: The cardiac malpositions. In Perloff JK (ed): Clinical Recognition of Congenital Heart Disease, 5th ed. Philadelphia, WB Saunders, 2003, pp 17–45.
10. Perloff JK, Hart EM, Greaves SM, et al: Proximal pulmonary arterial and intrapulmonary radiologic features of Eisenmenger syndrome and primary pulmonary hypertension. Am J Cardiol 92:182–187, 2003.
11. Broberg C, Jayaweera AR, Diller G, et al: The optimal relationship between resting oxygen saturation and hemoglobin in adult patients with cyanotic congenital heart disease can be determined and correlates with exercise capacity. American Heart Association Scientific Sessions, Atlanta, Ga, November 2006. Circulation 114:II-503, 2006.
12. Perloff JK, Rosove MH, Sietsema KE, Territo MC: Cyanotic congenital heart disease: A multisystem disorder. In Perloff JK, Child JS (eds): Congenital Heart Disease in Adults, 2nd ed. Philadelphia, WB Saunders, 1998, pp 199–266.
13. Oechslin E: Eisenmenger's syndrome. In Gatzoulis MA, Webb GD, Daubeney PEF (eds): Diagnosis and Management of Adult Congenital Heart Disease. London, Churchill Livingstone, 2003, pp 363–377.
14. Oechslin E: Hematological management of the cyanotic adult with congenital heart disease. Int J Cardiol 97(Suppl 1):109–115, 2004.
15. Bolger AP, Sharma R, Li W, et al: Neurohormonal activation and the chronic heart failure syndrome in adults with congenital heart disease. Circulation 106:92–99, 2002.
16. Colman J, Oechslin E, Taylor D: Glossary of terms, prepared for the CCS Consensus Conference 2001 update: Recommendations for the Management of Adults with Congenital Heart Disease. Available at http://www.achd-library.com/consensus/glossary.html.
17. Broberg CS, Ujita M, Prasad S, et al: Pulmonary arterial thrombosis in Eisenmenger syndrome is associated with biventricular dysfunction and decreased pulmonary flow velocity. J Am Coll Cardiol 50:634–642, 2007.

18. Niwa K, Perloff JK, Kaplan S, et al: Eisenmenger syndrome in adults: Ventricular septal defect, truncus arteriosus, univentricular heart. J Am Coll Cardiol 34:223–232, 1999.

19. Silversides CK, Granton JT, Konen E, et al: Pulmonary thrombosis in adults with Eisenmenger syndrome. J Am Coll Cardiol 42:1982–1987, 2003.

20. Birnbacher R, Proll E, Kohlhauser C, et al: Echocardiographic evidence of aortopulmonary collaterals in premature infants after closure of ductus arteriosus. Am J Perinatol 15:561–565, 1998.

21. Ing FF, Laskari C, Bierman FZ: Additional aortopulmonary collaterals in patients referred for coil occlusion of a patent ductus arteriosus. Cathet Cardiovasc Diagn 37:5–8, 1996.

22. Daliento L, Somerville J, Presbitero P, et al: Eisenmenger syndrome: Factors relating to deterioration and death. Eur Heart J 19:1845–1855, 1998.

23. Deanfield J, Thaulow E, Warnes CA, et al: Management of Grown-Up Congenital Heart Disease. Eur Heart J 24:1035–1084, 2003.

24. Oechslin EN, Harrison DA, Connelly MS, et al: Mode of death in adults with congenital heart disease. Am J Cardiol 86:1111–1116, 2000.

25. Therrien J, Warnes C, Daliento L, et al: Canadian Cardiovascular Society Consensus Conference 2001 update: Recommendations for the management of adults with congenital heart disease—part III. Can J Cardiol 17:1135–1158, 2001.

26. Vongpatanasin W, Brickner ME, Hillis LD, Lange RA: The Eisenmenger syndrome in adults. Ann Intern Med 128:745–755, 1998.

27. Somerville J: How to treat the Eisenmenger syndrome. Int J Cardiol 63:1–8, 1998.

28. Ammash N, Warnes CA: Cerebrovascular events in adult patients with cyanotic congenital heart disease. J Am Coll Cardiol 28:768–772, 1996.

29. Perloff JK, Marelli AJ, Miner PD: Risk of stroke in adults with cyanotic congenital heart disease. Circulation 87:1954–1959, 1993.

# Pulmonary Artery Thrombosis and Recurrent Hemoptysis in Eisenmenger Syndrome

**Craig S. Broberg**

**Age: 18 years**
**Gender: Male**
**Occupation: Student**
**Working diagnosis: Down syndrome with unrepaired atrial septal defect**

## HISTORY

The patient was known to have a congenital heart defect at birth. His parents remember being told that there were no means available to repair the defect safely. The child grew typically for one with Down syndrome. He had become a happy, energetic young man. He participated regularly at a special education facility and enjoyed theater and sports.

Cyanosis had been noted since his early childhood in both hands and feet, but otherwise he had no specific complaints. After an attack of gout he was started on allopurinol.

Eighteen months prior to presentation he coughed up a large volume of blood while resting at home. He collapsed unconscious onto the floor but regained consciousness soon thereafter. He was rushed to a nearby hospital, where intermittent hemoptysis continued over the next several hours. However, the bleeding subsided, and eventually he was sent home. Imaging showed a severely dilated pulmonary artery. Echocardiography demonstrated a large ASD, and a hypertrophied RV with normal function.

Over the ensuing months, the patient experienced several more episodes of hemoptysis. The episodes usually occurred while at home, and not in association with significant exertion or medical illness. On several of these occasions he was again observed to lose consciousness temporarily. On each occasion he was watched closely in either his local hospital or the regional tertiary care center, and bleeding subsided with bed rest and oxygen.

He was seen in the outpatient setting for consultation about how to best resolve the recurring hemoptysis.

**Comments:** Down syndrome, or trisomy 21, is the most common chromosomal abnormality occurring in roughly 1 in 700 live births.[1] Early mortality can be as high as 10% to 20%, and is nearly always attributable to CHD.[2]

Although Down syndrome should never be considered a rationale to not offer a patient a surgical correction of a heart defect, surgical correction was not always offered to these patients.

The patient has probably developed Eisenmenger physiology. However, his only known shunt is an ASD, which would not necessarily be expected to cause Eisenmenger syndrome at all or this early.[3] One therefore should be suspicious that there may be another shunt.

High uric acid levels can be seen in cyanotic heart disease. Allopurinol is indicated as chronic therapy only if episodes of acute gout occur (for secondary prevention) but is not recommended otherwise.

The acute management of hemoptysis is discussed elsewhere (see Case 73). Hemoptysis in a pulmonary hypertensive patient should prompt a focused search for a specific and treatable cause. The patient should receive oxygen and blood products (latter not usually necessary) if needed. Bronchoscopy should be avoided. The loss of consciousness here was felt to have been vagal, rather than reflecting an arrhythmia. No evidence of sustained arrhythmia was ever noted.

## CURRENT SYMPTOMS

The patient had fairly good exercise tolerance. He would complain to family members of dyspnea only after walking for 20 minutes or so on flat ground. Otherwise, he pursued any activity he wished, including climbing steps. He had mild joint aches on occasion. He denied palpitations or syncope other than during hemoptysis.

NYHA class: I–II

**Comments:** Bouts of hemoptysis are usually not predictable by any premonitory symptoms.

## CURRENT MEDICATIONS

Allopurinol 300 mg daily

## PHYSICAL EXAMINATION

BP 112/70 mm Hg, HR 93 bpm, oxygen saturation 82% (finger), 83% (toes)

Height 160 cm, weight 56 kg, BSA 1.58 m$^2$

Surgical scars: None

Neck veins: Jugular venous waveform was normal. There was no elevation of the central venous pressure.

Lungs/chest: Clear in all fields

Heart: Regular rate and rhythm with normal first heart sound and a loud pulmonary component of the second heart sound. There was a right ventricular lift. No systolic or diastolic murmurs were audible.

Abdomen: Soft, not tender, with no organomegaly present

Extremities: Clubbing and cyanosis were visible in all nail beds. The skin was warm and dry.

**Comments:** The findings here are all consistent with a stable patient with Eisenmenger syndrome, namely cyanosis, clubbing, an RV lift, and a loud second heart sound.

## LABORATORY DATA

| | |
|---|---|
| Hemoglobin | 16 g/dL (13.0–17.0) |
| Hematocrit/PCV | **55%** (41–51) |
| MCV | 84 fL (83–99) |
| Platelet count | **75 × 10⁹/L** (150–400) |
| Sodium | 141 mmol/L (134–145) |
| Potassium | 4.2 mmol/L (3.5–5.2) |
| Creatinine | 1.1 mg/dL (0.6–1.2) |
| Blood urea nitrogen | **6.9 mmol/L** (2.5–6.5) |

### OTHER RELEVANT LAB RESULTS

| | |
|---|---|
| Iron | **8.5 µmol/L** (12.6–26.0) |
| Ferritin | **19 µg/L** (30–233) |
| Transferrin sat | **18%** (20–45) |

**Comments:** Although the hemoglobin and hematocrit are high, they are inappropriately low for the level of hypoxemia in this patient, whose hemoglobin should be in the 20 to 22 range. A reasonable prediction of optimal hemoglobin would in this case give an estimate of 21 g/dL. Despite the normal MCV, the patient has iron deficiency. MCV is not a reliable screening tool for iron deficiency in cyanotic heart disease.[5] Serum ferritin for a stable patient and transferrin saturation under most circumstances are better markers of iron deficiency and should be routinely requested for patients with chronic cyanosis and secondary erythrocytosis.

Frequent hemoptysis is likely to be contributory to both iron deficiency and the relatively low hematocrit. It is advisable to have baseline laboratory values for all patients for comparison during an acute episode such as hemoptysis; blood products to correct abnormalities during an acute episode may occasionally be required.

## ELECTROCARDIOGRAM

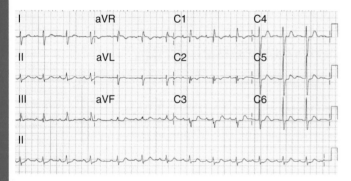

Figure 74-1 Electrocardiogram.

### FINDINGS
Heart rate: 76 bpm

QRS axis: +147°

QRS duration: 119 msec

Sinus rhythm with first-degree AV block. Right-axis deviation with RV hypertrophy.

**Comments:** These are typical findings of Eisenmenger syndrome, with right-axis deviation and RV hypertrophy. There is no evidence of left-axis deviation as might be expected in the AVSD most typically seen in Down syndrome (a superior axis is present in 95% of patients with AVSD).

## CHEST X-RAY

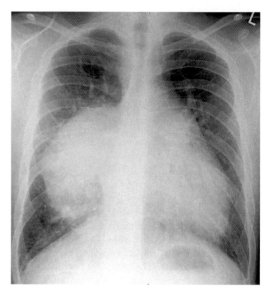

Figure 74-2 Posteroanterior projection.

### FINDINGS
Cardiothoracic ratio: 63%

Note the RA border, seen better at its mid/lower part, against the massive dilatation of the right pulmonary artery.

Cardiomegaly is present. There is enlargement of the main pulmonary artery. The discrete bulge in the right chest, the inferior aspect of which is calcified, is the giant right pulmonary artery.

**Comments:** This dramatic CXR reflects mostly a giant aneurysm of the right pulmonary artery. Sometimes seen in patients with PAH, in the Eisenmenger setting one may suspect the presence of thrombus within the aneurysm, as in this case.[6] (See Fig. 74-5.)

The cardiothoracic ratio can be difficult to determine in cases such as this, but the right atrial border in this instance is still visible.

## EXERCISE TESTING

Not performed

**Comments:** Recurrent hemoptysis may be considered a relative contraindication to exercise testing. Although the risk is unproven, fear of inducing further hemoptysis by increased ventilation may deter clinicians from ordering the test, at least until the patient is stable.

# ECHOCARDIOGRAM

## OVERALL FINDINGS

There was a large ASD with predominant right-to-left shunting. The RV was severely hypertrophied with preserved systolic function. The LV had mildly reduced systolic function. There was no VSD. There was no significant mitral or tricuspid regurgitation.

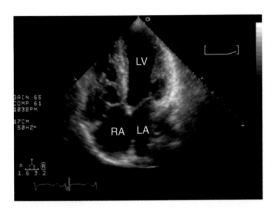

Figure 74-3 Apical four-chamber 2D echo.

## FINDINGS

Severe RV hypertrophy and a large ASD were seen.

**Comments:** There is no evidence of an AVSD as is commonly seen in Down syndrome. Note the normal alignment ("offset") of the tricuspid and mitral valve planes.

Although large, the size of the atrial defect here would not normally be expected to cause pulmonary hypertension,[3] as defects of this size are frequently encountered in older adults (see Case 2). On the other hand, patients with Down syndrome have a greater likelihood of developing pulmonary hypertension in general, even due to other causes such as obstructive sleep apnea. Furthermore, the presence of another cause of PAH such as a large PDA must be excluded.

# MAGNETIC RESONANCE IMAGING

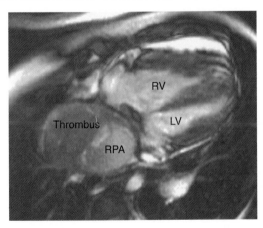

Figure 74-4 Oblique axial plane steady-state free precession cine, four-chamber view.

## Ventricular Volume Quantification

|  | LV | (Normal range) | RV | (Normal range) |
|---|---|---|---|---|
| EDV (mL) | 138 | (77–195) | 126 | (88–227) |
| ESV (mL) | 83 | (19–72) | 68 | (23–103) |
| SV (mL) | 55 | (51–133) | 58 | (52–138) |
| EF (%) | 40 | (57–74) | 46 | (48–74) |
| EDVi (mL/m²) | 87 | (68–103) | 80 | (68–114) |
| ESVi (mL/m²) | 53 | (19–41) | 43 | (21–50) |
| SVi (mL/m²) | 35 | (44–68) | 37 | (40–72) |
| Mass index (g/m²) | 100 | (59–93) | 85 | (23–50) |

## FINDINGS

The RV was hypertrophied with preserved systolic function. The LV was normal in size with mildly to moderately reduced systolic function. There was no VSD. Within the right pulmonary artery a large thrombus was seen adherent to the vessel wall. The Qp/Qs ratio was 1.06. The exam was complicated by the patient's difficulty with breath-holding instructions.

**Comments:** Quality MR imaging requires good patient cooperation with breath holding, which can occasionally be a limitation for this imaging modality in a patient with developmental delay. Nevertheless, many patients do fine. Ventricular volumes here are consistent with the echocardiographic findings.

Causes of LV dysfunction in Eisenmenger syndrome are not well understood and are likely multifactorial. LV dysfunction has been found to correlate with the presence of large pulmonary artery thrombi.[7] The Qp/Qs ratio of essentially 1 is not uncommon in Eisenmenger syndrome, although with advanced age it tends to fall as the right-to-left shunt increases. The RV and LV tend to be similar in ventricular volumes and size in stable Eisenmenger patients before clinical decompensation ensues.[7]

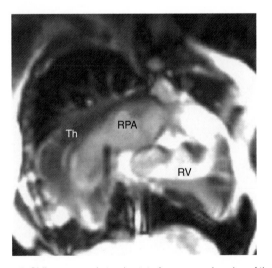

Figure 74-5 Oblique coronal steady-state free precession cine of the right pulmonary artery (RPA). Th, thrombus.

## FINDINGS

The right pulmonary artery was aneurysmal, and a large thrombus was seen adherent to the vessel wall.

**Comments:** Varying signal within the thrombus suggested layered thrombus of different ages. Typically, these thrombi organize in situ, rather than originating from an embolic source.

## COMPUTED TOMOGRAPHY

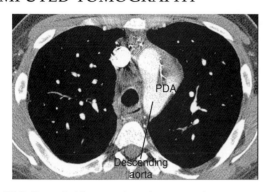

Figure 74-6 Computed tomography pulmonary angiogram.

### FINDINGS

A large PDA is present.

**Comments:** A CT angiogram should demonstrate unequivocally the presence of a PDA. PDA is one of many common congenital defects encountered in Down syndrome patients, occurring in as many as 29% of cases.[8]

In this case, it clearly explains the PAH and the development of Eisenmenger physiology. The absence of differential cyanosis is not surprising because bidirectional shunting occurs at the atrial level, and the patient is relatively young and thus the degree of right-to-left shunting at the PDA level has not reached its "peak."

Furthermore, there is evidence of an extensive bronchial collateral vessel network.

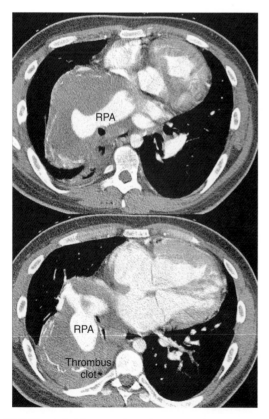

Figure 74-7 Computed tomography pulmonary angiogram.

### FINDINGS

The right pulmonary artery was severely dilated, and a large laminar thrombus occupied approximately two thirds of the lumen.

**Comments:** Large thrombi have been described in roughly one fourth of patients with Eisenmenger syndrome,[6,7,9,10] which is a much higher prevalence than in patients with other forms of PAH. Risk factors for this are not well understood. The size of the pulmonary artery is a risk factor for in situ thrombosis, as in this dramatic example, as it is associated with deceleration of blood flow.[7] In addition, LV and RV dysfunction are associated with thrombosis.

What impact these thrombi have on overall prognosis is not certain, although one remains fairly concerned about their presence and the patient's longer-term prospects.

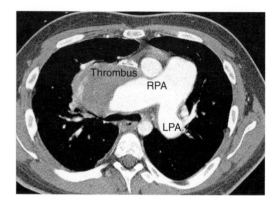

Figure 74-8 Computed tomography pulmonary angiogram.

### FINDINGS

The main and left pulmonary arteries were only mildly enlarged compared to the right. The wall of the pulmonary artery appeared calcified. Outside the artery a rim of radiopaque material was seen, likely thrombus.

**Comments:** The dilatation is mainly of the right pulmonary artery. Usually the right pulmonary is slightly larger than the left and carries slightly more flow. Theoretically, because of the relationship between radius and wall stress according to La Place's law, early dilatation of the right pulmonary artery may lead to further dilatation in the same artery despite equal pressure in both right and left, causing a positive feedback loop for further dilatation. Unpublished observations show that laminar thrombi tend to occur more often in the right than the left pulmonary artery.

The presence of possible thrombus outside the wall of the vessel lumen indicates that microrupture may be a possible cause of the patient's hemoptysis, although this is speculative.

## CATHETERIZATION

Not performed

### FOCUSED CLINICAL QUESTIONS AND DISCUSSION POINTS

1. **What is the relationship between thrombus and hemoptysis in this patient?**

   *Both thrombus[6,10] and hemoptysis[9,11] are common in Eisenmenger syndrome, and even described in Dr. Eisenmenger's original* case.[3] Generally it is believed that the cause of hemoptysis is pulmonary infarction due to occlusive thrombi. However, it has been difficult to demonstrate such infarctions in vivo on a macroscopic level with our current imaging modalities. Such infarctions may be microvascular. Alternatively, hemoptysis may be related to rupture of thin-walled arterioles under high pressure, or bronchial collaterals that develop in response to chronic cyanosis.

2. Should this patient be taking warfarin?

There are no controlled studies to guide us as to whether warfarin should or should not be given to patients with Eisenmenger syndrome for thromboprophylaxis. Since even the pathophysiology is poorly understood, it is difficult to make strong recommendations either way.

Dr. Paul Wood, in 1958, several years before warfarin was in widespread clinical use, believed that "treatment aims at preventing secondary thrombo-obstructive lesions by means of permanent anticoagulants, such as phenindione."[3] Based on the presumed pathophysiologic relationship between thrombus and hemoptysis, anticoagulation seems rational[11] although not all authors endorse its use.[9]

The arguments against routine anticoagulation in Eisenmenger syndrome include the following:
1. There are known abnormalities of clotting factors in cyanotic patients.
2. Hemoptysis may be exacerbated when patients are either taking or started on anticoagulation.[12]
3. Warfarin dose adjustment is problematic because of the relatively low plasma volumes in the presence of erythrocytosis. Before the blood sample is drawn careful adjustment of citrate in the sample tube needs to be made based on a premeasured hematocrit. Finger-stick home monitoring devices have not been formally tested in cyanotic patients.
4. Deaths from warfarin have been reported,[13] usually from INR levels that were out of control.
5. Though warfarin may be safely tried in a patient with infrequent, scant hemoptysis, in a patient such as this, the frequency and severity of the hemoptysis would make many clinicians wary of full anticoagulation.

3. Are there any mechanical options for preventing further hemoptysis?

This patient's options were discussed at length at multidisciplinary conferences during these months of recurring hemoptysis. Though bleeding was suspected to occur around the large aneurysmal right pulmonary artery, a discrete focus that might be amenable to embolization could not be completely excluded. Surgical thrombectomy and aneurysmectomy were judged to be excessively high risk with unproven benefit, and pneumonectomy was not felt to be rational given the patient's severity of PAH. Heart-lung transplantation was also considered. The option of empiric coil embolization of the bronchial arteries was thus revisited, and the family agreed to pursue it.[14] Though this would require general anesthesia, a risk in itself, it would otherwise be feasible and relatively straightforward. It was made clear that there are no published data about the overall clinical utility of this technique in general, particularly in Eisenmenger patients.

4. What is the risk of pulmonary artery rupture in severely dilated pulmonary arteries?

Noniatrogenic rupture of an aneurysmal pulmonary artery in the setting of Eisenmenger syndrome has not been widely reported. Although the size of the aneurysm in this patient seems to make rupture a real risk, it is also possible that the large, slowly organizing thrombus may actually be protective from catastrophe. Regardless of possible risks, however, one is limited in terms of safe treatment options to try to avoid rupture.

# FINAL DIAGNOSIS

Down syndrome

Atrial septal defect

Patent ductus arteriosus

Eisenmenger syndrome with recurrent hemoptysis

Aneurysmal right pulmonary artery with large mural thrombus

Inappropriately low hemoglobin due to iron deficiency

# PLAN OF ACTION

Empiric coil embolization of the bronchial arteries

Iron supplementation to facilitate secondary erythrocytosis

# INTERVENTION

Given the recurrence of hemoptysis, its dramatic and potentially life-threatening nature, and the lack of alternative low-risk approaches to address the patient's problem, bronchial arterial embolization was pursued. The procedure and its empiric nature were fully explained to the patient and his parents. It was understood that there was no guarantee the procedure would be successful in preventing further bleeding, and that the risks of general anesthesia were relatively high.

The patient was taken to the catheterization laboratory and general endotracheal anesthesia induced carefully by a team familiar with the perioperative management of cyanotic heart patients. Through the right femoral artery, the right and left bronchial arteries were located. Contrast injections failed to show any significant extravasation to suggest bleeding. The largest right bronchial artery was embolized successfully. The family was told it was unlikely that this had been the true cause of bleeding.

# OUTCOME

Following the embolization under general anesthesia the patient developed atrial flutter with a rapid ventricular rate. He was cardioverted within 24 hours, without TEE, under minimal sedation and with intravenous heparin. While still sedated, his blood pressure dropped to 60/40 with oxygen saturations in the 60s for several minutes after cardioversion, probably due to reduced afterload from anesthesia. With reversal of anesthesia and volume replacement the blood pressure returned to normal and oxygen saturation returned to baseline. Atrial arrhythmia did not recur.

A few months following the procedure the patient developed symptoms of an upper respiratory infection, which resolved over a few weeks. A CXR showed shadowing of the right lower lobe with loss of the right costophrenic corner, likely a pleural effusion, even though his symptoms had improved and he had no further hemoptysis by that point. One month later, at a follow-up visit, a repeat CXR showed a large, semiloculated right-sided pneumothorax (see Fig. 74-9). He was admitted for observation, but had no clinical decompensation and his oxygen saturation remained stable. A CT scan showed no change to the right pulmonary aneurysm and no focal pneumonia or empyema. The effusion was left to resorb physiologically. Over the next several weeks the lung reexpanded fully. No clear etiology was found, and overall it was felt this was unlikely to be related to his embolization.

Twelve months postprocedure the patient has had no further episodes of hemoptysis. Bouts of hemoptysis in patients with Eisenmenger syndrome often resolve for some time by them-

selves, so it is difficult to say with certainty that the embolization was the reason for improved symptomatic status. Still, the
temporal relationship between embolization and resolution of
the problem was noteworthy.

One year later, the patient had another bout of large-volume
hemoptysis. He was admitted to intensive care and stabilized,
as before. Twenty-four hours later, however, another large
bleed occurred. He suffered cardiovascular collapse and could
not be resuscitated. No post-mortem was performed. The
patient's history serves as a dramatic reminder of the frailty of
those with Eisenmenger syndrome.

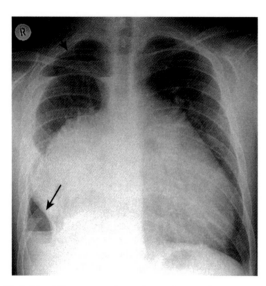

Figure 74-9 Chest X-ray several months post procedure.

## FINDINGS

Six months after coil embolization of a bronchial artery, CXR
showed a right pneumothorax (*arrows*) including an air fluid
level from a small effusion, which resolved slowly without
intervention. Coils were not easily seen.

**Comments:** Despite the potential for catastrophe from
poor ventilation in an Eisenmenger patient with a pneumothorax, the patient remained clinically stable, and no intervention
was necessary. The etiology of the pneumothorax was not

certain. Because of the 6-month span between the interventional
procedure and the finding here, it was felt unlikely that the
pneumothorax was related to the coil embolization.

## Selected References

1. Hoffman JI, Kaplan S: The incidence of congenital heart disease.
   J Am Coll Cardiol 39:1890–1900, 2002.
2. Frid C, Drott P, Lundell B, et al: Mortality in Down's syndrome in
   relation to congenital malformations. J Intellect Disabil Res 43(Pt
   3):234–241, 1999.
3. Wood P: The Eisenmenger syndrome or pulmonary hypertension
   with reversed central shunt. BMJ 2:701–709, 755–762, 1958.
4. Broberg CS, Jayaweera AR, Diller GP, et al: The optimal relationship between oxygen saturation and hemoglobin in adult patients
   with cyanotic congenital heart disease can be determined and
   correlates with exercise capacity. Circulation 114(Suppl):II-503,
   2006.
5. Kaemmerer H, Fratz S, Braun SL, et al: Erythrocyte indexes,
   iron metabolism, and hyperhomocysteinemia in adults with
   cyanotic congenital cardiac disease. Am J Cardiol 94:825–828,
   2004.
6. Perloff JK, Hart EM, Greaves SM, et al: Proximal pulmonary arterial and intrapulmonary radiologic features of Eisenmenger syndrome and primary pulmonary hypertension. Am J Cardiol
   92:182–187, 2003.
7. Broberg CS, Ujita M, Rubens M, et al: Pulmonary artery thrombosis in Eisenmenger syndrome is associated with ventricular
   dysfunction, neurohormonal activation, and poorer exercise
   capacity. J Am Coll Cardiol 50:634–642, 2007.
8. Vida VL, Barnoya J, Larrazabal LA, et al: Congenital cardiac
   disease in children with Down's syndrome in Guatemala. Cardiol
   Young 15:286–290, 2005.
9. Niwa K, Perloff JK, Kaplan S, et al: Eisenmenger syndrome in
   adults: Ventricular septal defect, truncus arteriosus, univentricular heart. J Am Coll Cardiol 34:223–232, 1999.
10. Silversides CK, Granton JT, Konen E, et al: Pulmonary thrombosis
    in adults with Eisenmenger syndrome. J Am Coll Cardiol 42:
    1982–1987, 2003.
11. Daliento L, Somerville J, Presbitero P, et al: Eisenmenger syn-
    drome: Factors relating to deterioration and death. Eur Heart J
    19:1845–1855, 1998.
12. Broberg C, Ujita M, Babu-Narayan S, et al: Massive pulmonary
    artery thrombosis with haemoptysis in adults with Eisenmenger's
    syndrome: A clinical dilemma. Heart 90:e63, 2004.
13. Somerville J: How to manage the Eisenmenger syndrome. Int J
    Cardiol 63:1–8, 1998.
14. Yoon W, Kim JK, Kim YH, et al: Bronchial and nonbronchial sys-
    temic artery embolization for life-threatening hemoptysis: A com-
    prehensive review. Radiographics 22:1395–1409, 2002.

# Pregnant Patient with Unoperated Truncus Arteriosus

**Anselm Uebing, Steve M. Yentis, and Philip J. Steer**

**Age:** 24 years
**Gender:** Female
**Occupation:** Housewife
**Working diagnosis:** Pregnancy in cyanotic heart disease

## HISTORY

The patient was cyanotic at birth and in infancy, but only a limited workup was possible in her native country. She and her family were told she had "a hole in the heart" but no surgical intervention was possible. She received no cardiologic follow-up. She recalls being told that pregnancy would be safe despite her heart condition.

She immigrated to the United Kingdom at the age of 15. Though still cyanotic, she felt generally well and thus did not consult a health care provider. She then married and became pregnant. She was referred at 23 weeks' gestation to a high-risk obstetric clinic.

**Comments:** It is not uncommon for unrepaired or even nonpalliated patients born in countries with limited medical care to present in adulthood without a clear diagnosis.

All female patients with ACHD should be given prepregnancy counseling after a complete medical evaluation. Patients should optimally be provided with information about how pregnancy may affect the mother and the fetus well before conception.[1] (See Case 83.)

Women with cyanotic heart disease and normal pulmonary artery pressure carry a moderate risk of death or other major complications during pregnancy (1%–5%) depending largely on ventricular function. The risk of fetal death increases with the degree of cyanosis. If prepregnancy maternal oxygen saturation is less than 85% the chance of a live birth is only 12%, compared to 92% if the saturation is greater than 90%.[2] If pulmonary vascular disease is present (Eisenmenger syndrome) the risk of maternal death becomes very high (approximately 40%),[3] and pregnancy is contraindicated.

## CURRENT SYMPTOMS

The patient complained of shortness of breath increasing gradually from the beginning of her pregnancy. At presentation she could walk only 50 m on level ground and was limited to climbing one flight of stairs without stopping for rest.

She had occasional palpitations but no chest pain, lightheadedness, or ankle swelling.

NYHA class: III

**Comments:** Significant cardiovascular changes occur during pregnancy, including an increase in plasma and blood volume, an increase cardiac output, a reduction in systemic vascular resistance, and an increase in oxygen consumption.

Shortness of breath is common in pregnant women without heart disease. But in a patient with cyanosis, pulmonary blood flow is usually relatively fixed, whereas systemic vascular resistance falls during pregnancy. Thus an increase in right-to-left shunting may well occur, aggravating cyanosis.

## CURRENT MEDICATIONS

None

## PHYSICAL EXAMINATION

BP 120/60 mm Hg, HR 90 bpm, oxygen saturation 80% on room air (right hand and left foot)

Height 156 cm, weight 59 kg, BSA 1.58 m²

Surgical scars: None

Neck veins: JVP was elevated to 6 cm above sternal angle with a normal waveform.

Lungs/chest: Chest was clear.

Heart: The heart was in a regular rhythm. There was a left parasternal lift. The first heart sound was normal, and the second heart sound was single and loud. There was a grade 2/3 ejection systolic murmur at the left sternal edge and a grade 2 high-pitched early diastolic murmur in the same area. A continuous murmur was heard in her left anterior chest.

Abdomen: No hepatomegaly

Extremities: Moderate digital clubbing was seen in both fingers and toes. High amplitude pulses of similar intensity were palpable at radial and femoral arteries.

**Comments:** The oxygen saturation of 80% should be compared to prepregnancy levels if available, as pregnancy usually worsens cyanosis.

If the patient has pulmonary hypertension, the single second heart sound rules out an unrestrictive VSD, transposition of the great arteries, or an aortopulmonary window, where a loud pulmonary component would be expected. In pulmonary atresia or truncus arteriosus the VSD does not cause a loud systolic heart murmur, as pressures are equal in both ventricles. If the diagnosis is truncus arteriosus, the systolic murmur in this patient could be due to either stenosis of a truncal valve or stenosis of the pulmonary artery at its origin from the ascending aorta.

The high pulse pressure and high-pitched diastolic murmur indicate an incompetent aortic valve or an incompetent truncal valve. The high-pitched diastolic murmur could also be seen in pulmonary hypertensive pulmonic regurgitation, but this would not explain the wide pulse pressure.

Since we know that no aortopulmonary shunts have been created (such as a BT shunt), a continuous murmur in the left chest may indicate blood flow to the left lung via aorto-pulmonary collateral arteries to lung segments without severe pulmonary hypertension, or another cause of a continuous murmur.

## LABORATORY DATA

| | |
|---|---|
| Hemoglobin | **13.6 g/dL** (9.5–12.0 in mid pregnancy) |
| Hematocrit/PCV | 38% (36–46) |
| MCV | 89 fL (83–99) |
| MCH | 31.9 pg (27–32.5) |
| Platelet count | $256 \times 10^9$/L (150–400) |
| Sodium | 139 mmol/L (134–145) |
| Potassium | 4.2 mmol/L (3.5–5.2) |
| Creatinine | 0.64 mg/dL (0.6–1.2) |
| Blood urea nitrogen | 4.5 mmol/L (2.5–6.5) |
| Iron | 22.1 µmol/L (12.6–26) |
| Ferritin | 25 µg/L (20–186) |
| Transferrin saturation | 27% (20–45) |

### OTHER RELEVANT LAB RESULTS

| | |
|---|---|
| Total protein | **58 g/L** (62–82) |
| Albumin | **27 g/L** (37–53) |

Fluorescence in situ hybridization test for chromosome 22 region q11.2: No evidence of deletion that would suggest DiGeorge syndrome.

***Comments:*** Cyanosis should result in secondary erythrocytosis, which is notably absent here. One would expect physiologic adaptation to saturations of 80% to produce a hemoglobin of at least 18 g/dL to maintain adequate oxygenation. The patient did not have iron deficiency and there had been no bleeding. An alternative explanation is that during pregnancy the anticipated expansion in plasma volume has resulted in diluted hemoglobin levels, the patient's hemoglobin being still relatively high for mid pregnancy (it normally ranges from 9.5–12 g/dL). The relatively low levels of total protein and albumin would also support this.[4]

Several lesions, including truncus arteriosus and pulmonary atresia, are associated with DiGeorge syndrome (deletion of chromosomal segment 22q11). The inheritance of DiGeorge syndrome is autosomal dominant and therefore carries a recurrence risk of 50%.[5] Therefore, any patient with these lesions should be offered screening before pregnancy. DiGeorge syndrome manifests as infantile hypocalcemia, thymic hypoplasia with immune deficiency, psychiatric disorders such as depression and schizophrenia, various degrees of mental retardation, and ACHD (most commonly truncus arteriosus, interrupted aortic arch, and TOF).

## ELECTROCARDIOGRAM

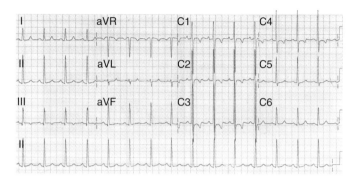

Figure 75-1 Electrocardiogram.

### FINDINGS

Heart rate: 90 bpm

PR interval: 152 msec

QRS axis: +65°

QRS duration: 90 msec

Sinus rhythm with normal AV conduction. High amplitude R-waves in leads V1–3 with inverted T-waves in these leads.

***Comments:*** The high amplitude R-waves and discordant T-waves in leads V1–3 suggest RV hypertrophy. There is no RA overload or right-axis deviation. LV hypertrophy may also be present.

## CHEST X-RAY

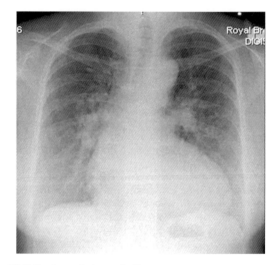

Figure 75-2 Posteroanterior projection.

### FINDINGS

Cardiothoracic ratio: 66%

The cardiac silhouette was enlarged with an elevated apex. The aortic arch was left-sided with a prominent aortic knuckle. The main pulmonary artery was not seen, but the central pulmonary arteries were prominent.

***Comments:*** A prominent aortic knuckle is compatible with chronically high flow in the proximal aorta, seen in a significant PDA or with important aortic regurgitation or extensive aortopulmonary collaterals.

An absent pulmonary artery segment is a typical finding for truncus arteriosus, transposition, and pulmonary atresia. Elevation of the apex may result from right ventricular hypertrophy. The combination of both elevation of the apex and absence of the main pulmonary artery segment ("empty pulmonary artery bay") results in the so-called boot-shaped silhouette seen in tetralogy of Fallot with pulmonary atresia, and truncus arteriosus.

Central pulmonary arteries are visible, but their origin is uncertain. Thus, in this patient, truncus arteriosus or pulmonary atresia with VSD both remain possibilities. The prominence of central pulmonary arteries may suggest the presence of elevated pulmonary artery pressure in this cyanotic patient.

Because radiation exposure presents potential harm to a developing fetus, nonradiating modalities, such as echo and MRI should be obtained instead. Hence a CXR is not usually necessary. Exposure to a fetus from a single CXR is well below the threshold for teratogenicity.[6] Thus, when desired, a CXR can be obtained without undue risk.

## EXERCISE TESTING

Not performed

## ECHOCARDIOGRAM

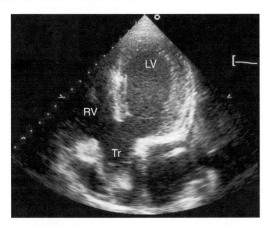

Figure 75-3 Four-chamber view.

### FINDINGS

Both left and right ventricles were present in the correct anatomical location and functioned well.

There was a large nonrestrictive VSD.

There was no significant mitral or tricuspid regurgitation.

The atria were of normal size.

The left and right ventricles were connected by the VSD. A single great artery (Tr) arose from both ventricles overriding the crest of the VSD.

*Comments:* To distinguish truncus arteriosus from pulmonary atresia, the origin of the pulmonary artery or arteries needs to be delineated, a task that can be challenging with echocardiography. To this point in this case, their origin remained uncertain.

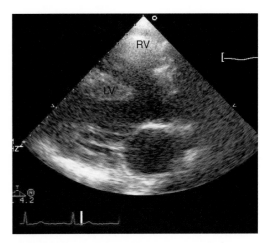

Figure 75-4 Parasternal long-axis view.

### FINDINGS

This parasternal long-axis view again showed the LV and RV in the correct anatomic location and functioning normally.

The semilunar valve overrode the ventricular septum.

*Comments:* In this view it is not possible to differentiate between truncus arteriosus and TOF with pulmonary atresia (also called complex pulmonary atresia due to a combination of pulmonary atresia, VSD, and multiple aortopulmonary collaterals).

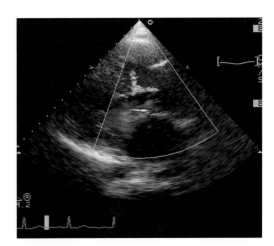

Figure 75-5 Long-axis color view.

### FINDINGS

This parasternal long-axis view showed mild regurgitation of the semilunar valve (truncal valve) with the regurgitant jet diverted at the crest of the VSD.

*Comments:* Regurgitation of the semilunar valve is common in both lesions, truncus arteriosus and complex pulmonary atresia. In truncus arteriosus it is often related to an intrinsic abnormality of the valve itself and may be present from birth. In complex pulmonary atresia it can be a consequence of aortic root dilatation and manifest itself later on in life.

# MAGNETIC RESONANCE IMAGING

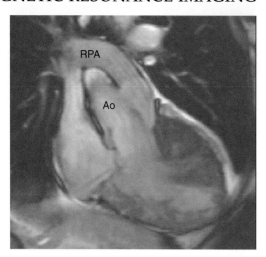

Figure 75-6 Oblique coronal plane aligned with the bifurcation of the arterial trunk. Ao, aorta.

## FINDINGS

There was a large truncal vessel giving rise to the right pulmonary artery as well as the aorta. A left pulmonary artery was not seen.

The RV was hypertrophied with preserved systolic function. The tricuspid valve showed no regurgitation. The SVC drained normally into the RA, which was not enlarged.

*Comments:* MRI has particular value in defining the relationship of the great vessels and the anatomy of aortopulmonary collateral arteries, and is safe during pregnancy.

In this case, the right pulmonary artery originated from the ascending aorta, which is consistent with truncus arteriosus. The left pulmonary artery is not yet accounted for in this view.

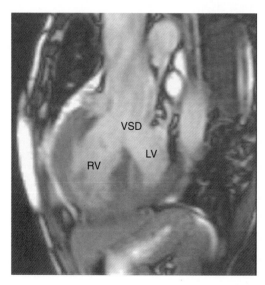

Figure 75-7 Sagittal oblique plane aligned with the truncal vessel and the ventricular septal defect.

## FINDINGS

The truncal vessel overrode a large, unrestrictive VSD. RV hypertrophy was present.

*Comments:* All arterial blood exits the ventricles via the VSD and the truncal valve. The VSD is not restrictive, and therefore pressure in both ventricles is equal and at systemic level. Systemic pressure in the RV has induced the hypertrophy.

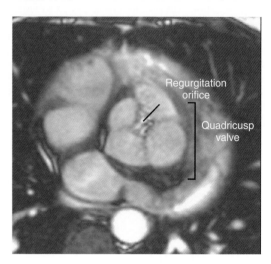

Figure 75-8 Oblique transaxial slice aligned with the truncal valve.

## FINDINGS

The truncal valve consisted of four leaflets, and there was moderate central regurgitation (regurgitant fraction 28%).

*Comments:* The truncal valve is tricuspid in 69% of cases, quadricuspid in 22%, and bicuspid in 9%. Truncal valve incompetence or stenosis is common.

Severe truncal valve incompetence is a common cause of heart failure and death in infants with truncus arteriosus. In adults, however, it is less likely to be a major problem.

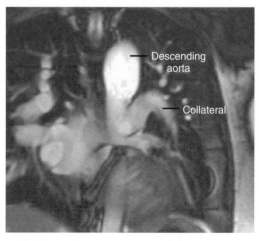

Figure 75-9 Left collateral image.

## FINDINGS

No left pulmonary artery could be identified.

A large aortopulmonary collateral artery arising from the descending aorta and supplying the left lung was seen. There were also smaller collaterals to the left lung from bronchial and intercostal arteries.

*Comments:* In combination with echocardiography, MRI confirmed the diagnosis of truncus arteriosus type A3 (Fig. 75-10). In this form the truncal vessel gives rise only to the right pulmonary artery. Blood flows to the left lung via aortopulmonary collateral arteries arising from the thoracic aorta.

At times these vessels, particularly collateral arteries that have a tortuous course and cannot be viewed in a single plane, are best seen using gadolinium enhancement, which is contraindicated during pregnancy. However, these findings were confirmed by MR angiography following pregnancy.

## FOCUSED CLINICAL QUESTIONS AND DISCUSSION POINTS

1. What is the diagnosis?

*This patient has truncus arteriosus communis (or common arterial trunk). There is only one single, large arterial vessel and one semilunar valve overriding both ventricles. Truncus arteriosus is almost always associated with an unrestrictive VSD located below the truncal valve; blood mixing at the level of the VSD results in cyanosis. Because blood flow to the lungs is usually not restricted, pulmonary vascular disease inevitably develops unless surgery is performed. Surgical repair, consisting of separation of the pulmonary arteries from the truncal vessel and connection of the pulmonary arteries to the right ventricle using a conduit and closure of the VSD, must be carried out in infancy to prevent the development of pulmonary vascular disease.*

2. How is truncus arteriosus classified?

*Truncus arteriosus communis is a rare congenital heart lesion (1%–4% of all congenital heart malformations). Two classifications exist based on the origin of the pulmonary arteries.[7,8] This patient has type A3 according to the Van Praagh classification (Fig. 75-10). The "A" indicates the presence of a VSD. If no VSD is present a "B" is given, but this condition is extremely rare and incompatible with life. The other classification scheme according to Collett and Edwards considered four types of truncus arteriosus based on the origin of the pulmonary arteries.*

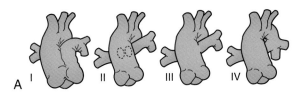

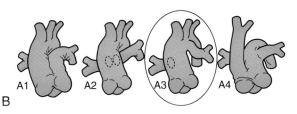

Figure 75-10 Classification schemes of truncus arteriosus. **A,** Collett and Edwards. **B,** Van Praagh. The schemes are similarly based on the origins of the pulmonary arteries.

3. What is the risk of pregnancy in women with cyanotic heart disease and pulmonary vascular disease?

*Pregnancy in women with cyanotic heart lesions and pulmonary vascular disease (Eisenmenger syndrome) carries a risk of maternal death as high as 40% to 50%. The risk of fetal death is also high (between 8% and 40%).[3,9] Ventricular function is one of the major determinants for maternal outcome and must be monitored carefully throughout pregnancy, delivery, and the postpartum period. Women die from heart failure, thromboembolic events, and bleeding complications, often in the postpartum period.*

*Right-to-left shunt increases during pregnancy, and oxygen extraction is increased because of placental-fetal exchange. Both of these factors worsen maternal cyanosis. The risk for fetal loss increases with the degree of cyanosis.[2] This patient was given wrong advice prior to conception, as pregnancy is high risk and thus should be avoided in women with Eisenmenger syndrome. It is crucial that the patient is aware of the risks involved. Prepregnancy counseling must provide this information along with advice on available types of contraception (see Case 83).*

4. Should therapeutic termination be advised in this patient because of the risk associated with pregnancy?

*The decision as to whether to proceed with the pregnancy must be made by the patient and the couple, not the physician. The role and responsibility of the latter is to provide appropriate counseling regarding maternal risks (both short and long term) and fetal risks related with either option. In general, therapeutic termination should be strongly recommended in patients with cyanosis and pulmonary vascular disease, as should timely sterilization. However, the patient should also know that the risk of termination rises as pregnancy proceeds. This patient presented at 23 weeks gestation, which is generally considered beyond the acceptable window in which to offer a low-risk therapeutic abortion.*

5. What is the optimal management of a pregnant woman with cyanosis and pulmonary vascular disease through gestation, labor, delivery, and the postpartum period?

*Close cardiovascular monitoring is mandatory throughout pregnancy, delivery, and the postpartum period. This is often done as an inpatient throughout the third trimester, where bed rest, anticoagulation, and continuous oxygen supplementation can be provided. Women should lie in the lateral position during labor and delivery to avoid supine hypotension from compression of the vena cava and the aorta.[10] In extreme circumstances, additional pulmonary vasodilator treatment (nitric oxide, prostacyclin) should be offered particularly in later gestation if heart failure develops or cyanosis becomes extreme. Growth of the fetus should be monitored frequently.*

*Decisions on the mode of delivery should be made by obstetricians and anesthetists with expertise in ACHD. Vaginal delivery should be the aim, as it usually carries the lowest risk of complications such as hemorrhage, thromboembolism, or infection. The key principle in the management of either method of delivery is to avoid pain and anxiety, as both lead to an additional increase in cardiac output. In this regard, epidural anesthesia should be used early, as it has minimal effects on hemodynamic performance. Close and continuous monitoring of the mother and the fetus is crucial to avoid emergency situations.*

*After delivery, fatal events can occur up to 7 to 10 days postpartum, thus hospitalization and monitoring ought to continue as long as is felt reasonable, with close outpatient follow-up thereafter.*

## FINAL DIAGNOSIS

Truncus arteriosus communis type A3 (Van Praagh classification)

Left lung perfused via a large aortopulmonary collateral arising from the descending aorta

Twenty-three weeks pregnant

## PLAN OF ACTION

Counsel the patient regarding maternal and fetal risks of pregnancy.

Continuation of pregnancy with close cardiovascular monitoring, bed rest, anticoagulation, and oxygen supplementation.

Close monitoring of fetal growth. Encourage sterilization after pregnancy.

## INTERVENTION

None

## OUTCOME

The patient was hospitalized from the 23rd week of gestation onward until delivery. She was maintained with bed rest, low molecular weight heparin (Dalteparin 12,500 units daily), and continuous nasal oxygen administration (2–4 L/min). Fetal growth was closely monitored with weekly ultrasounds.

At 34 weeks, fetal growth stagnated, and thus an elective cesarean section was planned. Low molecular weight heparin was stopped 12 hours before cesarean section and reinstated 6 hours after delivery. The patient had epidural anesthesia by a team with experience with cyanotic heart patients. Endocarditis prophylaxis was given.

The procedure was performed uneventfully. The patient gave birth to a healthy baby boy. Echocardiography of the newborn showed normal cardiac anatomy and function.

The patient recovered fully from delivery. She was supervised for 3 days in the intensive care unit and for 7 days on a regular ward thereafter. Anticoagulation was finally stopped 6 days after delivery when the patient was fully mobilized. As serious events often occur up to 10 days postpartum continuous monitoring continued throughout this period.

At the day of discharge the oxygen saturation was 89% at rest on room air. The grade 2 early diastolic murmur at the left sternal edge remained. The continuous murmur in her left anterior chest was present as well. Laboratory results 12 months after discharge showed:

| | | |
|---|---|---|
| Hemoglobin | **16.7 g/dL** | (11.5–15.0) |
| MCV | 93 fL | (83–99) |
| MCH | 31.8 pg | (27.0–32.5) |
| Hematocrit | **49%** | (36%–46%) |

The patient is scheduled for cardiac catheterization with reversibility studies as a prelude to potential PAH disease targeting therapy. We note that this patient presumably has systemic pressures in the right lung, and lower pressures in some or all of the left lung, permitting the continuous murmur to be present.

## Selected References

1. Steer PJ: Pregnancy and contraception. In Gatzoulis MA, Swan L, Therrien J, Pantley GA (eds): Adult Congenital Heart Disease: A Practical Guide. Oxford, BMJ Publishing Group, Blackwell, 16–35, 2005.
2. Presbitero P, Somerville J, Stone S, et al: Pregnancy in cyanotic congenital heart disease: Outcome of mother and fetus. Circulation 89:2673–2676, 1994.
3. Yentis SM, Steer PJ, Plaat F: Eisenmenger's syndrome in pregnancy: Maternal and fetal mortality in the 1990s. Br J Obstet Gynaecol 105:921–922, 1998.
4. Chesley LC: Plasma and red cell volumes during pregnancy. Am J Obstet Gynecol 112:440–450, 1972.
5. Baldini A: DiGeorge syndrome: An update. Curr Opin Cardiol 19:201–204, 2004.
6. Timins JK: Radiation during pregnancy. N Engl J Med 98:29–33, 2001.
7. Collett RS, Edwards JE: Persistent truncus arteriosus: A classification according to anatomic types. Surg Clin North Am 29:1245–1270, 1949.
8. Van Praagh R, Van Praagh S: The anatomy of common aortico-pulmonary trunk (truncus arteriosus communis) and its embryologic implications: A study of 57 necropsy cases. Am J Cardiol 16:406–425, 1965.
9. Avila WS, Grinberg M, Snitcowsky R, et al: Maternal and fetal outcome in pregnant women with Eisenmenger's syndrome. Eur Heart J 16:460–464, 1995.
10. Siu SC, Colman JM: Heart disease and pregnancy. Heart 85:710–715, 2001.

# Special Topics

# Part I

# Coronary Anomalies

Case 76

# Left Coronary Artery Arising from the Right Coronary Sinus

**Anselm Uebing**

**Age: 29 years**
**Gender: Female**
**Occupation: Housewife**
**Working diagnosis: Aberrant origin of the left coronary artery and aortic valve disease**

## HISTORY

The patient was diagnosed with congenital aortic stenosis (bicuspid aortic valve) in early infancy and underwent balloon dilatation of the aortic valve at the age of 13 years. Thereafter, she was well until the age of 20 years, when she developed chest pain on exertion. A cardiac catheter was performed and documented recurrent aortic stenosis with a peak-to-peak pressure gradient of 88 mm Hg and moderate aortic regurgitation.

In addition, the diagnosis of a coronary artery anomaly was made. Coronary angiography showed an aberrant origin of the left coronary artery from the right coronary artery. The left coronary showed an abnormal course crossing the RVOT anteriorly.

The patient underwent homograft aortic root replacement with reimplantation of the single right coronary ostium into the root of the homograft. Her chest pain improved after the operation, but 1 year later it recurred with increasing intensity.

She is a nonsmoker without a family history of coronary artery disease.

The patient now wanted to become pregnant.

**Comments:** Congenital aortic stenosis accounts for approximately 5% of congenital heart defects. By far the most common morphologic abnormality in the context of this lesion is a bicuspid valve (~ 95%).[1] A bicuspid aortic valve is usually an isolated anomaly but can be associated with coarctation, VSD and PDA.[2]

Recommended treatment of aortic valve stenosis depends on the severity of stenosis and the presence of symptoms (chest pain, syncope, heart failure). Asymptomatic patients with severe aortic stenosis should be referred for aortic valve replacement with the first signs of LV dysfunction, when there is evidence of rapid progression of the degree of stenosis, and if there are anticipated delays in proceeding with surgery.[3]

An ectopic origin of the left coronary artery from the right coronary artery is rare. This anomaly is not known to be associated with aortic valve disease.[4]

Balloon aortic valvotomy is the procedure of choice in childhood, as it effectively decreases the pressure gradient across the valve with a low mortality, but restenosis can occur and often requires surgery.[5] In this patient, the presence of moderate aortic regurgitation precluded a second attempt at balloon valvuloplasty.

Homograft aortic valve replacement is an alternative to the Ross procedure especially in women of reproductive age, as anticoagulation is not necessary following either operation. As the left coronary artery crossed the RVOT, a Ross procedure could not be performed, and homograft aortic valve replacement was chosen. The Ross procedure consists of pulmonary valve autograft replacement of the aortic valve, combined with pulmonary valve replacement using a homograft. It therefore involves an incision in the RVOT and was considered too risky for this specific patient, given her coronary artery anatomy.

## CURRENT SYMPTOMS

The patient did not have any symptoms of heart failure but had angina-like chest pain. She was limited in her exercise capacity by chest tightness radiating to the left shoulder and arm.

She never experienced any palpitations or syncope.

NYHA class: II

***Comments:*** The diagnosis of an aberrant origin and course of a coronary artery must be considered in the differential diagnosis of angina-like chest pain in adolescents and young adults.

Apart from chest pain this anomaly can present with syncope or even sudden cardiac death. In fact, coronary anomalies are the second most common cause of sudden, unexpected, and exercise-related death in young athletes, after hypertrophic cardiomyopathy.[6]

## CURRENT MEDICATIONS

None

## PHYSICAL EXAMINATION

BP 130/80 mm Hg, HR 75 bpm, oxygen saturation 99% on room air

Height 165 cm, weight 72 kg, BSA 1.82 m$^2$

Surgical scars: Scar from median sternotomy

Neck veins: JVP was not elevated and showed a normal waveform.

Lungs/chest: Chest was clear.

Heart: Precordial examination was normal. The apex was not displaced. There was a normal first and a physiologically split second heart sound and a grade 2–3/6 fairly short systolic ejection murmur audible at the upper right sternal border. There was no diastolic murmur.

Abdomen: Normal

Extremities: There was no peripheral edema, and normal peripheral pulses were palpable in all the extremities.

***Comments:*** The aortic pulse pressure suggests that there is no significant aortic regurgitation. This is supported by the lack of a diastolic murmur.

A 2–3/6 fairly short systolic ejection murmur and a physiologically split second heart sound indicate mild-to-moderate aortic stenosis, which would not explain the patient's chest pain.

Bicuspid aortic valves can be associated with aortic coarctation, but normal peripheral pulses and normal arterial blood pressure make this diagnosis highly unlikely.

## LABORATORY DATA

| | |
|---|---|
| Hemoglobin | 13.0 g/dL (11.5–15.0) |
| Hematocrit/PCV | 39% (36–46) |
| MCV | 88 fL (83–99) |
| MCH | 29.3 pg (27–32.5) |
| Platelet count | $305 \times 10^9$/L (150–400) |
| Sodium | 140 mmol/L (134–145) |
| Potassium | 4.3 mmol/L (3.5–5.2) |
| Creatinine | 0.75 mg/dL (0.6–1.2) |
| Blood urea nitrogen | 4.5 mmol/L (2.5–6.5) |
| Cholesterol | 4.9 mmol/L (<5) |
| HDL cholesterol | 1.4 mmol/L (1.1– 2.0) |

***Comments:*** Normal cholesterol levels make premature coronary artery disease an unlikely cause of the patient's exertional chest discomfort.

## ELECTROCARDIOGRAM

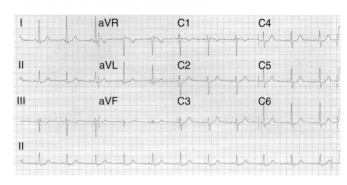

Figure 76-1 Electrocardiogram.

### FINDINGS

Heart rate: 67 bpm

PR interval: 136 msec

QRS axis: +8°

QRS duration: 107 msec

There was normal sinus rhythm with normal P-waves and normal AV conduction. The QRS axis was leftward with an R-wave in aVL of 12 mm, but without other signs of LV hypertrophy.

In particular, there were no signs of previous myocardial infarction or myocardial ischemia at rest.

***Comments:*** The pertinent negative findings are that no LV hypertrophy is seen, nor is there any evidence of myocardial ischemia or infarction.

## CHEST X-RAY

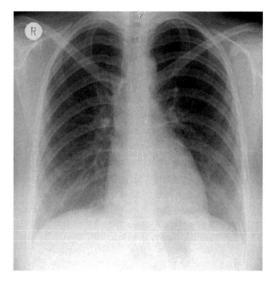

Figure 76-2 Posteroanterior projection.

### FINDINGS

Cardiothoracic ratio: 47%

The cardiac silhouette was not enlarged. There was no evidence of atrial or ventricular enlargement. The bulging of the right upper border of the mediastinum indicated some enlargement of the ascending aorta. The pulmonary vascular markings were normal. Sternal wires were present.

**Comments:** An ascending aortopathy is frequently associated with a bicuspid aortic valve and is related to structural abnormalities of the aortic wall. In severe cases, aortic dissection can occur.[7]

## EXERCISE TESTING

| Exercise protocol: | Modified Bruce |
|---|---|
| Duration (min:sec): | 7:28 |
| Reason for stopping: | Chest pain |
| ECG changes: | 2–3 mm ST depression |

| | Rest | Peak |
|---|---|---|
| Heart rate (bpm): | 75 | 151 |
| Percent of age-predicted max HR: | | 79 |
| $O_2$ saturation (%): | 99 | 98 |
| Blood pressure (mm Hg): | 130/80 | 180/80 |
| Double product: | | 27,180 |
| Peak $Vo_2$ (mL/kg/min): | | 15.6 |
| Percent predicted (%): | | 36 |
| $Ve/Vco_2$: | | 38 |
| Metabolic equivalents: | | 5.7 |

### FINDINGS

Exercise was stopped due to central chest pain radiating to the left arm accompanied by ST segment depression in the inferolateral leads.

**Comments:** Exercise-induced myocardial ischemia was clearly suggested by treadmill exercise testing. The chest pain induced was identical to the pain the patient had been experiencing.

## ELECTROCARDIOGRAM

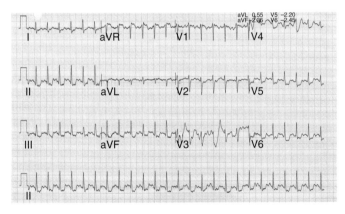

Figure 76-3 Electrocardiogram during stress.

### FINDINGS

The ECG during dobutamine stress showed ST segment depression in the inferolateral leads similar to those recorded during the exercise test.

## ECHOCARDIOGRAM

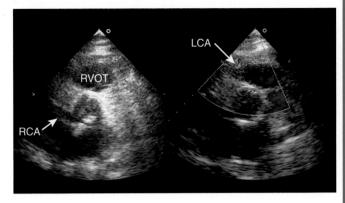

Figure 76-4 Parasternal short-axis view with 2D color Doppler.

### FINDINGS

This showed the enlarged origin of the right coronary artery (RCA). There was no other vessel detectable arising from the ascending aorta. The left coronary artery (LCA) arose from the right coronary artery and crossed the RVOT anteriorly.

The aortic valve (homograft valve) was mildly thickened with mild stenosis. A peak gradient of 23 mm Hg was measured on continuous-wave Doppler (not shown). LV and RV size and function were normal.

**Comments:** This echocardiogram is typical for the diagnosis of an aberrant origin and course of the left coronary artery. If the anatomy of the coronary artery system is normal, the origin of both coronary arteries from the ascending aorta can be demonstrated. Normally, no major coronary vessel crosses the RVOT.

As both the right and left coronary arteries have to be fed from the proximal right coronary artery, its proximal portion is enlarged.

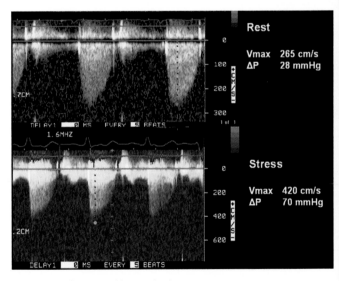

Figure 76-5 Parasternal long-axis view.

Stress echocardiography was performed with dobutamine infusion starting with 5 μg/kg/min and gradually increased to 20 μg/kg/min.

Her heart rate increased from 63 bpm to 107 bpm, and her blood pressure increased from 125/70 mm Hg to 186/62 mm Hg.

The patient's chest pain was reproduced.

## FINDINGS

No regional wall motion abnormalities were detected during stress. The transaortic flow velocity increased from 2.65 to 4.2 m/sec, indicating an increase in peak pressure gradient across the aortic valve from 28 to 70 mm Hg.

*Comments:* There was mild aortic stenosis at rest but a significant increase of the peak pressure gradient during dobutamine stress. Because no regional wall abnormalities could be seen, an ischemic basis could not be confirmed for her chest pain and the ECG changes suggestive of exercise-induced myocardial ischemia.

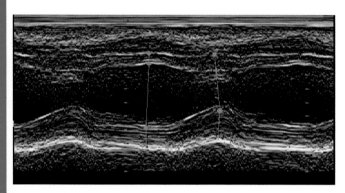

Figure 76-6  Parasternal long-axis view.

## FINDINGS

The parasternal long-axis M-mode documented normal size and function of the LV without wall motion abnormalities.

There was mild concentric LV hypertrophy.

The LVEDd was 4.6 cm, the LVESd was 2.9 cm, and the estimated LV ejection fraction was 63%.

*Comments:* Mild concentric hypertrophy of the LV was in keeping with the diagnosis of mild aortic valve stenosis.

# MAGNETIC RESONANCE IMAGING

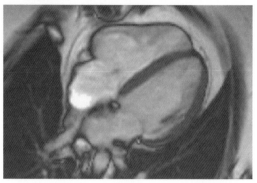

Diastole

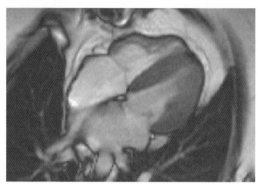

Systole

Figure 76-7  Oblique axial steady-state free precession cine, four-chamber view.

## FINDINGS

Both ventricles were of normal size and function. The LV was mildly hypertrophied. Both AV valves were competent.

### Ventricular Volume Quantification

|  | LV | (Normal range) | RV | (Normal range) |
|---|---|---|---|---|
| EDV (mL) | 121 | (52–141) | 102 | (58–154) |
| ESV (mL) | 51 | (13–51) | 31 | (12–68) |
| SV (mL) | 70 | (33–97) | 71 | (35–98) |
| EF (%) | 58 | (56–75) | 70 | (49–73) |
| EDVi (mL/m²) | 67 | (65–99) | 56 | (65–102) |
| ESVi (mL/m²) | 28 | (19–37) | 17 | (20–45) |
| SVi (mL/m²) | 39 | (42–66) | 39 | (39–63) |
| Mass index (g/m²) | 80 | (47–77) | 34 | (22–42) |

Stress

Rest

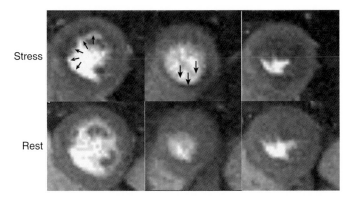

Figure 76-8 Myocardial perfusion magnetic resonance image, short-axis views.

## FINDINGS

Three consecutive short-axis planes of the apical portion of the LV were obtained early after injection of gadolinium both at rest (*lower panel*) and at hyperemia from adenosine administration (140 μg/kg/min) (*upper panel*).

There was homogeneous distribution of gadolinium at rest leading to a bright and homogeneous coloring of the LV myocardium. With hyperemia, there was reduced gadolinium enhancement in subendocardial areas of the anterior, lateral, and mid inferior wall of the LV (*dark areas, arrows*).

During hyperemia the patient developed her typical symptoms of chest pain radiating to the left shoulder and left arm.

**Comments:** Early after injection of gadolinium, the dye enhances in normally perfused tissue (bright coloring). As there was homogeneous enhancement in all areas of the LV after injection of the dye at rest (*lower panel*), previous myocardial infarction and impaired myocardial perfusion at rest could be excluded.

Reduced gadolinium enhancement with stress indicates limited myocardial perfusion (*upper panel; dark areas, arrows*).

MRI perfusion imaging, though still somewhat investigational at the time of this study, again confirmed limited myocardial perfusion at stress but not only in areas perfused behind the left anterior descending artery. There was evidence for ischemia in the mid inferior wall of the LV as well (*upper row, center*).

Absence of late gadolinium enhancement excluded previous myocardial infarction.

## PERFUSION SCAN

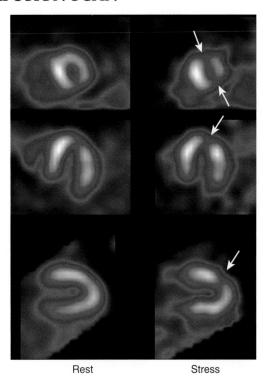

Rest          Stress

Figure 76-9 Tetrofosmin myocardial perfusion scan.

## FINDINGS

The myocardial perfusion scan was performed using dynamic exercise to 75 Watts. As the patient did not achieve the target heart rate, adenosine was added with continued exercise. A pulse rise was achieved from 69 bpm to 150 bpm, and the blood pressure increased from 130/80 mm Hg to 190/90 mm Hg.

This showed a normal uptake of tetrofosmin at rest without any evidence for myocardial infarction but a reduction of counts mainly in the apex of the left ventricle after exercise (*arrows*).

Myocardial perfusion was found to be normal elsewhere.

**Comments:** Again, this test confirmed the diagnosis of exercise-induced myocardial ischemia compatible with a limitation of flow to the left coronary artery at exercise.

# CATHETERIZATION

## HEMODYNAMICS

Heart rate    72 bpm

|  | Pressure | Saturation (%) |
|---|---|---|
| LV | 148/2 ED 8 | |
| Aorta | 125/68 mean 92 | 98 |

## FINDINGS

Cardiac catheterization was performed to obtain coronary angiograms. Limited hemodynamic data were obtained at the same time.

The study demonstrated a mild stenosis of the aortic valve (homograft valve) with a systolic pressure gradient of 23 mm Hg. The end-diastolic pressure in the LV was normal.

***Comments:*** The hemodynamic data confirmed the echocardiographic finding that there was no significant aortic valve stenosis at rest. Additionally, there was no evidence for irreversible damage of the LV myocardium potentially leading to diastolic dysfunction and in turn elevation of the end-diastolic pressure.

# ANGIOGRAM

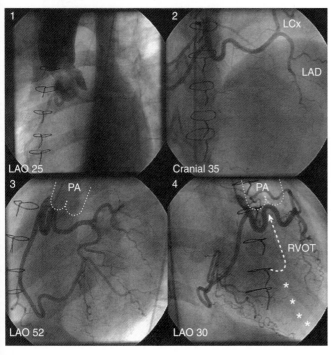

Figure 76-10 Coronary angiogram.

## FINDINGS

Coronary angiography was performed to exclude a discrete stenosis of the coronary arteries. Additionally, the origin and course of the coronary artery system could be delineated.

Contrast injection into the ascending aorta (*panel 1*) showed a normally functioning aortic valve prosthesis with no aortic regurgitation. There was a mild narrowing at the side of the anastomosis between the homograft valve and the native ascending aorta. There was mild dilatation of the ascending aorta (see also Fig. 76-2).

Repeated contrast injections into the right coronary artery (*panels 2–4*) showed a normal and unobstructed orifice of this vessel and no obstruction at the origin of the left coronary artery from the right.

The left coronary artery takes a long and tortuous course alongside the RVOT before branching to the circumflex (LCx) and left anterior descending artery (LAD).

The coronary angiogram demonstrates overall small peripheral coronary arteries that taper quickly, leaving relatively large areas underperfused (*panel 4, asterisks*).

***Comments:*** This investigation clearly excluded obstruction of the coronary arteries related to previous surgery or atherosclerosis. It demonstrated a rare variant of an aberrant origin and course of the left coronary artery with the vessel coursing anteriorly around the RVOT. In addition there was remarkable paucity of the peripheral coronary arteries of both the left and right coronary artery systems (*panel 4, asterisks*).

## FOCUSED CLINICAL QUESTIONS AND DISCUSSION POINTS

1. How common is an aberrant origin and course of the left coronary artery?

   *An aberrant origin of the left coronary artery is rare but must be considered in patients with exertional chest pain especially if they are young and without risk factors for acquired coronary artery disease. The exact incidence of this congenital anomaly in the general population is unknown. It was diagnosed in 0.6% of patients of a general cardiac catheterization laboratory population.[4] Males and females are equally affected. Recognition of this anomaly in childhood is rare and is more common in adolescence or young adult life possibly related to increased physical exertion.[8]*

2. What are the different anatomical types of anomalous coronary arteries?

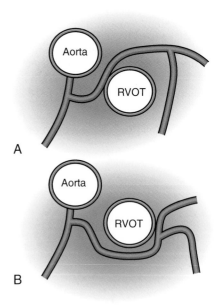

Figure 76-11 Schematic representation of two types of anomalous origin of the coronary artery (as viewed from the superior aspect).

*Both coronary arteries can arise ectopically from the aorta.*

*The ectopic left coronary artery may arise from the right sinus of valsalva, either from its own ostium or from a common ostium with the right coronary artery, or from the proximal right coronary artery. This distinction can be important to a surgeon attempting to remedy the problem, since an unroofing procedure may be performed for the former but not the latter. In either case,* the aberrant left coronary artery then usually passes posteriorly between the aorta and the RVOT to divide into the circumflex and anterior descending arteries (Fig. 76-11A).[4] In this patient, the aberrant left coronary artery crosses the RVOT anteriorly (Fig. 76-11B). This variant is rare.

The right coronary artery can arise aberrantly from the left coronary sinus and passes anteriorly between the aorta and the RV infundibulum. Similar to the ectopic left, the ectopic right coronary artery can arise from a separate ostium or from a common ostium with the left coronary artery or even from the proximal left coronary artery. The aberrant right coronary artery then passes anteriorly between the aorta and the pulmonary artery.

3. **What causes ischemia in patients with an aberrant left coronary artery?**

*Many mechanisms have been implicated and discussed by which an aberrant coronary artery can cause myocardial ischemia:*

*The ostium of the aberrant artery can be hypoplastic with a slit-like ostium or an ostium obstructed by excessive tissue within the tunica media of the aorta. This is usually associated with an isolated ectopic origin of the coronary artery (typically the left) from its own ostium off the aorta.*

*Obstruction of the coronary artery may also be explained by compression of the vessel by its abnormal course and acute takeoff or secondary to external compression (e.g., between the aorta and the RVOT; see panel A of Fig. 76-11).*

4. **Is an aberrant coronary artery necessarily of clinical significance?**

*Aberrant coronary arteries are sometimes an incidental finding. The aberrant artery does not necessarily cause ischemia and chest pain and therefore it is not always of clinical relevance. When the anomaly is identified, a related perfusion abnormality has to be ruled out.[9] The investigations suitable for this task are exercise ECG, myocardial perfusion scan, or MRI. All these modalities were employed in our patient.*

5. **What is considered to be the mechanism of stress-induced myocardial ischemia in this patient?**

*The patient has exercise-related ischemia, and none at rest. The mechanism of ischemia in this patient is not entirely clear. Several possibilities must be considered.*

**Aberrant Origin and Course of the Coronary Artery**
*It is possible that the aberrant left coronary artery becomes slightly compressed on exercise between the RVOT and the sternum. This compression may have become more significant after sternotomy, and subsequent scar tissue may have formed in the space between the left coronary artery and the sternum. This might explain the onset of symptoms late after aortic valve replacement.*

**Homograft Valve Stenosis**
*Even though this patient has only mild aortic (homograft) stenosis at rest, the pressure gradient across the valve increases significantly during exercise (though this was felt unlikely to be the single causative mechanism here).*

**Paucity of Distal Coronary Arteries**
*Lack of tertiary coronary arteries on coronary angiography and poor coronary blood supply in areas not perfused by the left coronary artery raise the possibility of insufficient coronary microvasculature.*

**Combination of Mechanisms**
*The combination homograft valve stenosis with increasing myocardial oxygen consumption on exercise and limited coronary blood flow at the level of the proximal left coronary artery and/or of the distal coronary arteries may provoke myocardial ischemia in this patient.*

*This case exemplifies a new major challenge in the care of patients with complex congenital heart lesions, namely the assessment of angina-like symptoms and myocardial ischemia. A common pitfall is to relate all symptoms to a single known congenital abnormality, when in reality several problems (acquired or congenital) may coexist. Because of complex etiology of symptoms, the results of intervention based on expected benefit are more difficult to predict.*

6. **What are the therapeutic options for this patient?**

*In general, therapy for symptomatic patients with an aberrant coronary artery should aim to avoid episodes of myocardial ischemia and hence to reduce the risk of ischemia-related complications like ventricular tachycardia and sudden cardiac death and to improve the symptoms of the patient.*

*Medical treatment with beta-blockers or calcium-channel blocking agents is recommended to limit heart rate increase on exercise.[8] It seems sensible to advise patients to limit their physical activities if necessary. Risk factors for atherosclerosis must be avoided or treated.*

*Mechanical interventions such as coronary artery bypass grafting and coronary ostioplasty do not seem appropriate interventions for this patient.*

*The indication for homograft replacement must be considered to reduce myocardial oxygen demand to the absolute minimum. This seems particularly important, as the patient wants to become pregnant. Pregnancy with its increase in blood volume and cardiac output can be seen as a state of continuous moderate exercise and may induce myocardial ischemia. In this patient, pregnancy may increase the patient's risk for ischemia-related complications like ventricular tachycardia and even sudden cardiac death. Although it may be tempting, the alternative of a mechanical valve would complicate future pregnancy a great deal because of the need for anticoagulation. After lengthy discussions, the multidisciplinary team felt there was not a clear risk:benefit ratio that would justify aortic valve replacement. The golden rule "first do no harm" prevailed, and the patient was prescribed medical therapy only.*

## FINAL DIAGNOSIS

Congenital aortic valve stenosis

Previous homograft aortic valve replacement

Mild stenosis of the homograft valve

Aberrant origin and course of the left coronary artery from the right coronary artery

## PLAN OF ACTION

Medical treatment with HMG-CoA reductase inhibitor (statin), beta-blockers, nitroglycerin, and aspirin for possible microvascular coronary artery disease, and modification of lifestyle to avoid exertional angina as much as possible

## OUTCOME

The patient was advised to avoid more than moderate exercise.

She was commenced on treatment with beta-blockers (metoprolol 25 mg twice daily), atorvastatin 10 mg once daily, isosorbide mononitrate 30 mg once daily, and aspirin 75 mg once daily.

Her symptoms improved on medical treatment, although mild angina still occurred at times.

The option of homograft replacement was discussed emphasizing that improvement of symptoms after surgery could not be guaranteed. The patient was not keen to undergo surgery but would reconsider this in case her symptoms worsened or when the function of the homograft valve deteriorated, as expected, with time. She is still anxious to have a child, and there is uncertainty as to what her current cardiovascular state means in terms of risks to herself, and whether aortic valve replacement would reduce that risk.

Continued clinical follow-up of the patient will focus on the function of the homograft valve to pick up any deterioration in valve function with time. It was felt that both resting and stress echocardiography in the first instance could guide management.

## Selected References

1. Brickner ME: Valvar aortic stenosis. In Gatzoulis MA, Webb G, Daubeney PEF (eds): Diagnosis and Management of Adult Congenital Heart Disease. Philadelphia, Churchill Livingstone, 2003, pp 213–221.
2. Ward C: Clinical significance of the bicuspid aortic valve. Heart 83:81–85, 2000.
3. Bonow RO, Carabello B, de Leon AC, et al: ACC/AHA guidelines for the management of patients with valvular heart disease. Exec- utive summary. A report of the American College of Cardiology/ American Heart Association Task Force on Practice Guidelines, Committee on Management of Patients with Valvular Heart Disease. J Heart Valve Dis 7:672–707, 1998.
4. Liberthson RR, Dinsmore RE, Fallon JT: Aberrant coronary artery origin from the aorta: Report of 18 patients, review of literature and delineation of natural history and management. Circulation 59:748–754, 1979.
5. Rocchini AP, Beekman RH, Ben Shachar G, et al: Balloon aortic valvuloplasty: Results of the Valvuloplasty and Angioplasty of Congenital Anomalies Registry. Am J Cardiol 65:784–789, 1990.
6. Liberthson RR: Sudden death from cardiac causes in children and young adults. N Engl J Med 334:1039–1044, 1996.
7. Niwa K, Perloff JK, Bhuta SM, et al: Structural abnormalities of great arterial walls in congenital heart disease: Light and electron microscopic analyses. Circulation 103:393–400, 2001.
8. Liberthson RR: Congenital anomalies of the coronary arteries. In Gatzoulis MA, Webb G, Daubeney PEF (eds): Diagnosis and Management of Adult Congenital Heart Disease. Philadelphia, Churchill Livingstone, 2003, pp 425–431.
9. Liberthson RR, Zaman L, Weyman A, et al: Aberrant origin of the left coronary artery from the proximal right coronary artery: Diagnostic features and pre- and postoperative course. Clin Cardiol 5:377–381, 1982.

# Anomalous Left Coronary Artery from the Pulmonary Artery

**Isabelle F. Vonder Muhll, Jonathan B. Choy, and Ivan M. Rebeyka**

**Age: 69 years**
**Gender: Female**
**Occupation: Retired office worker**
**Working diagnosis: Congestive heart failure**

## HISTORY

Although well throughout her life, the patient had been managed for angina and congestive heart failure with significant mitral regurgitation by her internist for the past 5 years. She presented to the hospital with a 3-month history of progressive nocturnal dyspnea and angina, relieved by sitting up.

**Comments:** In elderly patients presenting with heart failure symptoms, the underlying etiology usually relates to common acquired cardiac conditions: coronary artery disease, hypertensive heart disease, valvular heart disease, or idiopathic dilated cardiomyopathy.

At times, however, more rare causes may be encountered. This patient presented at an unusually advanced age with angina and heart failure symptoms caused by an anomalous left coronary artery from the pulmonary artery (ALCAPA).

## CURRENT SYMPTOMS

The patient could walk only 10 feet before becoming short of breath and was having paroxysmal nocturnal dyspnea. On the day of presentation to the emergency room she had experienced 2.5 hours of central chest pressure at rest that had not been relieved with nitroglycerin.

NYHA class: III

## CURRENT MEDICATIONS

Lisinopril 20 mg daily

Digoxin 125 µg daily

Metoprolol 25 mg twice daily

## PHYSICAL EXAMINATION

BP 110/70 mm Hg, HR 90 bpm, oxygen saturation 86% on room air and 91% on 5 L by nasal prongs

Height 170 cm, weight 74.4 kg, BSA 1.87 m²

Surgical scars: None

Neck veins: 10 cm above sternal angle, A-wave dominant

Lungs/chest: Chest exam had scattered bibasilar crepitations.

Heart: The pulse was regular. The apex was displaced to the anterior axillary line and enlarged. There was a single second heart sound and a prominent S3 gallop at the apex. A grade 2/6 pan-systolic murmur could be heard over the apex, along with a continuous murmur over the left second interspace.

Abdomen: Unremarkable

Extremities: No pedal edema was present, and distal pulses were palpable.

**Comments:** On presentation, this patient had findings of decompensated congestive cardiac failure, namely, low oxygen saturation, distended neck veins, a third heart sound, and pulmonary edema.

In ALCAPA, the LV clinically may show signs of dilatation with a displaced and enlarged apical impulse. Mitral regurgitation is common with ALCAPA, leading to a pan-systolic murmur. Mitral regurgitation in this condition relates to annular dilatation associated with ischemic remodeling of the LV, as well as papillary muscle ischemia and dysfunction. If mitral regurgitation is severe, a diastolic rumble due to increased flow may occur.

A continuous murmur is one that is heard in systole and continues without interruption into diastole. Such a murmur may be audible in ALCAPA due to high flow in coronary collaterals from the right coronary system to the low-pressure left coronary artery and pulmonary artery. Other possible causes of a continuous murmur (other than ALCAPA) include PDA, ruptured sinus of Valsalva, coronary fistulae to right-sided cardiac chambers, aortopulmonary collaterals, arteriovenous malformations, mammary souffle in pregnancy and lactation, venous hums, combined aortic regurgitation and VSD (not really continuous), and combined ASD with mitral stenosis (not really continuous).

## LABORATORY DATA

| | |
|---|---|
| Hemoglobin | 11.9 g/dL (11.5–15.0) |
| Hematocrit/PCV | **34%** (36–46) |
| MCV | 98 fL (83–99) |
| Platelet count | 226 × 10⁹/L (150–400) |
| Sodium | 142 mmol/L (134–145) |
| Potassium | 3.7 mmol/l (3.5–5.2) |
| Creatinine | 0.64 mg/dL (0.6–1.2) |
| Blood urea nitrogen | 5.4 mmol/L (2.5–6.5) |
| Cardiac troponin I | <0.2 µg/L (<0.2 µg/L) |

**Comments:** Normal hematology and chemistry panels were seen in this patient. With decompensated congestive cardiac failure, hyponatremia and impaired renal function might be expected but were not present.

Cardiac troponin is a useful marker of acute myocardial necrosis. Although it was not elevated in this patient on presentation, this does not rule out chronic ischemia or previous myocardial infarction.

## ELECTROCARDIOGRAM

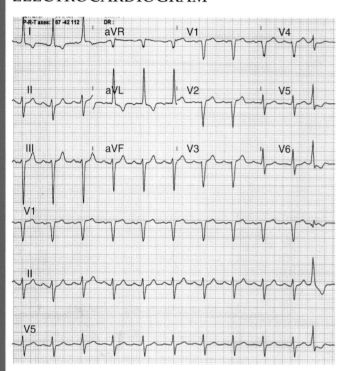

Figure 77-1  Electrocardiogram.

### FINDINGS

Heart rate: 87 bpm

QRS axis: –42°

QRS duration: 128 msec

The rhythm was sinus with a first-degree AV block and an interventricular conduction delay. There were occasional premature beats. There was left-axis deviation and probable LV hypertrophy with repolarization abnormalities (the ECG is not standardized).

**Comments:** The poor progression of the R-wave across the precordial leads suggests a possible old anterior wall infarction.

## CHEST X-RAY

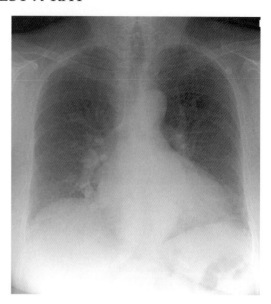

Figure 77-2  Posteroanterior projection.

### FINDINGS

Cardiothoracic ratio: 58%

Cardiomegaly was present as well as subtle vascular redistribution. No pleural effusions. LA dilatation was suspected because of the widened carinal angle.

**Comments:** These findings are in keeping with decompensated congestive cardiac failure. The elevated "horizontal" course of the left main bronchus is a sign of LA enlargement.

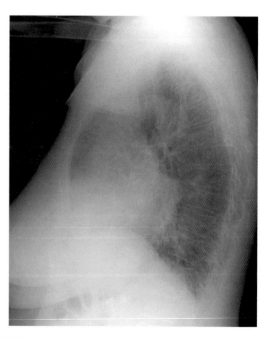

Figure 77-3  Lateral view.

## FINDINGS

On the lateral film, there was again evidence of LA enlargement with a prominent bulge at the upper posterior aspect of the main cardiac shadow.

***Comments:*** LA enlargement suggests the presence of underlying mitral valve disease.

# ECHOCARDIOGRAM

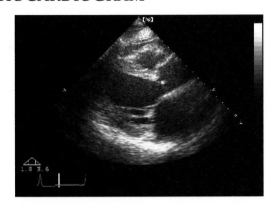

Figure 77-4 Parasternal long-axis view.

## FINDINGS

Initial transthoracic echocardiogram demonstrated poor LV systolic function with an ejection fraction of 20%. The parasternal long-axis view showed a dilated LV in diastole and systole with regional wall motion abnormalities consisting of anteroseptal akinesis and severe posterobasal hypokinesis.

***Comments:*** Impaired LV systolic function is common in ALCAPA due to chronic myocardial ischemia, and can be well demonstrated echocardiographically. Multiple short- and long-axis views of the LV are necessary for a complete wall motion assessment.

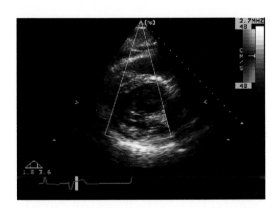

Figure 77-5 Color Doppler short-axis view.

## FINDINGS

On color Doppler imaging in short axis, prominent color flow was seen within the interventricular septum. Moderately severe mitral regurgitation was also present.

***Comments:*** The echocardiographic examination in ALCAPA should include an assessment of the severity of the mitral regurgitation. Prominent color flow within the interventricular septum and the epicardial surface of the heart is due to flow within large coronary collaterals.

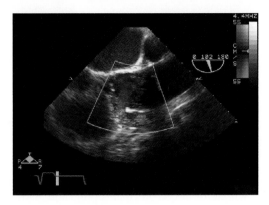

Figure 77-6 Long-axis view of the aortic root.

## FINDINGS

TEE identified a severely dilated right coronary artery (with aneurysmal appearance) seen on this long-axis view of the aortic root.

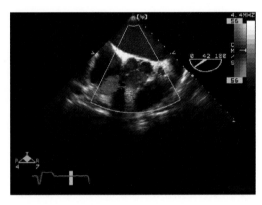

Figure 77-7 Transesophageal echocardiogram of short axis of aortic root.

## FINDINGS

In short axis of the aortic root by TEE, the dilated right coronary artery measured more than 10 mm in diameter. There was no left main coronary artery from the left coronary cusp.

***Comments:*** Echocardiography can be used to image the proximal coronary arteries. If normal origins of coronary arteries from their respective coronary sinus cannot be identified, anomalous origin should be suspected. The right coronary enlargement here is due to increased flow, as it connects via collaterals to the left coronary system and hence to the low-pressure pulmonary artery.

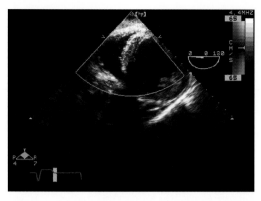

Figure 77-8 Transesophageal echocardiogram of short axis of left ventricle.

## FINDINGS

On the short axis of the LV by TEE, an extensive vascular network of dilated collateral vessels with prominent color flow was seen within the interventricular septum and on the epicardial surface of the heart. LV views also showed severely reduced systolic function.

## NUCLEAR IMAGING

Note: Nuclear images not available.

### FINDINGS

A resting thallium scan of the heart showed a small anterior wall infarct, although the remainder of the LV was viable.

***Comments:*** Although this patient had been subject to the effects of chronic ischemia, there was only a small area of infarcted myocardium, suggesting the patient had reversible myocardial dysfunction that might improve with revascularization.

## CATHETERIZATION

### HEMODYNAMICS

Heart rate  79 bpm

|        | Pressure       | Saturation (%) |
|--------|----------------|----------------|
| SVC    | 8              | 71             |
| IVC    | 8              | 60             |
| RA     | 8              | 68             |
| RV     | 37/9           | 67             |
| PA     | 35/10 mean 21  | 78             |
| PCWP   | 6              | 97             |
| LV     | 138/12         | 97             |
| Aorta  | 133/61 mean 89 | 97             |

### Calculations

| | |
|---|---|
| Qp (L/min) | 5.79 |
| Qs (L/min) | 3.92 |

| | |
|---|---|
| Cardiac index (L/min/m$^2$) | 2.09 |
| Qp/Qs | 1.48 |
| PVR (Wood units) | 2.59 |
| SVR (Wood units) | 20.64 |

### FINDINGS

Intracardiac pressures were normal after treatment of her heart failure. There was a significant step-up in oxygen saturation between the RV and the pulmonary artery, and the left-to-right shunt was calculated to be 1.5:1.

***Comments:*** Cardiac catheterization is indicated in patients presenting with symptoms of angina and heart failure, especially to assess for the presence and severity of acquired coronary artery disease.

A step-up in oxygen saturation between the right ventricle and the pulmonary artery suggests a shunt at the great vessel level: PDA, aortopulmonary window, and aberrant coronary artery origin should be considered. This patient had enough shunting of blood through the right coronary artery via fistulous collateral connections to the left coronary artery and retrograde to the pulmonary artery to produce a measurable step-up in oxygen saturation at the pulmonary artery level. This shunt contributed to a coronary steal syndrome from the myocardium, further affecting myocardial perfusion as well as increasing the workload of the LV.

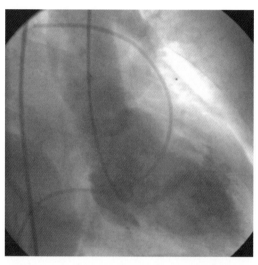

Figure 77-9 Left ventricular angiogram in anteroposterior projection.

### FINDINGS

The angiogram showed moderately severe LV dysfunction, particularly affecting the anterior and posterobasal walls of the LV.

***Comments:*** If contrast load was a concern, the LV angiogram could have been omitted since data about LV function were already available from the echocardiograms.

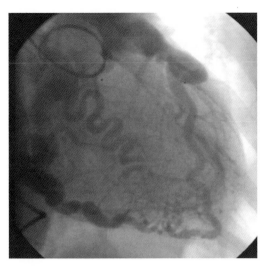

Figure 77-10 Right anterior oblique view.

## FINDINGS

The angiogram demonstrated the presence of an extensive network of collaterals from a hugely dilated right coronary artery draining through the left anterior descending and left main coronary into the pulmonary artery.

**Comments:** The goal of coronary angiography is to demonstrate the anatomy of the coronary arteries. A power injection was needed in this case to adequately opacify the right coronary. A gigantic right coronary artery supplied the entire left ventricle through a network of collaterals to the left anterior descending artery, which in turn drained into the main pulmonary artery. The main pulmonary artery could be recognized by its bifurcation into right and left pulmonary arteries.

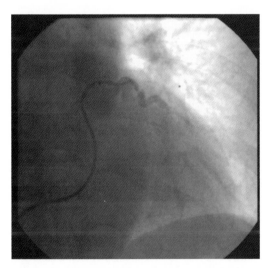

Figure 77-11 Right anterior oblique view as seen in pulmonary arteriography.

## FINDINGS

Pulmonary arteriography revealed the origin of the left main coronary artery from the pulmonary artery. In the RAO view shown here, selective injection of the left coronary artery showed the vessel to be tortuous and small relative to the right coronary artery.

**Comments:** Localizing the left coronary artery and its relationship to the aorta is helpful in planning a surgical inter-

vention. The ALCAPA anatomy can also be demonstrated non-invasively by contrast CT (best resolution) or CMR scan (lower resolution).

### FOCUSED CLINICAL QUESTIONS AND DISCUSSION POINTS

1. **What is the typical presentation of ALCAPA?**

*The clinical presentation of ALCAPA (sometimes also referred to as Bland-White-Garland syndrome) varies tremendously and depends on pulmonary arterial pressures and the adequacy of collateral coronary flow. In utero, the perfusion of the fetal heart is maintained due to high pulmonary arterial pressures, allowing the heart to develop normally. However, when pulmonary arterial pressures fall after birth, perfusion pressure in the left coronary artery starts to fall, which—in the absence of adequate collaterals—results in LV ischemia, leading to overt heart failure or sudden death in infancy. Without treatment, more than 80% of infants die in the first year of life.*

*Due to the stimulus of ischemia or perhaps because of innate potential, collaterals from the right coronary artery develop to supply left coronary flow. These are often incomplete resulting in zones of ischemic or infarcted myocardium. Typically, the LV remodels with dilatation, leading to significant mitral regurgitation. LV scar may lead to malignant ventricular arrhythmias. For those with collaterals who survive into childhood, presentation may be related to the murmur of mitral regurgitation, heart failure, chest pain on exertion, ventricular tachycardia, or sudden death.*

*If an extensive collateral coronary circulation is present, as in this patient, asymptomatic survival to adulthood is possible. Decompensation eventually occurred due to significant shunting of coronary blood through fistulous collaterals from the right coronary artery via the left coronary artery to the pulmonary artery, resulting in presumed myocardial steal with myocardial ischemia and dysfunction.*

2. **What management options are available in ALCAPA?**

*Medical management consists of standard therapies for heart failure such as diuretics for congestion, ACE inhibitors for afterload reduction, as well as beta-blockers. For symptoms of myocardial ischemia, nitroglycerin and beta-blockers can be used. Antiarrhythmic medications may be necessary. However, medical management is only adjunctive, as the diagnosis of ALCAPA is an indication for surgery if the needed skills and experience are available.*

*Surgical options include coronary reimplantation, bypass of the anomalous coronary artery with ligation of its origin, and simple ligation of the left coronary artery.[1] Concomitant mitral regurgitation is usually not addressed with initial repair of ALCAPA, although this is still an area of controversy. In children, as ventricular contractility recovers postoperatively, valve function usually improves.[2] In the event of severe LV dysfunction, heart transplantation may be required.*

3. **What are the risks and benefits of the various surgical options?**

*The goal of surgery is to improve myocardial perfusion, ideally by restoring a two-coronary arterial system. Surgical relocation of the anomalous left coronary onto the aorta is the procedure of choice, especially in infants and children.[3] This may be technically difficult depending on the position of the anomalous origin relative to the aorta, hence various surgical procedures have been developed to baffle the left coronary artery back to the aortic root, either through[4] or around[5] the pulmonary artery. Outcomes after restoration of a two-coronary system (at least in children) are very favorable with normalization of ventricular function and exercise capacity and amelioration of symptoms being the norm.[6] Moreover, earlier patient age at surgery has been associated with better recovery of LV function.[7]*

*Unfortunately, coronary tissue in the adult patient with ALCAPA may be friable and thin, making surgical relocation of the left coronary artery a challenge. Bypass grafting using left internal mammary artery or saphenous vein graft to the left coronary artery in combination with ligation of its origin from the pulmonary artery is advocated by some surgeons for adult patients; however, myocardial perfusion may be inadequate when collaterals from the right coronary artery are large, leading to competitive flow.*

*Ligation of the left coronary artery alone to alleviate the coronary steal syndrome and improve perfusion pressure of the myocardium was first performed in 1959 by Sabiston. Since publication of several cases demonstrating increased mortality and late complications in children after coronary ligation compared to reimplantation,[8] the ligation technique has largely been abandoned.*

*Unlike surgery in children, there is no definite consensus on which operative technique is superior in the adult patient with ALCAPA—reimplantation, ligation with bypass grafting, or ligation alone—as no clear benefit has been demonstrated for one technique over the other in adults.[9] The surgical approach should take into consideration patient factors (age, coronary anatomy, ventricular function, and viability), and local expertise.*

*Cardiac transplantation should be reserved for those with intractable heart failure and irreversible ventricular dysfunction.*

**4. What long-term complications need to be considered in follow-up?**

*There is potential for ongoing ventricular dysfunction, mitral regurgitation, and arrhythmias. Hence, clinical follow-up and serial echocardiography are indicated. Holter monitoring and stress testing with or without perfusion imaging may be useful to assess arrhythmia or ischemia, if clinically indicated.*

*Patients with conduits or baffles to support their left coronary circulation should be followed for potential late complications including conduit leaks or stenosis, supravalvular pulmonary stenosis, and aortic insufficiency.*

*Adult patients who were repaired in childhood with simple ligation should be monitored for ongoing ischemia and are at risk for sudden death. Consideration should be given to elective surgery to establish a two-coronary circulation.*

## FINAL DIAGNOSIS

ALCAPA with severe LV systolic dysfunction and moderate mitral regurgitation

## PLAN OF ACTION

The range of surgical options was considered in this case. However, mitigating factors against reimplantation of the left coronary artery were the extensive collateral system of coronary perfusion that had developed in this patient and the location of the left coronary, which would have made it technically challenging to relocate. The presence of ventricular dysfunction made the avoidance of cardiopulmonary bypass and cardioplegic arrest desirable. Given the age of the patient, a simple surgical solution was chosen, and the decision was made to ligate the left coronary artery at its origin from the pulmonary artery.

## INTERVENTION

Ligation of the left coronary artery was performed without complication, and the patient made a good postoperative recovery.

## OUTCOME

After ligation of the anomalous left coronary artery, there was a sustained improvement in symptoms. The patient remained free of angina, and her functional status improved to NYHA class I. A postoperative nuclear perfusion scan with exercise stress showed the previously seen small anterior wall infarct and no residual ischemia.

Postoperatively, she developed paroxysmal atrial fibrillation, requiring rate control with digoxin and beta-blockers as well as anticoagulation.

***Comments:*** Although ligation of the left coronary artery would not be recommended for children or younger adults because of the availability of better surgical techniques, this case illustrates a potential role for coronary ligation in selected older patients for amelioration of symptoms.

Patients with ALCAPA are at risk for the development of arrhythmias at any time in their clinical course. Supraventricular arrhythmias, such as atrial fibrillation, which occurred in this case, may arise due to atrial dilatation associated with ventricular dysfunction and/or mitral regurgitation.

Ventricular arrhythmias may be related to myocardial scarring due to previous infarction. With the current trend toward device implantation to prevent sudden cardiac death, if ventricular arrhythmias, complex ventricular ectopy, or persistently depressed LV function (EF < 30%) was documented postoperatively, consideration should be given to implantation of an automated cardioverter-defibrillator.

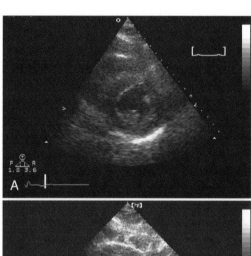

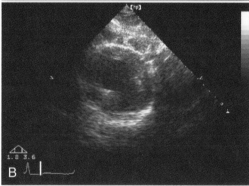

Figure 77-12 Short-axis view of the left ventricle. **A,** Postoperative echocardiography. **B,** Comparison preoperative image.

### FINDINGS

Follow-up echocardiography performed 6 months postoperatively revealed an improvement in anteroseptal wall motion seen on short-axis view of the LV (preoperative image is also shown for comparison). Overall LV function was significantly improved compared to preoperatively, albeit still depressed with an ejection fraction estimated to be 35%. The degree of mitral regurgitation after surgery was moderate, but improved.

***Comments:*** The degree of postoperative improvement in ventricular function can be predicted to some extent on the amount of viable myocardium from preoperative studies such as thallium scanning, stress echocardiography, or CMR with gadolinium hyperenhancement. Recovery of LV function will depend on the patient's age, the duration and severity of pre-operative ischemia, and the effectiveness of coronary perfusion after surgery.

## Selected References

1. Dodge-Khatami A, Mavroudis C, Backer CL: Anomalous origin of the left coronary artery from the pulmonary artery: Collective review of surgical therapy. Ann Thorac Surg 74:946–955, 2002.
2. Huddleston CB, Balzer DT, Mendeloff EN: Repair of anomalous left main coronary artery arising from pulmonary artery in infants: Long-term impact on the mitral valve. Ann Thorac Surg 71: 1985–1989, 2001.
3. Backer CL, Hillman ND, Dodge-Khatami A, et al: Anomalous origin of the left main coronary from the pulmonary artery: Suc-cessful surgical strategy without assist devices. Semin Thorac Cardiovasc Surg Pediatr Card Surg Ann 3:165–172, 2000.
4. Takeuchi S, Imamura H, Katsumoto K, et al: New surgical method for repair of anomalous left coronary artery from pulmonary artery. J Thorac Cardiovasc Surg 78:7–11, 1979.
5. Barth MJ, Allen BS, Gulecyuz M, et al: Experience with an alterna-tive technique for the management of anomalous left coronary artery from the pulmonary artery. Ann Thorac Surg 76:1429–1434, 2003.
6. Cochrane AD, Coleman DM, Davis AM, et al: Excellent long-term functional outcome after an operation for anomalous left coronary artery from the pulmonary artery. J Thorac Cardiovasc Surg 117:332–342, 1999.
7. Michielon G, Di Carlo D, Brancaccio G, et al: Anomalous coronary artery origin from the pulmonary artery: Correlation between sur-gical timing and left ventricular function recovery. Ann Thorac Surg 76:581–588, 2003.
8. Bunton R, Jonas RA, Lang P, et al: Anomalous origin of left coro-nary artery from pulmonary artery: Ligation versus establishment of a two coronary artery system. J Thorac Cardiovasc Surg 93: 103–108, 1987.
9. Moodie DS, Fyfe D, Gill CC, et al: Anomalous origin of the left coronary artery from the pulmonary artery (Bland-White-Garland syndrome) in adult patients: Long-term follow-up after surgery. Am Heart J 106:381–388, 1983.

# Coronary Artery Fistulae and Their Significance

Sabrina D. Phillips

**Age:** 63 years
**Gender:** Female
**Occupation:** Homemaker
**Working diagnosis:** Endocarditis

## HISTORY

The patient was well until approximately 4 months prior to presentation, when she developed exercise intolerance, fever, cough, and generalized malaise. She was evaluated and subsequently treated for presumed pneumonia.

The patient had no improvement after a 2-week course of oral erythromycin. The patient was reevaluated.

CXR revealed cardiomegaly, and an ECG demonstrated LA enlargement and first-degree AV block. Cardiology evaluation was recommended. Prior to the evaluation, the patient developed symptoms consistent with a urinary tract infection. After finishing a complete course of antibiotics, her urinary symptoms resolved. Her cough also improved, as did her feeling of malaise.

She was a lifetime nonsmoker, with no prior history of significant infection. She reported excellent exercise tolerance throughout her life, with no perceived limitations. She had had two pregnancies, which were uncomplicated.

*Comments:* The prolonged nature of this episode should prompt an evaluation for subacute infections or noninfectious causes of fever.

Cardiomegaly with clear lung fields raises the concern for either pericardial effusion or cardiac disease. First-degree AV block can be seen in age-related degeneration of the conduction system, but can also be related to intracardiac anomalies such as a primum atrial septal defect. A new first-degree AV block can be seen in aortic valve endocarditis with extension of infection into the perivalvular area.

## CURRENT SYMPTOMS

The patient complains of generalized fatigue and dyspnea on exertion.

NYHA class: II

## CURRENT MEDICATIONS

None

## PHYSICAL EXAMINATION

BP 135/80 mm Hg, HR 66 bpm, oxygen saturation 100%

Height 166 cm, weight 62 kg, BSA 1.69 m$^2$

Surgical scars: None

Neck veins: Normal

Lungs/chest: Clear to auscultation and percussion

Heart: The heart rhythm was regular. There was a normal left ventricular impulse with a 2+ RV impulse. There was a continuous murmur heard best at the left sternal border in the fourth intercostal space. P2 was soft.

Abdomen: No hepatosplenomegaly was present, or other masses palpated.

Extremities: Peripheral pulses were 4/4 throughout with no radiofemoral delay.

*Comments:* The pulse pressure was normal, and keeping with a good stroke volume.

Elevated JVP is seen in conditions resulting in increased RV and RA pressure, such as pulmonary hypertension, and RV outflow or inflow obstruction. Volume loading, especially chronic, does not necessarily cause JVP elevation because of increased compliance of the RA and the systemic venous bed.

A prominent right ventricular impulse implies RV volume or pressure overload. A soft P2 implies normal pulmonary artery systolic pressure. This patient likely has a lesion that has resulted in RV volume overload. A continuous murmur can be heard in an adult with PDA, ruptured sinus of Valsalva aneurysm, and coronary arteriovenous fistula. Of these, only ruptured sinus of Valsalva aneurysm and arteriovenous fistula might result in RV volume overload. A ruptured sinus of Valsalva aneurysm with significant shunt would be associated with a wide pulse pressure. Acutely, this could also result in cardiac decompensation. While both of these entities could be associated with endocarditis, given the clinical signs here the most likely underlying lesions would be a form of arteriovenous fistula.

## PERTINENT NEGATIVES

No cyanosis, clubbing, or edema. No Osler nodes or Janeway lesions. Normal funduscopic exam.

# LABORATORY DATA

| Leukocytes | $6.2 \times 10^9$/L (3.5–10.5) |
|---|---|
| Differential: | |
| Neutrophils | 58% (42–75) |
| Lymphocytes | 31% (16–52) |
| Monocytes | 9% (1–11) |
| Eosinophils | 1% (0–7) |
| Basophils | 1% (0–4) |
| Hemoglobin | **10 g/dL** (11.5–15.0) |
| Hematocrit/PCV | **31%** (36–46) |
| MCV | 90 fL (83–99) |
| Platelet count | $359 \times 10^9$/L (150–400) |
| Sodium | 138 mmol/L (134–145) |
| Potassium | 4.3 mmol/L (3.5–5.2) |
| Creatinine | 0.8 mg/dL (0.6–1.2) |
| Blood urea nitrogen | 3.0 mmol/L (2.5–6.5) |

***Comments:*** The leukocyte count and differential are normal. This does not exclude subacute bacterial endocarditis, as only 20% to 30% of cases will have a leukocytosis.[1]

A normocytic anemia is demonstrated, likely representing anemia of chronic disease, such as with a chronic infection.

## OTHER RELEVANT LAB RESULTS

Erythrocyte sedimentation rate (ESR): **92**
Blood cultures: No growth

***Comments:*** There is a significant elevation in erythrocyte sedimentation rate. This is a nonspecific marker, but consistent with the suspected diagnosis of endocarditis. Negative blood cultures are common in patients with endocarditis who have been recently treated with antibiotics. There are also several organisms that cause culture-negative endocarditis. These include *Coxiella burnetii*, Bartonella, nutritionally variant streptococci, and fungi. Of course, noninfectious causes of endocarditis (marantic endocarditis, Libman-Sacks endocarditis, and antiphospholipid antibody-related vegetation) should be considered in a patient with vegetation and persistently negative cultures while off antibiotics.

# ELECTROCARDIOGRAM

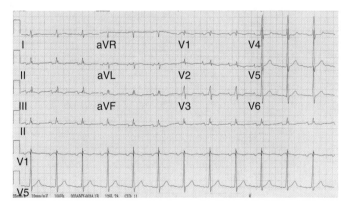

Figure 78-1 Electrocardiogram.

# FINDINGS

Heart rate: 73 bpm

QRS axis: +73°

QRS duration: 104 msec

Normal sinus rhythm with first-degree AV block. LA overload. Nonspecific T-wave abnormality.

***Comments:*** There is no specific diagnosis that can be supported by this surface ECG.

# CHEST X-RAY

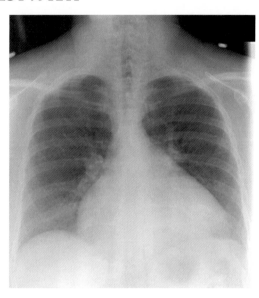

Figure 78-2 Posteroanterior projection.

# FINDINGS

Cardiothoracic ratio: 67%

Marked cardiac enlargement with somewhat prominent pulmonary arteries and a small aortic knuckle.

***Comments:*** The cardiac silhouette suggests enlargement of the RA. The rounded left cardiac border is consistent with RV enlargement. The pulmonary vasculature demonstrates pulmonary plethora (overcirculation) with central pulmonary artery enlargement and prominence of the peripheral pulmonary vessels. These findings are consistent with a long-standing left-to-right shunt.

# ECHOCARDIOGRAM

## Overall Findings

There was normal LV size and systolic function, with normal function of the aortic and mitral valves.

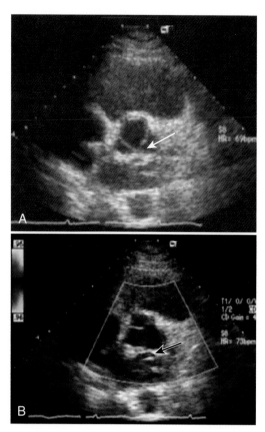

Figure 78-3 Parasternal short-axis view (**A**) with 2D color mapping (**B**).

## Findings

There was an unusual echolucent area near the aortic valve (*arrow*). Color flow mapping showed a bidirectional flow pattern within this space (*B*).

**Comments:** Abnormal fluid-filled areas seen around the aortic valve can be due to dissection, pericardial fluid in large pericardial recesses, abscess formation, or coronary fistulae. Visible color flow makes coronary fistulae the most likely diagnosis.

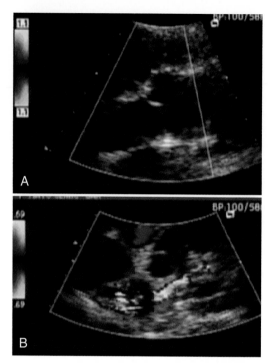

Figure 78-4 Parasternal long-axis view of aortic root (**A**) with 2D color mapping (**B**).

## Findings

A jet of turbulent color was present just behind the aortic root where the left coronary artery usually arises.

With further angulation of the transducer a long line of color flow within this region was visible throughout the cardiac cycle.

**Comments:** Typically, turbulent flow in the coronary arteries is never seen, and in this case must be consistent with a coronary fistula containing high-volume flow at high pressure, which persists throughout systole and diastole.

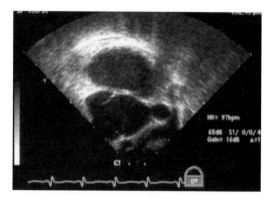

Figure 78-5 Upper esophageal view at 0 degrees.

## Findings

The view demonstrates a diffusely enlarged left main coronary artery with normal aortic origin. There are two segments of a large vessel seen posterior to the aorta.

**Comments:** Diffuse enlargement of the coronary arteries should prompt a search for a cause of increased flow through the artery. Examples include anomalous coronary artery origin from the pulmonary artery, a single coronary artery, and coronary artery fistula/arteriovenous malformation. In contrast, focal enlargement of the coronary arteries or aneurysm formation can be the result of atherosclerosis, vasculitis, or trauma. This image demonstrates diffuse enlargement of the left main and proximal left anterior descending artery, implying increased flow.

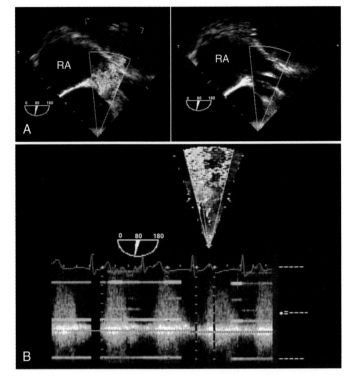

Figure 78-6 Midesophageal view at 80°, with and without 2D color (**A**). Continuous-wave Doppler interrogation of the turbulent flow (**B**).

## FINDINGS

This interrogation demonstrates continuous turbulent flow into the RA from two separate orifices, which originate from an anomalous vessel.

**Comments:** The RA normally has three major sources of inflow: the SVC, the IVC, and the coronary sinus. Flow into the RA near the SVC-RA junction could represent anomalous pulmonary venous return, an ASD, or a coronary artery fistula. The atrial septum appears intact in this view. Furthermore, the abnormal flow clearly arises from a vessel. Tracing the vessel to its origin and interrogating the flow with Doppler is necessary to correctly identify the anomaly. This vessel can be traced back to the left main coronary artery. This longitudinal view corresponds to the cross-sectional view of the tortuous vessel posterior to the aorta shown in Figure 78-3. The Doppler flow pattern demonstrates continuous flow. Continuous flow into the RA implies that both the systolic and diastolic pressures of the anomalous vessel are higher than the RA pressure.

## CATHETERIZATION

### HEMODYNAMICS

Heart rate    73 bpm

|  | Pressure | Saturation (%) |
|---|---|---|
| SVC | 6 | 54 |
| IVC | 6 | 66 |
| RA | 6 | 78 |
| RV | 26/9 | |
| PA | 27/10 mean 17 | 74 |
| PCWP | mean 13 | |
| LA | | 98 |
| LV | 116/14 | |
| Aorta | 115/58 mean 72 | 98 |

Calculations
| | |
|---|---|
| Qp (L/min) | 4.79 |
| Qs (L/min) | 2.80 |
| Cardiac index (L/min/m²) | 1.66 |
| Qp/Qs | 1.71 |
| PVR (Wood units) | 0.84 |
| SVR (Wood units) | 23.54 |

### FINDINGS

A left-to-right shunt at the atrial level is demonstrated, with a pulmonary-to-systemic flow ratio of 1.7:1. Pulmonary artery pressures are normal.

**Comments:** Right and left heart catheterization was performed to evaluate pulmonary artery pressures and to quantify the intracardiac shunt.

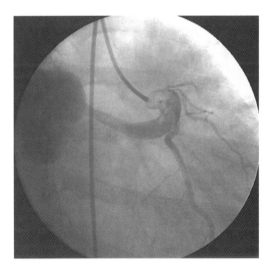

Figure 78-7 Coronary angiogram, 24 caudal 15 right anterior oblique view.

### FINDINGS

Contrast injection into the left main coronary artery showed a large fistula connecting the left main coronary artery to the RA.

**Comments:** Coronary angiography confirms the coronary artery fistula and demonstrates the remainder of the coronary artery. This information is helpful in planning surgical or catheter intervention.

## Focused Clinical Questions and Discussion Points

### 1. What is the anatomical diagnosis?

*The patient has a coronary artery fistula, with connection from the left main coronary artery to the RA. This results in a left-to-right shunt, with subsequent RA and RV volume overload. The incidence of coronary artery fistula in the adult population referred for coronary angiography is between 0.1% and 0.2%.[2] However, coronary artery fistulae are the most common hemodynamically significant congenital coronary artery anomalies.[3]*

### 2. Why was the patient febrile?

*Coronary artery fistulae can result in endocarditis,[4] with this being the presenting complaint of the patient. This patient likely had endocarditis, which was partially treated by the 4 weeks of antibiotics that she received before completing her evaluation.*

### 3. Should the fistula be ligated?

*Coronary artery fistulae with significant shunting can result in congestive heart failure, coronary ischemia from a "steal" phenomenon, aneurysmal dilation and fistula rupture, and arrhythmia.[5] This patient has a large left main coronary artery fistula with a significant left-to-right shunt and RA/RV volume overload. Furthermore, the fistula seems to have been complicated with endocarditis. Therefore, this fistula should be interrupted to avoid further complications.*

*Closure of nearly all coronary artery fistulae has been advocated by some authors to avoid fistula-related complications and mortality. Closure of fistulae that result in symptoms, right heart enlargement, or complications should be seriously considered.[6] Fistulae can be surgically ligated, or occluded with a transcatheter approach and coil placement. Coil occlusion has been recommended in patients with the following characteristics: access to the coronary artery supplying the fistula, a single narrow drainage site, absence of large branch vessels, and absence of multiple fistulae.[7]*

## FINAL DIAGNOSIS

Coronary artery fistula, left main to RA

## PLAN OF ACTION

Completion of full course of intravenous antibiotics, followed by elective surgical repair

## INTERVENTION

Ligation and division of the fistula was performed via median sternotomy. Two entry sites into the RA were visualized, and the fistulous attachments were ligated.

Catheter-based intervention was not considered since there was not a single narrow drainage site and the fistula was coming off directly from the left main coronary artery.

Cardiopulmonary bypass is not necessary in coronary fistula ligations, but is necessary in cases where intracardiac patching is performed. Large fistulae with multiple connections to a cardiac chamber may be best treated with an intracardiac approach.

## OUTCOME

There was no residual shunt after surgical ligation. The patient did develop atrial flutter postoperatively. She failed initial direct current cardioversion, but had successful cardioversion after the initiation of therapy with propafenone.

On 6-month follow-up the RV size had reduced, but the RA remained enlarged. There was no evidence of residual shunt on transthoracic echocardiography imaging, and no evidence of residual or recurrent endocarditis.

## Selected References

1. Infective endocarditis. In Kasper DL, Braunwald E, Fauci AS (eds): Harrison's Principles of Internal Medicine. New York, McGraw Hill Medical Publishing, 2004.
2. Vavurunakis M, Bush CA, Boudoulas H: Coronary artery fistulas in adults: Incidence, angiographic characteristic, natural history. Cathet Cardiovasc Diagn 35:116–120, 1995.
3. Levin DC, Fellows KE, Abrams HL: Hemodynamically significant primary anomalies of the coronary arteries: Angiographic aspects. Circulation 58:25–34, 1978.
4. Kasravi B, Reid CL, Allen BJ: Coronary artery fistula presenting as bacterial endocarditis. J Am Echocardiogr 17:1315–1316, 2004.
5. Liberthson RR, Sagar K, Berkoben JP, et al: Congenital coronary arteriovenous fistula: Report of 13 patients, review of the literature and delineation of management. Circulation 59:849–854, 1979.
6. Hong G, Lin C, Lee C, et al: Congenital coronary artery fistulas: Clinical considerations and surgical treatment. A NZ J Surg 74: 350–355, 2004.
7. Mavroudis C, Backer CL, Rocchini AP, et al: Coronary artery fistulas in infants and children: A surgical review and discussion of coil embolization. Ann Thorac Surg 63:1235–1242, 1997.

# Long-Term Management of Kawasaki Disease

**Etsuko Tsuda, Hideki Uemura, and Toshikatsu Yagihara**

**Age: 19 years**
**Gender: Female**
**Occupation: Student**
**Working diagnosis: Kawasaki disease**

## HISTORY

The patient presented acutely with Kawasaki disease at the age of 20 months and was treated with aspirin. At age 23 months, she experienced chest pain with ST elevation seen in ECG leads II, III, and aVF, and had an inferior myocardial infarction. The infarction was followed by mild mitral regurgitation and impaired LV systolic function.

At 3 years of age, coronary angiography showed complete occlusion of the right coronary artery, with a giant aneurysm at the bifurcation of the left coronary artery. Repeat coronary angiography at age 10 showed in addition segmental stenosis of the left circumflex artery, though the patient was clinically stable. Segmental stenosis, which is a typical characteristic lesion as sequelae after Kawasaki disease, implies the development of several new small vessels representing recanalization after coronary artery occlusion.

By age 15, the patient had signs of heart failure due to ischemic cardiomyopathy. LV end-diastolic volume was increased. Multifocal premature ventricular contractions, as well as non-sustained ventricular tachycardia, were noted. Within a year she underwent coronary artery bypass grafting to the left anterior descending artery using the left internal mammary artery concomitantly with conventional reduction of the mitral valve annulus (by means of the so-called Kay-Reed method). The patient was said to be in NYHA class III in the early postoperative period. Warfarin was meticulously given for 1 year after surgery, in addition to aspirin.

One year after bypass surgery her functional class had improved to NYHA class II. A beta-blocker was added to her medications. She had no chest pain. Catheterization showed that the LV end-diastolic volume had decreased. The left internal mammary graft remained patent, but was extremely slender ("string sign").

*Comments:* Kawasaki disease is an infantile acute febrile mucocutaneous lymph node syndrome. The inflammatory process can cause arteritis and, in a large proportion of patients, involves the coronary arteries in particular. This frequently leads to the formation of large aneurysms in the proximal coronaries, eventually with calcification of the wall of the aneurysm. Giant aneurysms (>8 mm) are likely to occlude with thrombosis, and this can lead to acute myocardial infarction. Acute myocardial infarction occasionally causes sudden death or impairs LV function, a major determinant of outcome in this population.

In this patient, mitral regurgitation worsened the LV dilatation and vice versa. Although surgical mitral valvuloplasty improved the regurgitation, LV dysfunction persisted.

In children undergoing coronary revascularization for Kawasaki disease, it is not rare for the bypass graft to become narrow and atretic.[1] This likely reflects competition from native coronary flow. This phenomenon indicates the importance of a justifiable indication for coronary artery bypass grafting. It should be performed only when the native flow is severely impaired.

## CURRENT SYMPTOMS

Mild exertional dyspnea. The patient was finding it more difficult to keep up with the demands of her full-time university education.

NYHA class: II

## CURRENT MEDICATIONS

Aspirin 200 mg daily

Furosemide 40 mg daily

Spironolactone 50 mg twice daily

Metoprolol 25 mg twice daily

*Comments:* Today, anticoagulation with warfarin is routinely recommended for patients with Kawasaki disease,[2] since giant aneurysms may become thrombosed, often within the first year after the acute phase of the disease. This was not known in the past, however, and this is the reason that this patient was not on warfarin at the time.

## PHYSICAL EXAMINATION

BP 104/60 mm Hg, HR 60 bpm, oxygen saturation 95%

Height 159 cm, weight 41 kg, BSA 1.35 m$^2$

Neck veins: Normal waveform, not elevated

Lungs/chest: Clear

Heart: The heart had a regular rhythm. The second heart sound was normally split. There was a grade 2/6 holo-systolic murmur at the apex. Peripheral pulses were normal.

Abdomen: Liver was not palpable.

Extremities: Normal, no edema was present

**Comments:** The murmur is consistent with mitral regurgitation.

## LABORATORY DATA

| | |
|---|---|
| Hemoglobin | 13.5 g/dL (11.5–15.0) |
| Hematocrit/PCV | 39% (36–46) |
| Sodium | 140 mmol/L (134–145) |
| Potassium | 3.5 mmol/L (3.5–5.2) |
| Creatinine | 0.6 mg/dL (0.6–1.2) |
| Blood urea nitrogen | 2.8 mg/dL (2.5–6.5) |

### OTHER RELEVANT LAB RESULTS

| | |
|---|---|
| Protein | 6.5 g/dL (6.5–8.2) |
| Albumin | 3.9 g/dL (3.6–5.5) |
| Total bilirubin | 1.0 mg/dL (0.2–1.2) |
| AST | 5 U/L (0–40) |
| ALT | 7 U/L (0–35) |
| LDH | 102 U/L (100–225) |
| CPK | 34 U/L (30–200) |
| T-chol | 130 mg/dL (130–220) |
| TG | 38 mg/dL (30–130) |
| hANP | **87 pg/mL** (<40) |
| BNP | **84.1 pg/mL** (<20.0) |

## ELECTROCARDIOGRAM

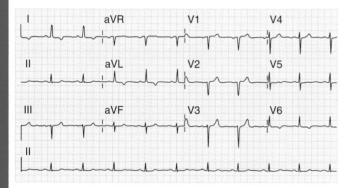

Figure 79-1 Electrocardiogram.

### FINDINGS

Heart rate: 60 bpm

QRS axis: −10°

QRS duration: 80 msec

Sinus rhythm. Leftward axis. Probable prior posterolateral infarction. T-wave inversion in the anterolateral leads.

## CHEST X-RAY

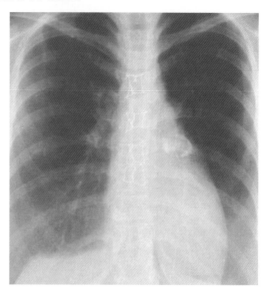

Figure 79-2 Posteroanterior projection.

### FINDINGS

Cardiothoracic ratio: 47%

Previous sternotomy. Normal cardiac size. There was a heavily calcified left coronary artery aneurysm, seen in cardiac silhouette.

**Comments:** The calcification seen is in the wall of the aneurysmal left coronary artery, indicative of a giant coronary aneurysm.

Another round and calcified lesion is vaguely seen around the third sternal wire from the top, which outlines the aneurysmal right coronary artery. This lesion is not as vivid as the one from the left coronary artery, probably because the right coronary one was more hidden between the sternum and vertebrae.

## EXERCISE TESTING

| | |
|---|---|
| Exercise protocol: | Modified Bruce |
| Duration (min:sec): | 5:05 |
| Reason for stopping: | Dyspnea |
| ECG changes: | Multifocal PVCs |

| | Rest | Peak |
|---|---|---|
| Heart rate (bpm): | 60 | 175 |
| Percent of age-predicted max HR: | | 87 |
| O₂ saturation (%): | 95 | 97 |
| Blood pressure (mm Hg): | 104/60 | 122/74 |
| Double product: | | 22,400 |
| Peak Vo₂ (mL/kg/min): | | 15.3 |
| Percent predicted (%): | | 31 |
| Ve/Vco₂: | | 48 |
| Metabolic equivalents: | | 4.2 |

**Comments:** The patient's exercise performance was poor. She reached anaerobic threshold at a very low level (10.3 mL/kg/min) indicating a substantial cardiac limitation. The blood pressure response was fairly flat, consistent with a poor myocardial response to exercise stress. However, the patient did not complain of exercise-induced chest pain.

# ECHOCARDIOGRAM

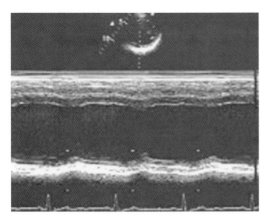

Figure 79-3 M-mode echocardiogram of the left ventricle in parasternal long-axis view.

## FINDINGS

Dilated LV with severely reduced LV systolic function.

There was only mild mitral regurgitation. LVEDD was 61 mm (for a constitutionally small patient), with a LV fractional shortening of only 8%.

***Comments:*** From this M-mode tracing one can appreciate that the posterior wall is thin and does not thicken. Overall LV systolic function is markedly impaired.

# COMPUTED TOMOGRAPHY

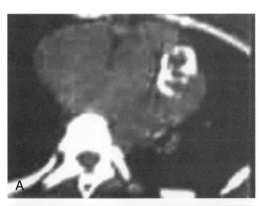

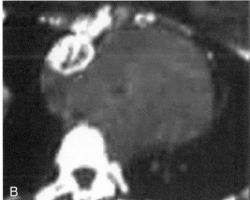

Figure 79-4 Electron beam computed tomography scan.

## FINDINGS

Severe calcification of the aneurysm at the bifurcation of the left coronary artery (*A*). Severe calcification of the right coronary artery aneurysm (*B*).

***Comments:*** Calcification has been reported to be exceedingly common when coronary artery aneurysms are larger than 6 mm at baseline angiography, and calcification becomes very common over time (12% at 5 years, 44% at 10 years, and 94% at 20 years).[3]

# CATHETERIZATION

## HEMODYNAMICS

Heart rate    60 bpm

|  | Pressure | Saturation (%) |
|---|---|---|
| SVC | 4 | 68 |
| IVC |  | 77 |
| RA | 3 |  |
| RV | 29/4 |  |
| PA | 27/10 mean 18 | 73 |
| PCWP | 8 |  |
| LV | 86/13 | 99 |
| Aorta | 88/54 mean 69 | 96 |

**Calculations**

| | |
|---|---|
| Qs (L/min) | 3.56 |
| Cardiac index (L/min/m²) | 2.41 |
| PVR (Wood units) | 1.63 |
| SVR (Wood units) | 18.52 |

***Comments:*** There was some elevation of LV end-diastolic pressures as expected. Overall resting hemodynamics were surprisingly normal, however, given the poor exercise capacity and the LV dysfunction previously seen on TTE.

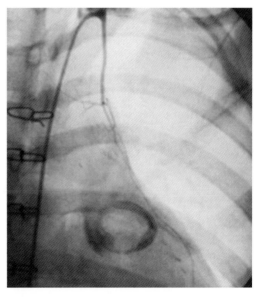

Figure 79-5 Coronary angiography, left internal mammary graft.

## FINDINGS

Selective injection in the internal thoracic artery anastomosed to the left anterior descending artery.

**Comments:** The left internal mammary artery had no anastomotic obstruction to the left anterior descending artery, but the graft had become very slender before reaching the coronary artery. Calcification at the proximal aneurysmal portion was clearly seen.

## FOCUSED CLINICAL QUESTIONS AND DISCUSSION POINTS

1. **What is the current optimal treatment for children with Kawasaki disease?**

*Treatment strategies have evolved over the past few decades. Today, intravenous immunoglobulin is administered early in the course of the disease to minimize damage to the coronary arteries and subsequent sequelae. Following the acute phase, giant aneurysms may still form, although the prevalence is lower. There is a relatively high risk for acute myocardial infarction during the first year. The use of warfarin can reduce this risk[2] and should be offered to all patients with giant aneurysms.*

*Coronary artery bypass venous grafting was first employed in the mid 1970s, improving symptoms and prognosis for children with severely obstructed coronary arteries. Later, the employment of arterial grafts has improved outcome further.[4,5] Arterial grafts remain patent longer and have the potential to grow with the child. Graft patency has been shown to decrease the risk of sudden death and improve quality of life.[6]*

*In cases where coronary artery obstruction is modest, bypass grafting is more controversial. The presence of an aneurysm alone does not constitute an indication for bypass surgery, since competitive blood flow through the native coronary artery can lead to occlusion of or damage to the graft. However, the majority of cases of acute myocardial infarction in Kawasaki disease are caused by acute thrombosis within giant aneurysms without necessarily significant stenoses. Prophylactic coronary artery bypass grafting in patients without severe ischemia should be avoided. Thus, the decision of whether to offer surgical interventions, and when to do so, remains challenging if not controversial.*

2. **What is the optimal medical treatment for this patient following her myocardial infarction?**

*As with adult patients after myocardial infarction, patients with Kawasaki-related infarcts are usually treated with ACE inhibitors and beta-blockers to prevent deleterious remodeling of the LV. Patients remain at risk of sudden death, and the multifocal premature beats and nonsustained ventricular tachycardia seen in this patient should not be ignored.*

3. **Should this patient undergo a second attempt at revascularization?**

*Despite the obvious abnormalities of her coronary arteries, this patient had no chest pain during exercise testing. Accordingly, it is uncertain whether further revascularization was indicated. The previous left internal mammary graft stenosis was most likely secondary to good competitive flow through the aneurysm of the left coronary artery.*

*Nonetheless, when considering her moderately severe myocardial dysfunction with multivessel disease, if there are areas of poor perfusion to viable areas of myocardium, revascularization should be performed in an effort to preserve or restore ventricular function.[7-9]*

*Revascularization in this patient would mean further bypass surgery, probably involving the right internal mammary artery. Balloon angioplasty or stenting is rarely an option in Kawasaki disease because of substantial rigid calcification and excessive intimal thickening. A rotational ablation catheter approach may be appropriate in selected cases, but experience in this setting remains limited at present.[9] We think a rotational ablation should be avoided for the last patent coronary artery.[10]*

4. **What is the patient's risk for sudden cardiac death?**

*Patients with Kawasaki disease are at risk for sudden cardiac death from previous myocardial infarction and scarring.[6] Since the premature ventricular contractions in this patient were multifocal, it was felt unlikely that catheter radiofrequency ablation or even surgical cryoablation would offer definitive therapy.*

*A patient such as this, today, would be considered a candidate for an ICD; however, this is a case from before the ICD era, and the patient was empirically covered with beta-blockers.*

## FINAL DIAGNOSIS

Kawasaki disease with aneurysmal dilatation of the proximal coronary arteries

Ischemic cardiomyopathy

"Occlusion" of prior coronary bypass graft

## PLAN OF ACTION

Repeat coronary arterial bypass grafting

## INTERVENTION

Coronary arterial bypass grafting was carried out to the left anterior descending artery. This time the right internal mammary artery was employed. The anastomosis between the graft and the coronary artery was constructed proximal to the previous bypass anastomosis using a 7-0 Prolene suture. The left anterior descending artery was not severely calcified there, though its wall was thick and stiff. The patient recovered from surgery uneventfully.

## OUTCOME

The patient remained stable for several months and was able to return to her studies.

Postoperative angiography 1 year after repeated coronary artery bypass grafting showed the string sign again. Nonetheless, her ventricular function and general condition had improved with the patient being maintained on ACE inhibitors and beta-blockers.

Six years after her second cardiac surgery, she developed frequent episodes of palpitations without syncope; runs of non-sustained ventricular tachycardia were detected on 24-hour ECG monitoring. An implantable defibrillator was still not an option.

Six months later, the patient experienced sudden-onset central chest pain, and she collapsed and died soon after. She was 27 years old. The family declined a postmortem examination. Whether the cause of sudden cardiac death was acute myocardial infarction or ventricular arrhythmia remains unknown. Her warfarin was within therapeutic levels, when tested 1 week prior to her demise.

When this patient was diagnosed with acute Kawasaki disease, there was uncertainty at the time as to whether intravenous immunoglobulins and/or steroids should be given as a primary treatment, so she received neither. Unfortunately, the patient went on to develop giant coronary artery aneurysms, further complicated with time by complex coronary artery stenoses.

Her coronary artery disease was periodically investigated with coronary angiograms (Figs. 79-6 to 79-8) and exercise testing according to institutional policy. The decision to proceed with coronary artery bypass surgery twice was based on the evidence of ischemic dilated cardiomyopathy, and it seemed to have conveyed short- to midterm benefits to the patient, in terms of LV function and management of heart failure.[1,8,9] Alternatively, catheter interventions,[10] such as rotational ablation or laser intervention for ischemic myocardium, could have been considered, had those techniques been established.

To prevent sudden cardiac death, many centers would have proceeded today with elective implantable cardiac defibrillator implantation. In retrospect, if available and offered, it might have prevented this patient's demise. Moreover, aggressive treatment with intravenous immunoglobulins at the time of acute presentation with Kawasaki disease, followed by full anti-coagulation with warfarin and aspirin immediately afterward, would have conveyed a much better cardiovascular outcome, but this body of knowledge was not present at the time. The case illustrates some of the ongoing challenges inherent in the management of Kawasaki disease.[11]

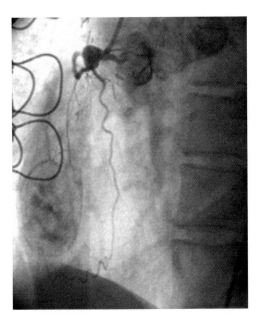

Figure 79-6 Postoperative coronary angiography, right coronary artery injection.

## FINDINGS

The right coronary artery appeared rather hypoplastic, though no obvious focal stenosis was identified. Complete occlusion at segment 1 of the right coronary artery is shown. Giant aneurysm with severe calcification at the right coronary artery is seen.

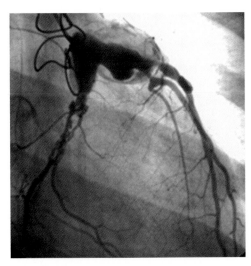

Figure 79-7 Postoperative coronary angiography, left main coronary artery injection.

## FINDINGS

The proximal left anterior descending artery and its oblique marginal branch appear to have localized stenoses. The left circumflex artery also shows segmental stenosis. Note giant aneurysmal dilatation of the whole proximal left coronary artery system.

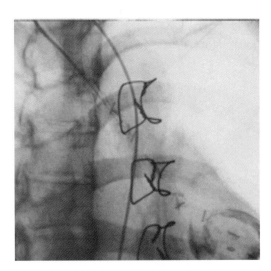

Figure 79-8 Postoperative coronary bypass graft angiography. The right internal thoracic artery to the left anterior descending artery is shown.

## FINDINGS

The right internal mammary artery had become extremely slender, and the left anterior descending artery is not well filled from this injection.

***Comments:*** It appears that, again, little has been gained to improve flow to the vulnerable areas, and the right internal mammary graft has occluded.

## Selected References

1. Yoshikawa Y, Yagihara T, Kameda Y, et al: Results of surgical treatments in patients with coronary-arterial obstructive disease after Kawasaki disease. Eur J Cardio-Thoracic Surg 17:515–519, 2000.
2. Newburger JW, Takahashi M, Gerber MA, et al; Committee on Rheumatic Fever, Endocarditis, and Kawasaki Disease, Council on Cardiovascular Disease in the Young, American Heart Association: Diagnosis, treatment, and long-term management of Kawasaki disease: A statement for health professionals from the Committee on Rheumatic Fever, Endocarditis, and Kawasaki Disease, Council on Cardiovascular Disease in the Young, American Heart Association. Circulation 110:2747–2771, 2004.
3. Kaichi S, Tsuda E, Fujita H, et al: Acute coronary artery dilation due to Kawasaki disease and subsequent late calcification as detected by electron beam computed tomography. Pediatr Cardiol 29:568–573, 2008.
4. Kitamura S: The role of coronary bypass operation on children with Kawasaki disease. Coron Artery Dis 13:437–447, 2003.
5. Tsuda E, Kitamura S: National survey of coronary artery bypass grafting for coronary artery lesions caused by Kawasaki disease. Circulation 110:II61–II66, 2004.
6. Tsuda E, Arakaki Y, Shimizu T, et al: Sudden death in patients with coronary arterial lesions due to Kawasaki disease: Changes in cause of death by decades. Cardiol Young 15:481–488, 2005.
7. Kitamura S, Kawachi K, Oyama C, et al: Severe Kawasaki heart disease treated with an internal mammary artery graft in pediatric patients. A first successful report. J Thorac Cardiovasc Surg 89:860–866, 1985.

8. Tsuda E, Kitamura S, Kimura K, et al: Long-term patency of internal thoracic artery grafts for coronary artery stenosis due to Kawasaki disease: Comparison of early with recent results in small children. Am Heart J 153:999–1000, 2007.

9. Sugimura T, Yokoi H, Sato N, et al: Interventional treatment for children with severe coronary artery stenosis with calcification after long-term Kawasaki disease. Circulation 96:3928–3933, 1997.

10. Tsuda E, Miyazaki S, Yamada O, et al: Percutaneous transluminal coronary rotational atherectomy for localized stenosis caused by Kawasaki disease. Pediatr Cardiol 27:447–453, 2006.

11. Kawasaki T, Kosaki F, Okawa S, et al: A new infantile acute febrile mucocutaneous lymph-node syndrome (MLNS) prevailing in Japan. Pediatrics 54:271–276, 1974.

Part II

# Marfan Syndrome

Case 80

# Recurrent Aortic Dissection
# in Marfan Syndrome

**Maarten Groenink, Gary D. Webb, and Barbara J.M. Mulder**

**Age: 30 years**
**Gender: Male**
**Occupation: Photographer**
**Working diagnosis: Marfan syndrome**

## HISTORY

Since age 10, this patient has been known to have the familial form of Marfan syndrome. Several family members had an aortic dissection.

For regular follow-up of his aortic root diameters, he visited a cardiologist once a year. Slow progression of the aortic root diameter was observed up to a diameter of 49 mm by the time he was 22 years old.

At the age of 23, he underwent an emergency aortic root replacement because of a type A aortic dissection, limited to the ascending aorta. A Bentall procedure was performed with a mechanical Medtronic Hall tilting disc aortic valve prosthesis. His postoperative course was uneventful.

When the patient was 29 years old, he underwent MR imaging for the first time as part of his routine follow-up. The aortic arch was aneurysmal with a diameter of 55 mm. He therefore underwent an elective aortic arch replacement soon thereafter. The procedure was complicated by persistent hoarseness due to vocal cord paralysis.

One year later (at age 30 years), a routine MR scan was performed and showed a descending thoracic aorta dimension of 38 mm. Six days later, he presented with acute severe interscapular pain.

***Comments:*** Recommendations for prevention of aortic dissection in patients with Marfan syndrome include (1) lifelong beta-adrenergic blockade, (2) maintenance of low normal blood pressure, (3) periodic routine imaging of the aorta, and (4) moderate restriction of physical activity.[1,2] Monitoring of the aortic root with echocardiography is very important, but the rest of the aorta should also be visualized, for example, with MRI or CT (MRI is preferable for recurrent imaging because it does not use radiation).

Indications for elective aortic root replacement in Marfan syndrome are (1) aortic root diameter of 55 mm; (2) aortic root of 50 mm if there is a family history of aortic dissection, if there is aortic growth of more than 2 mm per year, or if valve-sparing surgery is planned; (3) aortic root of 45 mm if valve-sparing

surgery is planned, or—for female patients—when pregnancy is contemplated.[2]

In this patient a type A dissection occurred at an aortic root diameter of around 50 mm. His risk of such an occurrence was high given his family history. Aortic root diameters should be monitored more frequently when diameters come close to 50 mm in these high-risk patients (every 3 to 6 months), or elective surgery should be planned.

Before and after aortic root replacement, regular imaging of the entire aorta should take place every 1 to 3 years with MRI or CT.

## CURRENT SYMPTOMS

While the patient was watching television, he suddenly felt a severe sharp pain in his interscapular area. The pain persisted and increased, and he was brought to the hospital. He had no syncope or paralysis.

NYHA class: I (excluding acute presentation)

***Comments:*** Despite the only slight dilatation of the descending aorta, a dissection may occur in patients with Marfan syndrome. There are no clear guidelines for elective replacement of the descending aorta. Usually, a diameter of 50 mm or more is considered an indication for preventive replacement.[2] In Marfan syndrome, especially in high-risk patients (previous aortic dissection, family history of dissections, rapid aortic growth), surgery should be considered at smaller diameters.

The incidence of reoperation in patients with Marfan syndrome is significantly higher in patients who present initially with an acute type A aortic dissection than in those with dilation only.[3] However, aortic rupture may occur in the downstream aorta even following uncomplicated elective aortic root surgery despite a normal-sized aorta.[4] Close follow-up of all Marfan patients is necessary to detect asymptomatic changes requiring surgery because complex *elective* redo operations can be performed with a relatively low perioperative risk.[4]

## CURRENT MEDICATIONS

Atenolol 100 mg daily

Coumadin (target INR of 2.5–3.5)

## PHYSICAL EXAMINATION

BP 190/110 mm Hg (both arms), HR 100 bpm, oxygen saturation 100%

Height 205 cm, weight 102 kg, BSA 2.41 m²

Surgical scars: Midline sternotomy after ascending aorta and arch replacement

Neck veins: Jugular veins were not dilated.

Lungs/chest: Chest was clear.

Heart: There was a grade 2/6 ejection systolic ejection murmur at the upper left sternal border. Loud aortic second heart sound. No diastolic murmur was heard.

Abdomen: No hepatosplenomegaly

Extremities: Pulsations of the femoral arteries were weak. A systolic bruit was heard over both femoral arteries.

***Comments:*** Typically, aortic dissection may be associated with hypertension.

## LABORATORY DATA

| | |
|---|---|
| Hemoglobin | 13.2 g/dL (13.0–17.0) |
| Hematocrit/PCV | **39** (41–51) |
| Platelet count | **123 × 10⁹/L** (150–400) |
| Sodium | 135 mmol/L (134–145) |
| Potassium | 3.7 mmol/L (3.5–5.2) |
| Creatinine | 0.8 mg/dL (0.6–1.2) |
| Blood urea nitrogen | 5.4 mmol/L (2.5–6.5) |

***Comments:*** Nonspecific thrombocytopenia is present; otherwise there are no abnormalities.

## ELECTROCARDIOGRAM

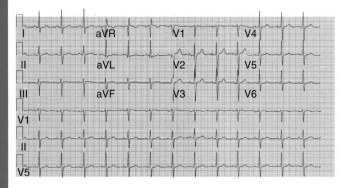

Figure 80-1 Electrocardiogram.

### FINDINGS

Heart rate: 80 bpm

QRS axis: –50°

QRS duration: 80 msec

Sinus rhythm. Left-axis deviation. No evidence of pericarditis, myocardial infarction, or ischemia.

***Comments:*** While there is weak voltage evidence of LV hypertrophy (R1 plus S3 > 25 and R aVL > 11 mm), this may well be falsely positive in the context of left-axis deviation.

## CHEST X-RAY

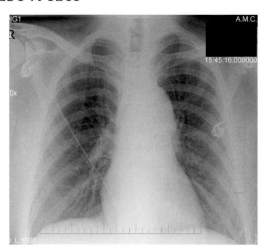

Figure 80-2 Anteroposterior projection at the time of presentation.

### FINDINGS

The mediastinum was widened with prominence of the descending thoracic aorta. The heart size was normal. No pleural effusions or signs of heart failure were noted.

***Comments:*** The contour of the aorta is of obvious importance in this case. Images should be compared to prior anteroposterior chest radiographs to look for evidence of new mediastinal widening.

## ECHOCARDIOGRAM

### OVERALL FINDINGS

The ventricles had normal dimensions, normal systolic function, and normal function of the mechanical aortic valve.

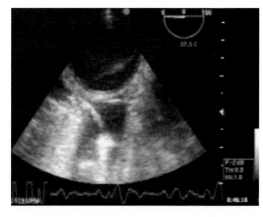

Figure 80-3 Transesophageal echocardiogram at the time of presentation.

### FINDINGS

There was dissection in the thoracic descending aorta.

***Comments:*** The sensitivity and specificity of TEE for the diagnosis of aortic dissection are comparable to those for CT or

MRI.[5] However, for assessment of the extent of the dissection, CT or MRI is usually required.[1]

# MAGNETIC RESONANCE IMAGING

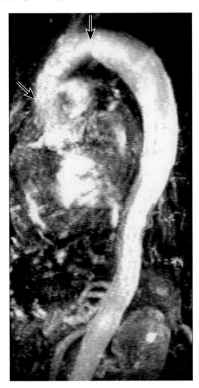

Figure 80-4 Gadolinium-enhanced 3D aortogram at 6 days before presentation.

## FINDINGS

The Bentall prosthesis and the aortic arch graft (*arrows*) were visible. Mild dilation of the descending thoracic aorta was seen with a maximal diameter of 38 mm.

**Comments:** These findings do not generally require specific interventions. It is advised to repeat MRI investigation annually to monitor changes.

There are no clear guidelines for elective replacement of the descending aorta. Usually, a diameter of 50 mm or more is considered an indication for preventive replacement.[2] In Marfan syndrome, especially in high-risk patients (previous aortic dissection, family history of dissections, rapidly expanding aortic diameters), surgery should be considered at smaller diameters.

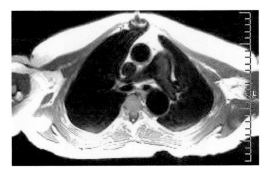

Figure 80-5 Axial spin-echo image showing the ascending and descending aorta.

## FINDINGS

The study 6 days prior to presentation showed no aortic dissection. There was a slight dilation (38 mm) present in the descending thoracic aorta. Distensibility of the descending aorta was decreased ($2.4 \times 10^{-3}$ mm Hg$^{-1}$).

**Comments:** Distensibility can be calculated from diastolic and systolic aortic diameters and pulse pressure by the equation:

(systolic diameter − diastolic diameter)/

(diastolic diameter × pulse pressure)

Normal values of distensibility in the descending aorta are $4.6 \pm 1.5 \times 10^{-3}$ mm Hg$^{-1}$.

Decreased descending thoracic aortic distensibility below $3.1 \times 10^{-3}$ mm Hg$^{-1}$ (which is the lower limit of normal) has been associated with future aortic complications in Marfan patients.[6]

For optimal risk assessment and monitoring of patients with Marfan syndrome, both aortic elasticity and diameters should be assessed regularly, every 1 to 3 years.

Note also the Marfan chest deformity (pectus carinatum).

# COMPUTED TOMOGRAPHY

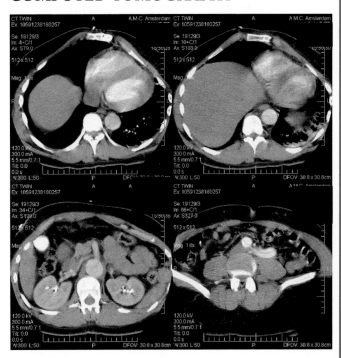

Figure 80-6 Spiral contrast-enhanced computed tomography at the time of presentation.

## FINDINGS

A type B aortic dissection is shown from the descending thoracic aorta (*upper left*) to the iliac arteries (*lower right*). No obstruction of major side branches was shown.

**Comments:** Note that the dissection occurred in an only slightly dilated descending aorta with decreased distensibility.

Two mechanisms may cause obstruction of side branches in aortic dissection: static narrowing and dynamic narrowing of a branch artery. Static narrowing occurs when the line of dissection intersects the vessel origin and the aortic hematoma propagates into the vessel wall, stenosing the side branch lumen. In dynamic obstruction the dissection flap is positioned across the vessel origin and collapses across the vessel origin, covering it like a curtain. Obstruction of a major side branch may be an indication for surgery or intervention. The indications for intervention in Marfan syndrome, however, need to be established. Vessels compromised by dynamic obstruction may be treated by percutaneous balloon fenestration.

## CATHETERIZATION

Not performed

### FOCUSED CLINICAL QUESTIONS AND DISCUSSION POINTS

1. **What is the clinical diagnosis?**

   *This patient with Marfan syndrome has a type B aortic dissection. Six days prior to the dissection a routine MR image showed a slightly dilated descending aorta (upper limit of normal is approximately 28 mm).[7] Local distensibility was clearly decreased. This is a high-risk patient. However, clear guidelines for prophylactic surgery of the descending aorta in patients with Marfan syndrome are lacking.*

2. **What information is essential to determine how best to treat an acute aortic dissection?**

   *The specific goals of imaging include confirmation of diagnosis, tear localization, determination of the extent of dissection, and identification of indicators of an emergency, namely fluid extravasation in the pericardium, pleural space, and/or mediastinum, and important visceral branch compromise.*

3. **What is the first-choice treatment in this patient?**

   *For type B aortic dissection, the initial therapy is medical. Careful monitoring of heart rate and blood pressure should be ensured. Beta-blocking therapy and blood pressure lowering medications should be started promptly, as well as sedation and analgesic therapy. In patients with significant hypertension, additional vasodilator therapy should be initiated (e.g., intravenous sodium nitroprusside to titrate the systolic blood pressure to 100 to 120 mm Hg).*

   *Survival for all patients with type B dissection is 70% to 80% at 1 year, decreasing to 50% to 60% at 5 years, and is similar for patients treated medically or surgically. Reoperation and late aortic complications are more frequent in patients with Marfan syndrome than in patients with aortic dissection due to other underlying pathology (most commonly systemic hypertension).*

4. **When is surgery indicated for dissection of the descending aorta?**

   *Surgery in patients with type B aortic dissection is indicated when aortic diameters are rapidly expanding, when there is persistent or recurrent pain, when there is persistent hypertension despite maximal antihypertensive medical treatment, when there are visceral or peripheral ischemic complications, or when there is rupture.*

   *Indications for operative intervention on postdissection aneurysms are similar to those for nondissecting aneurysms.[1] The role of covered stents in the treatment of aortic complications in patients with Marfan syndrome has yet to be established. Currently, results are not very satisfactory (Nienaber, personal communication).*

## FINAL DIAGNOSIS

Type B aortic dissection after previous aortic root and aortic arch replacement in a patient with Marfan syndrome

## PLAN OF ACTION

Medical treatment

## OUTCOME

The patient was admitted to intensive care and treated with sodium nitroprusside intravenously, labetolol, nifedipine, and morphine sulfate for pain relief.

Despite maximal antihypertensive treatment the patient developed recurrent pain attacks within the first 4 weeks. Moreover, his blood pressure could not be stabilized at acceptable levels.

A repeat CT scan showed no changes compared to the first CT images.

A decision was made to send him for surgery, and he underwent a replacement of the thoracic and abdominal aorta, including the proximal iliac arteries. The procedure was uncomplicated.

After his third aortic operation, the entire aorta had been replaced from the aortic valve to the proximal iliac arteries. His blood pressure remained well controlled for several years after.

He still uses beta-blocking therapy, although the use of beta-blockers after entire aortic replacement is questionable. Beta-blockers may increase vascular resistance in the peripheral vessels, thereby increasing wave reflections in the aorta, which may have a negative effect. However, heart rate reduction might still be useful for protection of aortic sites where main side branches have been reimplanted.[8] The long-term outcome of patients with Marfan syndrome and entire aortic replacement is unknown.

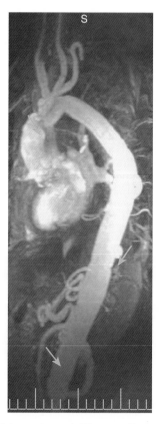

Figure 80-7 Gadolinium-enhanced 3D magnetic resonance aortogram (sagittal view) after replacement of the entire aorta.

## Findings

Main side branches have been reimplanted at various sites in the aorta (*arrows*).

***Comments:*** Aortic sites where main side branches have been reimplanted remain vulnerable and are at risk for dilatation. Regular (once yearly) MR follow-up should take place to identify such complications at an early stage.

## Selected References

1. Erbel R, Alfonso F, Boileau C, et al; Task Force on Aortic Dissection, European Society of Cardiology: Diagnosis and management of aortic dissection. Eur Heart J 22:1642–1681, 2001.
2. Therrien J, Gatzoulis M, Graham T, et al: Canadian Cardiovascular Society Consensus Conference 2001 update: Recommendations for the Management of Adults with Congenital Heart Disease—Part II. Can J Cardiol 17:1029–1050, 2001.
3. Finkbohner R, Johnston D, Crawford ES, et al: Marfan syndrome. Long-term survival and complications after aortic aneurysm repair. Circulation 91:728–733, 1995.
4. Carrel T, Beyeler L, Schnyder A, et al: Reoperations and late adverse outcome in Marfan patients following cardiovascular surgery. Eur J Cardiothorac Surg 25:671–675, 2004.
5. Nienaber CA, von Kodolitsch Y, Nicolas V, et al: The diagnosis of thoracic aortic dissection by noninvasive imaging procedures. N Engl J Med 328:1–9, 1993.
6. Nollen GJ, Groenink M, Tijssen JG, et al: Aortic stiffness and diameter predict progressive aortic dilatation in patients with Marfan syndrome. Eur Heart J 25:1146–1152, 2004.
7. Garcier JM, Petitcolin V, Filaire M, et al: Normal diameter of the thoracic aorta in adults: A magnetic resonance imaging study. Surg Radiol Anat 25:322–329, 2003.
8. Meijboom LJ, Westerhof BE, Nollen GJ, et al: Beta-blocking therapy in patients with the Marfan syndrome and entire aortic replacement. Eur J Cardiothorac Surg 26:901–906, 2004.

## Bibliography

De Oliveira NC, David TE, Ivanov J, et al: Results of surgery for aortic root aneurysm in patients with Marfan syndrome. J Thorac Cardiovasc Surg 125:789–796, 2003.

Nollen GJ, Mulder BJ: What's new in the Marfan syndrome? Int J Cardiol 97(Suppl 1):103–108, 2004.

Svensson LG, Kim KH, Blackstone EH, et al: Elephant trunk procedure: Newer indications and uses (Review). Ann Thorac Surg 78:109–116; discussion, 109–116, 2004.

Umana JP, Lai DT, Mitchell RS, et al: Is medical therapy still the optimal treatment strategy for patients with acute type B aortic dissections? J Thorac Cardiovasc Surg 124:896–910, 2002.

Umana JP, Miller DC, Mitchell RS: What is the best treatment for patients with acute type B aortic dissections—medical, surgical, or endovascular stent-grafting? Ann Thorac Surg 74:S1840–S1843; discussion, S1857–S1863, 2002.

# The Role of Pulmonary Vasodilators in Pulmonary Hypertension

**William Bradlow**

**Age: 26 years**
**Gender: Male**
**Occupation: Systems engineer**
**Working diagnosis: Pulmonary arterial hypertension**

## HISTORY

The patient had been diagnosed with a hemodynamically insignificant VSD at age 2 years. No further follow-up had been arranged, and his upbringing was unremarkable.

The patient was well until age 18 when he developed breathlessness, palpitations, and chest pain. After 3 years of symptoms, at age 21, he sought attention and a workup ensued.

TTE showed no VSD, but the right heart was enlarged. The estimated RV systolic pressure was 110 mm Hg. A right heart catheterization measured a mean pulmonary artery pressure of 97 mm Hg. Secondary causes of PAH were excluded. He was diagnosed with IPAH.

The patient was offered heart-lung transplant but declined. He also refused prostanoid therapy and was subsequently started on oxygen, warfarin, and sildenafil.

Initially, the patient noted marked improvement on sildenafil. At reassessment 3 months later, his myocardial oxygen consumption had increased from 15.2 mL/kg/min (predicted value, 42.9%) to 20.3 mL/kg/min, and he was able to manage 12 minutes of the Bruce protocol.

At age 26, the patient was admitted to his local hospital with a productive cough, breathlessness, coryzal symptoms, left-sided pleuritic chest pain, and groin pain. Antibiotics were started at his local hospital, and he was transferred to a tertiary care facility for further care.

***Comments:*** PAH is one of five causes of pulmonary hypertension (as outlined in the current classification from the 2003 Third World Symposium on Pulmonary Arterial Hypertension)[1] and is defined as a mean pulmonary artery pressure higher than 25 mm Hg at rest or higher than 30 mm Hg with exercise (in the context of an elevated pulmonary vascular resistance > 3 Wood units or > 240 dyn/sec/cm$^{-5}$). Known secondary causes include connective tissue disease, congenital left-to-right shunts, HIV, and drugs and toxins. Otherwise, it is termed idiopathic or familial (IPAH or FPAH, respectively). In this patient, the absence of a VSD now makes it unlikely that this was related to his pulmonary hypertension.

PAH is rare, and carries a poor prognosis (predicted median survival for IPAH patients is 2.8 years).[2] Although the condition is more common in women, men are also affected. Symptoms are nonspecific, and patients may appear deceptively well. Clinical detection therefore can be difficult and result in delay of appropriate treatment.

The velocity of the regurgitant jet through the tricuspid valve allows an assessment of RV systolic pressure (a value of > 2.8 m/sec is considered elevated). However, the predictive accuracy of the peak velocity diminishes in the setting of PAH.[3]

Calcium-channel blockers are used only in the small group of IPAH patients who demonstrate a positive response to short-acting vasodilators. Right heart failure is a contraindication to their use. Oxygen is used to reduce the pulmonary vasoconstrictor effect of hypoxia. Warfarin is used to attenuate the risks of in situ thrombosis and pulmonary thromboembolism (both resulting from stasis, procoagulability, and endothelin damage). Intravenous epoprostenol is the candidate of choice in IPAH given its rapid onset of action and favorable evidence base.[4] It aims to supplement circulating prostacyclin levels, which have been found, with nitric oxide levels, to be reduced.[5] Its effects are mediated via an intracellular second messenger (cAMP), and include vascular effects beyond vasodilatation. These reduce both platelet aggregation and vascular smooth muscle proliferation. Unfortunately, it requires long-term central venous access for continuous therapy. Attendant risks of infection and delivery failure are sources of morbidity and mortality. Prostanoids can be also be inhaled or given subcutaneously, though these forms have their own disadvantages.

As the suggested treatment options were not acceptable to the patient, sildenafil was used at the clinician's discretion. Sildenafil (given orally) inhibits phosphodiesterase 5, preventing breakdown of cGMP and indirectly that of cAMP. Sildenafil has a short half-life and must be taken three times a day. This augments the action of nitric oxide and prostacyclin. Current guidelines record a low level of evidence and weak recommendation (level of evidence C) for the use of sildenafil in patients with PAH who have failed or are not candidates for other therapy.[4,6,7]

## CURRENT SYMPTOMS

The patient noted a recent substantial deterioration in his exercise tolerance.

WHO class: III

***Comments:*** Often the World Health Organization classification is used as a rough gauge of the functional capacity of the patient, and is based on the NYHA format. It correlates with disease severity and prognosis and is useful in identifying those who require more advanced treatments.

## CURRENT MEDICATIONS

Sildenafil 25 mg orally three times daily

Warfarin (target INR of 2–3)

***Comments:*** The recommended dose of sildenafil for PAH is 20 mg by mouth three times daily, as a dose-response study did not show any further benefit at 50 or 100 mg.[8]

## PHYSICAL EXAMINATION

BP 126/60 mm Hg, HR 70 bpm, oxygen saturation 96% on room air

Height 169 cm, weight 65 kg, BSA 1.75 m$^2$

Neck veins: JVP was visible at the ears with the patient sitting upright. Prominent A-waves and CV-waves were noted.

Lungs/chest: Bronchial breathing and reduced percussion noted at the left base with a pleural rub in the same area

Heart: The rhythm was regular. There was a palpable left parasternal lift, a grade 1/6 pan-systolic murmur, and a grade 2/4 early diastolic murmur. Both murmurs were augmented on inspiration.

Extremities: Edema from the foot to the thighs, as well as over the sacrum

### PERTINENT NEGATIVES
There was no abdominal guarding, and no evidence of connective tissue disease.

***Comments:*** Neck vein distension reflects right heart failure and significant tricuspid regurgitation.

The lung exam suggests a respiratory cause for both the patient's pain and his deterioration.

Cardiac findings are consistent with severe RV pressure overload and systolic RV impairment with tricuspid and pulmonary regurgitation, and right heart failure.

## LABORATORY DATA

| | |
|---|---|
| Leukocyte count | $6.0 \times 10^9$/L (4.4–10.1) |
| Hemoglobin | 16.1 g/dL (13.0–17.0) |
| Hematocrit/PCV | 51% (41–51) |
| MCV | 89 fL (83–99) |
| Platelet count | **140 × 10⁹/L** (150–400) |
| Sodium | **132 mmol/L** (134–145) |
| Potassium | 4.1 mmol/L (3.5–5.2) |
| Creatinine | 0.97 mg/dL (0.6–1.2) |
| Blood urea nitrogen | 4.2 mmol/L (2.5–6.5) |

| | |
|---|---|
| Albumin | **2.3 g/dL** (35–50) |
| CRP | **106 mg/L** (0–10) |
| GGT | **89 IU/L** (11– 51) |
| ALT | **372 IU/L** (8–40) |

***Comments:*** Abnormal liver function tests should prompt consideration of liver congestion and sepsis. Anticoagulation should be monitored carefully in this setting.

Low albumin could be a sign of chronic illness and should prompt the involvement of a nutritionist. Raised CRP should prompt the exclusion of a significant source of infection.

## ELECTROCARDIOGRAM

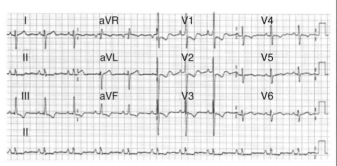

Figure 81-1 Electrocardiogram.

### FINDINGS
Heart rate: 85 bpm

QRS axis: +123°

QRS duration: 112 msec

Sinus rhythm, right-axis deviation, with an R/S ratio greater than 1 in V1. RA overload. RV strain pattern V1–5.

***Comments:*** These findings are typical for PAH. It has been shown that in patients with PAH, a P-wave height equal to or greater than 2.5 mm has a 2.8-fold greater risk of death over a 6-year period (1 mm increases thereafter corresponding to a 4.5-fold increased risk of death).[9]

## CHEST X-RAY

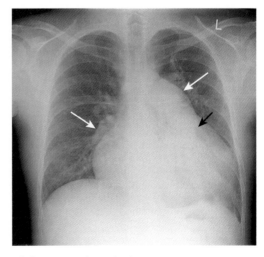

Figure 81-2 Posteroanterior projection.

## FINDINGS
Cardiothoracic ratio: 76%

Gross cardiomegaly, enlarged main (*white arrow*) and right descending (*white arrow*) pulmonary arteries. The left pulmonary artery is also dilated (*black arrow*) and is seen through the cardiac silhouette. Enlarged RA.

***Comments:*** Enlargement of the RV rotates the main pulmonary artery upward, contributing to its more prominent visibility on CXR. Dilatation of the left and right pulmonary arteries is also visible, though the distal pulmonary arteries do not appear abnormal.

## EXERCISE TESTING
Not performed.

## ECHOCARDIOGRAM

### OVERALL FINDINGS
RV dilatation and moderate-to-severe RV systolic impairment were noted.

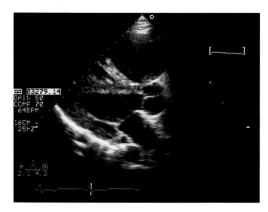

Figure 81-3 Echocardiogram.

***Comments:*** This patient's echocardiogram demonstrates two poor prognostic markers in PAH[10]—RA enlargement and moderate pericardial effusion (without evidence of tamponade). These both relate to elevated RA pressure. The interatrial septal position (bowed toward the LA) and the IVC dilatation (more than 20 mm with no change with respiration) support elevated RA pressure in this case. The RV Tei index (not measured here) is also an important prognostic marker.[11]

RV ejection time is prolonged, allowing the interventricular septum to impinge on the LV (small in comparison to the dilated and hypertrophied RV). The degree of interventricular septal displacement can be assessed by the eccentricity index. This deformation is most pronounced during early diastole, contributing to LV diastolic impairment (short filling time with high-filling velocities). The LV systolic impairment seen is a worrying sign. It is important to note that the severity of tricuspid regurgitation (moderate to severe in this case) should be considered independent of its velocity, since the latter is related to the driving force (RV systolic function) behind it.

No VSD was seen. It should be noted that in the presence of RV pressure overload (in this case from PAH) a VSD, if present, will have little or no shunt, since the RV-LV pressure gradient is dramatically reduced.

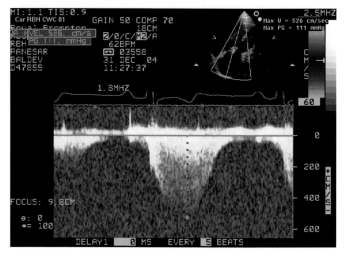

Figure 81-4 Tricuspid valve continuous-wave Doppler.

## FINDINGS
The tricuspid valve regurgitation velocity was 5.2 m/sec.

***Comments:*** Tricuspid valve regurgitation velocity is the best noninvasive test for assessing the presence of pulmonary hypertension, but may not accurately estimate the peak pressure in the setting of PAH.[3]

## MAGNETIC RESONANCE IMAGING

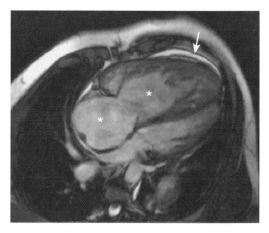

Figure 81-5 Four-chamber cine image.

***Comments:*** Gross RA and RV dilatation (*asterisks*) with RV hypertrophy was seen. A pericardial effusion (*arrow*) is also evident. Note the way in which the LV is displaced and deformed by the dominating RV. No VSD is present.

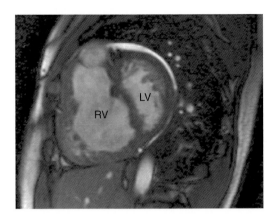

Figure 81-6 Short-axis stady-state free precession cine.

## FINDINGS

RV hypertrophy was seen, as well as RV dilatation. The septum was continuously deviated to the LV.

**Comments:** A persistently deviated septum is supportive of pressure overload of the RV. A septum that is deviated only in diastole is supportive of a volume overloaded RV.

## COMPUTED TOMOGRAPHY

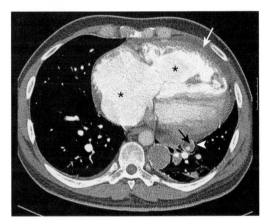

Figure 81-7 Chest scan with contrast.

## FINDINGS

Gross RA and RV dilatation (*asterisks*) with RV hypertrophy was seen. A pericardial effusion (*white arrow*) and severely dilated left lower lobe vessels with calcification of walls (*white arrowhead*) and thrombus (*black arrow*) within them were appreciated.

The CT scan also demonstrated opacification within the left lower lobe (not shown) reflecting consolidation and possibly pulmonary infarction.

## CATHETERIZATION

Not performed

### FOCUSED CLINICAL QUESTIONS AND DISCUSSION POINTS

1. **What are the potential hemodynamic mechanisms of decompensation in this patient?**

*In a retrospective multicenter review[12] of PAH patients receiving cardiopulmonary resuscitation following circulatory arrest,*

*significant intercurrent illness was identified in 54%. These are fragile patients with poor reserve. Sepsis reduces systemic vascular resistance through peripheral vasodilatation and elicits a tachycardia to maintain cardiac output (often already low). Coronary perfusion is threatened, and the RV (with an existing supply/demand imbalance because of RV hypertrophy and RV pressure overload) may become ischemic and may fail. Tissue acidosis results from low cardiac output. Hypoxia, induced by lung infection/infarction, promotes further pulmonary vasoconstriction.*

2. **After treatment of the underlying infection, what additional therapeutic options are available?**

*Rescue therapy at this stage consists of instituting measures to lower the pulmonary vascular resistance, treat sepsis, and correct hypoxia. The initial additional recommended therapy of choice is intravenous epoprostenol. Diuretics are indicated, as there is evidence of RV failure. Digoxin can also be used in those with refractory RV failure, though it should be noted that there is no significant evidence base and levels need monitoring.*

*Current recommendations state that combination therapy, or intravenous prostacyclin therapy, should be instituted in patients failing on existing treatment. In a manner analogous to the treatment of systemic hypertension, combination therapy offers the potential to target different pathways. The use of combination therapies in the treatment of PAH is under ongoing investigation; however, the combination use of bosentan and sildenafil has been investigated in a case series of nine patients[13] in which the combination was safely tolerated, and improved 6-minute walk and cardiopulmonary exercise testing resulted. Bosentan, the first oral therapy to receive FDA approval, is a nonselective endothelin receptor antagonist. It is thought to mitigate the potent vasoconstrictor and smooth muscle cell proliferation effect of endothelin-1.[5] Monthly liver function tests are mandatory given its potential for hepatotoxic side effects.*

## FINAL DIAGNOSIS

IPAH with deterioration

## PLAN OF ACTION

Addition of bosentan therapy

## INTERVENTION

None

## OUTCOME

After completing a full course of antibiotics, the patient was started cautiously on bosentan and the dose gradually increased. He was subsequently discharged and has been under follow-up. His symptoms and 6MWT have returned to their baseline at presentation, and he has returned to working full time.

This case reports the successful introduction of bosentan, during a clinical deterioration, to an existing treatment regime that included sildenafil. Bosentan is an endothelin-receptor blocker and was the first oral therapy to receive FDA approval in the treatment of PAH in November of 2001. Hepatotoxicity is a recognized side effect such that FDA approval stipulated monthly hepatic function tests; a practice supported in current guidelines.[4-6]

## Selected References

1. Simonneau G, Galie N, Rubin LJ, et al: Clinical classification of pulmonary hypertension. J Am Coll Cardiol 43(Suppl 12):S5–S12, 2004.

2. D'Alonzo GE, Barst RJ, Ayres SM, et al: Survival in patients with primary pulmonary hypertension. Results from a national prospective registry. Ann Intern Med 115:343–349, 1991.
3. Brecker SJ, Gibbs JS, Fox KM, et al: Comparison of Doppler derived haemodynamic variables and simultaneous high fidelity pressure measurements in severe pulmonary hypertension. Br Heart J 72:384–389, 1994.
4. Badesch DB, Abman SH, Ahearn GS, et al; American College of Chest Physicians: Medical therapy for pulmonary arterial hypertension: ACCP evidence-based clinical practice guidelines. Chest 126(Suppl 1):S35–S62, 2004.
5. Giaid A: Nitric oxide and endothelin-1 in pulmonary hypertension. Chest 114(Suppl 3):S208–S212, 1998.
6. Galie N, Seeger W, Naeije R, et al: Comparative analysis of clinical trials and evidence-based treatment algorithm in pulmonary arterial hypertension. J Am Coll Cardiol 43(Suppl 12):S81–S88, 2004.
7. Galie N, Torbicki A, Barst R, et al; Task Force: Guidelines on diagnosis and treatment of pulmonary arterial hypertension. The Task Force on Diagnosis and Treatment of Pulmonary Arterial Hypertension of the European Society of Cardiology. Eur Heart J Dec;25:2243–2278, 2004.
8. Galie N, Ghofrani HA, Torbicki A, et al; Sildenafil Use in Pulmonary Arterial Hypertension (SUPER) Study Group: Sildenafil citrate therapy for pulmonary arterial hypertension. N Engl J Med 353:2148–2157, 2005.
9. Bossone E, Paciocco G, Iarussi D, et al: The prognostic role of the ECG in primary pulmonary hypertension. Chest 121:513–518, 2002.
10. Raymond RJ, Hinderliter AL, Willis PW, et al: Echocardiographic predictors of adverse outcomes in primary pulmonary hypertension. J Am Coll Cardiol 39:1214–1219, 2002.
11. Tei C, Dujardin KS, Hodge DO, et al: Doppler echocardiographic index for assessment of global right ventricular function. J Am Soc Echocardiogr 9:838–847, 1996.
12. Hoeper MM, Galie N, Murali S, et al: Outcome after cardiopulmonary resuscitation in patients with pulmonary arterial hypertension. Am J Respir Crit Care Med 165:341–344, 2002.
13. Hoeper MM, Faulenbach C, Golpon H, et al: Combination therapy with bosentan and sildenafil in idiopathic pulmonary arterial hypertension. Eur Respir J 24:1007–1010, 2004.

# Pulmonary Hypertension after Repair of Congenital Diaphragmatic Hernia

**Astrid E. Lammers and Sheila G. Haworth**

**Age: 16 years**
**Gender: Female**
**Occupation: Student**
**Working diagnosis: Left-sided congenital diaphragmatic hernia**

## HISTORY

The patient was diagnosed antenatally with a left-sided congenital diaphragmatic hernia (CDH). She was delivered near term by elective cesarian section after an uneventful pregnancy. A cleft soft palate was noticed postnatally. Genetic studies showed a normal female karyotype.

The diaphragmatic hernia was repaired at 3 hours of age. The postoperative period was uneventful, she was weaned off the ventilator 10 days after repair, and was discharged home at the age of 3 weeks.[1-4]

The cleft palate was repaired at 15 months of age followed by a pharyngoplasty at the age of 4 years. She required speech and language therapy but had no symptoms referable to the CDH in infancy and early childhood.

At the age of 16, she experienced an episode of syncope after mild exertion. She also complained of increasing fatigue. She was referred for a cardiology review.

**Comments:** The incidence of CDH is 1 in 5000 live births, 1 in 2000 if stillbirths are included. Defects are more common on the left side (70%–85%). Occasionally there can be a bilateral defect (5%).[5] CDH is frequently associated with karyotypic abnormalities (34%).[6,7]

The optimal timing of repair of CDH has gradually shifted from "emergency repair" after birth to a strategy of delayed repair following stabilization with either conservative ventilation strategies or even the use of extracorporeal membrane oxygenation. No substantial advantage of either approach has been proven to date.

## CURRENT SYMPTOMS

The patient's main symptom has been fatigue. Throughout her life her exercise capacity had always been less than that of her peers, but there had been a marked deterioration over the previous 6 to 8 months. She was exhausted after each school day and had little energy. She admitted having had three dizzy spells, briefly losing consciousness on one occasion.

NYHA class: II

**Comments:** The symptoms experienced here should alert the physician to look for evidence of PAH. Pulmonary hypertension frequently accompanies CDH repair, which is associated with a hypoplasia of alveoli and their accompanying arteries and veins.

The clinical manifestations of pulmonary hypertension can often be subtle. Exertional dyspnea and effort intolerance are common. Patients can present with syncope related to exertion or in other settings. Other symptoms include chest pain and hemoptysis.

## CURRENT MEDICATIONS

None

## PHYSICAL EXAMINATION

BP 100/80 mm Hg, HR 70 bpm, oxygen saturation 98% on room air

Height 152 cm, weight 39.9 kg, BSA 1.3 m$^2$

Neck veins: JVP was not elevated and the waveform was normal.

Lungs/chest: Chest was symmetrical. On auscultation the lungs were clear with good air entry bilaterally.

Heart: There was a mild RV heave. The pulmonary component of the second heart sound was accentuated. There were no murmurs.

Abdomen: No hepatosplenomegaly

Extremities: There was no peripheral edema, pallor, no cyanosis at rest, and no clubbing.

Neurological examination was normal.

**Comments:** The patient is less than 0.4 percentile for weight, and less than 9 percentile for height.

Chest symmetry is an important finding in patients with prior repair of diaphragmatic herniation. The examiner should specifically look for signs of PAH. When the pulmonary artery pressure is elevated the pulmonary component of the second heart sound is loud. An RV heave may be present, due to hypertrophy and hyperactivity of the RV. Later in the disease there may be evidence of RV failure, such as hepatomegaly and peripheral edema.

## LABORATORY DATA

| | |
|---|---|
| Hemoglobin | 12.3 g/dL (11.5–15.0) |
| Hematocrit | 36% (36–46) |
| MCV | 90 fL (83–99) |
| MCH | 30.6 pg (27–32) |
| | |
| Sodium | 140 mmol/L (134–145) |
| Potassium | 3.9 mmol/L (3.5–5.2) |
| Creatinine | **59 mg/dL** (71–106) |
| Blood urea nitrogen | 5.0 mmol/L (2.5–6.5) |
| | |
| Total bilirubin | 7.0 μmol/L (0–17) |
| ALT | 9 IU/L (0–31) |
| Alkal. phosphatase | 66 IU/L (50–150) |
| Albumin | 46 g/L (35–50) |

Thyroid function tests were within normal limits.

***Comments:*** There were no significant abnormal findings in baseline laboratory tests.

## ELECTROCARDIOGRAM

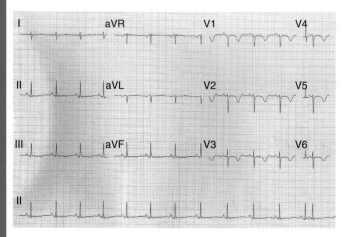

Figure 82-1 Electrocardiogram.

### FINDINGS

Heart rate: 85 bpm

PR interval: 140 msec

QRS axis: +95°

QRS duration: 75 msec

Sinus rhythm with normal intervals. There was borderline right-axis deviation. T-wave inversions were present throughout the precordial leads without voltage evidence of either RV hypertrophy or RA overload.

***Comments:*** In severe pulmonary hypertension, signs of RV hypertrophy are frequently seen. The P-wave amplitude may often be above 2.5 mv, consistent with RA hypertrophy. Neither one of these signs is present in our patient.

## CHEST X-RAY

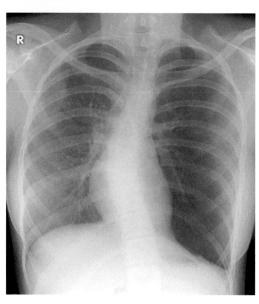

Figure 82-2 Posteroanterior projection.

### FINDINGS

Cardiothoracic ratio: 42%

Situs solitus, levocardia, left aortic arch.
   The cardiac size was normal. The translucency of the two lungs differed. The left lung appeared overinflated and hyper-translucent. The left hemidiaphragm was flattened. The patient had scoliosis.

***Comments:*** The abnormal left hemidiaphragm is explained by the previous history of CDH. The different opacification density of the right lung compared to the left is consistent with some degree of pulmonary hypoplasia. The pulmonary arteries are not enlarged, which would be expected in typical PAH.

## EXERCISE TESTING

### 6-Minute Walk Test Results

Distance walked: 350 m

Pretest $O_2$ saturation: 98% (room air)

Posttest $O_2$ saturation: 96% (room air)

| | |
|---|---|
| Exercise protocol: | Modified Bruce |
| Duration (min:sec): | 7:10 |
| Reason for stopping: | Dyspnea |
| ECG changes: | None |

| | Rest | Peak |
|---|---|---|
| Heart rate (bpm): | 70 | 150 |
| Percent of age-predicted max HR: | | 74 |
| $O_2$ saturation (%): | 95 | 87 |
| Blood pressure (mm Hg): | 100/80 | 160/80 |
| Peak $V_{O_2}$ (mL/kg/min): | | 22.9 |
| Percent predicted (%): | | 46 |
| Metabolic equivalents: | | 6.0 |

**Comments:** The 6MWT is commonly used as an "objective" measure of exercise capacity in patients with PAH.[8] In patients with IPAH the distance walked in 6 minutes is related to World Health Organization functional class and is predictive of mortality. In these patients a 6MWT distance of less than 300 m and a reduction in oxygen saturation of greater than 10% are associated with an increased mortality.[9]

Formal exercise testing gives additional objective information. In adult patients with IPAH peak $Vo_2$ has been found to be an independent strong predictor of survival.[10] Peak $Vo_2$ is also a useful parameter for objective longitudinal assessment of a patient's exercise capacity.

This patient has moderately impaired aerobic capacity, with measured desaturation.

## ECHOCARDIOGRAM

### OVERALL FINDINGS

Morphologically normal heart with evidence of mild pulmonary hypertension and possible obstruction of the pulmonary venous return from the right lung.

The LV is normal in size and function.

Mild tricuspid regurgitation with a maximum velocity of 3.4 m/sec was present, giving an estimated RV systolic pressure of 46 mm Hg + CVP. There was trivial pulmonary regurgitation. The RV appeared mildly dilated without evidence of hypertrophy, and systolic function was well preserved. The ventricular septum appeared slightly flattened during diastole.

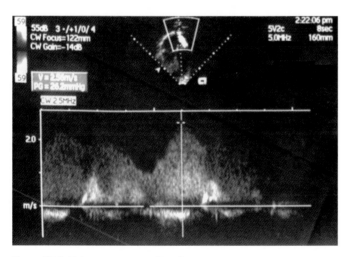

Figure 82-3 Pulmonary venous Doppler.

### FINDINGS

The venous return from the right pulmonary veins was prominent, turbulent, and accelerated. There was continuous flow signal with a maximum velocity of 2.6 m/sec (~26 mm Hg).

**Comments:** The heart is morphologically normal, with evidence of mild PAH. Despite this, the right ventricle is relatively normal, as we might have expected from the ECG and CXR. The more significant finding is elevated pulmonary venous velocity, which implies venous obstruction.

## VENTILATION-PERFUSION SCAN

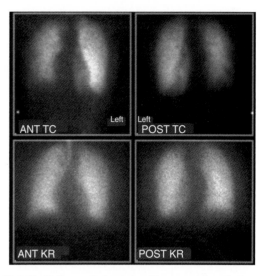

Figure 82-4 Ventilation-perfusion scan. *Upper panel*, perfusion, anterior view (*left*) and posterior view (*right*). *Lower panel*, ventilation, anterior view (*left*) and posterior view (*right*). KR, krypton; Tc, technicium.

### FINDINGS

A ventilation-perfusion scan and an MRI were performed to measure the relative flow and ventilation to each lung.

There was a normal distribution of isotope to both lungs.

The perfusion to the right lung was globally reduced, with segmental perfusion defects in the lower and mid zones. Perfusion to the left lung was greater, but was less in the lower than the upper lobe. The left lung received 64% of the cardiac output and contributed 50% to ventilation.

**Comments:** The left lung on the side of the diaphragmatic hernia had normal ventilation and only minimally reduced perfusion.

In contrast, the right lung showed markedly reduced perfusion despite normal ventilation. The findings are consistent with pulmonary venous obstruction.

## MAGNETIC RESONANCE IMAGING

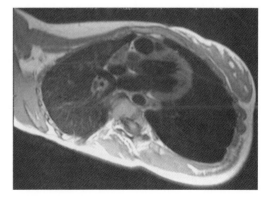

Figure 82-5 Black-blood spin-echo magnetic resonance image (MRI). Fast imaging with steady-state precession (FISP) cine phase contrast flow and gadolinium-enhanced MRI images of the heart and great vessels.

### FINDINGS

A discrete stenosis was seen at the orifice of the right middle and lower lobe pulmonary veins as they entered the LA. A membrane-like structure was present in the LA.

The right upper and left pulmonary veins appeared unobstructed.

More distally, the pulmonary veins had a normal caliber.

**Comments:** MRI is an excellent modality for visualizing pulmonary veins and measuring flow velocity. This study confirmed pulmonary venous stenosis of the right middle and lower lobe pulmonary veins.

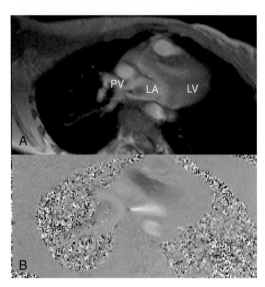

Figure 82-6 Oblique axial gradient echo magnetic resonance image (**A**) and in-plane velocity flow map (**B**).

## FINDINGS

Turbulence was noted, and a velocity of 2.3 m/sec across the membrane was measured.

**Comments:** An advantage of MRI over CT is the ability to both visualize turbulence and measure velocity in addition to visualizing anatomy. The jet of turbulence and high velocity shown here are confirmatory in this case.

### FOCUSED CLINICAL QUESTIONS AND DISCUSSION POINTS

1. **What is the relationship between repaired CDH and pulmonary artery hypertension?**

*Pulmonary hypertension is a common problem after diaphragmatic hernia repair as a consequence of the hypoplastic lungs and a rarefied cross-sectional area of the distal pulmonary vascular bed.[11] Retrospective studies suggest that approximately 14% of all patients who undergo repair of CDH have pulmonary hypertension at the time of discharge. However, in 87% of these patients the pulmonary hypertension resolves by the age of 12 months.[12] The strongest predictor of outcome is the relative ease with which the child can be weaned off the ventilator following repair, which is related to the degree of pulmonary hypoplasia.[13]*

*Our patient had experienced a relatively smooth postoperative course, with successful weaning from ventilation and discharge from the hospital 3 weeks after repair. It would appear that there was no evidence of pulmonary hypertension at that time.*

*However, long-term pulmonary morbidity still remains a problem in many survivors.[14] Ventilatory problems may occur. A mild restrictive pattern is described in approximately 25% of these patients, while 14% show an obstructive pattern.[15] Perfusion of the affected side can also be significantly reduced depending on the degree of hypoplasia.*

*Despite this, however, overall long-term survival rate is excellent and normalization of pulmonary artery pressures can be expected in most patients. Prolonged oxygen therapy beyond the age of 2 years is uncommon. All patients should be followed up by a respiratory physician who can refer to a cardiologist if necessary.*

2. **What is the etiology of pulmonary hypertension in this setting?**

*Historically, CDH was considered the primary anatomical defect, which resulted in displacement and compression of the developing lung by intra-abdominal organs and thus underdevelopment of the pulmonary parenchyma. This may be incorrect. In lungs of infants with CDH the number of airway and vascular generations is reduced bilaterally.[16,17] Morphologic and clinical studies demonstrate that abnormal lung development with resulting lung hypoplasia is present and may be the primary defect rather than secondary to mechanical forces as once believed.*

3. **What is the cause of syncope and pulmonary hypertension in this patient?**

*Syncope can be a presenting manifestation of PAH, as it may well have been here. Usually the cause is reduced cardiac output due to poor left atrial filling. In our case, pulmonary hypertension was present in the setting of obstruction to the right-sided pulmonary venous drainage. It is impossible to conclude that there is pulmonary vascular disease until after the mechanical obstruction is resolved. The case illustrates that a careful search for underlying anatomical reasons for this finding is mandatory.*

4. **Is further invasive assessment indicated in this case?**

*Cardiac catheterization remains the gold standard for establishing the diagnosis of pulmonary hypertension, especially for assessment of the pulmonary vascular resistance. In many institutions, presurgical hemodynamic assessment is carried out routinely. However, in this case, it was felt that no useful additional information would have been obtained from a cardiac catheterization study that would influence the decision to recommend surgical exploration and resection.*

## FINAL DIAGNOSIS

Repaired CDH

PAH secondary to pulmonary venous obstruction

Obstructive LA membrane

## PLAN OF ACTION

Surgical release of obstruction and resection of membrane

## INTERVENTION

The patient was brought to the operating room. Through a median sternotomy, the right pulmonary venous stenosis was repaired using an autologous patch. The LA membrane was resected.

Histological examination demonstrated a fibrous membrane with fragments of fibrous tissue containing hyaline and mucoid areas of degeneration.

## OUTCOME

There were no surgical complications, and the patient had an uneventful recovery.

Six months after the relief of the pulmonary venous obstruction the physical signs of pulmonary hypertension had resolved.

Subjectively, her exercise tolerance improved, and she was less tired. A repeated cardiorespiratory exercise test showed an improved peak $V_{O_2}$ of 25.2 mL/kg/min.

Echocardiography in follow-up showed that the maximum flow velocity in the right pulmonary veins had decreased from 2.6 m/sec to 1.2 m/sec. Trivial tricuspid regurgitation was present, with a maximum velocity of 2.2 m/sec.

## ACKNOWLEDGMENTS

The MRI images are courtesy of Dr. Andrew Taylor, Great Ormond Street Hospital for Children, London, United Kingdom.

## Selected References

1. Coughlin JP, Drucker DE, Cullen ML, et al: Delayed repair of congenital diaphragmatic hernia. Am Surg 59:90–93, 1993.
2. Nio M, Haase G, Kennaugh J, et al: A prospective randomized trial of delayed versus immediate repair of congenital diaphragmatic hernia. J Pediatr Surg 29:618–621, 1994.
3. Moyer V, Moya F, Tibboel R, et al: Late versus early surgical correction for congenital diaphragmatic hernia in newborn infants. Cochrane Database Syst Rev (3):CD001695, 2000.
4. Romiarek AJ, Qureshi FG, Cassidy L, et al: Factors influencing survival in newborns with congenital diaphragmatic hernia: The relative role of timing of surgery. J Pediatr Surg 39:821–824, 2004.
5. Hartman GE: Diaphragmatic hernia. In Behrman RE, Kliegman RM, Jenson HB (eds): Nelson Textbook of Pediatrics, 16th ed. Philadelphia, WB Saunders, 2000, pp 1231–1234.
6. Howe DT, Kilby MD, Sirry H, et al: Structural chromosome anomalies in congenital diaphragmatic hernia. Prenat Diagn 16:1003–1009, 1996.
7. Wilson RD, Chitayat D, McGillivray BC: Fetal ultrasound abnormalities: Correlation with fetal karyotype, autopsy findings, and postnatal outcome—five-year prospective study. Am J Med Genet 44:586–590, 1992.
8. Hoeper MM, Schwarze M, Ehlerding S, et al: Long-term treatment of primary pulmonary hypertension with aerosolized iloprost, a prostacyclin analogue. N Engl J Med 342:1866–1870, 2000.
9. Miyamoto S, Nagaya N, Satoh T, et al: Clinical correlates and prognostic significance of six-minute walk test in patients with primary pulmonary hypertension. Comparison with cardiopulmonary exercise testing. Am J Respir Crit Care Med 161:487–492, 2000.
10. Wensel R, Opitz CF, Anker SD, et al: Assessment of survival in patients with primary pulmonary hypertension. Importance of cardiopulmonary exercise testing. Circulation 106:319–324, 2002.
11. O'Toole SJ, Irish MS, Holm BA, Glick PL: Pulmonary vascular abnormalities in congenital diaphragmatic hernia. Clin Perinatol 23:781–794, 1996.
12. Iocono JA, Cilley RE, Mauger DT, et al: Postnatal pulmonary hypertension after repair of congenital diaphragmatic hernia: Predicting risk and outcome. J Pediatr Surg 34:349–353, 1996.
13. Dillon PW, Cilley RE, Mauger D, et al: The relationship of pulmonary artery pressure and survival in congenital diaphragmatic hernia. J Pediatr Surg 39:307–312, 2004.
14. Jaillard SM, Pierrat V, Dubois A, et al: Outcome at 2 years of infants with congenital diaphragmatic hernia: A population-based study. Ann Thorac Surg 75:250–256, 2003.
15. Stefanutti G, Filippone M, Tommasoni N, et al: Cardiopulmonary anatomy and function in long-term survivors of mild to moderate congenital diaphragmatic hernia. J Pediatr Surg 39:526–531, 2004.
16. Kitagawa M, Hislop A, Bozden EA, Reid L: Lung hypoplasia in congenital diaphragmatic hernia: A quantitative study of airway, artery, and alveolar development. Br J Surg 58:342–346, 1971.
17. Areechon W, Reid L: Hypoplasia of the lung with congenital diaphragmatic hernia. Br Med J 1:230–233, 1963.

# Contraception Counseling

**Lesley Jones, Craig Broberg, and Elisabeth Bédard**

**Age: 23 years**
**Gender: Female**
**Occupation: Housewife**
**Working diagnosis: Idiopathic pulmonary arterial hypertension**

## HISTORY

The patient was healthy at birth and through childhood without limitation, but at the age of 15 years she began to note exercise intolerance. Initially treated for asthma, she felt her symptoms progressed over the next several years. She developed Raynaud's phenomenon, oligomenorrhea, weigh loss, and anorexia. Gradually, she became unable to carry on with her education.

At age 20 she was transferred to a tertiary center with increasing exertional dyspnea. She was found to be profoundly hypoxic despite supplemental oxygen. Her oxygen saturations were as low as 75% on room air and 88% on 8 liters of oxygen. She had an ischemic infarct of one of her toes. Physically, she was unable to transfer from bed to chair.

The diagnosis of idiopathic pulmonary artery hypertension (IPAH) was made by echocardiography and confirmed by catheterization. The prognosis and therapeutic options were discussed with her and her family, and she was considered for lung transplantation.

She comes from a large family but had no affected siblings.

She was started on intravenous iloprost (prostacyclin). Within a week she noted a clinical improvement and was able to walk around the hospital ward without assistance. An indwelling central line was placed, and she was taught to care for her infusions herself. She was discharged home.

Over the next year she had two separate infections of her indwelling line requiring removal, intravenous antibiotics, and line replacement. After the third line infection, she was switched from intravenous to subcutaneous epoprostenol through a pump. Her exercise capacity remained improved and stable.

At age 22, the patient was married. She felt well and her clinical condition was stable. She and her husband were anxious to try to start a family, with the support and encouragement of both their extended families. The patient said "it would make her life complete." She did not want sterilization and hoped one day there might be a cure for her illness.

At an outpatient appointment pregnancy and contraception were discussed with her and her husband. She was told pregnancy would be a high-risk endeavor (see Case 75). The couple was using condoms as their contraceptive of choice. The merits and risks of various methods of contraception, including failure rates, were thoroughly discussed. A referral to a high-risk obstetrician/gynecologist was arranged to address further the patient's questions.

***Comments:*** The pathophysiology of PAH is poorly understood. An insult to the endothelium may occur (hormonal, mechanical, or other), resulting in a cascade of events characterized by vascular scarring, endothelial dysfunction, and intimal and medial smooth muscle proliferation. At least 10% to 15% of patients with PAH have the familial form, which has only recently been characterized. Some cases may be related to sporadic genetic defects.

Ischemic infarction of a systemic area (such as the patient's toe in this case) is very uncommon in PAH. The most plausible cause would be a venous thromboembolism through a PFO or other intracardiac shunt.

This patient is very young, and the impact of this chronic condition on her life is bound to be great. An individual's response to knowledge of chronic illness varies considerably. Involving close family members in discussions can help the patient come to terms with what the condition means in terms of planning the remainder of one's life.

The benefits of various pharmacotherapies in IPAH have become more evident (see Case 81), and, in general, patients now have much to hope for, compared to those afflicted in previous decades.

Depending on cultural and/or religious circumstances, patients may feel tremendous pressure to have a child soon after marriage. Health care providers ought to try to recognize such pressure, acknowledge it and its source, and help the patient to reconcile this with their individual health concerns.

Because of this, it is imperative to have in-depth discussions about pregnancy risk and contraception early on in a patient's care, even well before the opportunity for childbearing arrives.

## CURRENT SYMPTOMS

The patient had deteriorated in recent weeks. She now becomes short of breath on minimal exertion and has to stop twice when climbing one flight of stairs. She has not had any presyncope or syncope, nor has she had dependent edema or episodes of tachycardia.

NYHA class: III

## CURRENT MEDICATIONS

Warfarin (target INR of 2–3)

Sildenafil 100 mg three times daily

Ondansetron 8 mg three times daily

Intravenous prostacyclin

Spironolactone 25 mg daily

Amiodarone 200 mg daily

*Comments:* Pregnancy.

Anticoagulation is recommended in patients with primary PAH.[1]

Ondansetron in this patient was used for severe persistent nausea.

## PHYSICAL EXAMINATION

BP 85/55 mm Hg, HR 90 bpm, oxygen saturation 82% on room air and 88% on 8 L/min of supplemental oxygen

Height 156 cm, weight 46.9 kg, BSA 1.43 $m^2$

Surgical scars: None

Neck veins: JVP was elevated and showed prominent A-waves to about 5 cm above the sternal angle.

Lungs/chest: Chest was clear.

Heart: Regular rhythm with heart rate of 90 bpm, normal first heart sound and a loud pulmonary component to her second heart sound with no gallop or murmurs.

Abdomen: Abdominal exam revealed a smooth but tender liver edge 2 cm below the costal margin. No other masses or organs were palpable.

Extremities: Old ischemic infarct of her left fourth toe

*Comments:* The patient was markedly desaturated because of poor cardiac output as well as possible right-to-left shunting at the atrial level.

## LABORATORY DATA

| | |
|---|---|
| Hemoglobin | 13.4 g/dL (11.5–15.0) |
| Hematocrit/PCV | 39% (36–46) |
| MCV | **80 fL** (83–99) |
| Platelet count | $260 \times 10^9$/L (150–400) |
| Sodium | 136 mmol/L (134–145) |
| Potassium | 4.2 mmol/L (3.5–5.2) |
| Creatinine | 0.7 mg/dL (0.6–1.2) |
| Blood urea nitrogen | 5.9 mmol/L (2.5–6.5) |

*Comments:* Despite her low oxygen saturation, she had a low hemoglobin and hematocrit, with evidence of iron deficiency, which could contribute to her exercise intolerance.

## ELECTROCARDIOGRAM

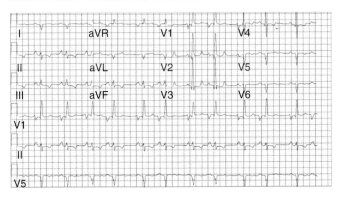

Figure 83-1 Electrocardiogram.

### FINDINGS

Heart rate: 70 bpm

QRS axis: +150°

QRS duration: 112 msec

Sinus rhythm with extreme axis deviation, RBBB, and evidence of RV hypertrophy. Biatrial enlargement. Nonspecific T-wave abnormalities.

*Comments:* ECG is consistent with PAH.

## CHEST X-RAY

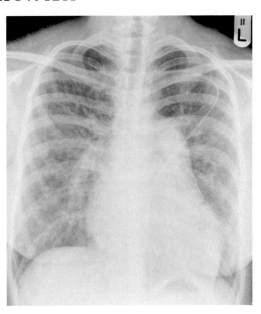

Figure 83-2 Posteroanterior projection.

### FINDINGS
Cardiothoracic ratio: 58%

Cardiomegaly, particularly right atrial enlargement, with a dilated main pulmonary artery and prominent central pulmonary arteries.

There is a diffuse pattern of interstitial thickening.

Note central line in the left subclavian vein (epoprostenol therapy via a pump).

*Comments:* The findings are all in keeping with her diagnosis of pulmonary hypertension.

## EXERCISE TESTING

Not performed

## ECHOCARDIOGRAM

### OVERALL FINDINGS
There was PAH with a severely dilated yet hypertrophied RV with severely impaired RV systolic function. The LV cavity was compressed with a dynamically narrowed LVOT.

The RA was severely dilated and was compressing the LA. There was no PFO. There was mild tricuspid regurgitation with a restrictive RV filling and an estimated pulmonary artery pressure of 110 to 120 mm Hg.

The RV dimension in this view was 3.5 cm.

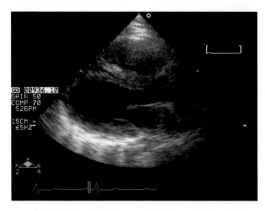

Figure 83-3  Parasternal long-axis view.

***Comments:*** The amount of RV visible in the parasternal long-axis view (Fig. 83-3) is indicative of RV enlargement. (Compare the CXR, which showed a prominent main pulmonary artery.) The RV rotates somewhat toward the left as it enlarges.

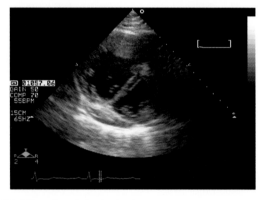

Figure 83-4  Parasternal short-axis view.

## FINDINGS

The RV was dilated and hypertrophied, and there was abnormal septal motion.

***Comments:*** Abnormal septal motion occurs when RV pressure is higher than LV pressure at any time during the cardiac cycle. Note that patients with pulmonary hypertension and a VSD, such as in Eisenmenger syndrome, do not exhibit this type of septal shift because the RV and LV pressures remain equal throughout the cardiac cycle.

## CT ANGIOGRAM

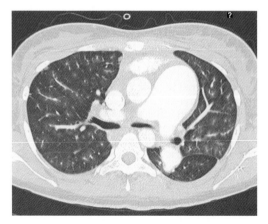

Figure 83-5  Computed tomography pulmonary angiogram.

## FINDINGS

The pulmonary arteries were enlarged. The central pulmonary artery measured 44 mm (upper normal = 27 mm). No thrombus was identified.

***Comments:*** Enlargement of the pulmonary arteries is the expected finding in pulmonary hypertension of any cause. The CT was helpful in excluding thromboembolic disease as the etiology of her pulmonary hypertension, and of her recent deterioration.

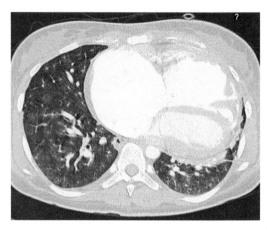

Figure 83-6  Computed tomography pulmonary angiogram.

## FINDINGS

RA enlargement, RV enlargement, prominent small branches of the pulmonary arteries.

***Comments:*** In this view the huge RA can be seen, as well as the dilatation of the RV. The lung fields themselves show heterogeneous changes and thickened, prominent small branch pulmonary arteries.

## CATHETERIZATION

### HEMODYNAMICS

Heart rate    90 bpm

|  | Pressure | Saturation (%) |
|---|---|---|
| SVC |  | 40 |
| IVC |  | 46 |
| RA | mean 17 | 42 |
| RV | 128/24 | 42 |
| PA | 127/66 mean 90 | 44 |
| PCWP | mean 18 |  |
| LV | 88/7 | 90 |
| Aorta | 94/64 mean 72 | 88 |

| Calculations | |
|---|---|
| Qp (L/min) | 1.66 |
| Qs (L/min) | 1.93 |
| Cardiac index (L/min/m²) | 1.36 |
| Qp/Qs | 0.86 |
| PVR (Wood units) | 49.86 |
| SVR (Wood units) | 22.77 |

### FINDINGS

There was a high transpulmonary gradient and severe elevation of pulmonary vascular resistance. Cardiac output was markedly reduced.

There was no change in her pulmonary artery pressures, cardiac output, or pulmonary vascular resistance after administration of pulmonary vasodilators (data not shown).

**Comments:** Catheterization was performed to assess pulmonary artery pressures and vasoreactivity prior to starting therapy with an epoprostenol infusion.

Pulmonary vasoreactivity still has a role in confirming the diagnosis and demonstrating vasoreactivity; when present, the latter provides prognostic information.

Our patient has systemic desaturation, is relatively anemic, and has a low cardiac output. All of these contribute to poor tissue oxygenation and symptoms.[2]

### FOCUSED CLINICAL QUESTIONS AND DISCUSSIONS POINTS

1. What should this patient be told about her risk of pregnancy?

*There is very little written specifically about primary pulmonary hypertension and pregnancy.[3,4] Most studies suggest a 30% to 50% maternal mortality risk in parturients with severe pulmonary hypertension in the context of Eisenmenger syndrome, with the mortality most often due to heart failure and/or hemorrhage.[5,6] There is an even higher risk of fetal death. Given these data it is widely accepted that pregnancy is contraindicated in severe pulmonary hypertension, irrespective of etiology.*

2. What is the safest form of contraception for this patient?

*No form of contraception is 100% effective and without side effects. The choice of contraception depends on personal preference, the underlying illness, its effectiveness, possible side effects, and its reversal potential for future desired pregnancies if the method is discontinued.*

*Estrogen-based contraception should be avoided in women with a high risk of thromboembolism, which includes patients with cyanosis. Barrier methods such as diaphragms and condoms do not increase thromboembolic risk but have a high failure rate.*

*Old-style intrauterine devices were associated with increased menstrual bleeding and an increased risk of pelvic inflammatory disease.*

*A newer hormone-releasing intrauterine device is very effective as a contraceptive. The hormone is mainly confined to the uterus, thus lowering the risk of infection and of thromboembolism. There is a risk of vagal response at time of implantation, so this should be used with caution in patients with a history of bradycardia or conduction defects. Infective endocarditis associated with these devices is rare but remains a concern in women in high-risk groups. Most providers will use prophylactic antibiotics at the time of implantation. Sterilization can be considered and is more than 99% effective (though not absolute) but carries an anesthetic risk,[7] which may not be inconsequential in a patient such as this.*

3. If the patient becomes pregnant, what counseling should she be given?

*For several reasons, the patient should be seen immediately if pregnancy is suspected or known. Because the risk of mortality in pregnancy is as high as 50% in a patient such as this, the expectant mother needs to know these statistics and make a decision of whether to continue. Obviously this is a difficult decision, and the caregiver must be considerate of the deep ethical/social/religious issues involved. Termination, if opted, carries its own risk, which increases as gestation continues. The preferred timing of termination is under 12 weeks' gestation.*

*Medical abortion using antiprogesterone agents and vaginally administered prostaglandin analogues is as effective as dilation and curettage if performed under 7 weeks. The patient would need a hospital stay until after expulsion, as the process is not controlled and systemic vasodilatation could be dangerous for women with pulmonary hypertension.*

*Since the patient is taking warfarin, which is the standard of care in patients with PAH, there is also a risk of teratogenicity and of fetal bleeding. This needs to be discussed with the patient if the couple chooses to go ahead with the pregnancy.*

## FINAL DIAGNOSIS

Idiopathic pulmonary arterial hypertension

## PLAN OF ACTION

Counseling regarding risks of pregnancy

Continue epoprostenol

## INTERVENTION

Recommend strongly against pregnancy. Arrange sessions with clinical nurse specialist, cardiologist, and high-risk obstetrician, together with the husband, to make sure that the perceived risks are clearly understood. Recommend barrier contraception with strong emphasis on compliance, or, even better, intrauterine device implantation.

## OUTCOME

Despite several attempts to formally schedule visits in the high-risk obstetrics clinic, the patient failed to attend her appointments. However, because of problems with her infusions, she was often seen in clinic or on the hospital ward, and the clinical nurse specialist repeatedly inquired about her marriage and their use of contraception. The patient still had difficulty accepting the fact that pregnancy was so discouraged.

Eighteen months after her marriage, the patient telephoned to say she had missed a menstrual cycle and thought she was pregnant. The patient also stated that she found walking upstairs more difficult and was having to stop more frequently.

She was told to come for evaluation immediately. On arrival urine and blood tests were sent and confirmed the patient's suspicion that she was indeed pregnant. She and her husband were both unsure of the date of her last period, so a fetal ultrasound was performed. The scan confirmed an intrauterine pregnancy of about 6 weeks gestation.

With the patient and husband seated in a comfortable private room, they were told they needed to make a decision about whether to continue with pregnancy. At no time during this 3-hour discussion were they advised to terminate the pregnancy. Rather, they were informed fully of the potential outcomes. They were reassured that no matter what their decision, they would be supported fully and given the best possible care by the medical staff.

The provider first questioned them about their own religious/ethical feelings about abortion. Then the full risks to both mother and fetus were reexplained, including the risk of death. There was also a risk that the child would be small for gestational age and/or premature.

It was explained that if the patient wanted to continue with the pregnancy, it may require altering her medication. The potential effects of warfarin were explained, but the patient was on a small dose, making the risk of teratogenicity much smaller. The uncertainties of prostacyclin therapy during pregnancy were mentioned, although epoprostenol has been used successfully in pregnancy for preeclampsia[8] and in select case reports in patients with pulmonary hypertension.[9,10]

The patient was also told that pregnancy would require a prolonged hospital stay on oxygen during the second and third trimesters. After delivery she would have to stay in the hospital for about 2 weeks.

It was suggested that they return home to talk to their families and return in 48 hours to talk again. The patient was told to discontinue her warfarin in the meantime, anticipating either continued pregnancy or termination.

Initially, the patient herself was adamant that she wanted to continue with the pregnancy. Seeing a copy of the fetal scan made the experience more heartfelt. On their return, however, their mutual decision had been reached. The husband did not want to risk losing his wife, and she felt okay about the decision not to continue. Termination of the pregnancy was arranged with the high-risk obstetrics team.

At the appointment for termination, a further scan found that there was no fetal heartbeat. The patient felt much more comfortable with this outcome and that the burden of having to make the decision not to carry the baby had been removed. After the successful dilatation and curettage procedure done at 9 weeks gestation, a hormone-releasing intrauterine device was inserted at the request of the patient and her husband, with prophylactic antibiotics given at the same time. She was started on her usual dose of warfarin thereafter.

## Selected References

1. Archer S, Rich S: Primary pulmonary hypertension: A vascular biology and translational research: Work in progress. Circulation 102:2781–2791, 2000.

2. Spence MS, Balaratnam, MS, Gatzoulis MA: Clinical update: Cyanotic adult congenital heart disease. Lancet 370:1530–1532, 2007.

3. Warnes CA: Pregnancy and pulmonary hypertension. Int J Cardiol 97(Suppl 1):11–13, 2004.

4. Kiely D, Elliot C, Webster V, Stewart P: Pregnancy and pulmonary hypertension: New approaches to the management of life-threatening condition. In Steer P, Gatzoulis M, Baker P (eds): Heart Disease and Pregnancy. London, RCOG Press, 2006, pp 211–229.

5. Kansaria JJ, Salvi VS: Eisenmenger syndrome in pregnancy. J Postgrad Med 46:101–103, 2000.

6. Avila WS, Rossi EG, Ramires JA, et al: Pregnancy in patients with heart disease: Experience with 1,000 cases. Clin Cardiol 26:135–142, 2003.

7. Connolly HM, Warnes C: Pregnancy and contraception. In Gatzoulis MA, Webb G, Daubeney PEF (eds): Diagnosis and Management of Adult Congenital Heart Disease. Philadelphia, Churchill Livingstone, 2003, pp 135–144.

8. Vainio M, Riutta A, Koivisto AM, Mäenpää J: Prostacyclin, thromboxane A and the effect of low-dose ASA in pregnancies at high risk for hypertensive disorders. Acta Obstet Gynecol Scand 83:1119–1123, 2004.

9. Bildirici I, Shumway JB: Intravenous and inhaled epoprostenol for primary pulmonary hypertension during pregnancy and delivery. Obstet Gynecol 103(5 Pt 2):1102–1105, 2004.

10. Badalian SS, Silverman RK, Aubry RH, Longo J: Twin pregnancy in a woman on long-term epoprostenol therapy for primary pulmonary hypertension. A case report. J Reprod Med 45:149–152, 2000.

# Part IV

# Isomerism

## Left Atrial Isomerism

**Jonathan Swinburn and Jan Till**

**Age: 40 years**
**Gender: Female**
**Occupation: Priest**
**Working diagnosis: Left atrial isomerism, partial atrioventricular septal defect**

## HISTORY

The patient presented at 3 years of age following recurrent attacks of bronchiolitis when a murmur was identified. Development had been normal until that time with no reported cyanosis. Clinical examination revealed a relative bradycardia, a fixed split second heart sound with a pulmonary ejection systolic murmur, and a pan-systolic murmur at the left sternal edge and apex.

Electrocardiography demonstrated a nodal rhythm with partial RBBB and left-axis deviation (–71°).

Cardiac catheterization demonstrated a single atrium with a persistent left SVC draining into the left side of the atrial chamber. There was severe regurgitation of the left AV valve.

At the age of 4 the patient underwent surgical septation of the atrium. At surgery the presence of a common atrium was confirmed, with separate orifices of bilateral SVCs. "Clefts" of the anterior cusp of the mitral valve and the septal cusp of the tricuspid valve were identified and repaired. A pericardial patch was used to divide the common atrium with separation of the systemic from the pulmonary venous return.

Postoperatively residual "mitral" regurgitation was noted clinically and progressed over the following years with an associated deterioration in exercise tolerance and a requirement for diuretic therapy.

At the age of 14 the patient underwent further septation of the atrium using a Dacron patch, the original patch having broken down allowing significant left-to-right shunting.

From the age of 31, she developed increasingly frequent and troublesome atrial tachycardia, requiring multiple DC cardioversions and amiodarone therapy. At this stage she had moderate left AV valve regurgitation, but this progressed over the ensuing 3 years. She underwent left AV valve repair. Postoperatively she was maintained in sinus rhythm with amiodarone.

Subsequent Holter monitoring demonstrated periods of atrial tachycardia and pauses in excess of 4 seconds. A pacemaker was therefore implanted on the left side, but it proved impos-

sible to advance a lead beyond the junction of the left SVC and the RA. Thus an AAI device was implanted.

Two years later, AV block was seen. Thus a new dual-chamber pacemaker was inserted on the right side. Subsequently atrial tachycardias were controlled with a combination of sotalol and occasional DC cardioversion, but atrial tachycardias were becoming more frequent and more symptomatic.

**Comments:** Recurrent lower respiratory tract infections may be common in children with ASDs.

The clinical features described combined with left-axis deviation on the ECG would suggest an ASD of the primum type (partial AV septal defect). The presence of a pan-systolic heart murmur supports this diagnosis, reflecting regurgitation of the left AV valve, which is an intrinsically abnormal trileaflet valve in this condition.

The presence of a nodal rhythm is surprising, since sinus rhythm would be expected with a primum ASD. This is a clue that the diagnosis may be more complex than it appears.

The finding of a common atrium indicates the possibility of a heterotaxy syndrome. The morphology of the atria and in particular of the atrial appendages then allows determination of LA or RA isomerism. This can usually be determined by echocardiography, although clues as to "sidedness" can be gained from analysis of the bronchial anatomy, pulmonary and systemic venous drainage, and the presence of asplenia or polysplenia.

In right atrial isomerism total anomalous pulmonary venous drainage is common, since pulmonary veins usually drain into the LA. In this situation pulmonary venous return is usually into the IVC or azygos system. Bilateral SVCs are common (50%–70%). RA isomerism is almost universally associated with bilateral right-sided bronchial anatomy and less consistently with asplenia.

In LA isomerism the IVC is usually interrupted, with azygos continuation of the IVC returning systemic venous blood from the lower half of the body into the SVC. In this situation the hepatic veins usually drain directly into the atrium.

Bilateral left bronchial anatomy is usual and polysplenia is common. Biliary atresia occurs in 11% and gut malrotation in 13% of patients.

An AVSD is seen in one third of patients with LA isomerism. Ventriculoarterial connections are normal in 60% of patients with LA isomerism, but double-outlet RV, TGA, pulmonary stenosis or atresia, and subaortic stenosis are all common.

Dysrhythmias are frequent (26%) in LA isomerism, related to the underlying anatomy and shunt, AV valve regurgitation, and atrial scarring from surgical repair.[1] Bradycardia occurs in 16% and is related to the lack of a sinus node (a right atrial structure absent in left isomerism) and consequent dependence on an ectopic atrial focus. Complete heart block is common, especially in patients with an AVSD. In 30% of patients with LA isomerism there is a dual AV node. Pacing was required in 12% of patients for a combination of sinus node disease and complete AV block.[1]

## CURRENT SYMPTOMS

The patient was able to walk on the flat without symptoms, but became breathless when climbing one flight of stairs. Short-lived palpitations still occurred with increasing frequency.

NYHA class: II

## CURRENT MEDICATIONS

Warfarin (target INR of 2.0–3.0)

Sotalol 160 mg morning and 80 mg evening

Amiloride/furosemide 5/40 mg daily

## PHYSICAL EXAMINATION

BP 139/82 mm Hg, HR 80 bpm, oxygen saturation 98%

Height 176 cm, weight 61 kg, BSA 1.75 m²

Surgical scars: Median sternotomy

Neck veins: JVP was 4 cm above the sternal angle, with a normal waveform.

Lungs/chest: Clear to auscultation

Heart: There was a midline cardiac impulse. A normal S1 was heard with fixed split S2. The pulmonary component was normal. A grade 2/6 pan-systolic murmur was audible at the apex.

Abdomen: Abdomen was soft. The liver edge and spleen tip were not appreciated.

Extremities: Peripheral pulses were all palpable. There was no peripheral edema.

## LABORATORY DATA

| | |
|---|---|
| Hemoglobin | 13.4 g/dL (11.5–15.0) |
| Hematocrit/PCV | 40% (36–46) |
| MCV | 93 fL (83–99) |
| Platelet count | 258 × 10⁹/L (150–400) |
| Sodium | 137 mmol/L (134–145) |
| Potassium | 3.9 mmol/L (3.5–5.2) |
| Creatinine | **58 mg/dL** (60–120) |
| Blood urea nitrogen | 4.0 mmol/L (2.5–6.5) |

| | |
|---|---|
| INR | 2.7 |
| Free T4 | 9.1 pmol/L (7.5–21) |

## ELECTROCARDIOGRAM

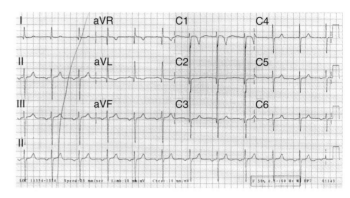

Figure 84-1 Electrocardiogram.

### FINDINGS

Heart rate: 68 bpm

QRS axis: –71°

P-wave axis: –78°

QRS duration: 96 msec

Ectopic atrial rhythm with left-axis deviation and incomplete RBBB.

***Comments:*** ECG before pacing shows an inferior P-wave axis consistent with a low atrial escape rhythm, since patients with LA isomerism have no sinus node (an RA structure). The (partial) RBBB and leftward axis raise the possibility of a primum ASD.

## CHEST X-RAY

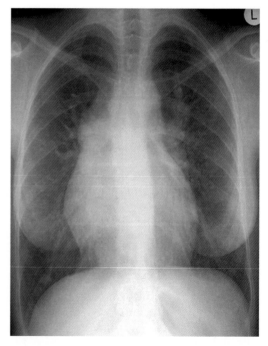

Figure 84-2 Posteroanterior projection.

## FINDINGS

Cardiothoracic ratio: 56%

CXR before permanent pacing. There is mesocardia (i.e., the heart is in the middle position), with a central liver and no visible gastric bubble. Bilateral left bronchial anatomy is evidenced by the lack of an upper lobe bronchus on the right. Note equal level of left and right pulmonary arteries (normally the left lies superior to the right).

*Comments:* Bronchial anatomy usually, but not always, correlates with atrial anatomy. Abdominal situs is less consistently related to atrial anatomy. Patients with heterotaxy may have levogastria, dextrogastria, or, as in this case, a central liver with no visible gastric bubble.

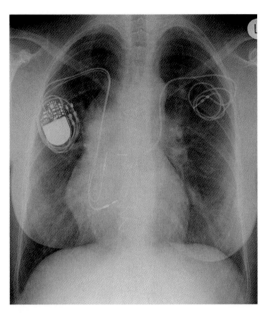

Figure 84-3 Posteroanterior projection.

## FINDINGS

This more recent posteroanterior CXR demonstrates pacing wires through both the left and right SVC.

# COMPUTED TOMOGRAPHY

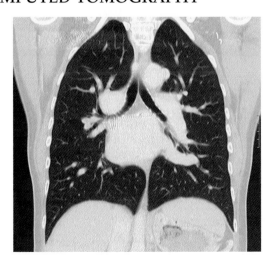

Figure 84-4 Coronal reconstruction, lung window.

## FINDINGS

This coronal plane section through the thorax confirms bilateral left bronchial anatomy with no right upper lobe bronchus visible.

*Comments:* The left main bronchus has a longer course before its first branch, roughly twice as long as the right main bronchus. Here both bronchi have a long course before branching, which is suggestive of and consistent with left atrial isomerism. Note the pulmonary branches above each bronchus. The aorta is left sided.

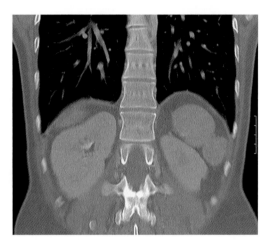

Figure 84-5 Coronal reconstruction, abdomen.

## FINDINGS

Coronal CT image demonstrates two spleens in the left hypochondrium.

*Comments:* In LA isomerism polysplenia is typically, but not invariably, present, while in right atrial isomerism patients are often asplenic, with Howell-Jolly bodies present on peripheral blood films.

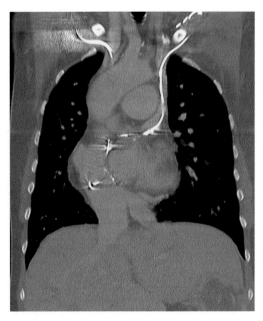

Figure 84-6 Coronal reconstruction.

## FINDINGS

This coronal section shows large hepatic veins draining directly into the lower floor of the atrial chamber.

***Comments:*** Typically, in LA isomerism the IVC is interrupted above the renal veins, and venous return from the lower half of the body drains via the azygos system into the SVC.

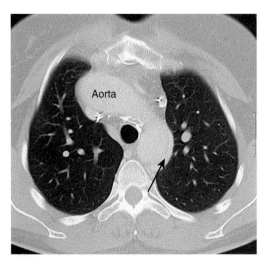

Figure 84-7  Axial plane.

## FINDINGS

This axial section shows the azygos vein (*arrow*) passing from the posterior aspect of the left hemithorax and around the aortic arch to the left SVC. Pacing wires are seen in both the left and right SVCs (to the front of this image).

### FOCUSED CLINICAL QUESTIONS AND DISCUSSION POINTS

1. Is there an ablative electrophysiological option to control recurrent atrial tachycardia?

*Ablation of atrial tachycardia is well established. However, several points specific to this case warrant comment. There are likely to be multiple reentrant atrial circuits given the atrial scarring from three previous atriotomies, and determining which of these are clinically significant can be difficult. Furthermore, even if one or more pathways are ablated, it is likely that further tachycardias will manifest in due course, and the ablation scars may even act as a substrate for further reentrant circuits.*

*More important, however, in this patient access can only be gained to the RA, since she has a Dacron interatrial septum. Given the history of left AV valve regurgitation and repair, the LA is perhaps the more likely chamber to be the origin of the arrhythmias, and this will not be amenable to percutaneous ablation.*

*If further left AV valve surgery is required in the future, the possibility of intraoperative ablation should be considered.*

2. What is the long-term outlook for this patient?

*Survival of patients with isomerism is related to the extent of underlying cardiac abnormalities, which vary considerably. Patients with no other congenital defects had a 20-year survival of 82%, those suitable for biventricular repair had a survival of 66%, while those with univentricular hearts had a survival of*

*only 37%.[1] The prognosis of this patient will be primarily related to the function of the left AV valve, and the impact of regurgitation on LV function.*

*She will require long-term anticoagulation because of atrial dysrhythmias.*

## FINAL DIAGNOSIS

LA isomerism

Partial AVSD

Recurrent atrial tachycardia

## PLAN OF ACTION

Electrophysiological study and possible ablation

## INTERVENTION

Electrophysiological study performed from the right femoral vein demonstrated a reentrant atrial tachycardia in the right-sided atrium. This was successfully ablated.

## OUTCOME

After 3 months the patient has had no recurrence of sustained tachycardia. She will remain under close follow-up, as one can anticipate further arrhythmias in the future.

## CATHETERIZATION

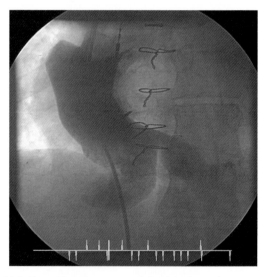

Figure 84-8  Femoral access may not lead to the atria except via the azygos system, complicating intervention.

## FINDINGS

This pump injection into the right-sided atrium performed at the time of electrophysiological study shows the pigtail catheter in the right atrium via the femoral vein. In this patient, fortunately, there was continuity between the IVC and hepatic veins, which is not always the case in heterotaxy.

## Selected References

1. Gilljam T, McCrindle BW, Smallhorn JF, et al: Outcomes of left atrial isomerism over a 28-year period at a single institution. J Am Coll Cardiol 36:908–916, 2000.

# Bibliography

Cohen MS, Anderson RH, Cohen MI, et al: Controversies, genetics, diagnostic assessment, and outcomes relating to the heterotaxy syndrome. Cardiol Young 17(Suppl 2):29–43, 2007.

Hassem Sobrinho S, Moscardini AC, Croti UA, et al: Sinus node dysfunction in a patient with left atrial isomerism. Arq Bras Cardiol 87:e122–e123, 2006.

Jacobs JP, Anderson RH, Weinberg PM, et al: The nomenclature, definition and classification of cardiac structures in the setting of heterotaxy. Cardiol Young 17(Suppl 2):1–28, 2007.

# Part V

# Cardiac and Yet Noncardiac

# Liver Dysfunction after the Mustard Procedure

**Peter J. Pugh**

**Age: 32 years**
**Gender: Female**
**Occupation: Radiographer**
**Working diagnosis: Transposition of the great arteries**

## HISTORY

The patient was cyanosed at birth and found to have TGA. She underwent reparative surgery at the age of 2 years, with the creation of a Mustard baffle. She subsequently enjoyed a normal childhood, with no physical limitation.

At age 21, her exercise capacity became markedly reduced. She was found to have obstruction of the IVC flow through the atrial baffle, which was treated successfully with balloon dilatation. This recurred 5 years later, and she was treated, again successfully, with balloon dilatation of the obstruction and insertion of a stent. Until recently, she exercised regularly at the gym, running 20 minutes a day and taking boxing classes. She continued taking a diuretic daily.

When she was 32 years old, her exercise capacity again declined. She reported significant ankle swelling if she missed her diuretic. Physical examination found no features of right or left heart failure. At exercise testing she completed 11 minutes of the Bruce protocol with the expected cardiovascular response. Echocardiography showed hypertrophy but good function of the systemic RV, normal valves, and widely patent systemic and pulmonary venous pathways.

She continued to deteriorate despite an increased dose of diuretics and was admitted to the hospital because of progressive dependent edema.

**Comments:** Atrial redirection surgery was the mainstay of treatment until the mid-1980s at most institutions3, when the arterial switch operation became the treatment of choice for TGA without pulmonary stenosis (see Case 52).

One of the complications of atrial redirection is obstruction of the low pressure venous return though the baffles. Often such obstruction can be tolerated for years because of runoff through the azygos system. Therefore, one should not routinely assume that the presence of obstruction is necessarily the cause of symptoms until other factors are excluded.

Deterioration in a Mustard patient should prompt investigation for systemic RV failure, regurgitation of the systemic AV valve (tricuspid valve), heart block, atrial arrhythmia, and obstruction or leak of the atrial baffle.

## CURRENT SYMPTOMS

The patient no longer attended the gym and had had to stop work. She was able to walk only 100 yards slowly. She also had abdominal bloating and swelling. She said she felt "exactly the same as when the baffle was obstructed." Her weight was considerably higher than it had been a year previously.

NYHA class: III

**Comments:** The history thus far is worrisome for further obstruction of her IVC flow.

## CURRENT MEDICATIONS

Furosemide 40 mg twice daily

Spironolactone 25 mg daily

## PHYSICAL EXAMINATION

BP 115/75 mm Hg, HR 92 bpm, oxygen saturation 98%

Height 160 cm, weight 59.2 kg, BSA 1.62 m$^2$

Surgical scars: None

Neck veins: JVP was visible 2 cm above the sternal angle with a normal waveform.

Lungs/chest: Chest was clear.

Heart: The pulse was regular. Heart sounds were normal with no added sounds; there was no heave, and peripheral pulses were all normal.

Abdomen: Smooth hepatomegaly (3 cm) and moderate ascites

Extremities: She was warm and well-perfused. Her ankles were free of edema, as were the upper extremities.

**Comments:** Features of baffle obstruction depend on the location of the obstruction. Obstruction within the SVC pathway usually manifests as upper body venous distension. Inferior baffle obstruction may result in abdominal swelling, hepato-splenomegaly, ascites, and lower limb edema. However, obstruction may go unnoticed if there is significant collateral drainage through the azygos vein.

Although ankle edema was absent due to her treatment, ascites and hepatomegaly were appreciable.

## LABORATORY DATA

| | |
|---|---|
| Hemoglobin | **9.8 g/dL** (11.5–15.0) |
| Hematocrit/PCV | **31%** (36–46) |
| MCV | 84 fL (83–99) |
| Platelet count | $305 \times 10^9$/L (150–400) |
| Sodium | 137 mmol/L (134–145) |
| Potassium | **3.3 mmol/L** (3.5–5.2) |
| Creatinine | 0.75 mg/dL (0.6–1.2) |
| Blood urea nitrogen | 4.3 mmol/L (2.5–6.5) |
| Bilirubin | **39 μmol/L** (3–24) |
| Alkaline phosphatase | **1364 U/L** (38–126) |
| γ-glutaryl transferase | **381 IU/L** (7–33) |
| Alanine transaminase | 37 IU/L (8–40) |
| Albumin | **29 g/L** (37–53) |
| C-reactive protein | **135 mg/L** (0–10) |
| Iron | **5.3 μmol/L** (12–26) |
| Ferritin | **195 μg/L** (20–186) |
| Transferrin saturation | **8%** (20–45) |
| Blood cultures | No growth |

***Comments:*** There is a normocytic anemia, normal renal chemistry, and marked elevation of hepatic enzymes. The pattern is not typical of either an obstructive or a hepatic picture.

## ELECTROCARDIOGRAM

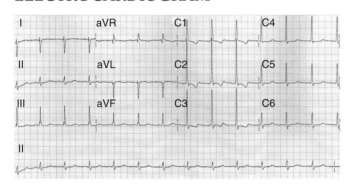

Figure 85-1 Electrocardiogram.

### FINDINGS
Heart rate: 70 bpm

QRS axis: +135°

QRS duration: 95 msec

Sinus rhythm with low-amplitude P-waves. There is marked right-axis deviation and tall dominant R-waves in the anteroseptal chest leads, with T-wave inversion in V1 and V2, reflecting the mandatory systemic RV hypertrophy.

***Comments:*** Maintenance of sinus rhythm is relatively uncommon in Mustard patients. Sinus rhythm is present in only 40% of patients 20 years after surgery.[4] Common rhythms include junctional rhythm and intra-atrial reentrant tachycardia. The other findings are as expected.

## CHEST X-RAY

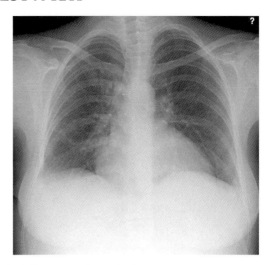

Figure 85-2 Posteroanterior projection.

### FINDINGS
Cardiothoracic ratio: 55%

There is cardiomegaly, with evidence of biatrial enlargement. Pulmonary vascular markings appear normal.

***Comments:*** The relatively narrow mediastinal window is due to the anteroposterior relationship of the great vessels. The stent placed in the IVC baffle cannot be seen in this view, likely because it overlies the spine.

## EXERCISE TESTING
Not performed

## ECHOCARDIOGRAM

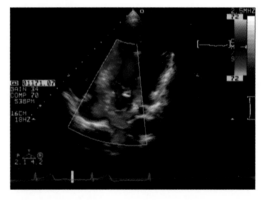

Figure 85-3 Four-chamber color Doppler.

### FINDINGS
There was a moderately dilated systemic RV with good systolic function. A normal systemic AV (tricuspid) valve was seen with mild regurgitation. The aortic valve was normal. The pulmonary venous pathway was widely patent.

Normal-sized subpulmonary LV with good function. Normal mitral valve. Normal pulmonary valve. Stent visible in the systemic venous pathway, with a peak velocity of 1.0 m/sec.

***Comments:*** Function of the systemic ventricle is not impaired, and there is no significant systemic AV valve regurgitation. The color flow map in this image shows no significant turbulence. The peak velocity of 1.0 m/sec is consistent with expected velocity for venous flow; thus it seems unlikely to be the cause of hepatic failure and ascites. Although at times the atrial pathways can be difficult to visualize echocardiographically, this study is reassuring on this point.

# MAGNETIC RESONANCE IMAGING

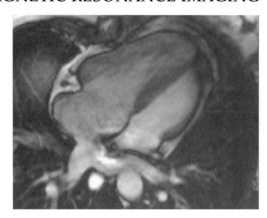

Figure 85-4 Oblique axial steady-state free precession cine, four-chamber view.

## FINDINGS

The systemic RV was hypertrophied, but with normal systolic function.

The pulmonary venous channels entering the systemic atrium were widely patent.

### Ventricular Volume Quantification

|  | LV | (Normal range) | RV | (Normal range) |
|---|---|---|---|---|
| EDV (mL) | 112 | (52–141) | 139 | (58–154) |
| ESV (mL) | 33 | (13–51) | 62 | (12–68) |
| SV (mL) | 79 | (33–97) | 77 | (35–98) |
| EF (%) | 71 | (57–75) | 55 | (51–75) |
| EDVi (mL/m²) | 69 | (62–96) | 86 | (61–98) |
| ESVi (mL/m²) | 20 | (17–36) | 38 | (17–43) |
| SVi (mL/m²) | 49 | (40–65) | 47 | (38–62) |

**Comments:** MRI can be a useful modality for imaging the atrial pathways and looking for obstruction. It also allows for a reliable means of quantifying the function of the systemic RV.

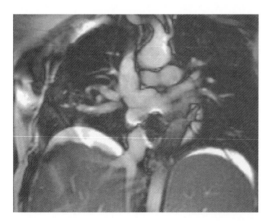

Figure 85-5 Oblique coronal plane steady-state free precession cine.

## FINDINGS

The metallic stent in the IVC channel produced artifact but pulsatility of IVC flow ruled out significant obstruction. In addition, there is no evidence of distal IVC dilatation.

**Comments:** As echocardiography can at times miss important baffle obstruction, this study was performed. The findings, however, illustrated normal venous flow. Stents give artifact but otherwise do not compromise image quality.

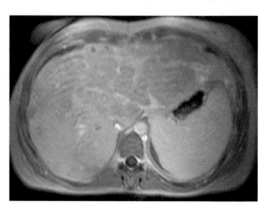

Figure 85-6 Axial plane through the upper abdomen after gadolinium injection.

## FINDINGS

The liver was markedly enlarged with a patchy, heterogeneous parenchymal enhancement. Ascites was present.

**Comments:** Although chronically elevated venous pressure can lead to hepatic congestion and liver failure, such as may be seen in Fontan patients, and nodules may be found, a diffuse, heterogeneous appearance should not be seen from venous congestion alone.

The problem now seems much more clearly to be intrinsic liver failure. Further imaging of the abdomen was therefore undertaken and blood tests sent for tumor markers.

# COMPUTED TOMOGRAPHY

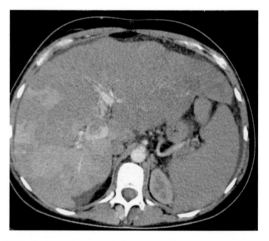

Figure 85-7 Abdominal computed tomography scan.

## FINDINGS

Abdominal ultrasound revealed an enlarged liver, with a heterogenous echo texture. There was no intrahepatic duct dilatation, but a thrombus was suspected in the hepatic and portal veins. The spleen was enlarged (16.8 cm), and there was a small amount of free fluid around the liver and within the pelvis. Kidneys were normal in size and appearance.

An abdominal CT scan was performed. This confirmed marked liver enlargement with irregular outline and diffusely uneven attenuation. Thrombus was confirmed in the portal vein but not the hepatic vein, excluding Budd-Chiari syndrome and suggesting the presence of intrinsic hepatic pathology. At this point, blood tests found α-fetoprotein level markedly elevated at 841,000 μg/L (normal < 13). Other tumor markers were not elevated.

**Comments:** Most cases of Budd-Chiari syndrome (hepatic vein thrombosis) are associated with a thrombophilic condition. Less commonly, it is associated with polycythemia or with the use of the oral contraceptive pill. A full thrombophilia screen demonstrated no specific thrombophilic abnormality.

This was not Budd-Chiari syndrome. The CT did not confirm hepatic vein thrombosis. Tumor markers established that the diagnosis was a primary malignancy.

There is now increasing recognition of hepatic cirrhosis and even hepatocellular cancer in Fontan patients, although still rare, but this has not been reported in Mustard patients, and a primary hepatocellular problem was thought unlikely.

## CATHETERIZATION

Not performed

### FOCUSED CLINICAL QUESTIONS AND DISCUSSION POINTS

1. What is the natural history of a patient after a Mustard or Senning atrial redirection procedure for TGA?

*Following an early postoperative mortality of around 5%, there remains a small ongoing attrition rate in patients with prior atrial redirection surgery. Twenty-year survival is 76% to 80%.[1,2]*

*Patients are often in NYHA class I or II until into their fourth or fifth decade when systemic ventricular dysfunction may become manifest. In the absence of ventricular dysfunction, mild exertional limitation, which is the norm,[3] is in part a reflection of almost universal chronotropic incompetence. Sinus node dysfunction is very common, with progression from sinus bradycardia to junctional rhythm in the majority of patients.[4] Symptomatic chronotropic incompetence responds well to rate-responsive pacing. Permanent pacing is required in 20% to 25% of adult Mustard or Senning patients.*

*Tachyarrhythmias are also common, occurring in up to 50% of patients. Most commonly, this is intra-atrial reentrant tachycardia, occasionally atrial fibrillation, and, rarely, ventricular tachycardia. Sudden death occurs in 7% to 15% of patients,[2] presumably due to dysrhythmia. The risk persists throughout life. Systemic ventricular dysfunction is observed in half of the patients, although this is severe in only 10%. Baffle obstruction occurs in 5% to 10% of patients, the majority involving the superior aspect. Obstruction of the pulmonary component occurs in 2%, and is particularly difficult to treat.*

2. Could this patient's diagnosis have been made sooner?

*As a rule, the most effective way of reaching a diagnosis in congenital heart disease is to ask the patient. Based on her own personal experience with IVC baffle occlusion, the patient felt her own symptoms were similar and thus indicative of recurrent baffle obstruction.*

*In retrospect, features were present here that did not fit with baffle obstruction, such as mild anemia, extreme liver function test abnormalities, and absence of lower extremity edema despite*

*ascites. On the one hand, such findings should never be relied on to exclude IVC obstruction; however, on the other, they should prompt a broader differential diagnosis.*

*The point has been made several times in this volume that these special patients should be cared for by those with special expertise in ACHD. In this case, perhaps the converse is more appropriate. Though impossible to say whether the diagnosis could have been made sooner in another setting, the patient was kept on a cardiology ward with investigations and treatment focusing on the suspected cardiologic problem, which most likely did delay her eventual referral to the appropriate professionals.*

*In a busy adult cardiology practice, presentations of noncardiac disease such as seen here are likely to occur on occasion. The case is an important reminder that patients with congenital heart disease can, of course, develop acquired disorders. However, these patients often look to their cardiologist to serve at their primary care physician. In the tertiary care center where ACHD patients are seen frequently, it is important that providers not become too fixated on the patient's cardiac disease.*

## FINAL DIAGNOSIS

Hepatic infiltration with elevated tumor markers, likely metastatic tumor

Uncomplicated Mustard correction for TGA

## PLAN OF ACTION

Oncologic workup and chemotherapy

## INTERVENTION

None

## OUTCOME

The patient was transferred to a regional liver unit. She underwent evaluation and liver biopsy, which revealed a primary hepatic germ cell tumor. She commenced chemotherapy, initially cisplatin, with a modest reduction in her α-fetoprotein level.

At 6-month follow-up her disease was in remission, and her ascites had improved. Her exertional tolerance remained poor, but there was no identifiable cardiovascular cause.

One year later on surveillance imaging there was a noted recurrence of her cancer. She was admitted for aggressive chemotherapy, but 6 months later died of complications related to her cancer.

This unfortunate case reminds us that patients with congenital defects are not immune to other illnesses that adults can develop. Providers should not be blinded by the cardiac diagnosis such that other diagnoses are not considered.

## Selected References

1. Gelatt M, Hamilton RM, McCrindle BW, et al: Arrhythmia and mortality after the Mustard procedure: A 30-year single-center experience. J Am Coll Cardiol 29:194–201, 1997.
2. Wilson NJ, Clarkson PM, Barratt-Boyes BG, et al: Long-term outcome after the Mustard repair for simple transposition of the great arteries. 28 year follow up. J Am Coll Cardiol 32:758–765, 1998.
3. Diller GP, Dimopoulos K, Okonko D, et al: Exercise intolerance in adult congenital heart disease: Comparative severity, correlates, and prognostic implication. Circulation 112:828–835, 2005.
4. Warnes CA: Transposition of the great arteries. Circulation 114:2699–2709, 2006.

# Appendix: Notes on Quantification

## OXYGEN SATURATION

Oxygen saturation herein is reported at rest while breathing ambient air (assumed sea level). Whenever oxygen saturation is measured, it is best done after a minimum of 5 minutes of rest. There may be differences between capillary beds as well, such as finger vs. earlobe, which tend to be higher, particularly in cyanotic individuals.

## VENTRICULAR VOLUMES AND NORMAL RANGE

Measured volumes of the RV or LV are as reported by each contributing center. Not every imaging laboratory uses identical methods in making these measurements, particularly regarding inclusion or exclusion of the trabeculations, which can be extensive in many forms of congenital heart disease. Differences between methods have been shown.[1]

Normal values for ventricular volumes in patients with congenital heart disease have not been defined, and interpretation of a "normal" systemic RV would not necessarily be expected to be similar to that of a pulmonary RV. The normal ranges provided herein for both LV and RV volumes and ejection fraction are from one of several sources now available.[2,3] These sources studied normal healthy subjects of both genders over a large age range, thus giving the ability to determine normal ranges based on age, gender, and body surface area. The techniques used in these studies were similar for both the RV and LV and incorporate a signal intensity–based algorithm for excluding trabeculation from blood pool. The reported values of ventricular volume therefore exclude papillary muscles and trabeculations, although such trabeculations were likely minimal in this healthy normal population. Our use of these normal value ranges is not necessarily an endorsement of one method over another.

At times we included these same normal values, quantified by CMR, in studies using CT or ventriculography for volume assessment. Significant differences in ventricular volume using different modalities are well recognized, even between CT and CMR,[4] with many likely explanations for these differences. Our inclusion here is strictly for comparative purposes and should be interpreted with this in mind, as is mentioned throughout the text.

## FLOW QUANTIFICATION FROM HEMODYNAMIC STUDIES

As slight differences exist in quantifying flow (Q) from a hemodynamic study, we performed these calculations uniformly throughout the book. Flow calculations are based on the Fick principle, namely the quotient of oxygen consumption divided by the difference in proximal versus distal oxygen content of the capillary bed in question. For these calculations, we used an estimated resting $V_{O_2}$ from existing algorithms based on gender, BSA, age, and resting heart rate.[5] Body surface area for each patient was calculated using the Mosteller formula.[6]

$O_2$ content is found by multiplying $O_2$ carrying capacity by oxygen saturation. $O_2$ carrying capacity is defined as Hgb (g/dL) × 1.36 (mL/g) × 10 (dL/L). Literature varies on the oxygen binding coefficient; 1.34, 1.36, and 1.39 mL/g have all been published.

Based on the above, we quantified the following whenever relevant:

$$Q_{pulmonic} = V_{O_2}/[O_{2capacity} \times (PV_{sat} - PA_{sat})/100]$$

$$Q_{systemic} = V_{O_2}/[O_{2capacity} \times (Ao_{sat} - MV_{sat})/100]$$

$$Q_{effective} = V_{O_2}/[O_{2capacity} \times (PV_{sat} - MV_{sat})/100]$$

where PV = pulmonary venous, PA = pulmonary arterial, Ao = aortic, and MV = mixed venous. $Q_{effective}$ represents blood flowing from one capillary bed to another, which is necessary to quantify shunt volumes. From the above, Qp/Qs can also be calculated using the abbreviated formula $(Ao_{sat} - MV_{sat})/(PV_{sat} - PA_{sat})$. There are many ways to estimate the true mixed venous oxygen saturation based on measured SVC and IVC saturations.[7] We used the formula $MV_{sat} = (3 \times SVC_{sat} + IVC_{sat})/4$.[8] Other methods have also been described.[9] We used an assumed pulmonary venous oxygen saturation of 98% unless specified.

We report standard vascular resistance in unindexed Wood units as the ratio of the pressure difference across the capillary bed to flow through the same bed. These calculations assume room air oxygen unless stated otherwise. Significant analgesia/anesthesia can affect hemodynamics and flows. Other sources of potential error include errors in oximetry, use of supplemental oxygen without calculation using $P_{O_2}$, or high or low flow states where small errors lead to larger differences. Many of these limitations are indicated throughout the book when relevant.

The electronic version of this volume includes a calculator based on the variables provided in each case, which can be manipulated to see the effects on calculations from alterations of each variable. This is meant to be an educational tool, not necessarily for clinical use.

## References

1. Winter MM, Bernink FJ, Groenink M, et al: Evaluating the systemic right ventricle by CMR: The importance of consistent and reproducible delineation of the cavity. J Cardiovasc Magn Reson 10:40, 2008.
2. Maceira AM, Prasad SK, Khan M, Pennell DJ: Normalized left ventricular systolic and diastolic function by steady state free precession cardiovascular magnetic resonance. J Cardiovasc Magn Reson 8:417–426, 2006.
3. Maceira AM, Prasad SK, Khan M, Pennell DJ: Reference right ventricular systolic and diastolic function normalized to age, gender and body surface area from steady-state free precession cardiovascular magnetic resonance. Eur Heart J 27:2879–2888, 2006.
4. Sugeng L, Mor-Avi V, Weinert L, et al: Quantitative assessment of left ventricular size and function: Side-by-side comparison of real-time three-dimensional echocardiography and computed tomography with magnetic resonance reference. Circulation 114:654–661, 2006.

5. LaFarge CG, Miettinen OS: The estimation of oxygen consumption. Cardiovasc Res 4:23–30, 1970.
6. Mosteller RD: Simplified calculation of body-surface area. N Engl J Med 317:1098, 1987.
7. Wilkinson JL: Haemodynamic calculations in the catheter laboratory. Heart 85:113–120, 2001.
8. Flamm MD, Cohn KE, Hancock EW: Ventricular function in atrial septal defect. Am J Med 48:286–294, 1970.
9. Pirwitz MJ, Willard JE, Landau C, et al: A critical reappraisal of the oximetric assessment of intracardiac left-to-right shunting in adults. Am Heart J 133:413–417, 1997.

# Index